Clinical Management of Sensorimotor Speech Disorders

Edited by

Malcolm R. McNeil, Ph.D.
Professor and Chair
Science and Disorders
Department of Communication
University of Pittsburgh
Pittsburgh, Pennsylvania

with 86 illustrations

1997

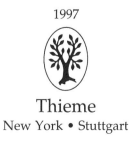

Thieme
New York • Stuttgart

Thieme Medical Publishers, Inc.
381 Park Avenue South
New York, NY 10016

Clinical Management of Sensorimotor Speech Disorders
Malcolm R. McNeil, Ph.D.

Library of Congress Cataloging-in-Publication Data

Clinical management of sensorimotor speech disorders / edited by
  Malcolm R. McNeil.
     p. cm.
  Includes bibliographical references and index.
  ISBN 0-86577-527-3
  1. Articulation disorders.   2. Speech disorders.   I. McNeil,
Malcolm Ray, 1947–   .
  [DNLM: 1. Speech Disorders—therapy.   2. Sppech Disorders—
diagnosis.   3. Dysarthria.   4. Speech—physiology.   WL 340.2 C641
1997]
RC424.7.C576   1997
616.85'5—dc20
DNLM/DLC
for Library of Congress   96-43579
                                                              CIP

Printed in the United States of America

5 4 3 2 1

TMP ISBN 0-86577-527-3
GTV ISBN 3-13-103771-7

Contents

Contributors

Scott G. Adams, Ph.D.
Assistant Professor
Department of Communicative Disorders
University of Western Ontario
London, Ontario
Canada

Richard D. Andreatta, A.B.D.
Speech and Hearing Center
University of Indiana
Bloomington, Indiana

Steven M. Barlow, Ph.D.
Professor
Speech and Hearing Center
University of Indiana
Bloomington, Indiana

Michael P. Cannito, Ph.D.
School of Audiology and Speech-Language
  Pathology
University of Memphis
Memphis, Tennessee

Donald S. Finan, A.B.D.
Speech and Hearing Center
University of Indiana
Bloomington, Indiana

Eileen M. Finnegan, M.A.
Department of Speech Pathology and
  Audiology
University of Iowa
Iowa City, Iowa

John W. Folkins, Ph.D.
Professor
Associate Provost
Department of Speech Pathology and
  Audiology
Wendell Johnson Speech and Hearing Center
University of Iowa
Iowa City, Iowa

Karen Forrest, Ph.D.
Assistant Professor
Speech and Hearing Center
University of Indiana
Bloomington, Indiana

Carlin F. Hageman, Ph.D.
Associate Professor
Department of Communicative Disorders
University of Northern Iowa
Cedar Falls, Iowa

Virginia A. Hinton, Ph.D.
Assistant Professor
Department of Communication and Theater
Division of Communication Disorders and
  Education of Deaf Children
University of North Carolina at Greensboro
Greensboro, North Carolina

Ray D. Kent, Ph.D.
Department of Communicative Disorders
University of Wisconsin-Madison
Madison, Wisconsin

Leonard L. LaPointe, Ph.D.
Professor
Department of Speech and Hearing Science
Arizona State University
Tempe, Arizona

Erich S. Luschei, Ph.D.
Department of Speech Pathology and
  Audiology
University of Iowa
Iowa City, Iowa

Thomas P. Marquardt, Ph.D.
Professor
Communication Sciences and Disorders
  Program
Department of Speech Communication
University of Texas at Austin
Austin, Texas

Malcolm R. McNeil, Ph.D.
Professor and Chair
Department of Communication Science
  and Disorders
University of Pittsburgh
Pittsburgh, Pennsylvania

Jerald B. Moon
Department of Speech Pathology and
  Audiology
Wendell Johnson Speech and Hearing Center
University of Iowa
Iowa City, Iowa

Bruce E. Murdoch, Ph.D.
Professor
Department of Speech and Hearing
Motor Speech Research Unit
The University of Queensland
Brisbane, Queensland
Australia

L. Ashley Paseman, M.A.
Speech and Hearing Center
University of Indiana
Bloomington, Indiana

Sheila R. Pratt, Ph.D.
Assistant Professor
Division of Communication Science and
   Disorders
Department of Communication
University of Pittsburgh
Pittsburgh, Pennsylvania

Donald A. Robin, Ph.D.
Associate Professor
Department of Speech Pathology and
   Audiology
Wendell Johnson Speech and Hearing Center
University of Iowa
Iowa City, Iowa

Anne Putnam Rochet, Ph.D.
Associate Professor
Department of Speech Pathology and
   Audiology
University of Alberta
Edmonton, Alberta
Canada

Richard A. Schmidt, Ph.D.
Professor
Department of Psychology
University of California, Los Angeles
Los Angeles, California

Nancy Pearl Solomon, Ph.D.
Research Associate
Department of Speech Pathology and
   Audiology
Wendell Johnson Speech and Hearing Center
University of Iowa
Iowa City, Iowa

Barbara C. Sonies, Ph.D.
Chief, Speech-Language Pathology Section
Director, Oral Pharyngeal Imaging
   Laboratories
National Institutes of Health Clinical Center
Bethesda, Maryland

Maureen Stone, Ph.D.
Departments of Electrical and Computer
   Engineering Cognitive Science
Johns Hopkins University
Baltimore, Maryland

Deborah G. Theodoros
Department of Speech and Hearing
Motor Speech Research Unit
The University of Queensland
Brisbane, Queensland
Australia

Elizabeth C. Thompson
Department of Speech and Hearing
Motor Speech Research Unit
The University of Queensland
Brisbane, Queensland
Australia

Nancy Tye-Murray, Ph.D.
Department of Speech Pathology and
   Audiology
Wendell Johnson Speech and Hearing Center
University of Iowa
Iowa City, Iowa

Anita Van der Merwe, Ph.D.
Professor
Department of Speech Pathology and
   Audiology
University of Pretoria
Pretoria, South Africa

Donald W. Warren, D.D.S., Ph.D.
Kenan Professor and Director
University of North Carolina Craniofacial
   Center
Department of Dental Ecology
School of Dentistry
Research Professor
Department of Otolaryngology
School of Medicine
University of North Carolina at Chapel Hill
Chapel Hill, North Carolina

Gary Weismer, Ph.D.
Professor
Department of Communicative Disorders
University of Wisconsin-Madison
Madison, Wisconsin

Richard I. Zraick, M.S.
Doctoral Candidate
Department of Speech and Hearing Science
Arizona State University
Tempe, Arizona

Foreword

Forewords should perhaps be called "Backwords" because the step forward represented by any important scholarly work can be recognized as such only in the context of the preceding footsteps. The valuable contents of *Clinical Management of Sensorimotor Speech Disorders* are no exception. They are the progeny of the past work of many individuals, including that of many of the book's contributing authors.

Disorders of speech have been part of the description of many neurologic diseases for centuries. But, in a 1983 Foreword to the book *Clinical Dysarthria* (Berry, 1983), Darley pointed out that "only in approximately the last 40 years have we seen people with clinical interests begin to cogitate on how to help the dysarthric patient" (p. xiv). The success of these early rehabilitation efforts were necessarily limited because only in the last 25 to 30 years have concerted efforts been made to understand the nature of sensorimotor speech disorders in a comprehensive way. The foundation for our current understanding of the dysarthrias has firm roots in two landmark articles by Darley, Aronson, and Brown in 1969. The term "apraxia of speech," and an appreciation for its characteristics and nature, emerged in the mid 1960s and early 1970s, again led by the strong influence of Darley and many of his colleagues. With the publication in 1975 of Darley, Aronson, and Brown's classic book, *Motor Speech Disorders*, the term "motor speech disorders" became the generic designation for disorders of speech production that include the dysarthrias and apraxia of speech.

A substantial body of knowledge about motor speech disorders had emerged over the last quarter century, with contributions from speech-language pathologists, speech scientists, and researchers from a number of other disciplines. The interest in these disorders has been at least partly motivated by the opportunity that such disorders provide to increase our understanding of how the brain is organized for speech, the fact that recognizing distinctions among the various motor speech disorders can help localize and diagnose neurologic disease, and the desire of clinicians to improve the communication ability of the many people with neurologic disease who have motor speech disorders.

Now, in the 1990s, the "Decade of the Brain," it is appropriate that Mick McNeil has brought together a group of highly respected individuals to comprehensively and critically address the state of the art in our understanding of sensorimotor speech disorders. The book will assist students, clinicians, and researchers who wish to learn about the nature, characteristics, and management of these disorders, and the methods and techniques that can be used to improve our understanding of them.

This book reflects the work of individuals whose diverse research and clinical contributions capture the range of sensorimotor speech disorders and methods for studying them. Perhaps because of this diversity, several important relationships emerge within and among the book's chapters. The reader may wish to keep them in mind. These include the notions that the study of sensorimotor speech disorders (1) is evolving in a way that reflects reliance on its historic foundations but needs to consider new approaches; (2) can have theoretical as well as clinical diagnostic and management implications; (3) can employ methods that are perceptual, acoustic, aerodynamic, kinematic, electromyographic, and imaging, each providing a different level of explanation, and each with its own advantages and shortcomings; (4) can both benefit from and contribute to what we know about the neurology and biomechanics of voluntary movement control in general; (5) may best be understood and managed through the collaborative efforts of clinicians and clinical and laboratory scientists.

To the reader desiring a broad overview of the disorders and the methods used to study them, you will find it here, but I urge you to attend to the contributors' attention to detail, and to their critical thinking about theory, method, the meaning of results, and directions for future study. It will help you know better the foundations upon which your own clinical or research activities are built. To the reader with narrow interests in a particular disorder or method of investigation, you will find chapters here to whet or satisfy your appetite, but I urge you also to appreciate the gestalt of the entire book. It will help you know better the important questions that still need to be addressed. To all readers of this book, you will find its attention to theory, methods of study, description, assessments, and management informative and thought provoking. What can be learned here may help shape the direction of our next steps in the understanding and management of these disorders that can so profoundly affect the ability to communicate.

Joseph R. Duffy, Ph.D., BC-NCD
Head, Section of Speech Pathology
The Mayo Clinic
Rochester, MN

References

Berry, W.R. (Ed.) (1983). *Clinical Dysarthria*. San Diego: College-Hill Press.

Darley, F.L., Aronson, A.E., & Brown, J.R. (1969). Clusters of deviant dimensions in the dysarthrias. *J. Speech Hear Res*, 12, 462–496.

Darley, F.L., Aronson, A.E., Brown, J.R. (1969). Differential diagnostic patterns of dysarthria. *J. Speech Hear Res.*, 12, 246–269.

Darley, F.L., Aronson, A.E., & Brown, J.R. (1975). *Motor Speech Disorders*, Philadelphia: WB Saunders.

Preface

Descriptions and formal definitions of dysarthria and other disorders of sensorimotor speech control are a matter of historical record and certainly preceded the 1969 work of Darley, Aronson, and Brown. However, no work has had a greater influence on research, measurement, or treatment of sensorimotor speech disorders. The theoretical foundation reflected in their classification system with its attempted integration of known anatomic, physiologic, and behavioral characteristics of neuromuscular disorders derived from classical clinical neurology, with the known speech production phenomenon, gave method and procedure to an area of neurology and speech-language pathology that had languished from a lack of order and systematicity. The fact that they were able to bring order to a disparate literature and provide a measure of support for it with their perceptually based cluster analysis gave sufficient structure to the area to promote research and offer clinicians enough organization to begin the tasks of developing appropriate assessment procedures and treatment paradigms. This book stands squarely on this foundation and provides a continuation of this journey into the theoretical bases, the assessment, the synthesis of relevant information about the pathologies of the central and peripheral nervous systems that cause sensorimotor speech disorders and into the state of the science for the treatment of these disorders. Each of the fifteen chapters is written by one or more internationally recognized authority(s) on the topic of the chapter. The book as a whole makes important advances into theory, assessment, and treatment beyond those that have preceded it. While accomplishing this, we recognize that these advances are possible only by standing on the firm foundation of those that have preceded us. To the degree that this book brings us closer to the advanced theory, assessment, and treatment of individuals with sensorimotor speech disorders, we gratefully acknowledge the important work of all whose contributions we have built upon, especially those contributors since 1969.

This book is organized into three major sections. The first section is addressed in a single chapter authored by Dr. Anita Van der Merwe from the University of Pretoria, Republic of South Africa. This chapter provides a broad theoretical account of speech sensorimotor control and its relationship to sensorimotor speech disorders. This inclusive theoretical account sets the floorplan for the second section of the book with seven chapters dedicated to assessment as well as for the third section with seven chapters allocated to the various sensorimotor speech disorders and to their management.

The second section begins with a chapter authored by Dr. Raymond D. Kent from the University of Wisconsin-Madison and addresses, with Dr. Kent's typical clarity and sophistication, the more traditional perceptual assessment of sensorimotor speech disorders. This chapter provides the motivation, techniques, reference data, and description of methods for the examination of the speech structures and the oralsensory system. Also discussed is the use of nonspeech dynamic tasks, simple speech and speech-like tasks, citation tasks; and the assessment of intelligibility, quality, fluency, prosody, as well as the classification of type and severity of speech disorders. This initial chapter is followed with a theoretical argument and suggested procedures for the use of non-speech behaviors as part of the assessment protocol for sensorimotor speech disorders. This unique clinically and theoretically important chapter, authored by Drs. Donald A. Robin from the University of Iowa, Nancy Pearl Solomon from the University of Minnesota and Jerald B. Moon and John W. Folkins from the University of Iowa, discusses traditional nonspeech behaviors used in the assessment of speech subsystems and ends with a detailed discussion of the Iowa Oral Performance Instrument (IOPI). The fourth chapter is authored by Drs. Karen Forrest from the Indiana University and Gary Weismer from the University of Wisconsin-Madison. This critical chapter provides the clearest and most user-friendly account to date of acoustic analyses for sensorimotor speech disorders. In this chapter, these speech scientists discuss the acoustic representations of speech, segmentation and measurement of the speech wave, the acoustic analysis of vowels including formant frequencies and transitions, imprecise consonants, hypernasality, and vocal dimensions. The fifth chapter is a complete discussion for the aerodynamic assessment of sensorimotor speech disorders and is authored by Drs. Donald W. Warren from the University of North Carolina at Chapel Hill, Anne Putnam Rochet from the University of Alberta, and Virginia A. Hinton from the University of North Carolina at Chapel Hill. In this chapter, these speech scientists discuss, in exquisite detail and with practical simplicity, the methods and procedures for the measurement of air pressure, flow, area, resistance and timing, as well as aerodynamic principles for assessing structural performance, postural/respiratory effort, and bilabial incompetence/closure. The sixth chapter is authored by Dr. Steven M. Barlow, D.S.

Finan, R.D. Andreatta and L.A. Paseman from Indiana University. Typical of these speech scientists' work, this chapter provides a complete discussion of the motivation, the anatomic, neurologic, and neurophysiologic substrates for the measurement of movements related to speech production. Descriptions of labial-mandibular strain gage transduction, X-ray Microbeam, magnetometry, glossometry, palatometry, and ultrasound movement measurement techniques are provided. In addition, the appropriate techniques for measuring velar, laryngeal and chest wall kinematics are discussed and illustrated. The seventh chapter is authored by Dr. Erich S. Luschei and Ms. Eileen M. Finnegan from the University of Iowa. This chapter provides the singularly best tutorial to date on electromyographic instrumentation and procedures used in the measurement of disordered speech production. In this chapter, these speech scientists describe the appropriate uses of EMG for speech, the basic source of the EMG signal, electrode type and configuration, amplifiers, monitors, recorders, and data acquisition and storage devices. It culminates with a concise description of the source and recognition of artifactual signals (e.g. movement) and methods for minimizing and dealing with them when they are unavoidable. The eighth chapter is authored by Drs. Barbara Sonies from the National Institutes of Health and Maureen Stone from The Johns Hopkins University and provides an up-to-date account of speech imaging procedures. This chapter provides a clear description of X-radiography, computerized tomography, magnetic resonance imaging, and ultrasound as well as their respective advantages and disadvantages.

This third section of the book, organized around the Darley, Aronson, and Brown classification of motor speech disorders, begins in Chapter 9 with a clearly written and comprehensive chapter on flaccid dysarthria authored by Dr. Carlin Hageman from the University of Northern Iowa. This chapter covers the motor unit including muscle innervation, contractile properties of muscle, breakdown of the motor unit, speech related cranial nerve distribution, function, pathologies, and symptoms. A clinically useful breakdown of cranial nerve syndromes, neural adaptation and behavioral compensation, general muscle training strategies, and those specifically appropriate for low motor neuron disorders is discussed with reference to speech process and behavioral, prosthetic, surgical, and pharmacological treatments. Chapter 10, authored by Drs. Michael P. Cannito from the University of Memphis and Thomas P. Marquardt from the University of Texas at Austin provides unparalleled coverage of ataxic dysarthria. This chapter provides an historical review of cerebellar and cerebellar pathway anatomy and neurophysiology with the integration of clinical signs and symptoms. These authors discuss the pathological conditions that give rise to ataxia, the nonspeech concomitants of ataxic dysarthria (e.g., hypotonia, hyporeflexia, asthenia, tremor, titubation, myoclonus, movement timing, dysmetria), and concomitant disorders such as abnormalities of stance and gate and oculomotor disorders. No finer coverage of the speech characteristics of ataxic dysarthria discussed by speech subsystem with specialized assessment considerations has been presented. The chapter culminates with a treatise on the various treatments of ataxic dysarthria that provides both the general principles of treatment and the specific methods and procedures that apply to individuals. Mr. Richard I. Zraick and Dr. Leonard L. LaPointe from Arizona State University, authored Chapter 11 on hyperkinetic dysarthria. These authors provide a thorough and clearly readable discussion of the dysarthrias resulting from disorders of the extrapyramidal system and provide an excellent neuroanatomic and neurophysiologic review of this complex system. Their definitions and differentiation among tremor, athetosis, chorea, myoclonus, tic disorders, dyskinesia, dystonia, and ballism provide the backdrop for their concise discussion of the evaluation and treatment of these hyperkinetic dysarthrias. Chapter 12 is dedicated to hypokinetic dysarthria in Parkinson's Disease and is authored by

Dr. Scott G. Adams from the University of Western Ontario. In this chapter Dr. Adams clearly and concisely reviews the history of Parkinson's Disease, its pathophysiology and the general symptoms associated with it. The review of the presenting perceptual, acoustic and physiologic speech signs and symptoms in hypokinetic dysarthria, arranged by speech process, speech subsystem and predominant features, provides the clinician with a well documented review and recipe for diagnosis and assessment. Dr. Adams' discussion of the treatment of hypokinetic dysarthria in Parkinson's Disease through pharmacological, surgical, biofeedback, prosthetic, assistive device, and behavioral procedures is second to none and offers the researcher and clinician a comprehensive review and a guidepost for managing specific deficits in specific individuals with hypokinetic dysarthria. Chapter 13 is authored by Dr. Bruce E. Murdoch, Ms. Elizabeth C. Thompson and Dr. Deborah G. Theodoros from the University of Queensland and provides a complete coverage of the complex topic of spastic dysarthria. As with the other chapters devoted to the clinical sensorimotor speech syndromes, this chapter provides a concise and superlative discussion of the basic neuroanatomy and neurophysiology of the nervous system responsible for this syndrome (upper motor neuron system) and the clinical features of spasticity and spastic dysarthria. The comprehensive review and rationale for the treatments arranged by speech process provide a state of the science inventory of what is known and how to implement it into the care of the person with spastic dysarthria. Chapter 14 is authored by Drs. Malcolm R. McNeil from the University of Pittsburgh, Donald A. Robin from the University of Iowa and Richard A. Schmidt from the University of California at Los Angeles. This chapter provides a theoretical account of apraxia of speech (AOS), reviewing the features differentiating AOS from dysarthria, and those differentiating AOS from phonemic paraphasia. Discussions of the phonologic, phonetic/motoric, force and position control, inter- and intra-articulator kinematic, prosodic and variability, consistency and target approximation, and effort characteristics of AOS motivate a formal redefinition of the disorder. A review of the current menu of treatments with a discussion of the principles of motor learning and their application to treatment provide heretofore unexplored principles for enhancing the effectiveness of AOS treatment. Chapter 15 represents a unique characterization of the speech of the deaf and hearing-impaired as one profitably considered as a sensorimotor disorder in the tradition of the dysarthrias and apraxia of speech. This chapter, authored by Drs. Sheila R. Pratt from the University of Pittsburgh and Nancy Tye-Murray from The Central Institute for the Deaf provide an exhaustive review of the speech characteristics of the deaf and hearing-impaired organized first by speech process and secondly by segmental (vowel and consonant), suprasegmental, and coarticulatory characteristics. A discussion of developmental speech characteristics, the role of audition in speech development, and concomitant non-speech characteristics set the stage for an encyclopedic review of evaluation procedures covering sensory, structural, perceptual, acoustic, kinematic, and aerodynamic techniques. The review and analysis of the multitude of treatment approaches and programs for the speech of the deaf and hearing-impaired is not only comprehensive, it is superlative in its scope and clarity of presentation.

The vitality of this volume began with the selection of contributors and is evident in the text they produced. The measures of its usefulness will be judged by the research it stimulates, the concepts it clarifies, and the clinicians it helps to organize and select appropriate assessment and treatment methods and procedures. The ultimate measure, however, will be the benefits it provides for persons with sensorimotor speech disorders.

Malcolm R. McNeil, Ph.D., BDNCD

Chapter *1*

A Theoretical Framework for the Characterization of Pathological Speech Sensorimotor Control

Anita Van der Merwe

Introduction

The need to work from a sound theoretical framework based on the normal process of speech and language production for both research and management of communication disorders has long been proclaimed by speech-language pathologists (Kent & McNeil, 1987; Marquart & Sussman, 1984; McNeil & Kent, 1990; West, Ansberry, & Carr, 1957). The almost overwhelming corpus of ever increasing data on the intricate detail of the speech production process and the neurophysiology of motor control and also unresolved issues concerning the nature of neurogenic speech disorders (McNeil & Kent, 1990) underscore the necessity of a comprehensive explanatory framework. Phenomenological models have great explanatory power (Scully & Guérin, 1991), and a comprehensive model can keep us from "making stabs in the dark" (Marquardt & Sussman, 1984, p 111). The practicing clinician can use a coherent model to put diagnosis, differential diagnosis, and management on a sound theoretical basis.

A functional model applicable to neurogenic speech disorders needs to explain the speech production process as fine sensorimotor skill (Netsell, 1982). Such a model should also be in line with current concepts, developments, and terminology in neuroscience. The neural basis of sensorimotor control is "a field in a wild flux of rapid evolution"

(Brooks, 1986, p ix), and the ever expanding theoretical framework based on animal movement studies, in particular, should be explored to enhance as far as possible our own insight into speech movements and movement disorders. Direct access to the human brain (which can produce speech) is for obvious reasons not possible. To be able to draw from this knowledge base, an important prerequisite, however, would be correspondence in terminology. Clinical intervention and interdisciplinary teamwork can only benefit as an additional advantage.

The theoretical framework proposed here portrays the transformation of the speech code from one form to another as seen from a brain behavior perspective. It poses a novel view on the phases involved during the transformation and stresses the importance of sensorimotor interface. This proposal represents a paradigm shift from the traditional three-stage speech production model (Itoh & Sasanuma, 1984) consisting of linguistic encoding, programming, and execution to one of four stages based on current neurophysiological data on sensorimotor control. McNeil and Kent (1990) state that assumptions underlying neurogenic pathologic populations need to be seriously reconsidered and that particular attention should be given to the motoric aspects of speech production. The proposed framework could be a step toward this goal. Before the different phases or levels of the proposed framework are fully explained, it is necessary to motivate the entries and to delineate the theoretical context within which it functions.

Background

Speech is the externalized expression of language, and speech sensorimotor control can be defined as "the motor-afferent mechanisms that direct and regulate speech movements" (Netsell, 1982, p 247). As a motor skill, speech is "goal-directed" and "afferent-guided," and it "meets the general requirements of a fine motor skill, viz, it (1) is performed with accuracy and speed, (2) uses knowledge of results, (3) is improved by practice, (4) demonstrates motor flexibility in achieving goals and (5) relegates all of this to automatic control, where 'consciousness' is freed from the details of action plans" (Netsell, 1982, p 250).

To appreciate the complexity of the speech production process, one only has to study the summary charts of events in respiration, voicing, and articulation during production of a short sentence, as summarized by Borden and Harris (1984). All of these motor events have to be coordinated and produced in such a way that the desired acoustic result is achieved. This process seems to occur in phases of processing.

Phases in the Transformation of the Speech Code

During the production of speech, the intended message has to be changed from an abstract idea to meaningful language symbols and then to a code amenable to a motor system. There is, in order words, a gradual appearance of new formations out of preexisting ones. The evolutionary change renders the code compatible with every level of processing (Schweiger & Browne, 1988). The identification of the phases involved in this process, however, remains problematic and debatable.

Most neurophysiologists recognize that the overall motor control process involves several phases or hierarchical levels of organ-ization (Jakobson & Goodale, 1991; Lacquaniti, 1989). The phases generally are identified as planning, programming, and execution (Brooks, 1986; Gracco & Abbs, 1987; Marsden, 1984; Schmidt, 1978). The control of movements is taken to be exerted through a command (or sensorimotor) hierarchy that can be portrayed as highest, middle, and lowest levels. The highest level is mediated by the association cortex (eg, prefrontal, parietal, and temporal lobes), which generates overall invariant motor plans. Motor plans are converted into motor programs at the middle level, which consists of the sensorimotor cortex, the cerebellum, and the putamen loop of the basal ganglia. At this level the specific parameters of the movement (eg, amplitude and speed) are defined. At the lowest level programs are translated into muscular activity and motor execution occurs (Brooks, 1986; Lacquaniti, 1989; Marsden, 1984; Schmidt, 1978).

In the literature on speech production, the deduction is usually made that the stage of motor planning referred to by neurophysiologists is equivalent to linguistic-symbolic planning. For example, Darley, Aronson, and Brown (1975) suggest that the phase of spatial-temporal planning of movement corresponds to syntactic planning during speech production. More often, however, the motor planning stage is equated to phonological planning during speech production. For example, Gracco and Abbs (1987, p 165) propose that motor programming and execution "would seem to lie immediately downstream from linguistic planning stages and hence reflect the implementation of phonological goals." The true nature of motor planning of speech movements is therefore not adequately contemplated and not differentiated from phonological planning.

The inadequate formulation of the process of speech motor planning is perhaps partially due to the impact of linguistic terminology within which the speech pathologist traditionally functions. Phonology as a linguistic term includes both the phonological and phonetic components (also referred to as covert and overt speech [Edwards &

Shriberg, 1983]), and, based on this premise, phonetic or motor planning of speech is assumed to be a linguistic function. It is true that speech needs to be "viewed within the superordinate behavior of language" (McNeil & Kent, 1990, p 352), but it is also imperative to view speech as a sensorimotor function of the human brain. A motor plan (not an abstract linguistic choice of a phoneme to be uttered) is necessary to guide speech movements. Motor planning of speech is a discernible process aimed at defining motor goals. In the formulation of a comprehensive theory on motor planning of speech, certain well-known speech phenomena may prove to be central. Data on the invariant and variant aspects of the spatial and temporal features of speech movements are particularly important, as will be explained later in the text.

An important consequence of the deduction that motor planning is a linguistic process and can be referred to as phonological planning is that the terms motor planning and programming are used interchangeably as if they constitute more or less the same process. From a neurophysiological viewpoint, however, motor planning and programming need to be differentiated. During the planning stage general decisions are made, which in the case of speech will probably be guided by phonologically based specifications such as manner and place of articulation. The details of the planned sequence of movements are fitted in later during the programming phase according to the circumstances of the moment (Brooks, 1986). Inadequate differentiation of planning and programming results in the three-level model described earlier.

The proposed theoretical framework postulates that linguistic-symbolic planning should be differentiated from phases in sensorimotor control and that sensorimotor control of speech movements comprises planning, programming, and execution phases. A clear differentiation among these processes or phases is necessary to comprehensively define the different sensorimotor speech disorders. A formulation of these phases also provides a theoretical framework for intervention and research in the field of neurogenic speech disorders.

Speech as Sensorimotor Skill

"Sensorimotor integration is the key to motor control" (Brooks, 1986, p 39). Most researchers today agree that sensory information or input is an integral part of movement control and coordination (Abbs & Connor, 1991; Brooks, 1986; Evarts, 1982; Gentil, 1990; Kawato & Gomi, 1992; Kent, 1990; Schmidt, 1982; Tatton & Bruce, 1981).

Early concepts postulated that movements were controlled by peripheral reafferent sensory input. Later research determined that movements could still be performed following deafferentation. This finding suggested central programming of movements. Research aimed at determining how central nerve cells generate so-called motor programs was then initiated. Two schools of motor control originated. The one emphasizes the importance of the central program and views afferent input as relatively unimportant (open-loop control), while the other school takes the position that afferent input is of great significance and that movements are under continuous control by feedback (closed-loop control; Evarts, 1982). For many years experiments addressed "a nul hypothesis and attempts were made to provide a general either-or solution" (Abbs & Cole, 1982, p 160). Today a more pragmatic approach is followed, and research is geared at defining the interaction and relative role of both feedback and feedforward control.

Auditory, tactile, and proprioceptive feedback arise as consequences of speech production. Proprioception is the most important sense from inside our bodies (as opposed to "exteroceptive" senses). Proprioception is "the sense of what the muscle itself is doing" (Brooks, 1986, p 11). This direct feedback from the muscles is faster than exteroceptive feedback (tactile and audition) and therefore presumably more involved in the control of speech movements (Borden & Harris, 1984). Sense organs (or mechanoreceptors) in the

3

tendons signal how hard the muscles are pulling and sense organs within the muscles; namely, muscle spindles signal how much and how fast the muscles are being stretched (Brooks, 1986). Striated muscles contract at will and muscle spindles are embedded in most striated muscles. Speech muscles are striated muscles, but not all have muscle spindles. Muscle spindles arranged in parallel with the extrafusal muscle fibers provide information about the length of the muscle and contribute to the stretch (myotatic) reflex. The stretch reflex can function as a servomechanism regulating muscle length (Gentil, 1990). Segmental and transcortical (via pyramidal tract neurons) proprioceptive reflexes exist. The major role of both is in small active movements and in active postural stability (Evarts & Fromm, 1981).

Golgi tendon organs, arranged in series with the extrafusal muscle fibers, inform the nervous system of the tension exerted by the muscle on its tendinous insertion to the bone (Gentil, 1990). Mechanoreceptors are present on the lips, oral mucosa, the jaw muscles, the periodontium, the temporomandibular joint, in the larynx, and in the respiratory apparatus (Landgren & Olsson, 1982). Distribution of different receptors in different structures, however, varies. Muscle spindles have been found in the lingual and laryngeal muscles. Concerning the jaw, the deep parts of the temporal and masseter muscles contain a high number of muscle spindles. Few spindles are observed in the lateral pterygoid muscle and only occasional ones in the anterior belly of digastric. There are no muscle spindles or Golgi tendon organs in facial muscles, including the lip muscles. Tendon organs are present in the jaw system (Gentil, 1990; Persson, 1982).

McClean (1991) reported that respiratory airways are supplied with mechanoreceptors capable of signaling pressure changes. He found that changes in oral pressure produced reflex responses in lip muscles and concluded that mechanoreceptor responses to intraoral pressure changes are involved in sensorimotor integration for speech production. (For further reading refer to Kent, 1990, who provides a summary of qualities, recep-

tors, and nerve innervation of oral sensation. Also see Sussman, 1972; Bowman, 1968; and Bowman and Combs, 1969a,b.)

In addition to information fed back from the periphery, the nervous system can handle information relayed from motor to sensory areas. Reciprocal connections between sensory and motor areas of the cerebral cortex substantiates the possibility of so-called internal feedback.

According to Kelso and Stelmach (1976), two sets of signals, both operating via feedforward mechanisms, are involved. The one is a downward discharge to effector organs, and the other is a simultaneous central discharge from motor to sensory systems that presets the sensory area for the anticipated consequences of the motor act. The neural response in the sensory system before the arrival of response-produced feedback is referred to as corollary discharge by Kelso and Stelmach (1976). This neural response is the result of an efference (reference) copy which tells the appropriate areas of the brain what to expect. The accuracy of the efferent command can thus be compared centrally with an internal model before the arrival of peripheral feedback. Apparently all levels of the nervous system can handle internally fed back information (Brooks, 1986; Evarts, 1971, 1982; Evarts & Fromm, 1981). According to Kawato and Gomi (1992), internal predictive models of the motor apparatus are developed during motor learning. One important function of these efference copies (reefference) is to prevent sensory feedback generated during movement from interfering with the intended movement (Brooks, 1986). Another function would be to detect and correct errors before movement commences.

Many studies have been conducted to determine the role of afferent feedback in speech production. The publication of the closed-loop speech production model of Fairbanks gave rise to many studies on the effect of disturbed tactile feedback (Ringel & Ewanowski, 1965; Ringel & Steer, 1963; Ringel, Burk, & Scott, 1968) and proprioceptive feedback (Abbs, 1973; Goodwin & Luschei, 1974). The fact that speech was slightly impaired by such interference was interpreted as an indication of closed-loop control. It was, however, later indicated that the methods used in the tactile studies caused motor interference too (Abbs, Folkins, & Sivarajan, 1976; Folkins & Abbs, 1977). The insubstantial effect of tactile and proprioceptive interference was also interpreted as an indication of open loop control (Borden, 1979; Folkins & Abbs, 1975; Putnam & Ringel, 1976).

In another line of experimentation designed to evaluate sensory information on speech production, the mandible is fixed by placing a bite block between the teeth (Folkins & Zimmerman, 1981; Lindblom, Lubker, & Gay, 1979). Formant patterns typical for the speaker are obtained even at the first glottal pulse before response feedback has occurred, indicating the operation of central feedback or predictive simulation.

The most recent research on the role of sensory feedback in articulatory movements has been performed by Gracco & Abbs (1986, 1988, 1989). Unanticipated perturbation of the movements of an articulator was studied. Significant magnitude compensations from the muscles and movements of the upper lip, lower lip, and jaw were observed. According to Gracco and Abbs (1987), these data suggest that sensory information is used not only to correct errors in individual movements, but also to make adjustments among the multiple movements involved in a given speech gesture. The latter observation is interpreted as evidencing that sensorimotor actions contribute to the coordination of speech movements.

Gracco and Abbs (1987) developed their theory further by introducing early (ie, well before agonist EMG onset) perturbations which would yield so-called autogenic (corrective or responsive) compensations indicative of a preexecution or programming process and later perturbations that would tap the stage of motor execution and reflect nonautogenic (predictive or projectional) sensorimotor processes. They assume that adjustments in the perturbed structure are "autogenic" while adjustments in a coactive but unperturbed structure, are "non-

autogenic." They prefer these terms because "they do not limit the conceptualization of the underlying neural processes to extant engineering control schemes" (Gracco & Abbs, 1987, p 168). Comparisons of nonautogenic (eg, upper-lip responses to a lower-lip load) and autogenic (lower-lip responses to a lower-lip load) compensation revealed different forms of multimovement coupling. Early perturbations to lower-lip movements resulted in a larger increase in the lower-lip response while later perturbations resulted in a larger increase in the upper-lip response. To them these observations suggest that voluntary speech production involves different sensorimotor actions during programming and execution. Their conclusion is that for complex voluntary behaviors such as speech, the control mode appears to involve both "corrective" and "predictive" sensorimotor actions.

Today it is generally accepted that sensorimotor interaction is integral to movement control and that the brain uses feed-forward and feedback information in a plastic and generative manner depending on task demands or context of motor performance. For example, studies of the activity of single cells in cerebral motor cortex of the monkey have shown that closed-loop control of a particular neuron can rapidly change to open-loop control (Evarts, 1982).

Different modes of interaction between centrally generated motor programs and sensory feedback may exist (Tatton & Bruce, 1981). During motor learning the control mode is presumably predominantly based on feedback control, which aids in optimizing accuracy. After that, feedback may only be vital when the brain's predictive model is changed by extraordinary circumstances (Brooks, 1986; Finocchio & Luschei, 1988; Grillner, 1982; Kelso & Stelmach, 1976). Sensory feedback is continually present, but the option of ignoring it seems to exist (Brooks, 1986).

During the time course of movement, progress, it seems, is assessed by an integration of peripheral sensory signals and corollary discharge (Brooks, 1986). During the production of speech, auditory feedback together with tactile and proprioceptive feedback might also be utilized for this purpose. Auditory feedback can provide information about completion of speech movements and might therefore play a role in speech timing. Auditory feedback can also monitor accuracy of articulation on a long-term basis. It cannot serve to monitor on-going skilled articulation as the information provided to the speaker arrives too late for on line speech motor control.

In the proposed framework, the presence of different feedback circuits is indicated. Feedback and feed-forward information is probably utilized at multiple levels of speech processing. The exact nature of sensorimotor interface during all of these phases is not yet known, but it is evident that sensory information is an integral part of speech motor control.

Contextual Sensitivity of Speech Sensorimotor Control

The proposed framework depicts speech production as being context-sensitive. The concept of context sensitivity is partially derived from the coalition model described by Kelso and Tuller (1981). Rather than seeing context as boundary conditions that specify exactly how the degrees of freedom of movement must be constrained, it is hypothesized in the present framework that contextual factors affect the dynamics of motor control by exerting an influence on the mode of coalition of neural structures involved during a particular phase and on the skill required from the planning, programming, and execution mechanisms. Certain variants of a specific contextual factor may require more complex control strategies than others. Differences in the level of activity of certain neural structures during different motor tasks (eg, self-initiated vs stimulus-induced) have been observed by neurophysiologists (Aizawa, Inase, Mushiake, Shima, & Tanji, 1991; Alexander and Crutcher, 1990a,b; Crutcher & Alexander, 1990; Lang, Beisteiner, Lindiner, & Deecke, 1992; Mushiake, Inase, & Tanji, 1990; Romo & Schultz, 1992; Romo, Scarnati,

& Schultz, 1992; Schultz & Romo, 1992). It also seems that precise fine or unfamiliar movements versus ballistic or well-learned movements require greater implementation of sensory input and thus greater involvement of sensory areas which again influence the coalition of neural areas (Brooks, 1986; Evarts, 1982; Evarts & Fromm, 1977; Kelso & Stelmach, 1976). Context therefore does influence the control system.

The contextual factors identified in the proposed framework are hypothetical and may be incomplete. A review of the literature, however, indicates that voluntary versus involuntary (or automatic) speech (Kelso & Tuller, 1981; Klein, 1976; Luria, 1966; Oberg & Divac, 1981), sound, or phonological structure (Calvert, 1980; Oller & MacNeilage, 1983; Edwards & Shriberg, 1983), motor complexity of the utterance (Calvert, 1980; Ladefoged, 1980), length of the utterance (Klapp, Anderson, & Berrian, 1973), familiar versus unfamiliar utterances (Allen & Tsukahara, 1974; Ashton, 1976; Kim & Corlew, 1979; Sharkey & Folkins, 1985), and rate of speech (Crompton, 1980; Gay, 1981; Kelso, Tuller, & Harris, 1983; MacNeilage, 1980) may be factors that influence the process of speech sensorimotor control. Research has already indicated that variation of factors such as sound structure may cause variation in the symptoms of apraxia of speech (Kent & Rosenbek, 1983; Van der Merwe & Grimbeek, 1990; Van der Merwe, Uys, Loots, & Grimbeek, 1987, 1988; Van der Merwe, Uys, Loots, Grimbeek, & Jansen, 1989). The role of all the identified contextual factors in the different phases of the speech act will have to be determined by research. Variation in contextual factors, however, will influence both treatment and research results.

The Proposed Framework of Speech Sensorimotor Control

The proposed theoretical framework of speech sensorimotor control is depicted in Figure 1–1. The hypothetical processes that

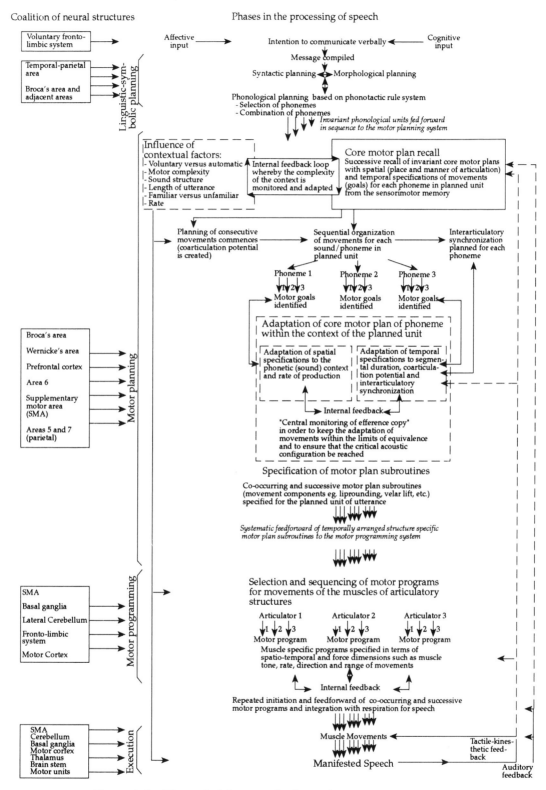

Figure 1–1. Theoretical framework of speech sensorimotor control.

occur during the different phases of the transformation of the speech code together with the different neural structures that are involved during a specific phase are indicated in the model.

The different phases are identified as linguistic-symbolic planning which is a nonmotor (or premotor) process, motor planning, motor programming, and execution. The differentiation of the three motor levels is in accord with the motor hierarchy as accepted by most neurophysiologists (Allen & Tsukahara, 1974; Brooks, 1986; Marsden, 1984; Schmidt, 1978). The concept of division of the events underlying the production of speech into phases may be somewhat simplistic, but it is useful in discussing brain behavior during speech production and in localizing levels of dysfunction. The serial analytic model is implicit in many contemporary theories of motor control (Alexander & Crutcher, 1990a). It would be wrong to assume multilevel processing as strictly hierarchical and thereby implying one-way information flow. It will be noticed in the framework that information flows in both directions and in loops, indicating sensorimotor interaction.

The different neural structures involved in speech production are portrayed as functioning in coalition as the exact function of each in relation to every other structure is highly complex and not yet fully known. Research in this field is abundant and often contradictory due to differences in subjects, experimental techniques, and nature of the movements studied. Indication of which neural structures are involved during a specific phase, however, is as essential for the speech pathologist charged with managing neurogenic communication disorders as it is for the speech researcher. This knowledge enhances our understanding of the level and nature of the breakdown.

Intention in Verbal Communication

Intention or readiness to commence intentional behavior is regulated by frontal-limbic formations of the forebrain (Kornhuber, 1977; Lamendella, 1977; Mogeson, Jones, & Yim, 1980; Pribram, 1976). The most basic function of the limbic system is to govern biological drives, but it also generates emotional motivation to act. Limbic drives are transformed into motor goals or general plans through corticocortical processing in the higher association cortex. Brooks (1986) further states that "motivational limbic influences are needed to enact motor plans and to assemble their programs and subprograms" (p 33).

In a discussion of motor behavior one should differentiate between the general intention to react and the initiation of movements. There is considerable evidence that limbic forebrain structures are important in "drives" and "motivational" processes contributing to the initiation of actions, but little is known about the neural mechanisms by which limbic processes gain access to the motor system. Mogeson et al (1980) provide a tentative model for limbic-motor inferface. They consider the nucleus accumbens to be the functional link between the limbic structures and the basal ganglia. More recently Nauta and Domesick (1984) also state that the limbic afferented striatal sector suggests itself as an interface between the motivational and the more strictly motor aspects of movement. There are indications that the supplementary motor area (SMA) too has a role in the initiation of movement including speech movements (Jonas, 1981; Orgogozo & Larsen, 1979). According to Ploog (1981), this area is functionally connected to the limbic cortex. Both the SMA and basal ganglia are involved in motor programming (see discussion later). It is proposed therefore that the frontolimbic system is involved not only in the initial intention to communicate but also in motor programming and most probably with regard to repeated initiation or feed-forward of motor programs for different muscles of the speech apparatus.

In the proposed framework the initial intention to communicate verbally closely links with affective input as the needs and motivation of the speaker influence the drive to communicate. Therefore, there has to be limbic support of sensorimotor processing. Brooks (1986) mentions that motivation of patients can be of great assistance in motor training and is therefore a clinically important factor to keep in mind.

Linguistic-Symbolic Planning

During verbal communication, semantic, syntactic, lexical, morphological, and phonological planning have to take place. This phase in the process of verbal communication requires linguistic-symbolic planning based on knowledge of the linguistic rules of the language. The term linguistic-symbolic planning indicates the nonmotor nature of this level of processing.

The intention to communicate verbally originates in the internal biological or cognitive needs of the person or in the external demands exerted by the environment. A message is compiled which reflects both the internal and external sources of input. The interaction between these arenas is indicated by double arrows in the framework.

Research indicates that planning of the complete utterance occurs simultaneously and not word for word (Holmes, 1984). Semantic construction of the message, recall and selection of lexical units, and syntactic, morphological, and phonological planning occur in coherence. The phonological plan is invariant (Linell, 1982), and changes therein influence the meaning or intelligibility of the utterance. Phonological planning, which is also referred to as the covert aspect of phonology (Edwards & Schriberg, 1983), entails the selection and sequential combination of phonemes in accordance with the phonotactic rules of the language, and it is portrayed as a linguistic-symbolic function in the proposed framework.

With regard to the neural structures responsible for linguistic-symbolic planning there are indications that the temporal-parietal area, particularly Wernicke's area, and also Broca's area are involved. Negative cerebral event-related potentials and regional cerebral blood flow indicate that activity is most prominent in the precentral and parietal regions while a person prepares to produce speech (Aschoff & Kornhuber, 1975; Fried, Ojemann, & Fetz, 1981; Grözinger, Kornhuber, & Kriebel, 1977; Lassen, Ingvar, & Skinhoj, 1978; Levy, 1977; Meyer, Sakai, Yamaguchi, Yamamoto, & Shaw, 1980). Grözinger et al (1977) find that with single-word production, the prespeech cerebral potentials are more pronounced over Broca's area than over Wernicke's area. The difference in amplitude between these two areas diminishes when full sentences are produced. In other words Wernicke's area becomes more active with an increase in semantic content while Broca's area remains active during any speech act. These data might indicate that these two areas are coactive during linguistic-symbolic and motor planning and that their relative roles change depending on the nature of the speech task and the phase of preparation of an utterance.

Motor Planning

During the planning phase of the production of articulated speech (vs for instance type-written language), a gradual transformation of symbolic units (phonemes) to a code that can be handled by a motor system has to take place. Motor planning entails formulating the strategy of action by specifying motor goals. In the proposed framework a hypothetical description of speech motor planning is presented.

Planning is mediated by the "highest" level of the motor hierarchy. It is widely accepted that the so-called association areas are responsible for motor planning (Allen & Tsukahara, 1974; Brooks, 1986; Evarts, 1982; Marsden, 1984; Schmidt, 1978). The motor association area, comprising the premotor cortex (lateral area 6) and the supplementary motor area (medial area 6) together with the prefrontal and parietal association areas are involved in motor planning (Brooks, 1986; Burbaud, Doegle, Gross, & Bioulac, 1991; Di Pellegrino & Wise, 1991; Guyton, 1981; Knight, Singh, & Woods, 1989; Mushiake et al, 1990; Romo & Schultz, 1992; Romo et al,

1992; Schultz & Romo, 1992), Broca's area can be considered as part of the premotor cortex. The anatomical location of inferior area 6, and in particular of F5 in the monkey, corresponds in large part to that of Broca's area in the human brain (Di Pellegrino, Fadiga, Fogassi, Gallese, & Rizzolatti, 1992). Brooks (1986) believes that the caudate circuit of the basal ganglia is part of the "higher" hierarchical level in that it enables the high-level plans to be translated into motor action.

A number of less recent studies have indicated the participation of most of these areas during the planning of speech movements. Negative cerebral event-related potentials and regional cerebral blood flow indicate that Broca's area in particular, but also other cortical motor association areas such as the premotor cortex (which includes area 6 and the supplementary motor area) and the prefrontal cortex together with the somatosensory cortex (which includes areas 5 and 7), become bilaterally active immediately prior to and during speech production (Darian-Smith, Johnson, & Goodwin, 1979; Halsen, Blauenstein, Wilson & Wills, 1980; Lassen et al, 1978; Levy, 1977; Marteniuk & MacKenzie, 1980; Weinrich, Wise, & Mauritz, 1984).

The prefrontal area seems to operate at a hierarchically superior level compared to the frontal areas (Di Pellegrino & Wise, 1991) and is necessary for formulating integrated behavior (Brooks, 1986). The association areas project to the premotor cortex and the SMA, which organize the principal output stage of the middle level (Brooks, 1986). The premotor cortex, SMA, and certain parts of the basal ganglia are richly interconnected and probably cooperate in neuronal processing directing planning (Burbaud et al, 1991).

The SMA receives a lot of attention in research. It is somatotopically organized and is not only a motor center controlling movements, but is also implicated in the initiation of movements (Aizawa et al, 1991; Kurata, 1992; Lang, Cheyne, Kristeva, Beisteiner, Lindinger, & Deecke, 1991; Luppino, Matelli, & Rizzolatti, 1990). Lang et al (1992) have

observed a *bereitschaftpotential* which starts about 2.5 sec prior to movement onset. Prior to single movements a shorter latency, of about 1.2 sec, was observed. There are indications that the SMA is involved in motor planning and initiation of speech movements, too (Jonas, 1981; Lassen et al, 1978).

It is, however, not only motor areas that become active prior to movement but also the parietal association cortex (in humans too) (Knight et al, 1989). Burbaud et al (1991) have found that the parietal association cortex is involved both in the integration of different sensory modalities and in the planning of movement. According to them it appears likely that various modes of sensorimotor interaction occur in the posterior parietal cortex.

The exact role of the posterior parietal areas in the planning of movement is not absolutely clear. Anatomic data point toward extensive connections with the frontal cortex, the cingulate gyrus, and the different motor areas (Brooks, 1986; Darian-Smith et al, 1979; Evarts, 1982). A possible explanation is that information from the sensory memory store is implemented during planning and that these areas are involved in internal feedback.

Posterior parietal areas, together with temporal areas and in particular Wernicke's, may play a similar role in speech production. Broca's and Wernicke's areas are extensively interconnected, and both are linked to other motor areas, with Broca's area more extensively so (Darian-Smith et al, 1979; Kornhuber, 1977; Ploog, 1981). The extensive connections between cortical motor and sensory areas suggest that the planning phase requires a complex coalition between these neural structures and thus between motor and sensory information. The involvement of temporal areas might imply that linguistic or covert phonological knowledge and rules are implemented during the initial phases of motor planning of speech. The participation of both Broca's and Wernicke's areas during motor and linguistic-symbolic planning seems realistic rather than a sharp distinction in function. It would suggest that gradual transformation of the code occurs.

In the proposed framework it is indicated that Broca's and Wernicke's areas are active during the planning phase together with the prefrontal cortex, Area 6, the SMA, and the parietal association areas 5 and 7. These areas are fed with a sequence of invariant phonological units from which motor plans have to be derived.

Motor planning is goal-orientated, and motor goals for speech production can be found in the spatial and temporal specifications of movements for sound production. A target-based model was first proposed by MacNeilage (1970). Underlying this approach is the assumption that the phoneme within the context of the utterance is the unit of planning.

The sounds or phonemes in every language can be described in terms of place and manner of articulation. Each sound has its own specifications, and these core features can be considered as invariant (Stevens & Blumstein, 1981). The core features determine the invariant core motor plan with spatial (place and manner of articulation) and temporal specifications for each sound. The specifications of movements constitute the motor goals. Invariance can therefore be found in the ultimate goals of production.

The core motor plan is attained during the development of speech and the motor specifications and sensory model (what it feels and sounds like) are stored in the sensorimotor memory. While mastering the core motor plan, proprioceptive, tactile, and auditory feedback is implemented. This feedback loop is indicated in the model.

During the production of speech, the core motor plans of the sequence of phonological units or phonemes are recalled from the sensorimotor memory. The context within which this motor plan has to be implemented is monitored and sometimes adapted if the complexity is found too high. Examples of such adaptation can be found in the phenomena of shorter chunks of utterances which are produced as units (eg, syllabic speech), phonological changes like shortening a word or duplicating sounds in a word, or slowed rate

of speech. Such compensatory strategies are often observed in sensorimotor speech disorders (Kent & Rosenbek, 1983; Van der Merwe et al, 1987, 1988, 1989, 1990; Wertz, La Pointe, & Rosenbek, 1984). The normal speaker will also decrease rate when an unfamiliar and long word is to be produced.

Following recall of the core motor plan, planning of the consecutive movements necessary to fulfill the spatial and temporal goals commences. The different motor goals for each phoneme are to be identified, and the movements that are necessary to produce the different sounds in the planned unit are then sequentially organized. It is important to point out that motor planning is articulator-specific and not muscle-specific. Motor goals such as lip rounding, jaw depression, glottal closure, or lifting of the tongue tip need to be specified. Interarticulatory synchronization is to be planned for the production of a particular phoneme.

At this stage the potential for coarticulation is created. When the different motor goals for the sounds in the planned unit, which presumably consists of a few words in the normal speaker, are specified, a certain movement such as lip rounding can be temporally prepositioned if there is no other, opposing movement prior to it.

An invariant core motor plan is recalled from the sensorimotor memory and the motor goals specified, but in the realization of speech we know that "speech violates what can be called the linearity and invariance conditions" (Wanner, Teyler, & Thompson, 1977, p 6). On the articulatory level speech movements are variant and context-dependent, and the boundaries between discrete phonological units fade away (Calvert, 1980; Kent & Minifie, 1977; MacNeilage, 1980; MacNeilage & De Clerk, 1969; Perkell & Klatt, 1986).

Variance manifested in the spatial and temporal aspects of speech movements originates from various sources. Adaptation of articulatory movements to the sound environment (Borden & Harris 1984), coarticulation of more than one articulator but for different phonemes (Borden & Harris, 1984;

Kent & Minifie, 1977), motor equivalence of speech targets with variations in the individual components (Abbs, 1986; Hughes & Abbs, 1976; Sharkey & Folkins, 1985), phonetic and linguistic influences on segmental duration (DiSimoni, 1974; Mitleb, 1984; Nishinuma, 1984; Walsh, 1984), and changes in speech rate (Gay, 1981; Kelso et al, 1983) are all factors that contribute to variance in speech production.

The core motor plan of the phoneme therefore has to be adapted to the context of the planned unit. Adaptation of spatial specifications to the phonetic (sound) context and to the rate of production has to occur. Adaptation of temporal specifications to segmental duration, coarticulation potential, and interarticulatory synchronization also takes place. The double arrows in the framework indicate that motor goals are identified in accordance with an adapted motor plan and a kind of parallel processing (Percheron & Filion, 1991) probably takes place. The same applies to interarticulatory synchronization. Temporal adaptation of the core plan might have implications for the synchronization of movements for a specific sound.

The adaptation of movements, however, has to be kept within certain limits of equivalence to ensure that the critical acoustic configuration is reached. The spatial and temporal differences between certain sounds are in many cases absolutely minimal, and if these boundaries or limits are violated, the sound will be perceived as being distorted or even substituted by another sound.

Adaptation of the core motor plan has to take place before articulation of a specific phoneme is initiated as adaptation determines the innervation of specific structures at particular points in time. Adaptation cannot be guided by response feedback, as the movement has not yet taken place at the moment of planning. It is, however, conceivable that internal feedback (Evarts & Fromm, 1981; Kelso, 1982; Teuber, 1974) or predictive simulation (Lindblom et al, 1979) guides adaptation. It is therefore proposed that internal feedback of an efference copy to the sensorimotor cortex is implemented to keep

adaptation of the core motor plan within the limits of equivalence. Numerous reciprocal connections between sensorimotor areas could support such a hypothesis (Burbaud et al, 1991; Brooks, 1986; Darian-Smith et al, 1979; Evarts, 1982).

Central monitoring of the efference copy implies that the speaker applies a kind of predictive simulation (Lindblom et al, 1979). Keller (1987, p 134) refers to "learned relations between specifications for the contraction of individual muscles." "Knowledge of results" of certain movements therefore is utilized during adaptation. Kawato and Gomi (1992) refer to an internal predictive model. They localize this model in the cerebellum, but there seems to be no reason why such internal models are not also present in cortical sensorimotor areas. Their concept of an inverse model, which they define as "a neural representation of the transformation from the desired movements of the controlled object (which can be an articulator) to the motor commands required to attain these movement goals" (p 446), seems to be an attractive theory for speech sensorimotor control. They contrast this inverse model to the forward model, which is "a neural representation of the transformation from motor commands to the resultant behavior of the controlled object" (p 445). More sophisticated feed-forward control can be achieved through an inverse model of the controlled object (Kawato & Gomi, 1992). An inverse model would require knowledge of results of movements, which seems to be present in the normal adult speaker.

It will be noticed in the proposed framework that peripheral tactile-kinesthetic feedback is available during the adaptation stage of motor planning. Under extraordinary conditions such as bite block (Folkins & Zimmerman, 1981) or weight perturbation (Gracco & Abbs, 1989) intervention, peripheral sensory feedback might be used to adapt movements. To a certain extent this process would be in accord with the notion of autogenic (or corrective) control proposed by Gracco & Abbs (1987).

Following the identification of motor goals

in accordance with the necessary adaptations to the core plan, the different subroutines that constitute the motor plan are specified. Co-occuring and successive subroutines such as lip rounding and velar lift are specified and temporally organized. Systematic feed-forward of temporally arranged structure-specific motor plan subroutines to the motor programming system then occurs.

Motor Programming

The intricacies of the programming of movement are being researched in abundance, but a comprehensive description of what programming entails remains enigmatic (Carpenter & Jayaraman, 1987; King, 1987; Strata, 1989). The term originated from the "centralist" view of motor control which proclaims the existence of a feedforward mechanism (Russell, 1976). In 1968 Keele defined the motor program as a "set of muscle commands that are structured before a movement sequence begins, and that follows the entire sequence to be carried out uninfluenced by peripheral feedback" (MacKay, 1980, p 98).

Many years of debate concerning the content of the program followed (Keele, 1982: Kelso, 1982; MacKay, 1980; Schmidt, 1976, 1982). Substantial evidence related to the minimal effect of unexpected perturbations and the negative effect of deafferentation on skilled movements stressed the functional importance of sensory updating and the need for a redefinition of the motor program (Brooks, 1986; Evarts, 1982; Kelso, 1982; Schmidt, 1982). The suggested redefinition of Marsden (1984) seems to capture the essential elements: "The motor program is a set of muscle commands that are structured before a movement sequence begins which can be delivered without reference to external feedback" (p 228). The implication seems to be that sensory feedback can be utilized to change or update a program should the need arise.

Gracco & Abbs (1987, p 175) state that in their view, "the motor program is an algorithm which sets up the system for a process whereby on-line sensory input and general motor command prespecifications are 'mixed' dynamically to yield appropriate intended goals."

Both these definitions reflect the generative and plastic nature of motor control in general. According to Gracco & Abbs (1987), who studied speech motor programming in particular, the ability to modify speech movements throughout the motor act indicates that movement control is "a real-time continuous process" and is sensitive to inputs during both preexecution and movement times. Interface between preplanned motor programs and real-time updating based on sensory input, therefore, seems to be intrinsic to the motor programming of movement, including speech movements.

Another major reason for the uncertainty that generally surrounded the nature of the motor program seems to be inadequate differentiation between motor plans and motor programs. To indicate central planning, terms such as preprogramming (Allen & Tsukahara, 1974), central programs (Evarts, 1982), and generalized motor programs (Schmidt, 1982) were used. Recent publications, however, do draw the distinction between motor plans mediated by cortical association areas and motor programs prepared by the middle level of the motor hierarchy (Brooks, 1986; Marsden, 1984; Wing & Miller, 1984). The same kind of confusion influenced the conception of levels or phases in speech motor control.

Brooks (1986) also uses the terms strategy and tactics to explain the plan-program relationship: "Strategies prescribe the general nature of plans and tactics give them particular specifications in space and time" (p 26). At the middle level of the motor hierarchy, strategy is converted into motor programs or tactics. Specific movement parameters are computed in the motor program (Schultz & Romo, 1992). Programs specify muscle tone, movement direction, force, range, and rate as well as mechanical stiffness of the joints (Brooks, 1986; Miall, Weir, & Stein, 1987) according to the requirements of the planned movement as it changes over time (Brooks,

1986). The timing and amount of muscle contraction in agonists, antagonists, synergists, and postural fixators need to be specified prior to movement onset (Marsden, 1984). The many degrees of freedom in the responding musculature are reduced by a structure or organization such as the motor program or the coordinative structure, as was also proposed by researchers such as Kelso et al (1983).

The quest for a better understanding of the process of programming is recently primarily geared toward a comprehensive formulation of the role of the different neural structures involved in the middle level (or programming phase) of motor processing. The neural areas involved in motor programming are indicated in the proposed framework and comprise the basal ganglia, the lateral cerebellum, the SMA, the motor cortex, and the frontolimbic system. It is generally accepted that the basal ganglia (Evarts & Wise, 1984; Marsden, 1980, 1984; McGeer & McGeer, 1987) and the lateral cerebellum (Allen & Tsukahara, 1974; Eccles, 1977; Houk & Gibson, 1987; Mano, Kanazawa, & Yamamoto, 1989; Miall et al, 1987) in particular are involved in programming and that these parts perform complementary functions. The exact role of each, however, is not known. There are indications that the basal ganglia has a more "sophisticated" role to play than the cerebellum (Bloxham, Mindel, & Frith, 1984; Brooks, 1986; Kornhuber, 1977).

The basal ganglia consist of three subcortical forebrain systems that are connected to the sensorimotor system and the limbic system. According to Brooks (1986), there are at least three circuits through the basal ganglia: the caudate one is linked to the higher level of the motor hierarchy, and the putamen circuit is linked to the middle level. The loop through the higher level is thought to control the assembly of overall motor plans, while the loop through the middle level is thought to update programs. Schultz and Romo (1992) have, however, found that both caudate and putamen appear to be involved in "setting and maintaining central preparatory states related to the internal generation of individual behavioral acts" (p 363). A third circuit through the ventral basal ganglia contains the ventral striatum, which has limbic innervations. The ventral basal ganglia contribute to the conversion of need-directed intentions into specific, goal-directed motor acts (Brooks, 1986).

Lidsky, Manetto, and Schneider (1985) have proposed a sensory-based model of basal ganglia functioning. They review data indicating that the basal ganglia have the potential to affect movement by gating sensory input into other motor systems that have more direct access to the final common path. It follows, then, that the basal ganglia's involvement in a given movement would vary with the role played by sensory stimulation in that movement. According to them the basal ganglia respond to somatosensory, auditory, and visual inputs and convert sensory data from a form that is receptor-oriented to a form that is relevant for guiding movement. According to Marsden (1980, 1984), all parts of the nervous system undertake sensorimotor integration, and he supports the traditional view of the basal ganglia as concerned with some aspect of motor function. He mentions that the striopallidal complex takes in processed sensory and other information from all areas of the cerebral cortex and midline thalamic nuclei and issues somatotopically organized motor instructions (Marsden, 1980). The basal ganglia have numerous afferent and efferent connections (Brooks, 1986; Evarts & Wise, 1984; McGeer & McGeer, 1987; Nauta & Domesick, 1984) and control by the basal ganglia might involve "comparisons of efference copies from successively linked areas of higher association cortex" (Brooks, 1986, p 313).

According to Marsden (1984), the negative symptoms of Parkinson's disease give the greatest clue to the normal function of the basal ganglia. Parkinson's disease causes delayed initiation, slowed execution, abnormal sequential complex movements, and an inability to automatically execute learned motor plans. The overall form of motor programs is preserved; however, the details of the number and frequency of motor neurons activated, at least in the first agonist burst, are inaccurate. There is a problem in switching from one program to another (Bloxham et al, 1984; Brooks, 1986; Marsden, 1984; Van den Bercken & Cools, 1982; Wing & Miller, 1984). Dysarthria due to Parkinson's disease also indicates that the basal ganglia may have a role to play in initiation, temporal synchronization, timing and automized production of speech (Kim & Corlew, 1979; Leanderson, Meyerson, & Persson, 1972; Leanderson, Persson, & Öhman, 1970; Nakano, Zubick, & Tyler, 1973).

The supplementary motor area (SMA) acts with the basal ganglia as part of an integrated system involved in the preparation of complex movements (Evarts & Wise, 1984; Romo & Schultz, 1992; Gaymard, Pierrot-Deseilligny, & Rivaud, 1990) in relation to conscious intention (Brooks, 1986). The SMA relays information to the basal ganglia via the association areas of the cortex (Brooks, 1986; Evarts & Wise, 1984; McGeer & McGeer, 1987), and the basal ganglia (globus pallidus and putamen) also send information back to the SMA (Brooks, 1986; Evarts & Wise, 1984; Mushiake et al, 1990; Romo & Schultz, 1992; Schultz & Romo, 1992) via the thalamus (Evarts & Wise, 1984). The exact role of the SMA at this middle level of motor processing is not known. However, both basal ganglia and SMA damage appears to cause deficits in spontaneously emitted motor acts and both are therefore implicated in the programming and control of movements (Evarts & Wise, 1984).

Cerebellar contributions lie in the tactical preparation of movements and postures needed for planned motor acts by making up appropriate programs. The lateral part of the cerebellum performs this "programming" task (Brooks, 1986). The cerebellum provides smoothness to the contraction of synergist and antagonist muscles (Gentil, 1990) by programming muscle length, force, and relations between them and also discharge rate (Houk & Gibson, 1987). Precise timing of movement is a function of the cerebellum

(Mano et al, 1989), but not only of the cerebellum (McNeil & Kent, 1990).

The cerebellum also performs a regulatory role for the middle level of the motor hierarchy (Brooks, 1986). The cerebellum receives input from the periphery, the brainstem, and the central cortex (Brooks, 1986; Gentil, 1990). The afferent and efferent connections of these zones form side loops that can function as comparators (Brooks, 1986).

Reports about motor commands and their execution reach the cerebellar cortex through "parallel" fibers. In addition, each microzone receives a small number of "climbing" fibers that convey information to indicate when the motor action is not being controlled optimally. Internal loops which allow for monitoring of the corollary motor commands, permit corrections to begin before movements are initiated (Brooks, 1986). The regulatory role of the cerebellum and a remarkable synaptic plasticity in the cerebellar cortex suggests that the cerebellum may play important functional roles in motor learning (Kawato & Gomi, 1992; Sanes, Dimitrov, & Hallett, 1990).

Cerebellar dysfunction can result in an inability to execute aimful movements correctly (dysmetria) and the failure to perform quick alternating movements (adiadochokinesia) (Glees, 1988). Cerebellar dysfunction decomposes intended movements into sequential constituents and causes errors of direction, force, velocity, and amplitude. Motor programs are thus degraded, because predictive control of trajectories is lost (Brooks, 1986; Larson & Sutton, 1978). Ataxic dysarthria is the result of a cerebellar lesion. Abnormalities of range, rate, force, timing, and coordination of speech movements are characteristic of this type of dysarthria (Darley et al, 1975; Joanette & Dudley, 1980; Kent & Netsell, 1975; Kent, Netsell, & Abbs, 1979). Available data suggest that the cerebellum may be involved, though not solely in the programming of spatiotemporal and force dimensions of speech movements.

The cerebellar and basal ganglia loops are separated from each other until they finally pool their influence through indirect paths via the thalamus on output neurons of the primary motor cortex (Brooks, 1986; Iversen, 1981; Marsden, 1984; McGeer & McGeer, 1987; Schmidt, 1978). The motor cortex, however, is not only a motor effector system (Brooks, 1986; Eccles, 1977; Kornhuber, 1977). It seems that sensory feedback to the motor cortex via at least two corticocortical pathways during ongoing movement provides a mechanism of sensorimotor integration (Porter, 1992). Sensory feedback continuously modulates motor cortex neuron discharge during accurate positioning and precise fine movements, whereas during ballistic movements such modulation is greatly attenuated (Evarts, 1982; Evarts & Fromm, 1977). The motor cortex therefore is important for the execution of learned, programmed movements (Brooks, 1986).

Motor cortex or upper motor neuron lesions cause spasticity and increased reflexes which can be considered to reflect a problem on the lowest level of the motor hierarchy. Brooks (1986) mentions that loss of corticospinal projection does not paralyze muscles but eliminates their use for skilled movements.

Extrapolating from available data, it appears that the programming of speech movements entails the selection and sequencing of motor programs of the muscles of the articulators (including the vocal folds) and specification of the muscle-specific programs in terms of spatiotemporal and force dimensions such as muscle tone, rate, direction, and range of movements. Updating of programs based on sensory feedback can occur, and programming is controlled by internal feedback mediated by all the neural structures involved at this stage. Repeated initiation and feed-forward of cooccurring and successive motor programs have to be controlled, and it is possible that the frontolimbic system, the SMA, and different sources of sensory feedback or input (even auditory feedback) might play a role in this process. The discussion is mainly geared toward movement control of the articulators and the vocal folds, but it is fully realized that the processes of articulation and phonation have to be integrated with breathing patterns for speech. Very little is known about supramedullary control (Von Euler, 1980, 1981) of breathing, but it seems logical that programming or control of inspiratory and expiratory muscles during speech would also be mediated at this level.

Execution

During the execution phase, the hierarchy of plans and programs is finally transformed into nonlearned automatic (reflex) motor adjustments. Successive specifications are relayed to the lower motor centers that control joints and muscles through the "final common path" (Sherrington's famous term). Programs are translated into activity of alpha and gamma motoneurons and reflexes that are under descending control of the middle level are modulated to meet the circumstances within which the movement occurs. Thus descending paths carry tactical instructions to the lowest level, where they are coordinated and finally translated into properly timed commands for muscle movements (Brooks, 1986).

The motor cortex is the last supraspinal station for conversion of the designs for movement arising in the association cortex into programs for movement. At the same time, it is the beginning of the chain of structures responsible for the execution of movement. The motor cortex, the lower motor neurones, peripheral nerves, and motor units in the muscles are the last neural structures in the hierarchical chain. However, it seems that control during movement is exerted by various structures also active during the premovement phases. Efferents from the cerebellum and basal ganglia pass primarily via the thalamus to the motor cortex, but there are also efferents passing directly to the motor centers of the brainstem, indicating control by these parts at this level (Allen & Tsukahara, 1974; Schmidt, 1978). Movement-related neuronal activity has been observed in the SMA, motor cortex, anterior striatum, and putamen (Crutcher & Alexander, 1990;

Luppino et al, 1990; Romo et al, 1992), which underscores the involvement of these areas during execution. Another implication of these observations is that multiple levels of motor processing proceed in parallel within all of these motor structures (Crutcher & Alexander, 1990). The relative role of each of the controlling centers remains unclear. Closed-loop, tactile-kinesthetic feedback as a possible means of control is also available during this phase of motor execution (Eccles, 1977) (see discussion above). During the manifestation of speech movements there is also an acoustic result which is fed back to the cortical areas, where it is implemented especially during speech development. This loop is indicated in the framework. The broken lines suggest that the different modes of feedback are available, though it is not necessarily constantly utilized. During speech development or in unfamiliar speech acts, a closed loop indicated by full lines may control execution.

The Characterization of Pathological Speech Sensorimotor Control

The proposed framework has implications for our current understanding of neurogenic speech and language disorders. The four-level framework modifies our traditional view of aphasia, apraxia of speech, and dysarthria as being disruptions on three diverse levels of a three-level model. The level and nature of breakdown in the different neurogenic communication disorders need some reconsideration within the context of this framework.

The differentiation between levels or phases of linguistic-symbolic planning, motor planning, motor programming, and execution would suggest that a distinct disorder (or disorders) on each of these levels is conceivable. A complicating factor, however, is the involvement of some neural structures on several levels of functioning. This would make cooccurring dysfunction in more than one phase of processing possible. Thus each specific disorder might exhibit deviances at more than one level of the speech production process. However, before contemplating this possibility it is necessary to delineate the nature of disruptions on a four-level model.

A dysfunction on the level of linguistic-symbolic planning would result in an inability in semantic, lexical, syntactic, morphological, and phonological planning, which are typical symptoms of aphasia. Deviant phonological planning will lead to disorders in the selection and sequential combination of phonemes, resulting in phoneme substitutions and transpositions which are characteristic of phonological (literal) paraphasias. Within the context of this framework, errors in phoneme sequencing and true sound substitutions (not distortions perceived as substitutions) would be assigned to a disorder in covert phonological ability.

The framework further proposes the possibility of a disorder in speech motor planning, which would imply that there can be an inability to:

- Recall the invariant core motor plans for specific phonemes
- Identify the different motor goals of specific phonemes
- Sequentially organize the movements for each phoneme and a series of movements for a sequence of phonemes
- Adapt the core motor plan to phonetic context
- Control interarticulatory synchronization
- Implement tactile-kinesthetic feedback from the periphery for adaptation (eg, adaptation to varying starting positions)
- Centrally monitor the efference copy
- Keep adaptation of movements within the limits of equivalence
- Systematically relay the structure specific motor plan subroutines to the motor programming system

Speech symptoms resulting from such problems in motor planning would be slow, struggling speech with distortion and even apparent substitutions. These are the symp-

17

toms that are ascribed to apraxia of speech. Distortion which is sometimes called the core symptom of apraxia of speech (Itoh & Sasanuma, 1984) can be the result of a number of the problems mentioned above. An inability to consistently make the necessary adaptations in movements, to synchronize the movements of the different articulators, to centrally monitor the parameters of all the necessary movements, and to keep these parameters within the limits of equivalence may result in sound distortion. An inability to plan consecutive movements at a high rate can lead to syllabic planning and slowed temporal flow of speech. The struggling behavior often observed in apraxic speakers may be the result of an inability to recall the core motor plan for the production of a phoneme or to identify and sequence the various motor goals of a planned unit. The framework thus not only offers an explanatory premise for apraxic symptoms but also suggests guidelines for principles of treatment in these cases.

The differentiation of phases as proposed in the framework not only has implications for apraxia of speech, but also complicates our traditional view of dysarthria as a motor execution problem. The role of structures such as the basal ganglia and the lateral cerebellum in both motor programming and execution suggests the possibility of dual symptomatology in certain types of dysarthria. Coexisting problems in both motor programming and motor execution would seem to be present in Parkinsonian (hypokinetic) dysarthria, hyperkinetic dysarthria, ataxic dysarthria (in which dysfunction of the lateral cerebellum occurs), and even spastic dysarthria. Dysarthria due to dysfunction of areas of the cerebellum other than the lateral cerebellum and dysarthria due to lower motor neurone disorders would be the only dysarthrias with a purely execution dysfunction. In these cases muscle tone problems such as hyper- and hypotonus and involuntary movements hamper accurate execution of movement. The possible masking role of symptoms such as spasticity will have to be considered when studying dysarthria where

coexisting programming and execution problems might be present.

Based on our current conceptualization of the programming of movement, a disorder at this level would result in an impairment of:

- The programming of muscle tone, rate, direction, and range of movements
- Repeated initiation and feedforward of co-occurring and successive motor programs

Theoretically speaking, such problems can occur in the absence of hyper- or hypotonia or involuntary movements, and indeed many classic symptoms of Parkinson's disease (see discussion above) in particular, do illustrate the nature of a programming disorder. The important implication for the speech pathologist is that pure programming speech defects do exist. Due to the involvement of different neural structures at this level, diverse programming defects is possible.

The symptoms resulting from a disorder at this level would probably be sound distortion, defects in speech rate, and/or problems in the initiation of movement. At first glance these symptoms seem to be similar to the symptoms characteristic of apraxia of speech, but there might be subtle differences. It is possible that these problems would be consistently present during all movements, as is the case with dysarthria. Distortion due to inaccurate movements in apraxic speakers, on the other hand, is not always present during repeated productions (Itoh & Sasanuma, 1984; Van der Merwe et al, 1989). It has been proposed that apraxia of speech due to a purely subcortical lesion can occur (Kertesz, 1984). This type of apraxia has not yet been extensively described, but it may represent one variety of a programming disorder. However, if the present neurophysiological conceptualization of the motor hierarchy is correct, apraxia of speech due to a purely cortical lesion would primarily be a disorder in motor planning.

Defects in speech rate may also result from programming disorders. A disruption on this level may lead either to a slowed rate of production or to an increased rate as sometimes observed in Parkinsonian speakers. Such primary disorders in speech rate, in contrast to compensatory changes in speech rate, can possibly differentiate between disruptions on a planning and programming level.

When contemplating the nature of motor programming speech disorders, we should perhaps also look beyond the traditional neurogenic problems. A three-level model cannot readily accommodate other disorders than the classic neurogenic pathologies. The four-level model, however, creates an expanded theoretical scope or field of reference. The fact that the limbic system, which is involved in volitional intent and emotional drives, gains access to the motor system via the basal ganglia at this level of the motor hierarchy (see discussion above), may prove to be most significant in the understanding of at least some of the speech defects not yet defined as motor programming disorders. Problems that come to mind is stuttering, cluttering, and even spasmodic dysphonia. The primary symptoms of stuttering seem to fit in well with a disorder in programming of speech rate and repeated initiation. Cluttering also exhibits defects in speech rate control and accurate articulation. According to Ploog (1981), the limbic system is directly linked to the vocal folds. The limbic —vocal structures—basal ganglia interface may be central to the precipitation of spasmodic dysphonia and may also play a role in some other programming disorders.

However, these are all merely hypotheses, but are worthy exploring. The theory on motor planning and programming of movement in general is not yet fully developed. The challenge of future research will be to define the different defects on different levels and to distinguish between motor planning and programming disorders. The localization of lesions may be a key concept. According to our current knowledge, a lesion in the SMA, basal ganglia, lateral cerebellum, motor cortex, and frontolimbic system and its interface with the basal ganglia in particular can lead to a programming disorder, while a planning disorder is caused by a lesion in the association areas.

The proposed theoretical framework not only offers explanations for neurogenic disorders, but it can also be implemented to clarify the nature of some other communication problems. Articulation problems and the speech of the hard-of-hearing can be used as examples to illustrate this point. The person with an articulation defect has a core motor plan for the production of that specific sound that differs from the core plan of the other speakers in his communication environment. The child born deaf, on the other hand, cannot develop motor plans for the different phonemes because of the lack of the reinforcing role of auditory feedback in building up sensorimotor memories. Linguistic-symbolic planning is not possible, and thus a motor plan will also not have any linguistic significance. The hard-of-hearing child who does learn to speak probably has to build up a sensorimotor memory of the production specifications of the core motor plan based mainly on tactile-kinesthetic feedback. Knowledge of the auditory results of productions and the ability to keep within the limits of equivalence will probably be influenced negatively by the changed or decreased auditory feedback. It is possible to continue speculating in this way, but research should rather address the issues raised by the framework.

In conclusion, we should remind ourselves that a theoretical framework or model is but a simple map to guide us in our quest for a better understanding of the nature of the phenomenon we are dealing with. The proposed framework posits a novel view on the neurogenic sensorimotor speech disorders and generates many new questions to be answered. These notions are to be pursued in future research. The ultimate goal, however, is that our gained insight will consequently assist in optimizing clinical assessment and intervention.

References

Abbs JH. (1973). The influence of gamma motor system on jaw movements during speech. *J Speech Hear Res* 16:175–199.

Abbs JH. (1986). Invariance and variability in speech production: a distinction between linguistic intent and its neuromotor implementation. In: Perkell JS, Klatt DH, eds. *Invariance and Variability in Speech Processes.* Hillsdale: Lawrence Erlbaum.

Abbs JH, Cole KJ. (1982). Consideration of bulbar and suprabulbar afferent influences upon speech motor coordination and programming. In: Grillner S, Lindblom B, Lubker J, Persson A, eds. *Speech Motor Control.* Oxford: Pergamon Press, vol. 36.

Abbs JH, Connor NP. (1991). Motorsensory mechanisms of speech motor timing and coordination. *J Phon* 19:333–342.

Abbs JH, Folkins JW, Sivarajan M. (1976). Motor impairment following blockade of the infraorbital nerve: implications for the use of anesthetization techniques in speech research. *J Speech Hear Res* 19:19–35.

Aizawa H, Inase M, Mushiake H, Shima K, Tanji J. (1991). Reorganization of activity in the supplementary motor area associated with motor learning and functional recovery. *Exp Brain Res* 84:668–671.

Alexander GE, Crutcher MD. (1990a). Preparation for movement: neural representations of intended direction in three motor areas of the monkey. *J Neurophysiol* 64:133–150.

Alexander GE, Crutcher MD. (1990b). Neural representations of the target (goal) of visually guided arm movements in three motor areas of the monkey. *J Neurophysiol* 64:164–178.

Allen GI, Tsukahara N. (1974). Cerebrocerebellar communication systems. *Physiol Rev* 54:957–997.

Aschoff JC, Kornhuber HH. (1975). Functional interpretation of somatic afferents in cerebellum, basal ganglia and motor cortex. In: Kornhuber HH, ed. *The Somatosensory System.* Stuttgart: Georg Thieme Publishers.

Ashton R. (1976). Aspects of timing in child development. *Child Dev* 47:622–626.

Bloxham CA, Mindel TA, Frith CD. (1984). Initiation and execution of predictable and unpredictable movements in Parkinson's disease. *Brain* 107:371–384.

Borden GJ. (1979). An interpretation of research on feedback interruption in speech. *Brain Lang* 7:307–319.

Borden GJ, Harris KS. (1984). *Speech Science Primer: Physiology, Acoustics and Perception of Speech,* ed 2. Baltimore: Williams and Wilkins.

Bowman JP. (1968). Muscle spindles in the intrinsic and extrinsic muscles of the rhesus monkey's *(Macaca mulatta)* tongue. *Anat Rec* 161:483–488.

Bowman JP, Combs CM. (1969a). The cerebrocortical projection of hypoglossal afferents. *Exp Neurol* 23:291–301.

Bowman JP, Combs CM. (1969b). Cerebellar responsiveness to stimulation of the lingual spindle afferent fibers in the hypoglossal nerve of the rhesus monkey. *Exp Neurol* 23:537–543.

Brooks VB. (1986). *The Neural Basis of Motor Control.* New York: Oxford University Press.

Burbaud P, Doegle C, Gross C, Bioulac B. (1991). A quantitative study of neuronal discharge in areas 5, 2 and 4 of the monkey during fast arm movements. *J Neurophysiol* 66:429–443.

Calvert DR. (1980). *Descriptive Phonetics.* New York: Thieme-Stratton.

Carpenter MB, Jayaraman A, eds. (1987). *The Basal Ganglia II: Structure and Function—Current Concepts.* New York: Plenum Press.

Crompton A. (1980). Timing patterns in French. *Phonetica* 37:205–234.

Crutcher MD, Alexander GE. (1990). Movement-related neuronal activity selectively coding either direction or muscle pattern in three motor areas of the monkey. *J Neurophysiol* 64:151–163.

Darian-Smith I, Johnson KO, Goodwin AW. (1979). Posterior parietal cortex: relations of unit activity to sensorimotor function. *Annu Rev Physiol* 41:141–157.

Darley FL, Aronson AE, Brown JR. (1975). *Motor Speech Disorders.* Philadelphia: W.B. Saunders.

Di Pellegrino G, Fadiga L, Fogassi L, Gallese V, Rizzolatti G. (1992). Understanding motor events: a neurophysiological study. *Exp Brain Res* 91:176–180.

Di Pellegrino G, Wise SP. (1991). A neurophysiological comparison of three distinct regions of the primate frontal lobe. *Brain* 114:951–978.

DiSimoni FG. (1974). Some preliminary observations on temporal compensation in the speech of children. *J Acoust Soc Am* 56:697–699.

Eccles JC. (1977). *The Understanding of the Brain.* New York: McGraw-Hill.

Edwards ML, Shriberg LD. (1983). *Phonology: Applications in Communicative Disorders.* San Diego: College-Hill.

Evarts EV. (1971). Activity of thalamic and cortical neurons in relation to learned movement in the monkey. *Int J Neurol* 8:321–326.

Evarts EV. (1982). Analogies between central motor programs for speech and for limb movements. In: Grillner S, Lindblom B, Lubker J, Persson A, eds. *Speech Motor Control.* Oxford: Pergamon Press, vol. 36.

Evarts EV, Fromm C. (1977). Sensory responses in motor cortex neurons during precise motor control. *Neurosci Lett* 5:267–272.

Evarts EV, Fromm C. (1981). Transcortical reflexes and servo control of movement. *Can J Physiol Pharmacol* 59:757–775.

Evarts EV, Wise SP. (1984). Basal ganglia outputs and motor control. In: *Ciba Foundation Symposium 107: Functions of the Basal Ganglia.* London: Pitman.

Finocchio DV, Luschei ES. (1988). Characteristics of complex voluntary mandibular movements in the monkey before and after destruction of most jaw muscle spindle afferents. *J Voice* 2:279–290.

Folkins JW, Abbs JH. (1975). Lip and jaw motor control during speech: responses to resistive loading of the jaw. *J Speech Hear Res* 18:207–220.

Folkins JW, Abbs JH. (1977). Motor impairment during inferior alveolar nerve blockade. *J Speech Hear Disord* 20:816–817.

Folkins JW, Zimmerman GN. (1981). Jaw-muscle activity during speech with the mandible fixed. *J Acoust Soc Am* 69:1441–1445.

Fried I, Ojemann GA, Fetz EE. (1981). Language-related potentials specific to human language cortex. *Science* 212:353–355.

Gay T. (1981). Mechanisms in the control of speech rate. *Phonetica* 38:148–158.

Gaymard B, Pierrot-Deseilligny C, Rivaud S. (1990). Impairment of sequences of memory-guided saccades after supplementary motor area lesions. *Ann Neurol* 28:622–626.

Gentil M. (1990). Organization of the articulatory system: peripheral mechanisms and central coordination. In: Hardcastle WJ, Marchal A, eds. *Speech Production and Speech Modelling.* Dordrecht, Kluwer Academic Publishers, vol. 55.

Glees P. (1988). *The Human Brain.* Cambridge: Cambridge University Press.

Goodwin GM, Luschei ES. (1974). Effects of destroying spindle afferents from jaw muscles on mastication in monkeys. *J Neurophysiol* 37:967–981.

Gracco VL, Abbs JH. (1986). Variant and invariant characteristics of speech movements. *Exp Brain Res* 65:156–166.

Gracco VL, Abbs JH. (1987). Programming and execution processes of speech movement control: potential neural correlates. In: Keller E, Gopnik M, eds. *Motor and Sensory Processes of Language.* Hillsdale, Lawrence Erlbaum.

Gracco VL, Abbs JH. (1988). Central patterning of speech movements. *Exp Brain Res* 71:515–526.

Gracco VL, Abbs JH. (1989). Sensorimotor characteristics of speech motor sequences. *Exp Brain Res* 75:586–598.

Grillner S. (1982). Possible analogies in the control of innate motor acts and the production of sound in speech. In: Grillner S, Lindblom B, Lubker J, Persson A, eds. *Speech Motor Control.* Oxford: Pergamon Press, vol. 36.

Grözinger B, Kornhuber HH, Kriebel J. (1977). Human cerebral potentials preceding speech production, phonation and movements of the mouth and tongue, with reference to respiratory and extracerebral potentials. In: Desmedt JE, ed. *Language and Hemispheric Specialization in Man: Cerebral Event-related Potentials, Progress in Clinical Neurophysiology.* Basel: S. Karger, vol. 3.

Guyton AC. (1981). *Textbook of Medical Physiology,* ed 6. Philadelphia: W.B. Saunders.

Halsey JH, Blauenstein UW, Wilson EM, Wills EL. (1980). Brain activation in the presence of brain damage. *Brain Lang* 9:47–60.

Holmes VM. (1984). Sentence planning in a story continuation task. *Lang Speech* 27:115–133.

Houk JC, Gibson AR. (1987). Sensorimotor processing through the cerebellum. In: King JS, ed. *New Concepts in Cerebellar Neurobiology, Neurology and Neurobiology,* vol. 22. New York: Alan R. Liss.

Hughes OM, Abbs JH. (1976). Labial-mandibular coordination in the production of speech: implications for the operation of motor equivalence. *Phonetica* 33:199–221.

Itoh M, Sasanuma S. (1984). Articulatory movements in apraxia of speech. In: Rosenbek JC, McNeil MR, Aronson AE, eds. *Apraxia of Speech: Physiology, Acoustics, Linguistics, Management.* San Diego: College-Hill.

Iversen SD. (1981). Motor control. *Br Med Bull* 37:147–152.

Jakobson LS, Goodale MA. (1991). Factors affecting higher-order movement planning: a kinematic analysis of human prehension. *Exp Brain Res* 86:199–208.

Joanette Y, Dudley JG. (1980). Dysarthria symptomatology of Friedreich's ataxia. *Brain Lang* 10:39–50.

Jonas J. (1981). The supplementary motor region and speech emission. *J Commun Disord* 14:349–373.

Kawato M, Gomi H. (1992). The cerebellum and VOR/OKR learning models. *TINS* 15:445–453.

Keele SW. (1982). Learning and control of coordinated motor patterns. In: Kelso JAS, ed. *Human Motor Behavior: An Introduction.* London, Lawrence Erlbaum.

Keller E. (1987). The cortical representation of motor processes of speech. In: Keller E, Gopnik M, eds. *Motor and Sensory Processes of Language.* Hillsdale: Lawrence Erlbaum.

Kelso JAS. (1982). Concepts and issues in human motor behavior: coming to grips with the jargon. In: Kelso JAS, ed. *Human Motor Behavior: An Introduction.* London: Lawrence Erlbaum.

Kelso JAS, Stelmach GE. (1976). Central and peripheral mechanisms in motor control. In: Stelmach GE, ed. *Motor Control: Issues and Trends.* New York: Academic Press.

Kelso JAS, Tuller B. (1981). Toward a theory of apractic syndromes. *Brain Lang* 12:224–245.

Kelso JAS, Tuller B, Harris KS. (1983). A "dynamic pattern" perspective on the control and coordination of movement. In: MacNeilage PF, ed. *The Production of Speech.* New York: Springer-Verlag.

Kent RD. (1990). The acoustic and physiologic characteristics of neurologically impaired speech movements. In: Hardcastle WJ, Marchal A, ed. *Speech Production and Speech Modelling.* Dordrecht: Kluwer Academic Publishers, vol. 55.

Kent RD, McNeil MR. (1987). Relative timing of sentence repetition in apraxia of speech and conduction aphasia. In: Ryalls JH, ed. *Phonetic Approaches to Speech Production in Aphasia and Related Disorders.* Boston: Little, Brown and Company.

Kent RD, Minifie FD. (1977). Coarticulation in recent speech production models. *J Phon* 5:115–133.

Kent RD, Netsell R. (1975). A case study of an ataxic dysarthric: cineradiographic and spec-

trographic observations. *J Speech Hear Disord* 40:115–134.

Kent RD, Netsell R, Abbs JH. (1979). Acoustic characteristics of dysarthria associated with cerebellar disease. *J Speech Hear Res* 22:627–648.

Kent RD, Rosenbek JC. (1983). Acoustic patterns of apraxia of speech. *J Speech Hear Res* 26:231–249.

Kertesz A. (1984). Subcortical lesions and verbal apraxia. In: Rosenbek JC, McNeil MR, Aronson AE, eds. *Apraxia of Speech: Physiology, Acoustics, Linguistics, Management.* San Diego: College-Hill.

Kim BW, Corlew M. (1979). Electromyographic-aerodynamic study of Parkinsonian speech. *Allied Health Behav Sci* 2:375–382.

King JS, ed. (1987). *New Concepts in Cerebellar Neurobiology, Neurology and Neurobiology,* vol 22. New York: Alan R. Liss.

Klein RM. (1976). Attention and movement. In: Stelmach GE, ed. *Motor Control: Issues and Trends.* New York: Academic Press.

Klapp ST, Anderson WG, Berrian RW. (1973). Implicit speech in reading reconsidered. *J Exp Psychol* 100:368–374.

Knight RT, Singh J, Woods DL. (1989). Premovement parietal lobe input to human sensorimotor cortex. *Brain Res* 498:190–194.

Kornhuber HH. (1977). A reconsideration of the cortical and subcortical mechanisms involved in speech and aphasia. In: Desmedt JE, ed. *Language and Hemispheric Specialization in Man: Cerebral Event-related Potentials, Progress in Clinical Neurophysiology.* Basel: S. Karger, vol. 3.

Kurata K. (1992). Somatotopy in the human supplementary motor area. *TINS* 15:159–160.

Lacquaniti F. (1989). Central representations of human limb movement as revealed by studies of drawing and handwriting. *TINS* 12:287–291.

Ladefoged P. (1980). Articulatory parameters. *Lang Speech* 23:25–30.

Lamendella JT. (1977). The limbic system in human communication. In: Whitaker H, Whitaker HA, eds. *Studies in Neurolinguistics.* New York: Academic Press, vol. 3.

Landgren S, Olsson KA. (1982). Oral mechanoreceptors. In: Grillner S, Lindblom B, Lubker J, Persson A, eds. *Speech Motor Control.* Oxford: Pergamon Press, vol. 36.

Lang W, Beisteiner R, Lindinger G, Deecke L.

(1992). Changes of cortical activity when executing learned motor sequences. *Exp Brain Res* 89:435–440.

Lang W, Cheyne D, Kristeva R, Beisteiner R, Lindinger G, Deecke L. (1991). Three-dimensional localization of SMA activity preceding voluntary movement: a study of electric and magnetic fields in a patient with infarction of the right supplementary motor area. *Exp Brain Res* 87:688–695.

Larson CR, Sutton D. (1978). Effects of cerebellar lesions on monkey jaw-force control: implications for understanding ataxic dysarthria. *J Speech Hear Res* 21:309–323.

Lassen NA, Ingvar DH, Skinhoj E. (1978). Brain function and blood flow. *Sci Am* 239:50–60.

Leanderson R, Meyerson BA, Persson A. (1972). Lip muscle function in Parkinsonian dysarthria. *Acta Otolaryngol* 74:350–357.

Leanderson R, Persson A, Ohman S. (1970). Electromyographic studies of the function of the facial muscles in dysarthria. *Acta Otolaryngol* 263:89–94.

Levy RS. (1977). The question of electrophysiological asymmetries preceding speech. In: Whitaker H, Whitaker HA, eds. *Studies in Neurolinguistics*. New York: Academic Press, 1977.

Lidsky, TI, Manetto C, Schneider JS. (1985). A consideration of sensory factors involved in motor functions of the basal ganglia. *Brain Res Rev* 9:133–146.

Lindblom B, Lubker J, Gay T. (1979). Formant frequencies of some fixed-mandible vowels and a model of speech motor programming by predictive simulation. *J Phon* 7:147–161.

Linell P. (1982). The concept of phonological form and the activities of speech production and speech perception. *J Phon* 10:38–72.

Luppino G, Matelli M, Rizzolatti G. (1990). Cortico-cortical connections of two electrophysiologically identified arm representations in the mesial agranular frontal cortex. *Exp Brain Res* 82:214–218.

Luria AR. (1966). *Higher Cortical Functions in Man.* New York: Basic Books.

MacKay WA. (1980). The motor program: back to the computer. *TINS* 3:97–100.

MacNeilage PF. (1970). Motor control of serial ordering of speech. *Physiol Rev* 77:182–196.

MacNeilage PF. (1980). Speech production. *Lang Speech* 23:3–23.

MacNeilage PF, De Clerk JL. (1969). On the motor control of coarticulation in CVC monosyllables. *J Acoust Soc Am* 45:1217–1233.

Mano N, Kanazawa I, Yamamoto K. (1989). Voluntary movements and complex-spike discharges of cerebellar Purkinje cells. In: Strata P, ed. *The Olivo-cerebellar System in Motor Control, Experimental Brain Research Series 17.* Berlin: Springer-Verlag.

Marquardt TP, Sussman H. (1984). The elusive lesion—apraxia of speech link in Broca's aphasia. In: Rosenbek JC, McNeil MR, Aronson AE, eds. *Apraxia of Speech: Physiology, Acoustics, Linguistics, Management.* San Diego: College-Hill.

Marsden CD. (1980). The enigma of the basal ganglia and movement. *TINS* 3:284–287.

Marsden CD. (1984). Which motor disorder in Parkinson's disease indicates the true motor function of the basal ganglia? In: Ciba Foundation Symposium 107: *Functions of the Basal Ganglia.* London: Pitman.

Marteniuk RG, MacKenzie CL. (1980). Information processing in movement organization and execution. In: Nickerson RS, ed. *Attention and Performance VIII.* New Jersey: Lawrence Erlbaum Associates.

McClean MD. (1991). Lip muscle reflex and intentional response levels in a simple speech task. *Exp Brain Res* 87:662–670.

McGeer PL, McGeer EG. (1987). Integration of motor functions in the basal ganglia. In: Carpenter MB, Jayaraman A, eds. *The Basal Ganglia II: Structure and Function—Current Concepts.* New York: Plenum Press.

McNeil MR, Kent RD. (1990). Motoric characteristics of adult aphasic and apraxic speakers. In: Hammond GR, ed. *Cerebral Control of Speech and Limb Movements.* Amsterdam: North-Holland.

Meyer JS, Sakai F, Yamaguchi F, Yamamoto M, Shaw T. (1980). Regional changes in cerebral blood flow during standard behavioral activation in patients with disorders of speech and mentation compared to normal volunteers. *Brain Lang* 9:61–77.

Miall RC, Weir DJ, Stein JF. (1987). Visuo-motor tracking during reversible inactivation of the cerebellum. *Exp Brain Res* 65:455–464.

Mitleb FM. (1984). Voicing effect on vowel duration is not an absolute universal. *J Phon* 12:23–27.

Mogeson GJ, Jones DL, Yim CY. (1980). From motivation to action: functional interface between the limbic system and the motor system. *Prog Neurobiol* 14:69–97.

Mushiake H, Inase M, Tanji J. (1990). Selective coding of motor sequence in the supplementary motor area of the monkey cerebral cortex. *Exp Brain Res* 82:208–210.

Nakano KK, Zubick H, Tyler HR. (1973). Speech defects of parkinsonian patients effects of levodopa therapy on speech intelligibility. *Neurology (Minneap)* 23:865–870.

Nauta WJH, Domesick VB. (1984). Afferent and efferent relationships of the basal ganglia. In: *Ciba Foundation Symposium 107: Functions of the Basal Ganglia.* London: Pitman, 1984.

Netsell R. (1982). Speech motor control and selected neurologic disorders. In: Grillner S, Lindblom B, Lubker J, Persson A, eds. *Speech Motor Control.* Oxford: Pergamon Press.

Nishinuma Y. (1984). Prediction of phoneme duration by a distinctive feature matrix. *J Phon* 12:169–173.

Oberg RGE, Divac I. (1981). Levels of motor planning: cognition and the control of movement. *TINS* 4:122–124.

Oller DK, MacNeilage PF. (1983). Development of speech production: perspectives from natural and perturbed speech. In: MacNeilage PF, ed. *The Production of Speech.* New York: Springer-Verlag.

Orgogozo JM, Larsen B. (1979). Activation of the supplementary motor area during voluntary movement in man suggests it works as a supramotor area. *Science* 206:847–850.

Percheron G, Filion M. (1991). Parallel processing in the basal ganglia: up to a point. *TINS* 14:55–56.

Perkell JS, Klatt DH, eds. (1986) *Invariance and Variability in Speech Processes.* Hillsdale: Lawrence Erlbaum.

Persson A. (1982). Some comments on the motor control of speech. In: Grillner S, Lindblom B, Lubker J, Persson A, eds. *Speech Motor Control.* Oxford: Pergamon Press, vol. 36.

Ploog D. (1981). Neurobiology of primate audio-vocal behavior. *Brain Res Rev* 3:35–61.

Porter LL. (1992). Patterns of projections from area 2 of the sensory cortex to area 3a and to the motor cortex in cats. *Exp Brain Res* 91:85–93.

Pribram KH. (1976). Mechanisms in transmission of signals for conscious behaviour. In: Desiraju T, ed. *Executive Functions of the Frontal Lobes.* Amsterdam: Elsevier Scientific Publishing Company.

Putnam AHB, Ringel RL. (1976). A cineradiographic study of articulation in two talkers with temporarily induced oral sensory deprivation. *J Speech Hear Res* 19:247–266.

Ringel RL, Burk KW, Scott CM. (1968). Tactile perception: form discrimination in the mouth. *Br J Disord Commun* 3:150–155.

Ringel RL, Ewanowski SJ. (1965). Oral perception: two point discrimination. *J Speech Hear Res* 8:389–397.

Ringel RL, Steer MD. (1963). Some effects of tactile and auditory alterations on speech output. *J Speech Hear Res* 6:369–378.

Romo R, Scarnati E, Schultz W. (1992). Role of primate basal ganglia and frontal cortex in the internal generation of movements. II. Movement related activity in the anterior striatum. *Exp Brain Res* 91:385–395.

Romo R, Schultz W. (1992). Role of primate basal ganglia and frontal cortex in the internal generation of movements. III. Neuronal activity in the supplementary motor area. *Exp Brain Res* 91:396–407.

Russell DG. (1976). Spatial location cues and movement production. In: Stelmach GE, ed. *Motor Control: Issues and Trends.* New York: Academic Press.

Sanes JN, Dimitrov B, Hallett M. (1990). Motor learning in patients with cerebellar dysfunction. *Brain* 113:103–120.

Schmidt RA. (1976). The schema as a solution to some persistent problems in motor learning theory. In: Stelmach GE, ed. *Motor Control: Issues and Trends.* New York: Academic Press.

Schmidt RA. (1982). *Motor Control and Learning: A Behavioral Emphasis.* Champaign: Human Kinetics Publishers.

Schmidt RF. (1978). Motor systems. In: Schmidt RF, ed. *Fundamentals of Neurophysiology.* New York: Springer-Verlag.

Schultz W, Romo R. (1992). Role of primate basal ganglia and frontal cortex in the internal generation of movements. I. Preparatory activity in the anterior striatum. *Exp Brain Res* 91:363–384.

Schweiger A, Browne JW. (1988). Minds, models and modules. *Aphasiology* 2:531–543.

Scully C, Guérin B. (1991). Speech production: models, methods and data. *J Phon* 19:249–250.

Sharkey SG, Folkins JW. (1985). Variability of lip and jaw movements in children and adults: implications for the development of speech motor control. *J Speech Hear Res* 28: 8–15.

Stevens KN, Blumstein SE. (1981). A search for invariant acoustic correlates of phonetic features. In: Eimas PD, Miller JL, eds. *Perspectives on the Study of Speech.* Hillsdale: Lawrence Erlbaum.

Strata P, ed. (1989). *The Olivocerebellar System in Motor Control, Experimental Brain Research Series 17.* Berlin: Springer-Verlag.

Sussman HM. (1972). What the tongue tells the brain. *Psychol Bull* 77:262–272.

Tatton WG, Bruce JC. (1981). Comment: A schema for the interactions between motor programs and sensory input. *Can J Physiol Pharmacol* 59:691–699.

Teuber HL. (1974). Concluding session: panel discussion on key problems in the preprogramming of movements. *Brain Res* 71:533–568.

Van den Bercken JHL, Cools AR. (1982). Evidence for a role of the caudate nucleus in the sequential organization of behaviour. *Behav Brain Res* 4:319–337.

Van der Merwe A, Grimbeek RJ. (1990). A comparison of the influence of certain contextual factors on the symptoms of acquired apraxia of speech and developmental apraxia of speech (title translated). *S Afr J Comm Dis* 37:27–34.

Van der Merwe A, Uys IC, Loots JM, Grimbeek RJ. (1987). The influence of certain contextual factors on the perceptual symptoms of apraxia of speech (title translated). *S Afr J Comm Dis* 34:10–22.

Van der Merwe A, Uys IC, Loots JM, Grimbeek RJ. (1988). Perceptual symptoms of apraxia of speech: indications of the nature of the disorder (title translated). *S Afr J Comm Dis* 35:45–54.

Van der Merwe A, Uys IC, Loots JM, Grimbeek RJ, Jansen LPC. (1989). The influence of certain contextual factors on voice onset time, vowel duration and utterance duration in apraxia of speech (title translated). *S Afr J Comm Dis* 36:29–41.

Von Euler C. (1981). The contribution of sensory inputs to the pattern generation of breathing. *Can J Physiol Pharmacol* 59:700–706.

Von Euler C. (1980). Central pattern generation during breathing. *TINS* 3:275–277.

Walsh T. (1984). Modelling temporal relations within English syllables. *J Phon* 12:29–35.

Wanner E, Teyler TJ, Thompson RF. (1977). The psychobiology of speech and language—an overview. In: Desmedt JE, ed. *Language and Hemispheric Specialization in Man: Cerebral Event-Related Potentials, Progress in Clinical Neurophysiology.* Basel: S. Karger, vol. 3.

Weinrich M, Wise SP, Mauritz KH. (1984). A neurophysiological study of the pre-motor cortex in the Rhesus monkey. *Brain* 107:385–414.

Wertz RT, La Pointe LL, Rosenbek JC. (1984). *Apraxia of Speech in Adults: The Disorder and Its Management.* Orlando: Grune and Stratton.

West RW, Ansberry M, Carr A. (1957). *The Rehabilitation of Speech.* New York: Harper and Brothers, p 43.

Wing AM, Miller ED. (1984). Basal ganglia lesions and psychological analyses of the control of voluntary movement. In: Ciba Foundation Symposium 107: *Functions of the Basal Ganglia.* London: Pitman.

Chapter 2

The Perceptual Sensorimotor Examination for Motor Speech Disorders

Ray D. Kent

Introduction

The term "perceptual sensorimotor examination" is intended to include assessment procedures that can be performed with little or no equipment except for a tape recorder and miscellaneous low-cost items. These procedures rely on the eyes, the ears, and, to some extent, the tactile skills of the clinician. It is not assumed that an examination protocol can be used invariantly with every client in every clinical setting. Inevitably, modifications need to be considered to account for client characteristics, purpose of examination, and time or resources available. The protocol described here is a general-purpose examination, components of which could be omitted, shortened, elaborated, or otherwise modified for a given client. The intention is not to present an inflexible examination protocol but rather a menu from which individually tailored examinations can be developed. In keeping with this objective, the chapter is written not so much to provide detailed information on all components of the examination as to indicate general choices to be made in planning an examination. The details of a given component will vary according to client characteristics and scope of the examination.

Information on the examinaton of the speech production system is available in the following sources: (1) assessment issues with an emphasis on children (Robbins and Klee, 1987; Hodge, 1991); (2) assessment issues with an adult or general emphasis (Mason & Simon, 1977; Ruscello et al., 1982). In addition, several report forms are reprinted in Kent (1994).

Basic Components of the Examination

Information from Client History and Referral

This information is important in planning the examination. Examinations often must be tailored to an individual's sensory, motor, and cognitive capabilities. History and referral letters are a source of information in these areas. Client characteristics should be considered in advance of the examination because this information (1) may determine restrictions on performance in certain tasks, (2) helps in the selection of suitable test procedures and materials, and (3) guides the examiner to answer specific questions that may have been raised in a referral or are frequently of issue for a certain disorder. To take a simple example, if the client's referral information indicates diplopia, right hemiplegia, and a history of vestibular problems, the clinician should be careful to select tasks that do not rely critically on visual acuity, right-sided limb movements or unsupported postures.

Structural (Static) Examination of the Speech Structures

Structure refers to anatomy, but anatomy in a living person is not inert. In many respects, anatomy is a performance anatomy—that is, a set of structural features and relations that permit functions (actions) and are in turn influenced by these functions. It is therefore helpful to conceptualize a structural examination as a set of "snapshots" of a dynamic system. Each snapshot represents one configuration or function of that system. In the following description, structural examination is carried out in reference to specific functions of a rather static nature, such as resting state and sustained phonation. But even "at-rest" or static positions have a functional significance and reflect the dynamics of a living system. Systems at rest are not truly resting; there is always some level of muscle activity (tone). "Resting" systems normally are working at low levels of activation. In some pathological conditions, the resting state may be highly active (for example, fasciculations, tremors, or other involuntary movements). In other conditions, the resting state may have a reduced tone—leading to drooping of facial features, for example. Although the heading of this section emphasizes static as opposed to dynamic features, the distinction is not a hard one. The term static denotes postures that can be maintained for a considerable time if desired.

Observations During Initial Conversation
These observations are typically performed during the initial meeting with the individual to be examined. What may appear to be simply a "small talk" is in fact an opportunity to gather information on a variety of characteristics, such as balance and general body control, posture and its variations, size and general appearance of body structures, and asymmetries of the orofacial complex. It is somewhat artificial to separate structure and function in observations of casual conversation, because they are inevitably intertwined. However, some general observations can be made of structural features. Of course, conversation in inherently dynamic, but it is mentioned here because (1) it is a useful beginning point in the examination, and (2) it does involve some static features, such as posture and pauses.

Observations During Rest State
Rest state is simply the state the individual assumes when asked to take a comfortable, resting position. It can be informative to observe different rest states, for example: a rest state with the lips closed, one with the mouth moderately open to permit observation of the anterior tongue, and one with the mouth widely open to make visible the blade of the tongue and more posterior features such as the pharyngopalatal arch. The examiner should look for asymmetry of size or shape, abnormal color, fasciculations, tremor, tics, or other abnormalities. Any suspicious feature should be noted and compared with other parts of the examination.

Observations of Vowel Phonation
In this task, the client is asked to phonate a vowel (typically /ɑ/) for a prolonged period with a comfortable effort level ("easy" or "natural" production). The vowel /ɑ/ is particularly suitable because it is produced with a wide mouth opening so that intraoral structures can be viewed.

Observations of Rest State (Repeated)
The examiner can elect to repeat any task, but the rest state in particular can be repeated to determine if the modest requirements of the intervening tasks have produced remarkable differences in the rest state. Sometimes, even moderate activity can elicit clinical signs that may not have appeared on the initial observation of the rest state. The second observation is also an opportunity to assess the reliability of an observation—for example, asymmetry of structures or presence of fasciculations. Concerning the latter, some individuals have active tongues, but the activity state frequently changes after tongue movements are performed in some of the tasks described above.

Orosensory Examination

Examination of orosensory function is probably one of the most neglected and uncertain areas in contemporary clinical assessment. Although it is true that careful, quantitative assessment of sensory function requires special-purpose equipment, the clinician can evaluate sensory function using inexpensive instruments and simple tasks. Some examples will be summarized in this chapter. But first, the clinician should be aware of certain neurologic disorders in which orosensory testing is especially warranted: trigeminal nerve damage, localized cerebral lesions, Parkinson's disease, oral apraxia, head injury, and any severe motor involvement of the orofacial system (Kent, Sufit, & Martin, 1990).

Some simple but informative assessment procedures are as follows:

1. Light static touch. The client is asked to respond whenever the clinician touches a monofilament to the client's skin. This is a static task insofar as the stimulation is one at location. Force of application can be controlled by using a monofilament that bends at a certain force. Sensory innervation of the face is supplied by the three branches of cranial nerve V (trigeminal nerve): ophthalmic (V_1), maxillary (V_2), and mandibular (V_3). Static touch is suitable to test the function of the slowly adapting mechanoreceptors. An advantage of testing light static touch is that no motor response is required of the client except for a report of when a stimulus is felt. The examination may identify abnormalities such as hypesthesia or asymmetrical sensitivity.

2. Kinetic touch. The client is asked to indicate either verbally or with gesture the direction of motion of a monofilament drawn across the skin or mucousal surface. This procedure is easily accomplished with stimulus to the lips or tongue. Kinetic touch is conveyed by rapidly adapting mechanoreceptors. This assessment complements light touch examination and is particularly relevant to the perception of motion. A degree of control over stimulus variables can be accomplished as follows: (a) traverse length: move the monofilament from the midline to the lateral aspects of a structure (or vice versa); (b) touch pressure: use a monofilament that bends as the desired force is applied; and (c) movement velocity: practice producing a smooth, steady motion in a specified time. The primary objective in testing kinetic sensitivity is to determine if the client can reliably determine the direction of a moving stimulus.

3. Temperature. Temperature sensitivity can be examined with test tubes filled with warm or cold water. Temperature sensitivity may be particularly important in the examination of dysphagia. Quanitative testing involves a number of considerations, as summarized in Kent, Sufit, and Martin (1990).

4. Double-simultaneous touch. The clinician touches either one part of the client's body or two parts. The client's task is to report whether one or two parts were touched. This task can be used with the speech structures by selecting pairs such as lip-tongue, right lip-left lip, right cheek-left cheek. Some neurologic disorders impair the ability to detect simultaneous stimulation, and poor performance on this task may indicate the need for a more detailed examination.

These and other procedures of the orosensory examination are discussed in a review article by Kent et al (1990). Even when quantitative assessment is not possible, the clinician may notice performance deficits that indicate the need for more definitive assessment.

Nonspeech Tasks

Opinions differ on the usefulness of various nonspeech tasks, but many clinicians believe that these tasks offer important opportunities to observe functional characteristics relevant to speech and other oral motor behaviors. A particular advantage that these tasks offer is observation of isolated muscle systems performing a specified action that is free of phonetic restrictions. They also can be used to evaluate the strength or endurance of a given motor system (Luschei, 1991). A number of tasks are listed in Table 2–1.

Simple Nonverbal Oral Movements

These movements are typically used to assess movements of selected structures. Movements can be examined in isolation (eg, a single protrusion of the tongue), in a repeti- tion sequence (eg, several tongue protrusions in a row), or in combination sequences (eg, a sequence of tongue protrusion, lip retraction, jaw opening). Impairments can indicate dysarthria (which may be evident as slow, inaccurate, or incomplete movements) or oral nonspeech apraxia (which may be evident as inaccuracy of movement or as a difficulty in sequencing of gestures).

Table 2–1. Tasks for the nonspeech motor examination.

Pulmonic function
    Maximum expiratory pressure
    Maximum inspiratory pressure
    Flow-volume loops
    Other pulmonic function measures (VC, IC, PEFR, etc)
    Respiratory maneuvers (eg, panting, checking, sniffing)
    Pressure regulation (eg, maintaining a specified intraoral pressure for a prescribed
        duration)
Laryngeal function
    Laryngeal maneuvers (eg, coughing, adduction of vocal folds)
Upper airway (articulatory system)
Compression/contraction force (maximal forces developed by muscles of the tongue,
    jaw, or lip)
Fine force regulation (eg, sustaining /s/ production)
Rapid alternating movement (various structures at maximum rate or prescribed rates)
Oral nonverbal gestures
    Scoring possibilities:
    Basic response scoring:
        No response / Fragmented / Distorted / Correct
    Elaborated response scoring (detailed description):
        Delay / Self-correction / Perseveration / Nonscorable
    Substitution responses (use of alternative body part):
        Oral / Verbal / Body / Noise
    Augmentation responses (accompanying behaviors)
        Oral / Body / Noise
Tasks:
    Tongue protrusion
    Baring teeth
    Smile
    Pucker lips
    Cough
    Puff cheeks
    Touch nose with tongue tip
    Touch chin with tongue tip
    Touch corner of mouth with tongue tip
    Blow
    Suck
    Bite lip
    Bite tongue
    Lick lips
    Move tongue from corner to corner of mouth
Other nonspeech oral motor function
    Mastication
    Swallow (wet and dry, different bolus sizes)

High-Effort Tasks (Maximum Performance Tasks)

High-effort tasks can be used to assess strength, endurance, and rate (Fig. 2–1). Although speech production for most communicative purposes places only modest demands on physiological support available to normal speakers, testing at high effort levels is performed for several reasons, most of them related to determining a speaker's physiological capacity. Some disorders, such as amyotrophic lateral sclerosis, may reduce physiological capacity before pronounced effects are noticed in speech production (DePaul, 1989). Even though early declines in physiological capacity may not impair

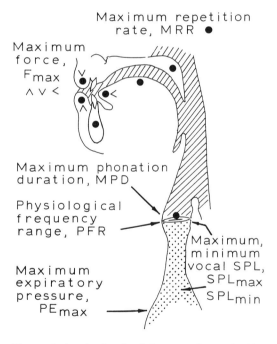

Figure 2–1. A sketch of the speech production system labeled with high-effort tasks at selected sites. Additional tasks are discussed in the text. The filled circles indicate some articulatory structures for which MRR can be tested: lips, jaw, tongue tip, tongue dorsum, velum, and vocal folds. The arrowheads indicate vectors for force assessment in the upper airway. Tasks that target the larynx are MPD and PFR. Respiratory or respiratory-laryngeal tasks include MPD, PE max, and the SPL measures.

speech, they can alert the clinician to the need for follow-up examinations, especially in the case of neurodegenerative conditions such as amyotrophic lateral sclerosis or Parkinson's disease. Evaluations of physiological capacity also can be informative regarding possible compensations available to the speaker. (See Kent, Rosenbek, & Kent, 1987, for a general review of maximal performance measures.)

Expiratory pressure. The basic procedure is to instruct the client to inspire maximally and then blow forcefully into a pressure-transducing system. A low-cost substitute for electronic equipment is a water manometer. Performance on this task can vary considerably from trial to trial, but practice and feedback can help to obtain reliable and valid estimates. But repeated performance should be attempted cautiously: a high-effort task carries health risks, especially to individuals who may not be robust. The clinician should consider the risk-benefit ratio: the value of the information to be obtained versus the possible hazards of the procedure. It is often possible to assess pulmonary sufficiency with less demanding tasks, such as sustained phonation for an age-appropriate interval, as discussed in a following section. Alternatively, respiratory driving pressure can be estimated with a small set of inexpensive items, as described by Hixon, Hawley, and Wilson (1982). Normative data for maximum expiratory pressure are compiled in Table 2–2.

Articulatory force. The procedure is to instruct the client to press hard against an appropriate device for force measurement. (Caution: maximal forces produced with the teeth, as in jaw clenching, can cause damage to dental or other tissues.) If force-transducing equipment is not available, the clinician can make general assessments by asking the client to press against an object such as a tongue depressor. For instance, labial strength can be assessed by inserting the depressor between the lips (not the teeth!) and then gently tugging on the depressor to withdraw it. If force transduction equipment is available, the normative data in Table 2–3

31

Table 2–2. Values of maximum expiratory pressure in cm H$_2$O and kPa for four subject groups: men, women, boys, and girls. Reprinted from Kent et al (1987, p 375), with permission from the American Speech-Language-Hearing Association. See original article for sources.

Subject group	Age range (years)		M	SD	Source
Men					
n = 60	20–54	cm H$_2$O	233	42	Black & Hyatt, 1969
		kPa	20.0	3.6	
n = 31	18–39	cm H$_2$O	167	37	Ptacek et al, 1966
		kPa	14.3	3.2	
n = 27	68–89	cm H$_2$O	124	43	Ptacek et al, 1966
		kPa	10.6	3.7	
n = 2,614	—	cm H$_2$O	177	—	Rahn et al, 1946, summary of six reports
		kPa	15.2	—	
n = 100	18–83	cm H$_2$O	237	46	Ringqvist, 1966
		kPa	20.3	3.9	
n = 48	19–65	cm H$_2$O	148	34	Wilson et al, 1984
		kPa	12.7	2.9	
Women					
n = 60	20–54	cm H$_2$O	152	27	Black & Hyatt, 1969
		kPa	13.0	2.3	
n = 31	18–38	cm H$_2$O	121	24	Ptacek et al, 1966
		kPa	10.4	2.0	
n = 36	66–93	cm H$_2$O	88	37	Ptacek et al, 1966
		kPa	7.5	3.1	
n = 100	18–83	cm H$_2$O	165	30	Ringqvist, 1966
		kPa	14.1	2.6	
n = 87	18–65	cm H$_2$O	93	17	Wilson et al, 1984
		kPa	8.0	1.5	
Boys					
n = 20	12 only	cm H$_2$O	96	23	Cerretelli, Brandi, & Brambilla, 1959
		kPa	8.2	2.0	
n = 66	6–14	cm H$_2$O	Range:	70–201	Inkley, Odenburg, & Vignos, 1974
		kPa	Range:	6–17.2	
n = 137	7–17	cm H$_2$O	96	23	Wilson et al, 1984
		kPa	8.2	2.0	
n = 11	7.4–8.6	cm H$_2$O	99	23	Gaultier & Zinman, 1983
		kPa	8.5	2.0	
n = 26	9.0–10.8	cm H$_2$O	123	27	Gaultier & Zinman, 1983
		kPa	10.5	2.3	
n = 23	11.0–13.0	cm H$_2$O	161	37	Gaultier & Zinman, 1983
		kPa	13.8	3.2	
Girls					
n = 20	12 only	cm H$_2$O	88	16	Cerretelli et al, 1959
		kPa	7.5	1.4	
n = 98	7–17	cm H$_2$O	80	21	Wilson et al, 1984
		kPa	6.9	1.8	
n = 15	7.1–8.9	cm H$_2$O	74	25	Gaultier & Zinman, 1983
		kPa	6.3	2.1	
n = 17	9.0–10.8	cm H$_2$O	108	39	Gaultier & Zinman, 1983
		kPa	9.2	3.3	
n = 27	11.7–13.3	cm H$_2$O	126	32	Gaultier & Zinman, 1983
		kPa	10.8	2.7	

Table 2–3. Normative data on maximum forces for tongue protrusion (anterior, left lateral, and right lateral), bilabial closure (pulling force), and upper and lower lips (vertical force). All values in newtons (N). Ages of children (in years) are shown in parentheses under subject description. Reprinted from Kent et al (1987, p 378), with permission from the American Speech-Language-Hearing Association. See original article for sources.

Force measure	Subjects	M	Range
Tongue-anterior Posen (1972)	Girls (8)	15.66	7.16–20.27
	Boys (8)	14.97	9.54–24.09
	Girls (10)	17.22	10.14–22.36
	Boys (10)	18.04	9.54–23.55
	Girls (12)	22.25	13.83–28.03
	Boys (12)	21.68	13.6–29.82
	Girls (16)	22.37	16.1–28.03
	Boys (16)	22.70	17.29–27.13
	Girls (18)	23.82	15.5–29.82
	Boys(18)	24.93	20.27–29.82
Dworkin, Aronson, &	Women	19.26	11.57–27.58
Mulder (1980)	Men	20.46	12.77–32.92
Dworkin & Culatta (1985)	Girls (M of 7.7 years)	19.69	—
	Boys (M of 8.1 years)	20.12	—
Tongue-left lateral			
Dworkin et al (1980)	Women	14.23	8.32–23.71
	Men	15.70	9.79–29.36
Dworkin & Culatta (1985)	Girls (M of 7.7 years)	16.06	—
	Boys (M of 8.1 years)	18.09	—
Tongue-right lateral			
Dworkin et al (1980)	Women	14.55	8.59–28.74
	Men	17.04	9.48–31.72
Dworkin & Culatta (1985)	Girls (M of 7.7 years)	15.38	—
	Boys (M of 8.1 years)	17.60	—
Bilabial closure Posen (1972)	Girls (8)	1.54	1.07–2.15
	Boys (8)	1.58	1.07–2.27
	Girls (10)	2.04	1.43–2.98
	Boys (10)	2.1	1.43–2.62
	Girls (12)	2.31	1.79–3.10
	Boys (12)	2.53	1.91–3.40
	Girls (16)	3.11	1.91–4.77
	Boys (16)	3.47	1.91–5.25
	Girls (18)	3.0	2.15–4.29
	Boys (18)	4.16	3.10–5.96
Ingervall & Janson (1981)	Girls and boys (7–13)	2.47	0.17–5.49
Upper lip Barlow & Rath (1985)	Women	3.35	1.15–5.07
	Men	4.44	1.85–6.87
Lower lip Barlow & Rath (1985)	Women	8.98	3.44–17.61
	Men	14.13	7.2–22.06

may be helpful guidelines in clinical assessment.

Repetitions of nonverbal oral movements. The client is asked to repeat as rapidly and evenly as possible selected oral movements, such as jaw opening and closing (muscles innervated by cranial nerve V), alternately pursing and retracting the lips (cranial nerve VII), alternatively starting and stopping phonation (cranial nerve X), and tapping the alveolar ridge with the tongue tip (cranial nerve XII). It is noteworthy that these four tasks are associated with four different cranial nerve innervations. Performance on this task typically is evaluated with respect to maximum rate and the quality of the repetitions. Maximum rate is influenced by client characteristics such as age (see following section on syllable repetition). In general, clients should be capable of at least three to five repetitions per second for up-and-down movements of the jaw and for tongue tip contacts with the alveolar ridge. Pursing and retracting movements of the lips tend to be slower. Clients should be able to perform these simple motor tasks with a regular cadence and uniform ranges of movement.

Sequences of nonverbal oral movements. Sequences of nonverbal oral movements are particularly informative if oral apraxia or apraxia of speech is suspected. The clinician can design movement sequences that challenge sequential abilities but that are within general motoric capability. For example, if a client has persistent difficulty with movements of the tongue tip but is capable of other oral movements, then sequential testing might be done with the movements that can be performed well individually.

Sequences of cross-modal movements (optional). Sequences of cross-modal movements are indicated in some situations where apraxia, agnosia, or sensory disorder is suspected. The basic idea of cross-modal movements is to select movements that are performed with different musculatures, or different cranial and spinal nerves. For example, a movement sequence that involves tongue protrusion, lip retraction, and jaw lowering requires an innervation sequence of cranial nerves XII, VII, and V.

Simple Speech or Speechlike Tasks

High-Effort (Maximal Performance) Tasks
High-effort tasks designed to assess strength, endurance, and rate can involve speech or speechlike maneuvers as well as nonspeech

maneuvers (Fig. 2–1). Normative data for many of the following tasks are available in the review by Kent et al. (1987) and the reference manual by Kent (1994). Particular attention should be given to effects related to age and gender, feedback and practice, and number of trials used to gauge performance.

Phonation duration. Maximum phonation duration is simply the maximum length of time that an individual can phonate a vowel after a maximal inspiration. This measure is commonly used as a global assessment of phonatory capacity but it should always be remembered that performance on this task reflects both pulmonary capacity and laryngeal efficiency. Decreased phonation duration can reflect a respiratory deficiency, a laryngeal dysfunction, or both to some degree. It is also important to note that age effects can be profound. It is inappropriate to use normative data from young adults in evaluating task performance for young children or geriatric individuals. See Table 2–4 for normative data on maximum phonation duration.

Frication duration. Maximum frication duration is analogous to maximum phonation duration as a task in which sound is produced following a maximal inspiration. Typically, a voiceless fricative such as /s/ is selected for sustained production. Performance on the task reflects both respiratory capacity and articulatory function. Table 2–5 summarizes normative results for /s/ and /z/ durations as well as the /s/-/z/ ratio.

Physiological voice frequency range. Physiological voice frequency range is the range of fundamental frequencies that can be produced by the client. This variable is also called fundamental frequency range (FFR) or pitch range (PR). In normal speakers, this range greatly exceeds the range of voice frequency used in speaking. Normative data are provided in Table 2–6.

Sound pressure range. The range of sound pressure level from softest to loudest is typically determined for the vowel /ɑ/. One caution is that phonation at maximum effort can be taxing to the subject and can carry

Table 2–4. Normative data on maximum phonation duration (in seconds except for the coefficient of variation, C, which is dimensionless) for vowel /ɑ/. M = male; F = female. Reprinted from Kent et al (1987, pp 370–371), with permission from the American Speech-Language-Hearing Association. See original article for sources. (Table continues on next page.)

Source	Subjects	Sex	M	SD	Range	C
Williams (1977)	8-year-olds	M	13.3	2.5	—	.19
	8-year-olds	F	13.6	5.2	—	.38
	11-year-olds	M	17.8	4.7	—	.26
	11-year-olds	F	15.8	4.1	—	.26
Child (1979)	10-year-olds	M	20.2	4.7	—	.23
	10-year-olds	F	15.1	4.3	—	.28
Reich et al (1986)	8.5–10.4 years	F	14.3	4.69	—	.33
Ptacek & Sander (1963)	Young adults	M	22.6	8.1	9.3–43.3	.36
		F	15.2	5.0	6.2–28.4	.33
Ptacek et al (1966)	Young adults	M	24.6	6.7	12.5–36.0	.27
		F	20.9	5.7	11.8–32.0	.27
Kreul (1972)	Young adults		18.2	4.3	—	.24
Hirano et al (1986)	Adults	M	34.6	—	15.0–62.3 (CR)	
		F	25.7	—	14.3–40.4 (CR)	
Inglis (1977)	Young adults	M	24.8	8.4	—	.34
		F	22.8	4.1	—	.18
Taylor (1980)	Young adults	M	28.0	8.9	—	.32
		F	22.9	5.8	—	.25
Neiman & Edeson (1981)	Young adults	M	29.0	5.5	—	.19
		F	19.6	4.7	—	.24
Yanagihara & Koike (1967)	Young adults	M	30.2	9.7	20.4–50.7	.32
		F	22.5	6.1	16.4–32.90	.27
Bless & Hirano (1982b)	Young adults	M	33.6	11.4	16.7–58.4	.34
		F	26.5	11.3	11.6–60.5	.43
Canter (1965)	Men (35–75 years)		20.6[a]	—	14.8–42.4	—
Kreul (1972)	Aged M (65–75 years)		14.6	5.9	—	.40
	F (66–93 years)		14.6	5.8	—	.40
Ptacek et al (1966)	Aged M (68–89 years)		18.1	6.6	10.0–37.2	.36
	F (66–93 years)		14.2	5.6	7.0–24.8	.39
Mueller (1971)	Aged M (51–65 years)		13.0	—	—	—
	F (49–72 years)		15.4	—	—	—
Mueller (1982)	Aged M (85–92 years)		13.0	—	7.0–12.0	—
	F (85–96 years)		10.0	—	6.0–18.0	—
Harden & Looney (1984)	6-year-olds	M	10.4	5.1	3.8–16.8	.49
		F	10.6	6.3	6.2–30.6	.59
Beckett et al (1971)	7-year-olds	M	14.2	3.3	12.0–22.0	.23
		F	15.4	2.7	9.0–19.0	.175
Finnegan (1984)	3-year-olds	M	7.9	1.81	4.38–11.46	.23
	3-year-olds	F	6.3	1.76	2.84–9.72	.28
	4-year-olds	M	10.0	2.51	5.08–14.90	.25
	4-year-olds	F	8.7	1.84	5.26–12.46	.21
	5-year-olds	M	10.1	3.05	4.15–16.09	.30
	5-year-olds	F	10.5	2.57	5.44–15.50	.24
	6-year-olds	M	13.9	2.98	8.06–19.74	.21
	6-year-olds	F	13.8	3.65	6.66–20.96	.26
	7-year-olds	M	14.6	2.82	9.11–20.15	.19
	7-year-olds	F	13.7	2.45	8.88–18.48	.18
	8-year-olds	M	16.8	4.51	7.98–25.64	.27
	8-year-olds	F	17.1	4.62	8.07–26.17	.27
	9-year-olds	M	16.8	6.07	4.94–28.72	.36
	9-year-olds	F	14.5	3.78	7.07–21.87	.26
	10-year-olds	M	22.2	4.74	12.91–31.49	.21

35

Table 2–4. *Continued*

Source	Subjects	Sex	M	SD	Range	C
	10-year-olds	F	15.9	5.99	4.14–27.62	.38
	11-year-olds	M	19.8	3.79	12.43–27.27	.19
	11-year-olds	F	14.8	2.06	10.73–18.79	.14
	12-year-olds	M	20.2	5.72	9.02–31.44	.28
	12-year-olds	F	15.2	3.87	7.58–22.74	.25
	13-year-olds	M	22.3	8.19	6.29–38.29	.37
	13-year-olds	F	19.2	4.58	10.27–28.21	.24
	14-year-olds	M	22.3	6.89	8.84–35.84	.31
	14-year-olds	F	18.8	5.15	8.76–28.94	.27
	15-year-olds	M	20.7	5.32	10.32–31.16	.26
	15-year-olds	F	19.5	4.66	10.40–29.93	.24
	16-year-olds	M	2.10	4.40	12.43–29.66	.21
	16-year-olds	F	21.8	4.47	13.09–30.61	.20
	17-year-olds	M	28.7	7.08	14.83–42.57	.25
	17-year-olds	F	22.0	6.30	9.65–34.33	.29
Lewis et al (1982)	8-year-olds	M	20.0	—	11.5–24.5	
	8-year-olds	F	19.1	—	11.9–23.0	
	10-year-olds	M	24.9	—	15.9–39.0	
	10-year-olds	F	16.5	—	12.9–21.8	

Note. CR = critical region.
[a]Median.

Table 2–5. Normative data on maximum /s/ and /z/ duration and the s/z ratio (all values in seconds). Reprinted from Kent et al (1987, p 372), with permission from the American Speech-Language-Hearing Association. See original article for sources.

Source	Subjects	Maximum /s/ duration			Maximum /z/ duration			s/z ratio	
		M	SD	Range	M	SD	Range	M	Range
Tait et al (1980)	Girls, 5 years	8.3	4.0	4.8–18.3	10.0	3.3	5.2–16.0	0.83	0.50–1.14
	Boys, 5 years	7.9	1.4	5.4–9.8	8.6	2.1	6.6–13.0	0.92	0.82–1.08
	Girls, 7 years	10.2	2.6	7.3–16.0	13.1	4.0	9.1–20.0	0.78	0.51–1.10
	Boys, 7 years	9.3	1.7	7.4–12.5	13.2	3.6	9.2–19.6	0.70	0.52–0.97
	Girls, 9 years	14.4	3.1	9.3–20.9	15.8	5.2	8.5–24.2	0.91	0.75–1.26
	Boys, 9 years	16.7	8.5	7.1–44.0	18.1	6.8	10.1–33.1	0.92	0.66–1.50
Eckel & Boone (1981)	Mixed ages, both sexes	17.7	7.6	5–38	18.6	7.0	5–37	0.99	0.41–2.67
Young & Bless (1983)	Sedate geriatrics	14.7	4.4	7.7–21.6	19.3	8.4	10.2–35.6	0.76	—
	Active geriatrics	20.2	13.4	6.4–51.3	24.5	8.0	14.7–36.6	0.82	—

some risks. For this reason, it is sometimes recommended that only the minimum sound pressure level be determined. This measure presents little risk or discomfort and may provide information on phonatory function. Normative data are given in Table 2–7 for maximum sound pressure levels of vowel production. The minimum sound pressure level of phonation is in the range of 45–66 dB SPL re 20 μPa.

Table 2–6. FFR (fundamental frequency range or pitch range) in semitones in several studies. Ramig and Ringel classified their subjects into good condition and poor condition groups based on resting heart rate, resting systolic and diastolic blood pressure, percentage of fat, and forced vital capacity. Reprinted from Kent et al (1987), with permission from the American Speech-Language-Hearing Association. See original article for sources.

Source	Subjects	M	SD	Range
Ptacek et al (1966)	Young men	34.5	5.2	23–47
	Geriatric men	26.5	6.5	11–35
Ptacek et al (1966)	Young women	32.8	4.4	20–40
	Geriatric women	25.1	7.9	9–41
Hollien et al (1971)	Young men	37.9	5.0	13–55
	Young women	37.0	5.3	23–50
Colton & Hollien (1972)	Male singers	34.9	—	—
	Male nonsingers	33.3	—	—
Coleman et al (1977)	Young men	37.1	—	28.9–43.8
	Young women	37.4	—	30.6–42.2
Ramig & Ringel (1983)	Young men (good cond.)	32.2	8.8	—
	Young men (poor cond.)	26.6	7.1	—
	Mid-age men (good cond.)	28.3	8.7	—
	Mid-age men (poor cond.)	26.8	3.6	—
	Geriatric men (good cond.)	31.4	4.4	—
	Geriatric men (poor cond.)	24.3	7.1	—
Pederson et al (1986)	Boys 8.7–12.9 years	34.4	—	—
	Boys 13–15.9 years	37.5	—	—
	Boys 16–19.5 years	41.4	—	—

Syllable repetition rates. Maximum repetition rate, or diadochokinesis, is a frequently-used test of a speaker's ability to perform rapid sequences of oral movements. The three syllables /pʌ/, /tʌ/, and /kʌ/ are commonly selected for this task, and a substantial set of normative data are available for these items (Tables 2–8, 2–9, and 2–10 for adults, and Table 2–11 for young children). The trisyllabic sequence /pʌtʌkʌ/ is often used as well (Table 2–12). One caveat is that some speakers, especially children, may have difficulty with complex nonsense strings such as /pʌtʌkʌ/ but perform satisfactorily with a similar word such as buttercup or pattycake. Failure on the nonsense trisyllable should not be immediately interpreted as evidence of a motor disorder. It is wise to use both nonsense utterances and real words in testing syllable repetition. It is also important to note that children can be highly

variable on the task of maximum syllable repetition. But in general, children should be able to produce at least four syllables per second in this task. Slower performance should be taken as an indication of the need for additional assessment to rule out motor difficulties.

Performance on syllable repetition can be compared with analogous movements in nonspeech tasks. For example, repetition of the syllable /pʌ/ can be compared with repetition of lip closing and opening, and repetition of the syllable /tʌ/ can be compared with elevation and lowering of the tongue tip to and from the alveolar ridge.

Sustained phonation with pitch or loudness change. The objective here is to determine if the speaker can modulate sustained phonation. Some possible tasks are (1) sustained phonation with rising pitch near the end of phonation; (2) sustained phonation

37

Table 2–7. Normative data on maximum sound pressure levels (dB re 20 µPa) for vowel production. The ages of the children studied by Susser and Bless ranged from 5 years, 4 months, to 11 years, 2 months. Tabled values are not corrected for differences in mike-mouth distance. Reprinted from Kent et al (1987, p 376), with permission from the American Speech-Language-Hearing Association. See original article for sources.

Source	Subjects	Measure	M	SD	Range
Canter (1965)	Men aged 35–75 years	SPL of syllable *no* measured 23.32 cm from lips with sound level meter on C-scale	100.4[a]	—	—
Ptacek et al (1966)	Young men	SPL of vowel /a/ with 30.48-cm mike-mouth distance	105.8	5.1	92–116
	Geriatric men		100.5	5.9	88–110
	Young women		106.2	3.0	99–112
	Geriatric women		98.6	4.5	90–104
Coleman et al (1977)	Young men	SPL of vowel /a/ with a 15.24-cm mike-mouth distance	126	—	—
	Young women		122	—	—
Colton (1973)	Young male nonsingers	SPL of vowel /a/ with a 22.86-cm mike-mouth distance	101	—	—
	Young male singers		102	—	—
Susser & Bless (1983)	Boys	SPL of vowel /a/ with a 15-cm mike-mouth distance	87	—	—
	Girls		84	—	—

[a]Median.

Table 2–8. Normative adult data on maximum repetition rate in syllables per second for [pʌ]. M = male; F = female; YA = young adult; A = adult with unreported or wide range of age; GA = geriatric adult. Reprinted from Kent et al (1987, p 381), with permission from the American Speech-Language-Hearing Association. See original article for sources.

Source	Subjects	M	SD	Range
Dworkin et al (1980)	M, A	6.5	—	4.5–7.5
	F, A	6.1	—	4.6–8.6
Kreul (1972)	M, YA	6.0	0.66	—
	F, YA	5.9	0.35	—
	M, GA	6.0	0.82	—
	F, GA	6.7	0.93	—
Lass & Sandusky (1971)	M, YA	6.3	0.53	5.2–7.4
	F, YA	6.2	0.61	5.0–7.8
Lundeen (1950)	M & F, YA	7.0	—	—
Ptacek et al (1966)	M, YA	7.0	1.0	5.4–9.4
	F, YA	6.9	0.6	5.8–7.8
	M, GA	5.4	1.2	2.8–8.2
	F, GA	5.0	1.2	1.3–7.0
Sigurd (1973)	8M & 1F, A	6.9	—	—
Tiffany (1980)	7M & 3F, A	7.1	0.7	—

Table 2–9. Normative adult data on maximum repetition rate in syllables per second for [tʌ]. M = male; F = female; YA = young adult; A = adult with unreported or wide range of age; GA = geriatric adult. Reprinted from Kent et al (1987, p 381), with permission from the American Speech-Language-Hearing Association. See original article for sources.

Source	Subjects	M	SD	Range
Dworkin et al (1980)	M, A	6.5	—	4.4–8.2
	F, A	6.0	—	4.3–8.5
Kreul (1972)	M, YA	6.0	0.96	—
	F, YA	5.8	0.37	—
	M, GA	5.8	0.69	—
	F, GA	6.5	0.44	—
Lass & Sandusky (1971)	M, YA	6.1	0.50	5.0–7.8
	F, YA	6.2	0.64	4.4–7.8
Lundeen (1950)	M & F, YA	7.1	—	—
Ptacek et al (1966)	M, YA	6.9	1.1	4.2–9.4
	F, YA	6.8	1.0	4.8–8.4
	M, GA	5.3	1.0	3.0–6.8
	F, GA	4.8	1.1	2.2–6.8
Sigurd (1973)	8M & 1F, A	6.9	—	—
Tiffany (1980)	7M & 3F, A	7.1	0.8	—

Table 2–10. Normative adult data on maximum repetition rate in syllables/second for [k^]. M = male; F = female; YA = young adult; A = adult with unreported or wide range of age; GA = geriatric adult. Reprinted from Kent et al (1987, p 381), with permission from the American Speech-Language-Hearing Association. See original article for sources.

Source	Subjects	M	SD	Range
Dworkin et al (1980)	M, A	6.1	—	4.4–7.5
	F, A	5.7	—	4.3–7.9
Kreul (1972)	M, YA	5.4	(0.54)	—
	F, YA	5.2	(0.60)	—
	M, GA	5.8	(0.62)	—
	F, GA	5.9	(0.83)	—
Lass & Sandusky (1971)	M, YA	5.8	0.55	4.6–6.8
	F, YA	5.6	0.75	4.0–7.4
Lundeen (1950)	M & F, YA	6.2	—	—
Ptacek et al (1966)	M, YA	6.2	0.8	5.0–8.2
	F, YA	6.2	0.8	4.6–8.2
	M, GA	4.9	1.0	2.6–6.8
	F, GA	4.4	1.1	2.2–6.4
Sigurd (1973)	8M & 1F, A	6.4	—	—
Tiffany (1980)	7M & 3F, A	6.2	0.8	—

Table 2–11. Maximum repetition rates in syllables/second for typically developing children. These values are based on mean data reported in the literature (Kent et al, 1987). Large intersubject and intrasubject variability can occur on this task.

Age (years)	[p^]	[t^]	[k^]
3	4.7	4.7	4.3
4	4.7	4.7	4.3
5	4.9	4.9	4.7
6	5.3	5.3	4.8

with loudness changes on demand from the examiner; and (3) sustained phonation with a gradual pitch change.

Syllable repetition with pitch or loudness change. The objective is similar to that for sustained phonation with pitch or loudness change. Syllable repetitions are combined with attempts at various pitch or loudness changes.

Table 2–12. Normative adult data on maximum repetition rate in syllables/second for [p^t^k^]. M = male; F = female; YA = young adult; A = adult with unreported or wide range of age; GA = geriatric adult; B = boy; G = girl. Reprinted from Kent et al (1987, p 381), with permission from the American Speech-Language-Hearing Association. See original article for sources.

Source	Subjects	M	SD	Range
Lass & Sandusky (1971)	M, YA	6.36	0.42	4.8–7.2
	F, YA	6.27	0.31	4.8–7.2
Tiffany (1980)	7M & 3F, A	7.5	1.1	—
Ptacek et al (1966)	M, YA	5.8	1.0	4.8–8.2
	F, YA	6.3	0.9	3.8–7.8
	M, GA	4.4	1.3	2.4–7.0
	F, GA	3.6	1.3	1.4–6.2
Blomquist (1950)	B-9	4.3	0.68	
	G-9	4.8	0.72	
	B-10	5.0	0.80	
	G-10	5.0	0.47	
	B-11	5.0	0.54	
	G-11	5.3	0.58	

Citation Tasks: Repetition, Routinized Speech

There is not a clear boundary between citation tasks and the simple speech tasks in the previous section. However, the term citation tasks is used here to designate speaking tasks that introduce a greater degree of phonetic or linguistic complexity. Citation tasks include monosyllabic or polysyllabic words, phrases, or sentences. Frequently, citation tasks include repetition of phonetic sequences that are selected to target basic articulatory functions and interarticulatory coordination. An example is the use of a word such as pamper to target nasal-nonnasal consonant sequences as part of an examination of velopharyngeal function. Another example is selection of a set of words that vary in syllabic length or complexity. These sets are often part of the examination for apraxia of speech, which tends to become more severe as the complexity of the phonetic sequence increases. Many clinicians also examine routine (automatic) speech, such as counting or simple greetings. These expressions sometimes are preserved when propositional speech is disturbed.

Tasks Requiring Language Formulation

These tasks go beyond simple repetition of a word or phrase to involve processes of language formulation as well as speech production. The objective is to evaluate speech production that is executed along with the various processes of utterance production, including syntactic, semantic, and phonologic processes. The specific tasks include confrontational naming, conversation, describing a picture or object, retelling a story, narrating a scene on video, or answering questions.

Special Issues in Assessment

This section considers intelligibility, quality, fluency, prosody, classification of motor speech disorder, and additional procedures for assessment.

Intelligibility Assessment

Two issues of primary concern in speech are intelligibility and quality. Despite their intrinsic value to speech, these two areas continue to be problematic both in respect to definition and assessment method. Most procedures for assessing intelligibility fall in one of the following categories (the emphasis of the assessment is explained in the parentheses following each category): phonetic contrast analysis (determines the accuracy with which selected phonetic contrasts are transmitted); phonological process analysis (analyzes transcribed speech in terms of phonological processes); word identification test (typically determines the number of words correctly identified by listeners); phonetic indices derived from continuous speech scoring (quantifies some aspect of transmitted speech—eg, number of consonants correct); scaling of continuous speech (represents speech intelligibility on some kind of global scale—eg, a 7-point equal-appearing interval scale); and traditional word-level analysis of continuous speech.

Each method has its advantages and disadvantages for various clinical populations and purposes of evaluation. For detailed discussion, see Kent, Weismer, Kent, and Rosenbek (1989), Kent (1992), and Kent, Miolo, and Bloedel (1994). A number of procedures for intelligibility assessment are included in Appendix A to this chapter. These procedures were developed for a variety of clinical populations, including individuals with dysarthria, individuals with hearing impairment, and children with phonological disorders. However, with some modification, each of them can be used to assess the intelligibility of adults or children with a variety of neurogenic speech disorders. Obviously, a wide variety of speech materials and measures have been proposed to assess speech intelligibility. There is no "gold standard" for clinical assessment across age and severity of disorder. Appendix A is another part of the menu from which the clinician can select client-appropriate methods of assessment.

Quality Assessment

There is no generally accepted method of evaluating speech quality. For that matter, there may not even be a generally accepted definition of speech quality. But for all the difficulties of definition and measurement, there is no question that quality is an important aspect of the perceptual sensorimotor examination. Quality disorders may include abnormalities in resonance, phonation, and prosody. A number of perceptual scales have been devised, but it is doubtful that any single scale will satisfy every application. For general purposes, a simple voice rating scale for dimensions such as hoarseness, roughness, and pitch level will suffice, but for some clinical populations, a more specialized scale may be needed. For example, a quality scale for Parkinson's disease might focus on certain aspects of prosody, such as speaking rate (including accelerated rate) and loudness decay. A highly detailed phonetic description of voice quality has been described by Laver (1980), and this approach may be suitable for the description of quality impairments in motor speech disorders. However, proper use of this system requires careful training. A simpler scale that might be generally useful for efficient clinical purposes is the GRBAS scale, included in Appendix B.

Fluency Assessment

Although the concept of fluency is not always included within the assessment of motor speech disorders, it can be a relevant dimension. Indeed, for some disorders, such as palalalia, the dimension of fluency is the most suitable to describe the disorder and its severity. Other disorders can also have a component that can be described as dysfluency. For example, some individuals with Parkinson's and some with apraxia of speech may have noteworthy dysfluencies that are part of the speech disorder. At the very least, the clinician should be prepared to recognize repetitions, pauses, prolongations, and other dysfluencies that contribute to the total picture of a speech impairment.

Prosody Assessment

Prosody refers to the suprasegmental aspects of speech, including stress, rhythm, melody, intonation, juncture, and rate. Prosody is receiving a new emphasis in motor speech disorders, especially in relation to the speech of individuals with right-hemisphere lesions, certain types of apraxia of speech, and the dysarthrias that are judged to have a remarkable dysprosodic component. Unfortunately, there is no commonly accepted method for the clinical assessment of prosody. However, the literature is rapidly developing in this area, so procedures should be better defined in the future. Interested readers are referred to Hargrove and McGarr (1993) for a book-length discussion of prosody in communication disorders, and to the chapters by Kent (1988) and Yorkston (1988).

Classification of Type and Severity of Speech Disorder

In the United States, classification of type of dysarthria is probably accomplished most often with the Mayo Clinic system described by Darley, Aronson, and Brown (1969a,b, 1975). The perceptual dimensions are listed in Appendix C. The research by Darley et al. identified the following major types of dysarthria: flaccid, spastic, mixed flaccid-spastic, ataxic, hypokinetic, hyperkinetic (chorea), and hyperkinetic (dystonia). This classification system for dysarthria appears to be the most frequently used in the United States. See Yorkston, Beukelman, and Bell (1988) for additional discussion of the system and its application, and see Zyski and Weisiger (1987) for concerns about the reliability of classification.

Other Assessment Alternatives

Additional information sometimes can be obtained by special modifications of the assessment procedure. The following are examples:

1. Postural adjustment can improve performance for some individuals.

Particularly if the client is slumped, postural support might be attempted to determine if such adjustment leads to improved speech performance. Caution should be observed when using binding to improve posture or enhance respiratory function.

2. Rate variations sometimes lead to changes in speech performance.
3. Pacing or stress patterns involve some kind of pacing procedure (such as tapping on a board) or prosodic patterns.
4. Physiologic adjustments can take a variety of forms, such as phonating during isometric contraction of the arms (as in pushing up from a chair).
5. Bite blocks inserted between the upper and lower molars are one way to minimize jaw movements, as might be desired in the examination of speakers who appear to rely on extensive movements of the jaw to aid lip or

tongue movements. Construction and use of bite blocks are described by Netsell (1985).

Summary

The results of the examination are written in a summary report that identifies sensorimotor impairments, describes major speech and voice dysfunctions, and suggests a prognosis. It may also offer management recommendations.

The different tasks and observations summarized in this chapter can be conceptualized in terms of the interpretive framework of Table 2–13. The table indicates how the major categories of the sensorimotor examination (nonspeech, simplified speech, citation, and formulation tasks) relate to potential conclusions in several areas of sensorimotor speech evaluation. For example, the nonspeech tasks yield information primarily on reflexes, tone, range of movement, speed, strength or

Table 2–13. Association matrix for assessment tasks and variables to be observed. ++ = good or preferred task; + = fair or adequate task; ? = questionable task; 0 = poor or inappropriate task.

Variable	Nonspeech	Simplified speech	Citation	Formulation
Reflexes	++	+	?	?
Tone	++	++	+	+
Range of movement	++	++	+	+
Speed	++	++	++	+
Strength, endurance	++	++	++	+
Initiation time	++	++	++	++
Stability over time	++	++	+	+
Coordination	++	++	++	+
Voice quality	?	+	++	++
Prosody	0	+	++	++
Fluency	0	+	+	++
Intelligibility	0	+	++	++
Communicative adaptability	0	?	+	++

Column group header: Type of task

endurance, initiation, stability, and coordination. However, these tasks are questionably informative about voice quality and provide no information about prosody or intelligibility. Verbal formulation tasks, such as composing a sentence to describe a picture are of questionable value in assessing reflex integrity (at least in contemporary practice), are often difficult to interpret in terms of speed but highly useful in evaluating prosody, fluency, and intelligibility. Communicative adaptability, the last entry in the matrix variables, pertains to the speaker's ability to make adjustments that enhance communicative success. Such adjustments can take several forms, including linguistic (eg, simplification of grammatical structure and reduction of utterance length), prosodic (eg, slowing of rate), articulatory (eg, using exaggerated oral movements), or cross-modal (eg, taking full advantage of visual and situational cues to enhance communication).

References

Boothroyd A. (1985). Evaluation of speech production of the hearing impaired: some benefits of forced-choice testing. *J Speech Hear Res* 28:185–196.

Bross R. (1992). An application of structural linguistics to intelligibility measurement of impaired speakers of English. In: Kent RD, ed. *Intelligibility in Speech Disorders: Theory, Measurement and Management.* Amsterdam: Benjamins, pp 35–65.

Darley FL, Aronson AE, Brown JR. (1969a). Differential diagnostic patterns of dysarthria. *J Speech Hear Res* 12:249–269.

Darley FL, Aronson AE, Brown JR. (1969b). Cluster of deviant speech dimensions in the dysarthrias. *J Speech Hear Res* 12:462–496.

Darley FL, Aronson AE, Brown JR. (1975). *Motor Speech Disorders.* Philadelphia: W.B. Saunders.

DePaul R. (1989). Orofacial muscle weakness and motor control for speech in amyotrophic lateral sclerosis. PhD dissertation, University of Wisconsin-Madison.

Hargove PM, McGarr, NS. (1993). *Prosody Management in Communication Disorders.* San Diego: Singular Publishing Group.

Hixon TJ, Hawley JL, Wilson KJ. (1982). An around-the-house device for the clinical determination of respiratory driving pressure: a note on making the simple even simpler. *J Speech Hear Dis* 47:413–415.

Hodge MM. (1993). Assessing early speech motor function. *Clin Commun Dis* 2:69–86.

Hodson BW, Paden E. (1983). *Targeting Intelligible Speech.* San Diego: College-Hill.

Kent RD, Kent JF, Rosenbek JC. (1987). Maximum performance tests of speech production. *J Speech Hear Dis* 52:367–387.

Kent RD, Martin RE, Sufit RL. (1990). Oral sensation: a review and clinical prospective. In: Winitz H, ed. Human Communication and Its Disorders, vol 3. Norwood, NJ: Ablex, pp 135–191.

Kent RD, Miolo G, Bloedel S. (1994). The intelligibility of children's speech: a review of evaluation procedures. *J Am Speech-Lang Pathol* 3:81–93.

Kent RD, Weismer G, Kent JF, Rosenbek JC. (1989). Toward phonetic intelligibility testing in dysarthria. *J Speech Hearing Dis* 54:482–499.

Kent RD. (1988). Prosody in the young child. In: Yoder DE, Kent RD, eds. *Decision Making in Speech-Language Pathology.* Toronto: Decker, pp 144–145.

Kent RD. (1992). Speech intelligibility and communicative competence in children. In: Kaiser AP, Gray DB, eds. *Enhancing Children's Communication: Research Foundations for Intervention,* Vol 2. Baltimore: Brookes Publishing Co, pp 223–239.

Kent RD. (1994). *Reference Manual for Communicative Sciences and Disorders.* Austin, TX: Pro-Ed.

Laver J. (1980). *The Phonetic Description of Voice Quality.* Cambridge: Cambridge University Press.

Ling D. (1976). Speech and the Hearing-Impaired Child: Theory and Practice. Washington, DC: Alexander Graham Bell Association for the Deaf.

Luschei ES. (1991). Development of objective standards of nonspeech oral strength and performance: an advocate's views. In: Moore CA, Mason RM, Simon C. (1977). An orofacial examination checklist. *Lang Speech Hear Serv Schools* 8:140–154.

Monsen RB, Moog JS, Geers AE. (1988). *CID Picture SPINE.* Central Institute of the Deaf.

Monsen RB. (1981). A usable test for the speech intelligibility of deaf talkers. *Am Ann Deaf* 126:845–852.

Netsell R. (1985). Construction and use of a bite-block for the evaluation and treatment of speech disorders. *J Speech Hear Dis* 50:103–106.

Osberger MJ. (1992). Speech intelligibility in the hearing impaired: research and clinical implications. In: Kent RD, ed. *Speech Intelligibility in Speech Disorders: Theory, Measurement and Management.* Amsterdam: John Benjamins, pp 233–264.

Robbins J, Klee T. (1987). Clinical assessment of oropharyngeal motor development in young children. *J Speech Hear Dis* 52:271–277.

Ruscello D, St. Louis K, Barry P, Barr K. (1982). A screening method for evaluation of the peripheral speech mechanism. *Folia Phoniat* 34:324–330.

Schiavetti N. (1992). Scaling procedures for the measurement of speech intelligibilty. In: Kent RD, ed. *Intelligibility in Speech Disorders: Theory, Measurement and Management.* Amsterdam and Philadelphia: John Benjamins, pp 11–34.

Shriberg LD, Kwiatkowski J. (1982). Phonological disorders. III. A procedure for assessing severity of involvement. J Speech Hear Disord 47:256–270.

Shriberg LD. (1993). Four new speech and prosody measures for genetics research and other studies in developmental phonological disorders. *J Speech Hear Res* 36:105–140.

Webb JC, Duckett B. (1990). The RULES Phonological Evaluation. Vero Beach, FL: The Speech Bin, 1766 Twentieth Avenue.

Weiss CE. (1982). *Weiss Intelligibility Test.* Tigard, OR: C.C. Publications.

Wilcox KA, Schooling TL, Morris SR. (1991). The preschool speech intelligibility measure. Paper presented at the Annual Meeting of the American Speech-Language-Hearing Association, Atlanta, GA, November.

Yorkston K, Beukelman DR, Traynor CD. (1984). *Computerized Assessment of Intelligibility and Dysarthric Speech.* Austin, TX: Pro-Ed.

Yorkston KM, Beukelman DR, Bell KR. (1988). *Clinical Management of Dysarthric Speakers.* Boston: Little, Brown.

Yorkston KM, Beukelman DR, eds. *Dysarthria and Apraxia of Speech: Perspectives on Management.* Baltimore: Brookes, pp 1–14.

Yorkston KM. (1988). Prosody in the adult. In: Yoder DE, Kent RD, eds. *Decision Making in Speech-Language Pathology.* Toronto: Decker, pp 146–147.

Zyski BJ, Weisiger BE. (1987). Identification of dysarthria types based on perceptual analysis. *J Commun Dis* 20:367–378.

Appendix A

Summaries of intelligibility assessments (Based on Kent et al, 1994). The following are representative of procedures used to assess intelligibility of speech production in children or adults. Some procedures are designed for a pediatric population, others for adults, and still others can be used across a large age range. The letter in parentheses after each title indicates the age level for which the test is most suitable: C—children, A—adults, G—general application across ages.

Procedures that Emphasize Word-Level Intelligibility

Assessment of Intelligibility in Dysarthric Speakers (AIDS) (A)
Material: Single-word task: 50 word pools, each consisting of 12 words; sentence task: pools of sentences of different lengths. **Measure:** Percentage of words correctly transcribed. **Source:** Yorkston, Beukelman, and Traynor (1984).

Preschool Speech Intelligibility Measure (P-SIM) (C)
Material: 50 words. **Measure:** Percentage of correctly identified words. **Source:** Wilcox et al (1991).

Weiss Intelligibility Test (C)
Material: Isolated words: 25 words elicited from picture naming; contextual speech sample collected while subject describes a set of 6 pictures. **Measure:** Isolated words: percent of words correctly identified from a set of 25 words. Contextual speech: percentage of words correctly understood by listeners. **Source:** Weiss (1982).

Procedures that Emphasize Phonetic Contrast Analysis

CID Word SPINE (C or G)
Material: 40 words (10 sets of 4 minally contrastive words) written on cards. **Measure:** Percentage of words correctly identified from total set. **Source:** Monsen (1981).

CID Picture SPINE (C or G)
Material: 100 words depicted pictorially on cards. **Measure:** Percentage of words correctly identified from total set. **Source:** Monsen, Moog, and Geers (1988).

Ling's Phonologic Level Speech Evaluation (C or G)
Material: 50 representative utterances. **Measure:** Percentage of utterances judged as unintelligible. **Source:** Ling (1976).

Ling's Phonetic Level Speech Evaluation (C or G)
Material: A range of sound patterns including vowels, diphthongs, CV, CCV and VCC syllables. **Source:** Ling (1976).

Qualitative Rating of Performance (PQR) (A)
Material: Segmental contrasts are examined in minimal-pair lexical contrasts in initial, medial, and final positions. Suprasegmental contrasts of pitch, stress, and juncture are examined for minimal-pair intonation patterns in phrases and sentences. **Measure:** QPR, overall numerical score. **Source:** Bross (1992).

Speech Pattern Contrast Test (SPAC) (C or G)
Material: Seven subtests, three for testing stress and intonation and four for testing phonetic contrasts. Short phrases or sentences are used in examining stress and intonation. A constant sentence frame and variable target word are used to examine the phonetic features. **Measure:** Percentage of correct contrast transmission. **Source:** Boothroyd (1985).

Procedures that Emphasize Phonological Analysis

Assessment of Phonological Processes-Revised (APP-R) (C or G)
Material: 50 words (names for three-dimensional stimuli). **Measure:** Frequency of process occurrence determined for 40 processes. **Source:** Hodson and Paden. (1983).

RULES: The RULES Phonological Evaluation (C)
Material: Screening test used 12 pictured stimulus words; phonological inventory uses 10 pictured stimulus words in two contexts, confrontation naming and self-generated sentences. **Measure:** Use of processes. **Source:** Webb and Duckett (1990).

Procedures that Derive an Index for Continuous Speech

Articulation Competence Index (ACI) (G)
Material: Continuous speech. **Measure:** Severity of articulation involvement, based on both consonants correct and relative distortion. **Source:** Shriberg (1993).

Percentage of Consonants Correct (PCC) (G)
Material: continuous speech. **Measure:** percentage of consonants correct. **Source:** Shriberg and Kwiatkowski (1982).

Procedures that use Scaling Methods

Meaningful Use of Speech Scale (MUSS) (C)
Material: Speech in everyday situations (assessed by parent/teacher interviews). **Measure:** Determination if child (1) uses speech without other communicative support, (2) adjusts speech to variations in listener familiarity, and (3) effectively uses clarification and repair strategies. **Source:** Osberger (1992).

NTID Rating Scale (G)
Material: A wide variety of material can be used. Samples are most often obtained from

spontaneous speech or oral reading of passages. **Measure:** A metric of speech intelligibility is computed as the arithmetic mean of the interval scale values assigned by the listeners for each speech sample. **Source:** Schiavetti (1992).

Appendix B: Voice rating scale.

GRBAS Voice Rating Scale

GRADE: degree of hoarseness or voice abnormality

0	1	2	3
Normal	Slight	Moderate	Extreme

ROUGH: auditory/acoustic impression of irregularity of vibration (jitter and shimmer)

0	1	2	3
Normal	Slight	Moderate	Extreme

BREATH: auditory/acoustic impression of degree of air leakage (related to turbulence)

0	1	2	3
Normal	Slight	Moderate	Extreme

ASTHENIC: weakness or lack of power (related to vocal intensity and energy in higher harmonics)

0	1	2	3
Normal	Slight	Moderate	Extreme

STRAINED: auditory/acoustic impression of hyperfunction (related to fundamental frequency, noise in high-frequency range, and energy in higher harmonics)

0	1	2	3
Normal	Slight	Moderate	Extreme

Check for presence of the following:
[ ] tremor [ ] pitch variation [ ] loudness variation
[ ] voice interruption [ ] other: specify _____

Appendix C. Perceptual dimensions used by Darley et al (1969a,b, 1975) (Mayo Clinic rating scales).

Dimension	*Dimension*
Pitch level	Pitch of voice sounds consistently too low or too high for an individual's age and sex.
Pitch breaks	Pitch of voice shows sudden and uncontrolled variation (falsetto breaks).
Monopitch	Voice is characterized by a monopitch or monotone. Voice lacks normal pitch and inflectional changes. It tends to stay at one pitch level.
Voice tremor	Voice shows shakiness or tremulousness.
Monoloudness	Voice shows monotony of loudness. It lacks normal variations in loudness.
Excess loudness variation	Voice shows sudden, uncontrolled alterations in loudness, sometimes becoming too loud, some times too weak.
Loudness decay	There is progressive diminution or decay of loudness.

Alternating loudness	There are alternating changes in loudness.
Loudness (overall)	Voice is insufficiently or excessively loud.
Harsh voice	Voice is harsh, rough, and raspy.
Hoarse (wet) voice	Wet, "liquid-sounding" hoarseness.
Breathy voice (continuous)	Continuously breathy, weak, and thin.
Breathy voice (transient)	Breathiness is transient, periodic, intermittent.
Strained-strangled	Voice (phonation) sounds strained or strangled (an apparently effortful squeezing of voice through glottis).
Voice stoppages	There are sudden stoppages of voiced airstream (as if some obstacle along the vocal tract momentarily impedes flow of air).
Hypernasality	Voice sounds excessively nasal. Excessive amount of air is resonated by nasal cavities.
Hyponasality	Voice is denasal.
Nasal emission	There is nasal emission of airstream.
Forced inspiration-expiration	Speech is interrupted by sudden, forced inspiration, and expiration sighs.
Audible inspiration	Audible, breathy expiration.
Grunt at end of expiration	Grunt as expiration terminates.
Rate	Rate of actual speech is abnormally slow or rapid.
Phrases short	Phrases are short (possibly due to fact that inspirations occur more often than normal). Speaker may sound as if he has run out of air. He may produce a gasp at the end of a phrase.
Increase of rate in segments	Rate increases progressively within given segments of connected speech.
Increase of rate overall	Rate increases progressively from beginning to end of sample.
Reduced stress	Speech shows reduction of proper stress or emphasis pattern.
Variable rate	Rate alternately changes from slow to fast.
Intervals prolonged	Prolongation of interword or intersyllable intervals.
Inappropriate silences	There are inappropriate silent intervals.
Short rushes of speech	There are short rushes of speech separated by pauses.
Excess and equal stress	Excess stress on usually unstressed parts of speech, e.g. (1) monosyllabic words and (2) unstressed syllables of polysyllabic words.
Imprecise consonants	Consonant sounds lack precision. They show slurring, inadequate sharpness, distortions, and lack of crispness. There is clumsiness in going from one consonant sound to another.
Phonemes prolonged	There are prolongations of phonemes.
Phonemes repeated	There are repetitions of phonemes.
Irregular articulatory breakdown	Intermittent nonsystematic breakdown inaccuracy of articulation.
Vowels distorted	Vowel sounds are distorted throughout their total duration.
Intelligibility (overall)	Rating of overall intelligibility or understandability of speech.
Bizarreness (overall)	Rating of degree to which overall speech calls attention to itself because of its unusual, peculiar, or bizarre characteristics.

Chapter **3**

Nonspeech Assessment of the Speech Production Mechanism

Donald A. Robin, Nancy Pearl Solomon, Jerald B. Moon, and John W. Folkins

Introduction

The assessment of nonspeech abilities has long been a part of the clinical examination of individuals with suspected speech problems, particularly those with potential motor speech disorders. The oral mechanism examination is replete with nonspeech tasks, as are other types of tests used by speech-language pathologists. For instance, Darley, Aronson, and Brown (1975), in their description of examination for dysarthria and apraxia of speech, recommend a number of nonspeech observations and maneuvers.

Recently, the use of nonspeech tasks for clinicians and researchers interested in speech motor control and its disorders has been challenged (eg, Weismer & Forrest, 1992; Weismer & Liss, 1991). By contrast, other speech researchers/clinicians have argued that there are good reasons to perform nonspeech tasks both clinically and in a research setting (eg, Folkins, Moon, Luschei, Robin, Tye-Murray, & Moll, 1995; Luschei, 1991; Moon, Zebrowski, Robin, & Folkins, 1993; Solomon, Robin, Lorell, Rodnitzky, & Luschei , 1994). However, the fact remains that data addressing the issue of using nonspeech tasks to assess the speech motor system are remarkably scarce. Moreover, the data that are available are open to numerous interpretations. For both clinical and research purposes, the use of any task should be driven by the questions one needs to answer. Thus, for any task (nonspeech or speech), we would urge clinicians to criti-cally question why they are using a given procedure. That is, for each and every task used, clinicians should be able to state the specific rationale for its use and whether or not data are available in the literature to support their rationale.

The purpose of this chapter is to present our philosophical approach to evaluation of the speech production system. Our philosophy of assessment of motor speech disorders mandates the use of nonspeech tasks in the clinic. The present chapter does not attempt to review all of the available nonspeech procedures available to the speech-language pathologist, but rather to provide examples of some tasks and to examine if they meet the needs of the clinician based on our beliefs about the utility of nonspeech tasks. We emphasize at the outset that we are not advocating the use of nonspeech tasks only. Rather, our position is that nonspeech tasks can provide useful information about the functioning of the motor system that is unique and aids in understanding a person's ability to communicate using the speech production system. Specifically, we believe the combined use of nonspeech and speech tasks are beneficial if one's goal is to determine the integrity of the speech motor system.

Nonspeech Assessment of the Speech Motor System: A Perspective

As clinicians, we must be able to distinguish problems of movement control (ie, of the motor system) during speech as separate from the linguistic demands placed on the system. Simply stated, we must be able to separate the contributions to the speech disorder arising from the motor system from contributions to the speech disorder arising from the linguistic system. The assessment of nonspeech and speech capabilities enhances our ability to evaluate the interaction between the motor and linguistic contributions to motor speech disorders.

Our basic philosophical position, which drives our clinical practice, is that it is not necessary to assume that the goals of the speech motor system are the same as the goals of other levels of the system (ie, the linguistic system). In fact, assuming that linguistic and motor goals are the same may impede our understanding of the underlying pathogenesis of motor speech disorders. One can assume that all behaviors are composed of a number of different behaviors. Moreover, each behavior may be part of some larger set of behaviors, which are probably part of still larger behavioral goals. As we have noted elsewhere (Folkins et al, 1995), regardless of the terminology used, goals or organizing principles of speech behavior operate on many different levels which include the motoric, phonologic, syntactic, semantic, and pragmatic domains. It is also clear that there is no consensus on how goals or units are organized relative to speech production. Some investigators prefer to define speech motor goals in terms of the linguistic system (eg, Browman & Goldstein, 1986; Fowler, Rubin, Remez, & Turvey, 1980). In these models of speech production, it is assumed that some linguistic unit (eg, the phoneme or the syllable) serves as the focus of the organizing principles of the motor system during speech. However, as has been pointed out by us and others, there is no need to assume that there exists an explicit or even implicit relationship between linguistic goals and the units of motor control during speech (Folkins, 1985; Folkins & Bleile, 1990; Folkins et al, 1995; Moll, Zimmerman, & Smith, 1977). The issues of task specificity and units of control

have been debated in the nonspeech motor control literature as well (Schmidt, 1988). As noted above, it is our contention that although formulation of linguistic messages must precede speech movements, the units of speech motor control are not necessarily related to the units of linguistic control. Furthermore, we contend that the confound of positing that linguistic constraints drive the speech motor system may impede our ability to understand and ultimately determine motoric contributions to speech and speech disorders.

This argument is particularly relevant for the assessment of motor speech disorders in which the impaired speaker may have an inability to adequately control the movements of the structures that produce speech in order to formulate perceptually accurate speech. Difficulty with speech production assessed during speech does not allow the clinician to isolate the motoric impairments from those that may be linguistic in nature. This argument is useful even if one assumes that the units of speech production derive from phonological or higher-order psycholinguistic behaviors (eg, Lindblom, 1982; Studdert-Kennedy, 1987). That is, when assessing a patient's motor abilities, one problem the clinician is faced with when using speech tasks is that speech production occurs in the context of constraints that produce motoric demands in conjunction with the linguistic demands of the task. It is important for the clinician to separate the motor processes and the linguistic levels of constraint. Ideally (though, unfortunately not presently practiced), the clinician should systematically vary the level of constraint (motoric and linguistic) and determine how they interact to affect speech production.

There is another powerful advantage in the use of nonspeech tasks to assess patients with motor speech disorders that has to do with the degrees of freedom during speech movements. Since speech production involves the interaction and coordination of all speech production subsystems (respiratory, phonatory, and supraglottal [velar and articulatory systems]) in an integrated manner, one cannot assess the relative contribution of a given speech production subsystem to the disorder without using nonspeech tasks. If the clinician wishes to determine the contribution of motor impairments of the lips or the respiratory system to the motor speech disorder, one must use nonspeech tasks. Using speech tasks does not allow the clinician to examine individual articulators without the interaction with and possible compensation from other speech production subsystems.

Netsell and Rosenbek (1985), among many others (eg, Darley et al, 1975), have promoted the consideration of differential subsystem involvement during the assessment and management of motor speech disorders. Netsell and Rosenbek (1985) note that each of the major speech production subsystems can be affected differentially following neurologic insult. Furthermore, there may even be differential involvement within a given major system (eg, upper lip versus lower lip). During speech production, the structures work together to achieve the goal of perceptually accurate speech. Thus, different combinations of movements can be used for the same speech task. Consequently, during speech, individuals with motor speech disorders often show compensations between and within the components of speech motor subsystems. As a result, the clinician does not know if the resultant movements are caused by primary motor involvement of a given structure, or if they result from compensation of a given structure for the motor impairment of a different speech structure.

Nonspeech tasks allow the clinician to assess individual structures in order to determine if there is a primary motoric involvement of that structure. Nonspeech tasks that utilize more than one structure can examine the coordination and interaction of multiple structures under controlled conditions, allowing for unambiguous interpretation of motor involvements and compensations. That is, nonspeech tasks allow for the systematic manipulation of combinations of a structure or structures that the clinician is interested in studying (Barlow & Netsell, 1986).

The concept of operating range is also important when considering the clinical utility of nonspeech tasks. One can consider the maximal limits of a given system as its envelope. The operating range is the part of the envelope that is typically used for a given task (eg, speech). For example, Zimmerman (1980) has suggested that nonfluency results when the motor system exceeds its operating range during speech and the speaker does not have the control to compensate for the excursions from the typical range of speech. As noted below, speech typically uses only a limited portion of the envelope and having a reduced envelope may not affect speech directly. Rather, factors that reduce the envelope (eg, low strength, rigid structures) may make speech gestures difficult to produce.

The concept of operating range is closely related to flexibility and compensations (see above) and has been discussed elsewhere in detail (Folkins, 1985). Physiologic parameters of speech vary when the same speech sample is reproduced repeatedly in the same context. As long as this variability remains within the operating range of the motor system, perceptually accurate speech can occur. Variability may be so great as to exceed the operating range. Speakers may be able to compensate, or be flexible enough, to handle the excessive variability and produce accurate speech. That is, speakers with good motor control can make up for limitations in the operating range of one or more structures. For instance, the insertion of a bite block, using a normal speaker, brings the operating range of the jaw to zero, but the lips, tongue, and velum can compensate for this in order to produce accurate speech. However, following motor impairments, the speaker may not have the flexibility to handle excessive variability or movements that fall outside of the operating range of the system, and speech will not be produced accurately.

We do not know the operating range of all of the systems of speech production. Some systems or structures may have very restricted ranges and therefore be more prone to disruption than others. The operating range of speech (at least in the laboratory) for some systems appears for many different areas to be about 10–25% of the maximal envelope. It is important for clinicians to know if the envelope is reduced, or if the operating range is shifted towards the maximum. Thus, for speech produced under conditions with little stress or demand, 10–25% of the range may well be adequate. However, in situations where the demands or stresses on the system are high and there is a need to exceed the typical operating range of speech, speakers with a reduced envelope may be prone to break down (ie, be more likely to produce speech errors). Thus, normal speakers have the flexibility to handle the inherent variability that occurs when producing the same speech in various contexts. A speaker with dysarthria who has a reduced envelope may function well under conditions of low demand but suffer a breakdown in speech accuracy when situational variability results in the need to use a larger physiological range. For instance, it is estimated that the amount of maximal strength of the articulators used during speech production is about 20% maximal strength during the quiet production of single words or simple phrases (Barlow & Burton, 1990). The speaker whose maximal strength is reduced by 50% due to neurologic involvement may produce adequate speech during word production at a relatively slow rate, but may not be able to produce perceptually accurate speech in utterances due to an inability to hit articulatory targets in the appropriate time frame because the shortening velocity of muscle fibers is directly related to muscle strength. Reduced strength decreases the shortening velocity and therefore reduces the speed of movement.

Depending on the speech-language pathologist's setting, the use of nonspeech tasks may vary. For instance, nonspeech tasks of the oral structures may provide information about the absence or presence of neurological diseases such as stroke, parkinsonism, myasthenia gravis and many others. As well, disease progression, treatment effects (drug or behavioral), and new neurological incidents may be quantified by nonspeech measures. Such measures may show change before associated changes in perceptually adequate speech occur.

Regardless of the rationale, nonspeech measures have long been part of the speech evaluation for people with sensorimotor involvement. Below we review selected nonspeech tasks typically used in evaluation of patients with sensorimotor impairments. Finally we review recent developments in assessment of the speech production and focus on fine force or position control tasks, visuomotor tracking tasks, and strength and fatigue tasks.

Examples of Tasks Typically Used in the Clinic

Respiratory System

The evaluation of the respiratory system may begin with pulmonary function testing. This may be accomplished by referral to a pulmonary function laboratory. However, many of the typical pulmonary function measures can be made by the speech-language pathologist. The measures that one obtains from pulmonary function testing are useful in defining the envelope of the respiratory system and its operating range. Measures that are obtained include the vital capacity (VC), total lung capacity (TLC), residual volume (RV), forced expiratory volume in 1 sec (FEV1), the flow-volume loop, the diffusion capacity, resting tidal volume (TV), and resting breathing rate. Of these measures, the SLP with access to a spirometer is equipped to measure VC, FEV1, TV, and breathing rate. The other measures must be obtained from a pulmonary function laboratory. The VC represents the total volume of air that can be expelled from the lungs following a maximal inspiration. Following maximum expiration, there is still a small portion of air remaining in the lungs which is referred to as the RV. The TCL is the addition of VC plus the RV.

The FEV1 is the volume of air that a person can expire in one second when asked to inspire maximally and expire as quickly as possible. The diffusion capacity represents the pulmonary gas exchange or amount of gas exchange from the alveoli to the blood. These pulmonary function measures inform the clinician about the basic status of the respiratory system. Pulmonary function abnormalities can affect the ability to speak in a number of ways. For instance, involvement of the respiratory system from some lung diseases can severely reduce the envelope or operating range of the respiratory system, which may affect a person's ability to produce speech. A severe reduction in vital capacity could potentially affect utterance length and phrasing during speech. As well, the effects of some lung diseases may render use of the respiratory system during speech more effortful which could potentially reduce the speaker's desire to communicate using speech. Neurologic disease also can affect the muscles of respiration and result in abnormal respiratory control during speech. Knowledge of the speaker's respiratory abilities should assist the clinician in designing appropriate intervention strategies.

Evaluation of breathing for speech involves assessment of tracheal (subglottal) pressure, lung volume, air flow, and chest-wall shape. Before considering how these parameters are controlled actively for speech, it is important to understand how passive forces (eg, elastic recoil and rebound, and gravity) affect the respiratory system. At the end of a resting expiration, the respiratory system is at a state of equilibrium. Passive forces acting on the chest wall and pulmonary system are equalized and pressure in the lungs is equal to atmospheric pressure. Active forces (ie, forces generated by muscle contraction) are required to stray from this resting expiratory level, and then passive and active forces may combine to achieve the desired volume, pressure, flow, and shape outcome. For resting breathing, the goal is adequate ventilation at the lowest possible effort, so passive forces are relied upon for expiration. For speech breathing, a relatively constant lung pressure is desired throughout a certain extent of lung volume expenditure (depending on the length of the utterance). The passive forces acting on the respiratory system depend on lung volume. Therefore, during speech we must contend with constantly changing passive pressures while trying to deliver relatively constant pressures to the larynx. We achieve this goal by varying the degree of muscle contraction provided by a variety of expiratory and some inspiratory muscles at different portions of an utterance. At high lung volumes, inspiratory forces are needed to hold back or brake against high recoil forces. At middle and low lung volumes, expiratory forces are needed to maintain adequate pressures and resist rebound forces. This is a delicate balancing act that our brains are designed to perform with little or no awareness by us.

The pressure delivered to the larynx by the lungs, necessary for phonation to occur, can be estimated by placing one end of a small tube in the mouth and connecting the other end to a pressure transducer. A U-tube manometer with a leak to simulate laryngeal resistance can also be used (Netsell & Hixon, 1978). An even simpler, more readily available, technique for measuring respiratory driving pressure was described by Hixon, Hawley, and Wilson (1982). It involves having the patient blow through a straw into a glass of water. Fix the straw so that its tip is 5 cm below the surface of the water, and have the patient blow just until bubbles come out. This indicates that the patient can generate 5 cm H_2O pressure. If she or he can sustain that pressure for 5 sec, the pressure is considered to be adequate for speech purposes. Perceptually, tracheal pressure is reflected in vocal loudness. Thus, prolonging phonation with adequate and steady loudness indicates good generation and control of tracheal pressure. However, laryngeal interactions make this assessment somewhat difficult to interpret.

Lung volume refers to how much air is used to speak (lung volume excursion), and where within the vital capacity speech occurs. Typically, we use approximately 20%

of the VC for speech, and speak in the mid-range of the vital capacity. Lung volume can be assessed with a spirometer, by integrating a flow signal obtained with a pneumotachograph, or by measuring motions of the chest wall and calibrating this to know volume measures. Lung volume excursion can be judged perceptually by the duration of speech phrases produced on one breath, assuming that air flow is within normal limits.

Air flow is a measure of the amount of lung volume expended over time, and can be assessed with a spirometer, pneumotachometer, or chest-wall kinematics. During phonation, high air flows may be perceived as breathiness. In many cases, breathy phonation may reflect laryngeal abnormalities rather than respiratory dysfunction. Assessing flow during nonspeech tasks can reveal characteristics of lower airway patency. Obstructive lung disease may lead to collapsing airways, and this can be detected during high-flow breathing tasks.

The shape and motions of the chest wall during speech can provide valuable insight regarding the muscular mechanisms used for speech. Motions of the rib cage and abdominal wall can be measured with respiratory inductive plethysmography or magnetometry. If these types of equipment are unavailable, assessment is still possible by watching or touching the patient's anterior torso during resting breathing, maximal breathing tasks, and speech. A normal pattern of resting breathing involves outward movement of both the rib cage and abdomen during inspiration, and inward movement of both parts of the chest wall during expiration. If this pattern is abnormal, important inferences regarding the passive and active forces that affect respiration can be made (eg, Putnam & Hixon, 1983; Solomon & Hixon, 1993). Demands for speech breathing are superimposed on these basic respiratory functions. Normal chest-wall shape for speech generally involves an inward displacement of the abdominal wall and an outward displacement of the rib cage from their resting position. Usually, but not necessarily, both parts of the chest wall move inward during the speech utterance.

The timing of breathing for speech involves a quick inspiration followed by a slow expiration. Having a patient produce this pattern of breathing without phonation can provide insight into respiratory control without the interactions of laryngeal and upper airway valving. Indeed, assessment of speech breathing aside from the rest of the speech production mechanism is possible and important for drawing conclusions regarding the respiratory system's contribution to a speech disorder and possible compensations for other disordered subsystems.

Phonatory System

Most measures used to evaluate the function of the phonatory system require the use of speech. Here we review measures related to vowel and single-consonant production. The stimuli discussed below are operationally defined as "nonspeech" measures since they do not have linguistic or communicative intent, and are generally not as multisystem demanding as the production of words and longer units of speech. However, producing a vowel or a consonant utilizes all of the speech production system in a manner that does not allow for as clear a distinction between speech subsystems and their compensations among structures.

One commonly used measure of phonatory function is airflow. Typically, airflow is measured during the production of an /a/ or an /i/. Airflow is most often measured using a pneumotachograph, an instrument that measures the pressure drop across a known resistance that is placed in the airstream. Some clinicians examine air flow over time to detect changes such as increased flow due to fatigue of the larynx. Netsell, Lotz, and Barlow (1989) suggest examination of airflow during production of /pa/ at a rate of 1.5/sec and 3.0/sec, /pi/ as described above for /pa/, sustaining /a/ and /i/ for 3 sec each, maximal phonation time, and possibly during different pitches, loudnesses, and both. Such tasks allow one to quantify airflow characteristics in a variety of contexts and gain information about the consistency of flow. Normal airflow for the consonants listed above is around 200 cc/sec.

While maximal prolongation times are not uniformly accepted indices of phonatory status, many voice clinicians believe them to be useful in the evaluation of phonatory function (Verdolini, 1994). One reason these measures may not be universally accepted is that, like other nonspeech tasks, they do not examine the operating range of the system when used for speech. However, they do provide information about the envelope of maximal performance which, as discussed above, has clinical utility. As well, the normative data on maximum phonation times varies with a number of factors including vital capacity, age, gender, and body stature (Kent, Kent, & Rosenbek, 1987). Thus, the clinician should be very careful as to the method used to obtain maximum phonatory times and the normative data used to interpret the times obtained on their patients. Maximal phonation times are considered to reflect membranous vocal fold closure patterns (Verdolini, 1994). That is, maximal phonation times are decreased when conditions are such that the vocal folds do not achieve complete closure such as during bowing or the presence of nodules. As well, sustained phonation is thought to provide information on some supraglottal control (Kent et al, 1987) such as the variability of formant frequency (Gerratt, 1983).

Maximal phonation time measurement requires the client to produce a vowel, typically /a/, for as long as possible. If the vocal folds do not achieve good closure during phonation, air leakage will occur and maximum phonation time will be reduced. Reduced maximal phonatory times may result from nonlaryngeal mechanisms such as respiratory insufficiency or leakage of the air downstream (eg, velopharyngeal incompetence). In general, normative values for sustained phonation for the vowel /a/ in children are approximately 10 sec and for adults 20 sec (see Table 2 in Kent et al, 1987,

for review of normative data from different studies).

The S:Z ratio was developed to assist the clinician in the differentiation between respiratory and laryngeal contributions to speech production problems (Boone, 1983). The patient is asked to produce the /s/ and /z/ for as long as possible. If the respiratory and phonatory systems are functioning normally, the S:Z ratio should be slightly less than 1. Normal /s/ durations are around 9 sec in children and 16 sec in adults (Kent et al, 1987). Normal durations for /z/ are around 11 sec in children and 19 sec in adults. The S:Z ratios reported in the literature range from .70–.99. S:Z ratios greater than 1 are interpreted as an indication of vocal fold involvement in that the /s/ should be produced with normal durations, but the /z/ is reduced in duration due to air leakage at the level of the vocal folds. Of course, reduction in both /s/ and /z/ tend to implicate respiratory system problems. They could also be indicative of ineffective vocal tract constriction. Thus, the isolation of one subsystem from another is not easily accomplished using these measures.

Verdolini (1994) suggests that laryngeal diadochokinesis, the rapid and repetitive production of glottal plosives, may serve as an index of neural integrity of the phonatory system. She recommends that clinicians obtain measures of the rate of production, strength (loudness/clarity) of plosives and the consistency of production over time. The procedure requires the client to repeat a vowel as rapidly as possible for 5 sec. The rate of production is typically 3.6–5.4/sec in children and around 5.0/sec in adults. Verdolini suggests that the clinician should perceptually rate the strength of the productions and their consistency. Strong consistent productions are indicative of normal phonatory functioning. Data on reliability of these ratings and their sensitivity in detecting phonatory problems are not currently available.

Other measures of phonatory range and control are sometimes used by clinicians. Measures of range relate to the envelope of the phonatory system. The pitch or frequency range (lowest to highest) is often used as an index of phonatory function. On average, the normal pitch range is approximately 35 semitones or approximately 3 octaves. Similarly, clinicians may gain an index of loudness or intensity range by asking patients to phonate as softly and as loudly as possible. On average, adults can produce approximately 100 dB SPL and have a minimum level of about 5 dB SPL (see Kent et al, 1987, for review). Children have a slightly lower average maximal intensity of 85 dB SPL and a similar minimal level.

Measures of control require the patient to modulate the voice in systematic ways. Clinicians frequently ask patients to sing the notes of the scale from the lowest to highest pitch. They may also ask patients to phonate at different loudness levels to assess control. Also, clients may be asked to vary pitch

variations (eg, high-low; low-high-low) or amplitude (eg, soft-loud). To gain further information about the control of the phonatory system some clinicians examine the ability to change pitch without changing loudness or to change loudness without changing pitch. One index of phonatory control is the phonetogram or voice range profile (see Titze, 1994, for detail). The phonetogram is a display of the intensity range versus the fundamental frequency range. To obtain a phonetogram the clinician has the patient produce the softest and loudest notes he or she can at each pitch across the frequency range. The plot of intensity-by-frequency has a characteristic shape and deviations from that shape may be indicative of phonatory difficulties (Titze, 1994). A phonetogram of a normal male speaker is shown in Figure 3–1. The figure is a plot of loudness level (dB) on the Y axis and

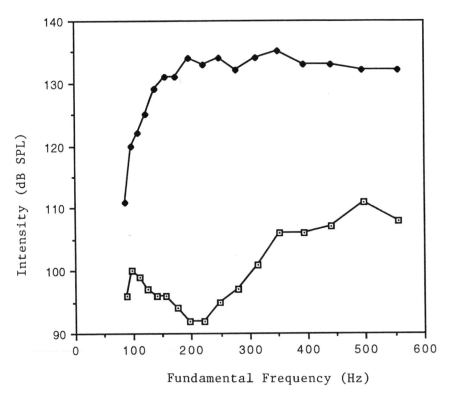

Figure 3–1. Phonetogram (voice range profile) of a normal male subject producing the vowel /a/. The X axis is the fundamental frequency, and the Y axis is the intensity in dB SPL at 0.5 m mike-to-mouth distance. The top and bottom lines represent maximum and minimum of the range, respectively.

fundamental frequency (Hz) on the X axis. Top and bottom lines represent the maximum and minimum of this normal subject's range.

Velar-Pharyngeal System

Like the phonatory system, there are few tasks of velar function used clinically that are truly nonspeech in nature. However, some tasks may allow for assessment of the envelope or maximal range. For instance, Kuehn and Moon (1995) assessed electromyographic (EMG) activity of the palate during blowing versus speech. The blowing task was performed at relatively low pressures (5 cm H_2O) and at maximal pressure generation. Blowing with maximal effort forced the levator muscle to its maximal activity level. Results showed that EMG activity during speech was about 10–30% of the maximal EMG activity as assessed during blowing. Patients with neurologic involvement of the palate that reduces their maximal range may produce perceptually accurate speech under nonstressful conditions. However, when placed in situations of increased demand, they may not have the range to accommodate the added stress and, as a result, speech accuracy will be adversely affected. Nonspeech tasks to evaluate the velar-pharyngeal system are relatively few in number. Clinicians may ask patients to blow with the lips sealed to determine if there is leakage of the velar-pharyngeal (VP) valve. As well, one might observe the patients while swallowing a liquid (typically water) to determine if water leaks around the VP valve and into the nasal cavities.

Articulatory System

There are more nonspeech tasks used in the clinic to assess the function of articulatory structures (ie, lips, tongue, jaw) than for the other speech subsystems. This is partially because these structures are more readily observed by the clinician than the other speech production systems. Hall (1995) has recently reviewed the oral mechanism ex-amination for nonspeech and speech function. Relative to lip function, the clinician frequently asks for a pucker, retraction (unilateral and bilateral), and sequential movements of the lips. Similar activities are also used to assess tongue function. The clinician may ask the client to protrude the tongue, move it from side to side, touch the nose or chin with the tip of the tongue or provide a series of movements in sequence. The purpose of these tasks is to assess the speed, symmetry, distance and accuracy of movements of the tongue, lips, and jaw. As well, observations by the clinician are used to determine if there are abnormal movements associated with the structure such as tremor, hyperkinesis or hypokinesis.

A common task used to assess nonspeech control of the articulators is diadochokinesis. The patient is required to move a given structure repeatedly as rapidly as possible for a given amount of time. For example, the patient may be asked to touch the tip of the tongue to the alveolar ridge as rapidly as possible repeating the movement until told to stop. Both the number of repetitions per unit time, and the accuracy of placement are noted. This task is designed to assess coordination and is thought to be indicative of the underlying neural integrity of the system.

While many of the above tasks are used in an everyday manner in many clinics, their relation to speech and speech breakdown are largely unknown. Weismer (1992) argues that motor tasks involve task-specific control strategies and that the generalization from one task to another is not possible. He goes on to argue that it is therefore inappropriate to use nonspeech tasks as a window into speech motor control processes and their disorders. However, even though many aspects of motor control are task specific, as noted earlier in this chapter, the tasks clinicians use should be specific to the control processes of the speech motor system, and not based on processes borrowed from the linguistic level of analysis. As we discuss in the next section, tasks can be developed that mimic the motor control demands of speech.

Another issue related to nonspeech tasks is that they are often "subjective" in nature and normative data are not well developed. For instance, Hall (1995) writes that having the patient circle the lips with tongue is an "excellent way to gain subjective judgements about the smoothness, accuracy and coordination of the tongue." However, there are no norms for many of these tasks. Moreover, the tasks are often unreliable in terms of intra- and interjudge measures. This is certainly the case with measures of maximal strength (discussed below) where the typical subjective measures (Hall, 1995, for discussion of typical strength assessment procedures) may be unreliable and insensitive to changes over time that occur as a result of treatment or disease progression (Robin, Somodi, & Luschei, 1991).

Recent Developments in the Assessment of Nonspeech Movements

In this section we report on a number of recently developed nonspeech tasks that we believe tap the motor demands of speech motor control processes. Two recently developed nonspeech tasks for the assessment of neuromotor speech disorders, require patients to control static position or isometric force (Barlow & Abbs, 1986; McNeil, Weismer, Adams, & Mulligan, 1990). A modification of the basic static force or position maneuvers is a dynamic ramp and hold force control task (Barlow & Burton, 1990). The rationale underlying the Barlow and colleagues task (and the visuomotor tracking task discussed below) is to use nonspeech movements that are closer to the control requirement during speech movements than those allowed by the traditional clinical nonspeech tasks. The basic force or position control paradigm requires the placement of a force or position transducer on the articulator of interest (eg, upper lip). A target level of force or a position is indicated on an oscillographic screen (or with a visual cue). The patient's transduced signal is also present on the screen. The patient is told to reach a given target force level, or a target

position, and hold it there as steadily as possible for a specific period of time (eg, 5 sec). One can test multiple force levels or positions. Motor control or stability is indexed by examination of the distance of the patient's force or position from the target level as well as the performance variance.

The dynamic ramp and hold force task is a modification of the above procedure in which subjects are asked to generate a given force level as rapidly and accurately as possible (Barlow & Burton, 1990). The duration of a trial has typically been about 5 sec. The rationale for this procedure is to make the nonspeech movement more speech like by having a dynamic, not a static task. Measures used to index articulatory stability include the reaction time, the peak rate of force change, the peak force during the ramping maneuver, and the mean and standard deviation for the force output during the hold phase.

Results from these tasks have shown utility in the evaluation of neuromotor involvement in speech disorders. For instance, McNeil et al (1990) showed that subjects with apraxia of speech or dysarthria performed abnormally on the static position and force tasks. Barlow and Abbs (1984) studied lip, jaw, and tongue force instability in subjects with spastic muscle conditions. They found that the subjects with spasticity had less stability than normal subjects. Moreover, their results showed that force instability correlated well with listener judgments of speech intelligibility ($r = .886$). Barlow and Burton (1987) reported data on four subjects who had suffered a traumatic brain injury. The four subjects with TBI performed more poorly than normal on the ramp and hold force task.

A different task that has great potential clinical utility, and has increased our understanding of motor involvement in speech disorders is the visuomotor tracking task, first described in the speech system by McClean, Beukelman, and Yorkston (1987). We (Moon et al, 1993; Hageman, Robin, Moon, & Folkins, 1994) have modified and expanded the visuomotor tracking task. Visuomotor tracking requires patients to follow a moving target on a screen with a given speech structure (eg, jaw, lower lip, voice). A transducer (eg, strain-gauge for the lips and jaw or a microphone for the voice) is placed on the appropriate structure(s) and the transduced signal appears as a dot on the screen. The target signal is represented on the screen by a horizontal bar that moves up and down. The patient is told to keep the dot in the bar as it moves. Targets are either predictable (sine wave motion) or unpredictable (random motion). Target speed and amplitude can be varied systematically. Dependent measures include the cross-correlation between the target signal and the signal produced by the patient, the phase relationship between the two signals, the gain ratio (an index of how closely in amplitude the two signals match), and the absolute difference between the target signal and the signal produced by the patient (eg, mm for lips and jaw, Hz for voice).

The advantages of the visuomotor tracking task are similar to some of those for the ramp and hold maneuver described above. The basic rationale is that the task better reflects some of the motor demands placed on the articulators during speech production than the traditional nonspeech tasks routinely used by clinicians. In addition to utilizing dynamic movements, the predictable tracking task requires a movement with the peak velocity approximately in the center of the movement, much like speech. Moreover, one can change the complexity of the task in a number of different ways. For instance, increasing the speed of tracking or the predictability of the target alters task complexity. Such changes in complexity may have potential for prognosis, treatment candidacy decisions, and monitoring changes due to treatment, or in the case of a progressive disease, decline.

Subjects with apraxia of speech show difficulty with the visuomotor tracking task (Hageman et al, 1994, in review). Specifically, subjects with apraxia of speech were shown to have poorer performance than subjects who were normal or had aphasia when

tracking predictable targets, but performed normally when tracking unpredictable targets. Subjects with conduction aphasia tracked both predictable and unpredictable targets normally. Subjects with ataxic dysarthria had difficulty tracking predictable and unpredictable targets (Hageman, Robin, Moon, & Folkins, 1993). Data from the tracking performance of subjects with apraxia of speech were correlated with perceptual judgments of speech. Results showed strong correlations between predictable target tracking and judgments of speech. Their correlations ranged from .82–.96, depending on the structure and speed of tracking.

The tracking data suggest that subjects with apraxia of speech have difficulty developing or executing a model of target motion. It has been suggested that the ability to track predictable signals is best performed based on an internal representation of target motion (Flowers, 1978). When tracking a predictable target, subjects typically are in phase or are phase advanced of the target signal. Thus, they are not following the target, but rather must be following an internal model of the target. Moreover, subjects can maintain tracking accuracy when the feedback is removed, suggesting an internal representation of the target movement pattern drives performance. The tracking of unpredictable signals requires feedback from the external signal, since one cannot develop a model of random motion. In the unpredictable conditions, subjects phase lag the target. That the subjects with AOS were able to track the unpredictable, but not the predictable target, seems reasonable since these speakers were chosen because they have difficulty with the development or execution of high level motoric planning. By contrast, speakers with ataxia have a disorder that affects the execution of movements and possibly the planning of movement patterns since they had difficulty with both predictable and unpredictable targets.

The motor control tasks described above allow the clinician to vary systematically the level of force or the distance traveled by the articulator. Each of the tasks allows assessment of individual articulators, and differential involvement is often found following neurologic disease. As well, each task provides insight into the motor system, without the constraints of the language system.

A final area of nonspeech research that has recently received attention in the literature has to do with articulatory strength and fatigability. Studies in our laboratory have used the Iowa Oral Performance Instrument (IOPI) (Breakthrough, Inc.) to assess strength and fatigue of the tongue in a variety of subject groups. The paradigm we use requires subjects to push on an air-filled bulb with the anterior portion of the tongue. The IOPI contains a digital readout of pressure as well as a series of lights that indicate how much pressure is being generated. There is also an analog output.

To test maximal strength using the IOPI, patients are required to push against the bulb with their tongue as hard as possible. Patients are encouraged through verbal cheerleading and expressive demeanor (eg, "PUSH PUSH REALLY HARD!!"). To test fatigue, patients are asked to hold 50% of their maximal pressure for as long as possible. Here the light display is utilized and patients are told to keep the middle light on, which is set to 50% of the maximal pressure. More recently developed fatigue tests include a sense of effort task (Somodi, Robin, & Luschei, 1995) and a task where patients are told to hold "effort" constant (Solomon, Robin, Mitchinson, VanDaele, & Luschei, 1996).

Results from a variety of patients groups have been promising. We have documented fatigue problems in children with apraxia of speech and adults with spastic dysarthria (Robin et al, 1991). We have found tongue strength, but not fatigue abnormalities, in adults with Parkinson's disease (Solomon, Lorell, Robin, Rodnitzky & Luschei, 1995). Additionally, we have documented a modest but significant correlation between perceptual rating of the speech of subjects with Parkinson's disease and tongue strength (Solomon et al, 1995). As well, we have found strength and fatigue abnormalities

in a group of subjects who had sustained a traumatic brain injury (Stierwalt, Robin, Solomon, Weiss, & Max, 1996). Perceptual ratings of the speech of the subjects with TBI were significantly correlated with strength and fatigue of the tongue.

In summary, some of the newer nonspeech tasks that assess strength, fatigue, or motor control of the speech production system appear to be promising as clinical tools. These procedures allow for evaluation of the integrity of a given structure without the constraint of the linguistic system, but with similar motor demands as found during speech. Further research will determine how well performance on these newer nonspeech tasks correlates with perceptual ratings of speech, how much utility these tasks ultimately have in the clinic, and if differential diagnosis, prognosis or the ability to monitor disease progress is enhanced by these methods.

References

Barlow SM, Abbs JH. (1984). Orofacial fine-motor control impairments in congenital spasticity: evidence against hyper-tonus related performance deficits. *Neurology* 34:145–150.

Barlow SM, Abbs JH. (1986). Fine force and position control of select orofacial structures in the upper motor neuron syndrome. *Exp Neurol* 94:699–713.

Barlow SM, Burton MK. (1990). Ramp-and-hold force control in the upper and lower lips: developing new neuromotor assessment applications in traumatically brain injured adults. *J Speech Hear Res* 33:660–675.

Barlow SM, Netsell R. (1986). Differential fine force control of the upper and lower lips. *J Speech Hear Res* 29:163–169.

Boone DR. (1983). *The Voice and Voice Therapy*, 3rd ed. Englewood Cliffs: Prentice-Hall.

Browman C, Goldstein LM. (1986). Towards an articulatory phonology. In Ewan C, Anderson J, eds. *Phonology Yearbook*. Cambridge: Cambridge University Press, pp 219–252.

Darley FL, Aronson A, Brown J. (1975). *Motor Speech Disorders*. Philadelphia: W.B. Saunders.

Flowers K. (1978). Some frequency response characteristics of parkinsonism on pursuit tracking. *Brain* 101:19–34.

Folkins JW, Bleile KM. (1990). Taxonomies in biology, phonetics, phonology, and speech motor control. *J Speech Hear Disord* 55:596–611.

Folkins JW, Moon JB, Luschei ES, Robin DA, Tye-Murray N, Moll KL. (1995). What can nonspeech tasks tell us about speech motor disabilities? *J Phon* 23:139–147.

Folkins JW. (1985). Issues in speech motor control and their relation to the speech of individuals with cleft lip and palate. *Cleft Palate J* 22:106–122.

Fowler CA, Rubin P, Remez RE, Turvey MJ. (1980). Implications for speech production of a general theory of action. In Butterworth B, ed. *Language Production*. New York: Academic Press, pp. 373–420.

Gerratt BR. (1983). Formant frequency fluctuation as an index of motor steadiness in the vocal tract. *J Speech Hear Res* 26:297–304.

Hageman C, Robin DA, Moon JB, Folkins JW. (1993). Visuomotor tracking in neurogenic disorders. Paper presented to the Annual Meeting of the American Speech-Language-Hearing Association, San Antonio, November.

Hageman C, Robin DA, Moon JB, Folkins JW. (1994). Visuomotor tracking abilities of speakers with apraxia. *Clin Aphasiol* 22:219–229.

Hageman C, Robin DA, Moon JB, Folkins JW. (In review). Visuomotor tracking abilities of persons with apraxia of speech versus conduction aphasia.

Hall PK. (1995). The oral mechanism. In: Tomblin JB, Morris HL, Spriestersbach DC, eds. *Diagnosis in Speech-Language Pathology*. San Diego: Singular Press, pp 67–97.

Hixon TJ, Hawley JL, Wilson KJ. (1982). An around-the-house device for the clinical determination of respiratory driving pressure: a note on making simple even simpler. *J Speech Hear Disord* 47:413–415.

Kent RD, Kent JF, Rosenbeck JC. (1987). Maximum performance tests of speech production. *J Speech Hear Disord* 52:367–387.

Kuehn D, Moon JB. (1995). Levator veli palatini muscle activity in relation to intraoral air pressure variation. *J Speech Hear Res* 37:1260–1270.

Lindblom B. (1982). The interdisciplinary challenge of speech motor control. In: Grillner S, Lindblom B, Lubker J, Persson A, eds. *Speech Motor Control*. New York: Pergamon Press, pp 3–18.

Luschei ES. (1991). Development of objective standards of nonspeech oral strength and performance: an advocate's view. In Moore CA, Yorkston KM, Beukelman DR, eds. *Dysarthria and Apraxia of Speech: Perspectives on Management*. Baltimore: Paul H. Brookes, pp 3–14.

McClean MD, Beukelman DR, Yorkston KM. (1987). Speech-muscle visuomotor tracking in dysarthric and nonimpaired speakers. *J Speech Hear Res* 30:276–282.

McNeil MR, Weismer G, Adams S, Mulligan M. (1990). Oral structure nonspeech motor control in normal, dysarthric, aphasic, and apraxic speakers: isometric force and static position control. *J Speech Hear Res* 33:255–268.

Moll KL, Zimmerman GN, Smith A. (1977). The study of speech production as a human neuromotor system. In Sawashima M, Cooper FS, eds. *Dynamic Aspects of Speech Production*. Tokyo: University of Tokyo Press, pp 107–127.

Moon JB, Zebrowski P, Robin DA, Folkins JW. (1993). Visuomotor tracking ability of young adult speakers. *J Speech Hear Res* 36:672–682.

Netsell R, Hixon TJ. (1978). A noninvasive method for clinically estimating subglottal air pressure. *J Speech Hear Disord* 43:326–330.

Netsell R, Lotz WK, Barlow SM. (1989). A speech physiology examination for individuals with dysarthria. In: Yorkston KM, Beukelman DR, eds. *Recent Advances in Clinical Dysarthria*. Boston: College-Hill Press, pp 3–33.

Netsell R, Rosenbek JC. (1985). Treating the dysarthrias. In: Darby J, ed. *Speech and Language Evaluation in Neurology: Adult Disorders*. Orlando: Grune & Stratton, pp 363–392.

Putnam AHB, Hixon TJ. (1983). Respiratory kinematics in speakers with motor neuron disease. In: McNeil M, Rosenbeck J, Aronson A, eds. *The Dysarthrias*. San Diego: College-Hill Press, pp 37–67.

Robin DA, Somodi L, Luschei ES. (1991). Measurement of tongue strength and endurance in normal and articulation disordered subjects. In: Moore C, Yorkston KM, Beukelman DR, eds. *Dysarthria and Apraxia of Speech: Perspectives on Management*. Baltimore: Paul H. Brookes Publishing, pp 173–184.

Schmidt RA. (1988). *Motor Control and Learning: A Behavioral Emphasis*, 2nd ed. Champaign: Human Kinetics Publishers.

Solomon NP, Hixon TJ. (1993). Speech breathing in Parkinson's disease. *J Speech Hear Res* 36:294–310.

Solomon NP, Lorell DM, Robin DA, Rodnitzky RL, Luschei ES. (1995). Tongue strength and endurance in mild to moderate Parkinson's disease. *J Med Speech-Lang Pathol* 3:15–26.

Solomon NP, Robin DA, Lorell DM, Rodnitzky RL, Luschei ES. (1994). Tongue function testing in Parkinson's disease: indications of fatigue. In: Till J, Yorkston K, Beukelman D, eds. *Motor Speech Disorders: Advances in Assessment and Treatment.* Baltimore: Paul H. Brookes, pp 147–160.

Solomon NP, Robin DA, VanDaele DJ, Luschei ES. (1996). Sense of effort and the effects of fatigue in the tongue and hand. *J Speech Hear Res* 39:114–125.

Somodi LB, Robin DA, Luschei ES. (1995). A model of "sense of effort" during maximal and submaximal contractions of the tongue. *Brain Lang* 51:371–382.

Stierwalt JAG, Robin DA, Solomon NP, Weiss AL, Max J. (1996). Tongue strength and endurance: relation to the speaking ability of children and adolescents following traumatic brain injury. In: Robin DA, Yorkston KM, Beukelman DR, eds. *Disorders of Motor Speech: Assessment, Treatment, and Clinical Characterization.* Baltimore: Paul H. Brookes Publishing Co., pp 241–258.

Studdert-Kennedy M. (1987). The phoneme as a perceptuomotor structure. In: Allport A, Mackay D, Prinz W, Scheerer E, eds. *Language Perception and Production.* London: Academic Press, pp 67–84.

Titze IR. (1994). *Principles of Voice Production.* Englewood Cliffs: Prentice-Hall.

Verdolini K. (1994). Voice disorders. In: Tomblin JB, Morris HL, Spriestersbach DC, eds. *Diagnosis in Speech-Language Pathology.* San Diego: Singular Press, pp 247–306.

Weismer G, Forrest K. (1992). Issues in motor speech disorders: a position paper. Paper presented at the Conference on Motor Speech: Motor Speech Disorders Track, Boulder.

Weismer G, Liss JM. (1991). Reductionism is a dead-end in speech research: perspectives on a new direction. In: Moore C, Yorkston KM, Beukelman DR, eds. *Dysarthria and Apraxia of Speech: Perspectives on Management.* Baltimore: Paul H. Brookes, pp 15–27.

Weismer G. (1992). Personal communication. Letter to John Folkins, Aug 9, 1992.

Zimmerman G. (1980). Stuttering: a disorder of movement. *J Speech Hear Res* 23:122–136.

Acknowledgments

Preparation of this chapter was supported by a center grant from the NIH-NIDCD (DC90076). As well, a portion of Dr Robin's effort was supported by a NIH-NINDS program project grant (PO NS19632). The authors also acknowledge many of their colleagues and students who have assisted with the work at the University of Iowa reviewed in the chapter. These individuals include Heather Clark, Carlin Hageman, Sara Mitchinson, Daryl Lorell, Erich S. Luschei, Dave Kuehn, Kenneth Moll, John Nichols, Wendy Edwards, Robert Rodnitzky, Sami Seddoh, Lori Somodi, Julie Stierwalt, Nancy Tye-Murray, and Patricia Zebrowski. Mary Jo Yotty is thanked for her superb secretarial support.

Chapter *4*

Acoustic Analysis of Dysarthric Speech

Karen Forrest and Gary Weismer

Introduction

Although perceptual analysis is the major tool used by speech-language pathologists to gather information concerning speech production characteristics of persons with various speech disorders, there is good reason to explore the potential of instrumental analyses for enhancing and refining this information. Especially in the case of motor speech disorders, where speech production characteristics may pose a particular challenge to the fragile stability of perceptual judgments, such as phonetic transcription (Shriberg & Kwiatkowski, 1982), or psychophysical scaling (Schiavetti, Metz, & Sitler, 1981), instrumental analyses may be particularly attractive. Among the different types of instrumental analysis (eg, aerodynamic, electromyographic) that could be used in speech disorders, acoustic analyses can be highly recommended for the following reasons.

First, there is a well-developed body of literature on acoustic characteristics of normal speech production (see summaries in Baken, 1987; Kent & Read, 1992; Klatt, 1987) and a growing literature concerning acoustic characteristics in various speech disorders, including those resulting from neurologic disease (see summaries in Kent, Weismer, Kent, & Rosenbek, 1989; Weismer & Martin, 1992; Weismer, in press). Second, the acoustic output of the vocal tract can be thought of as a bridge between speech production and perception and so is uniquely able to shed light on both the mechanism problems associated with disordered speech and the effect of those problems on speech intelligibility.

Third, the acoustic output of the vocal tract contains the product of the entire speech system's effort, rather than an isolated component of that effort. To the extent that a speech disorder is defined by its anomalous communication product, acoustic analysis may therefore prove to be valuable. Fourth, acoustic analysis is completely noninvasive, and last, computer-based analyses of speech acoustics have become highly sophisticated, accessible, and relatively cheap. Acoustic analysis of speech is therefore within the reach of many clinicians for diagnostic, data-keeping, and research purposes.

Exactly what can one expect to get from an acoustic analysis of a patient's speech? Information is available in the acoustic signal concerning such factors as speaking rate, articulatory configuration for vowels and consonants, rates of change in the overall configuration of the vocal tract, flexibility of articulatory behavior, and aspects of phonatory behavior. The measurements made to draw inferences about articulatory and phonatory behavior often reveal a pattern that partially explains why a speaker is unintelligible and how speech therapy may focus on a particular aspect of speech production to improve intelligibility. As with any instrumental analysis of speech production, a certain amount of training and sophistication are required to select the appropriate analyses for a given problem and to interpret the resulting data. The purpose of this chapter is to provide examples of the kinds of information one can obtain from acoustic analysis of selected motor speech disorders and to indicate the kinds of expertise required for gathering such information. We will begin by detailing procedures for acoustic analysis, as well as providing values of various acoustic parameters for normal speakers. Application of these acoustic measures to the study of motor speech disorders and the supplementation of perceptual data will then be discussed.

Acoustic Representations of Speech

There are a variety of ways that an acoustic signal can be displayed and, when it comes to the speech signal, the format of the display will impact the types of measures that can be made. In an attempt to quantify aspects of the speech signal, measures of temporal and spectral characteristics often are undertaken. Temporal characteristics reflect the duration of selected events, whereas spectral characteristics show how sound energy is distributed across frequency (ie, the pattern of resonances for a given sound). The precise nature of these temporal and spectral measures will vary with the utterance produced. Factors that influence the choice of acoustic measures include manner of production and voicing for consonants, as well as source characteristics and nasalization. This section will outline different types of acoustic displays, as well as measurement procedures and techniques used in the analysis of speech. These technical issues will be followed by a discussion of acoustic measures that relate to some well-known perceptual descriptions of motor speech disorders.

Segmentation and Measurement of the Speech Wave

The speech wave is a complex, time-varying signal from which temporal "pieces" must be selected for analysis. The selection of these pieces can be made from waveform displays, which show sound energy amplitude as a function of time (Fig. 4–1, top), and from spectrograms, which are three-dimensional displays of frequency, time, and relative amplitude (Fig. 4–1, bottom). The speech signal, such as that displayed in Figure 4–1, can be

segmented to identify measurement intervals that are relevant to the structure of the utterance. Boundaries between sentences, phrases, syllables, phonemes, and so forth must be determined before temporal measurements of specific intervals can be made. Because of the interaction of speech segments due to coarticulation, boundary identification is in some cases a difficult task. Operational definitions of the onset and offset of events must be provided, and consistent application of these definitions must be maintained throughout the analysis.

Specific criteria for segmenting the speech wave will be discussed in the context of measures that are relevant to motor speech disorders. Here we can note that the most common purposes for segmenting the speech wave are (1) to isolate segment durations, or pieces of the signal corresponding to durations of specific sounds, such as vowels, and consonants (see the segmentation in Fig. 4–1), and (2) to select a temporal "win-

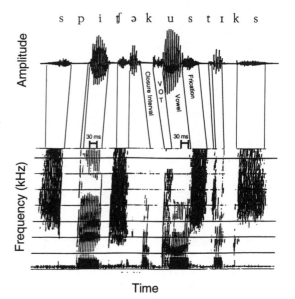

Figure 4–1. Waveform (top) and spectrogram (bottom) of the utterance "speech acoustics." Note the segmentation of the utterance into consonantal and vocalic elements and the correspondence between these segments on the waveform and spectrogram. Note the 30-msec window in the center of the vowel /i/ used for spectral analysis of formant frequencies.

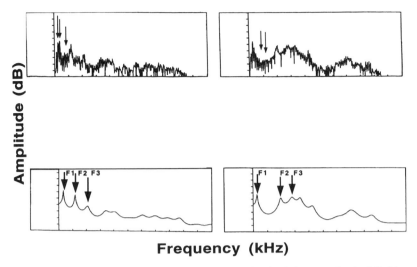

Figure 4–2. Fast Fourier Transform (FFT) displays (top) of the vowels /u/ (left) and /i/ (right). Each small peak in this display corresponds to a harmonic of the fundamental frequency associated with vocal fold vibration. The Linear Predictive Coded (LPC) spectra for the vowels /u/ and /i/ presented in the lower portion of the figure display the formant frequency peaks more clearly than can be seen in the FFT spectra, but do not provide information about the fundamental frequency.

dow" for spectral analysis. Segment durations have been studied extensively because they are thought to reflect principles of speech timing. Table 4–1 summarizes some of the factors that have an effect on segment durations. The acoustic evaluation of speech sound durations must take into account the relative nature of these measurements, because the durations depend on so many factors. Thus, when comparing speech segment durations from a clinical speech acoustic evaluation of a given patient to values found in the literature (either for neurologically normal or impaired speakers), care must be taken to ensure the equivalence of factors such as segment identity, stress, phonetic context, dialect group, and so forth (see Table 4–1). Summaries of segment duration data for normal speakers can be found in Crystal and House (1988a,b,c), Umeda (1975, 1977), and Kent and Read (1992). Issues concerning speaking rate characteristics in normal populations are discussed by Crystal and House (1982) and by Miller, Grosjean, and Lomanto (1982).

Spectral measures have also been studied extensively, because they can be related to vocal tract configurations, and by inference, articulatory positions, and movements. In general, spectral measures that are used to describe a given sound class (eg, vowels) are based on a rather small temporal window (30–50 msec). Because the resonances of the vocal tract are constantly changing, as a result of constantly varying articulatory move-

Table 4–1. Factors that influence segment durations and vowel formant frequencies. Factors marked with an asterisk (*) influence segment durations, and factors marked with a pound sign (#) influence formant frequencies.

*	Speaking rate
*	Phonetic Context
*	Position in utterance (eg, at end vs beginning of utterance)
*	Stress
*	Inherent characteristics (eg, vowel tongue height, advancement, lip rounding [#], consonant voicing [*])
*	Type of speech material (eg, isolated words vs connected speech, casual vs formal speech styles)
*	Idiosyncratic speaker characteristics (eg, dialect, age, gender, vocal tract length)

ments, a larger temporal window for spectral analysis might include too many varying acoustic features and thus "smear" the analysis. In many cases, however, the time-varying vocal tract resonances are the critical features of interest, and analysis of formant transitions (ie, changes in formant frequencies over time) is required. This is discussed in greater detail, below.

Fant (1960), in his classic work, showed that changes in vocal tract configuration have predictable influences on the acoustic output. Although strictly unique relations between vocal tract shape and acoustic output cannot be defined, general principles can be applied. For example, in the case of vowels (1) advancement of the tongue from a posterior to anterior location within the vocal tract results in an increase of the second formant (F2) frequency and a decrease of first formant (F1) frequency (Fant, 1960; Stevens & House, 1955, 1963); (2) lowering of the tongue from high (eg, /i/) to low (eg, /ae/) positions within the vocal tract increases the F1 frequency; and (3) elongation of the vocal tract by lip protrusion or larynx lowering tends to result in a decrease of all formant frequencies. The relationships between articulatory configuration and spectral characteristics are somewhat more complicated for consonants, but in general it can be stated that the pattern of resonances, or formants, associated with a stop, fricative, or affricate production is lawfully related to the size of the vocal tract cavity in front of the major constriction. For example, the spectrum of the stop burst for /t/ has a higher frequency representation than the spectrum for /k/, because of the smaller front cavity in /t/ articulation.

Because of these types of relationships, information about the spectral characteristics of speech can be extremely useful in the investigation of normal and disordered production. That is, insight about the articulatory bases of perceived speech abnormalities can be obtained by analysis of the spectral characteristics of the speech signal. The types of analyses that can be made and the information that they provide

will be reviewed in this and following sections.

A few limitations to interpretations of speech spectra need to be emphasized. First, comparisons of spectra across subjects need to be made with care. Differences in vocal tract size as well as relative sizes of the cavities comprising the vocal tract will result in changes in the speech spectrum. Because information about the physical dimensions of the vocal tract is difficult if not impossible to obtain directly, comparison between individual speakers needs to be made cautiously. Second, as in the case of segment durations, variations in the speech material will impact the spectra, so comparisons between speakers must be made using the same sample. Last, within speaker variation can be quite large so frequent repetition of the material is required to obtain a reasonable estimate of speaker characteristics (see Table 4–1).

Techniques for spectral analysis include computer-based Fourier and Linear Predictive analysis as well as spectrography. Fourier analysis, usually performed digitally by means of a Fast Fourier Transform (FFT), is based on the theorem that complex periodic waveforms can be decomposed into a series of sinusoidal components of certain amplitude and phase. Each sinusoidal component derived from the analysis of a complex periodic waveform is an integer multiple of a fundamental frequency, defined as the lowest common frequency in the complex. Fourier's theorem permits the transformation of a signal with amplitude that varies in time (ie, a waveform) into an spectrum in which the amplitude of each component frequency is represented. The importance of this theorem for speech analysis is that it provides a technique for extraction of the fundamental frequency and its associated harmonics, related to vocal fold vibration, as well as an approximation of the vocal tract resonances. As seen in the top of Figure 4–2, the many small peaks in the /u/ (left) and /i/ (right) vowel spectra represent the harmonics of the fundamental frequency. However, some peaks have higher amplitude than others because they are near a vocal tract resonance which acts to further amplify those frequencies. The regions of the awectrum where a group of harmonics is of relatively great amplitude, forming a coarser-grained spectral peak, are the formants.

Vocal tract resonances, that is, formant frequencies, can be measured more easily from Linear Predictive Coding (LPC) of the waveform, as seen in the lower part of Figure 4–2. Note that the peaks in the LPC spectra (arrows) match the peaks in the FFT spectra fairly well. LPC (Makhoul, 1975) is a procedure that derives a series of coefficients that describe the time-varying waveform. These coefficients, if properly calculated, correspond to the formant frequencies. CSpeech (Milenkovic, 1992), the computer program used to make these measurements, generates the LPC and Fourier spectra in fractions of a second using a few key strokes. A cursor can be placed on a peak in the spectrum and the value at that point—that is, the formant value—is reported on screen. Thus, the measurement of formant frequencies is simple and straightforward. Advantages of this procedure include the relative ease in estimating formant frequencies from the spectrum as well as the utility of the procedure with aperiodic signals. Because LPC can be applied to aperiodic signals, resonances associated with obstruent consonants can be derived. However, there are some disadvantages of the procedure. Primary among these is that LPC analysis is based on the assumption that there are no side-branch resonators in the vocal tract; that is, only resonant frequencies are assumed with no provision for antiresonances or zeroes in the signal. Antiresonances, most commonly associated with nasal coupling in speech, interact with resonances to affect the spectral output. When antiresonances are introduced, which may occur commonly in motorically impaired speakers, errors may be made in LPC estimates of formant frequency and bandwidth. A second limiting assumption of LPC analysis is that the vocal tract is modeled on the male speaker with a voiced source. In conventional LPC analysis, it is

assumed that the source is a series of pitch pulses, each of which decays in the vocal tract prior to the next series of pitch pulses. Any deviation from this assumption results in an interaction between the source and vocal tract which yields systematic errors of formant frequency and bandwidth. Although the LPC technique is powerful, easy to use, and informative, knowledge of its limitations, particularly for disordered speakers, is important.

Formant frequencies for vowels have been studied extensively (see summaries in Hillenbrand & Gayvert, 1993; Kent & Read, 1992) and, as summarized in Table 4–1, many factors can affect these measures. The same caution about comparing vowel durations from clinical settings to previously published data applies, therefore, to formant frequencies as well. Figure 4–3 shows an F1–F2 plot of the vowels of American English for men, women, and children. These formant measurements were obtained in the classical way (Peterson & Barney, 1952), using a narrow temporal window centered in the middle of the vowels, as displayed on spectrograms. Note that the first and second formant frequencies for these vowels are consistent with the rules relating vocal tract configuration and vocal tract output, stated above, and help to categorize vowels on the basis of

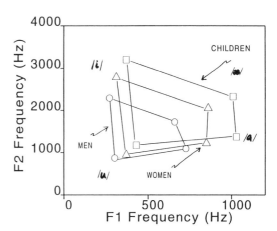

Figure 4–3. Vowel quadrilaterals for men (circles), women (triangles), and children (squares) from data reported by Peterson and Barney (1952).

formant frequencies. For example, the low F1 and high F2 of the high front vowel /i/ follows from the rules stating that (1) moving the tongue forward raises F2 and lowers F1, and (2) raising the tongue lowers F1. The reader may want to test the logic of these rules on the other vowels plotted in Figure 4–3 to prove the general utility of inferring vocal tract configurations from vowel formant frequencies.

As illustrated in Figure 4–4, consonant spectra are typically multipeaked with energy spread widely throughout the frequency range. Figure 4–4 shows a spectrum for a 20-msec window at the onset of the affricate /tʃ/ in "speech" (top), and a spectrum for the same-size window at the onset of the /k/ in "acoustics" (bottom). The peaks in consonant spectra are unlike the prominent, stable peaks in vowel spectra (see Fig. 4–2). The lack of stability of peaks in consonant spectra makes it difficult to quan-

tify the acoustic characteristics via a small group of formants (eg, the frequencies of the three most intense peaks in the spectrum), as was discussed above for vowels. The spectral shape of consonants depends on the overall distribution of energy across the frequency range of interest, rather than a few selected peaks. Description of acoustic characteristics of consonants, therefore, must include information about the shape of the spectrum, in addition to frequency. Quantification of spectral shape not only avoids the problem of finding stable peaks in the spectrum, but also seems to reflect the perceptual processing of consonant spectra (Tomiak, 1990). As in the case of vowels, spectral analysis for consonants requires the selection of some temporal window for the analysis; the actual size of this window may vary from 20 to 100 msec, depending on the type of sound and purpose of the analysis. Additional details of spectral measurement strategies for consonants are provided below, in the discussion of the acoustic correlates of "imprecise consonants." The spectral characteristics of English consonants have been reviewed by Forrest, Weismer, Milenkovic, and Dougall (1988), Kent and Read (1992), and Olive, Greenwood, and Coleman (1994).

Acoustic Analysis in Motor Speech Disorders

The classical departure point for understanding the speech production deficit in motor speech disorders is the Mayo classification system (Darley, Aronson, & Brown, 1969a,b; 1975). Darley et al listened to tape recordings of the "Grandfather Passage" read by patients with a variety of known neurological diseases, and generated psychophysical scalings of 38 selected dimensions of disordered speech (see Darley et al, 1975, pp 289-293). These perceptual dimensions were then combined in various ways to produce apparently unique clusters of dimensions for the different dysarthria types. Here we will introduce some general concepts of speech acoustic analysis in motor speech disorders by describing the likely acoustic correlates of

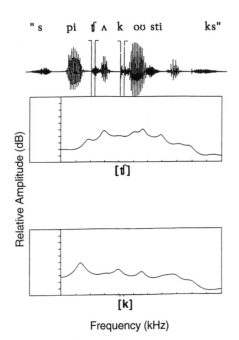

Figure 4–4. LPC spectra computed during the affricate /t/ (top) from the word "speech" and the stop /k/ (bottom) from the word "acoustics." Waveforms above each spectrum denote the segment that was included in the LPC analysis. Note the diffusion of peaks in the spectra for consonants.

some of the perceptual dimensions used in the Mayo system. We do not mean to suggest that the exemplar analyses described here are specific to the selected types of motor speech disorders; indeed, most of these analyses can be applied to any type of speech disorder.

Selected Perceptual Dimensions and Their Acoustic Correlates

Although the Mayo studies made use of 38 perceptual dimensions, a more limited set seemed to figure prominently in the descriptions of several different types of motor speech disorders. Some of these perceptual dimensions, along with their corresponding acoustic characteristics or measures, are listed in Table 4–2 and discussed below.

Distorted Vowels

Although the common view of speech intelligibility is that most of the "information-bearing" elements of speech are to be found in the consonants, there is accumulating evidence that vowel characteristics contribute

Table 4–2. Prominent perceptual dimensions from the Mayo studies (Darley et al, 1969a,b; 1975) and the likely acoustic correlates of these dimensions.

Perceptual dimension	Acoustic correlates
Distorted vowels	Vowel durations
	Formant frequencies
	Formant transitions
Imprecise consonants	Consonant durations
	Consonant spectra
	Formant transitions
Hypernasality	Low F1 frequency
	Low-intensity formants
	Spectral zeros
Monopitch	Flat f0 contour
Monoloudness	Flat SPL contour
Harsh voice	Jitter
	Decrease signal-to-noise ratio
Stress abnormalities	Limited f0 range
	Vowel duration
	Consonant duration

heavily to speech intelligibility deficits (Kent, Kent, Weismer, Sufit, Brooks, & Rosenbek, 1989; Ziegler & von Cramon, 1986). This contribution was probably reflected in the Mayo studies of dysarthria, where the perceptual dimension "distorted vowels" was a prominent component of several different dysarthrias. Acoustic measures relating to perception of distorted vowels include, but are not necessarily limited to, vowels durations, vowel formant frequencies, and characteristics of formant transitions.

Vowel Durations

Measures of vowel durations are fairly straightforward, especially when the vowels are located between obstruent consonants. In Figure 4–1 there are four vowel segments indicated. Note that the initial and final, "full" glottal pulses of the formant pattern are used to denote the vocalic's onset and offset, respectively. A full glottal pulse is one that shows energy at least through the first two formants, indicating that the vocal tract was still open at this point in time; this contrasts with the glottal pulses seen during the closure intervals of voiced stops and fricatives, which tend to have very low amplitude in waveform displays, and show energy only along the baseline in spectrograms.

Vowel durations are quite variable during speech production, ranging anywhere from about 40 to 300 msec for normal speakers. The variation in vowel duration is due to factors such as stress, vowel identity, speaking rate, dialect, and phonetic context, among others (see Crystal & House, 1988a–c, for a complete review). In speakers with neurological disease, variation in vowel duration is often greater than that observed in normal speakers. In addition, the contribution of abnormal vowel durations to the perception of distorted vowels may actually involve relational attributes of several vowels, rather than absolute durational characteristics of single vowels. In connected English, vowel durations are conditioned in large part by the stress patterns of the language and therefore tend to alternate between relatively long and short intervals.

When successive vowels in an utterance deviate from this pattern and have roughly equalized durations (see Kent, Netsell, & Abbs, 1979), the intended short (unstressed) vowel may sound distorted in relation to the sequence in which it is embedded. The Mayo dimension "equal and excess stress" partly reflects this loss of vowel duration contrast. For example, in Figure 4–5 note the variability of the vowel durations for /I/, /ə/, and /a/ (from " . . . is in the pot") produced by a normal speaker (top), but the greater similarity of these vowel durations in produced by a speaker with cerebellar disease (middle; note

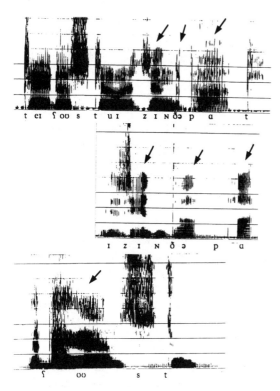

Figure 4–5. Spectrograms of portions of the utterance, "The potato stew is in the pot" spoken by a neurologically normal adult (top), a speaker with cerebellar disease (middle), and a person with spastic dysarthria (bottom). Note how these different speakers control vowel duration, with the normal speaker varying duration depending on the importance of the target word. By comparison, the speaker with cerebellar disease has similar durations for all vowels, whereas the spastic dysarthric prolongs the vocalic elements.

especially the long schwa in "the"). Finally, vowel duration measures can obviously serve as an index of the perceptual dimensions "slow rate" and "prolonged intervals," as shown in the bottom spectrogram of Figure 4–5, where the production of a spastic dysarthric individual's /oU/ and /s/ durations can be compared to the normal durations in the top spectrogram.

Formant Frequencies and Transitions
Vowel spectra can be used to make inferences about the vocal tract configuration. There are a rich tradition of measuring the formant frequencies of vowels as an index of vocal tract shape at a given instant in time (Peterson & Barney, 1952; summary in Kent & Read, 1992) and a more recent focus of using formant transitions (ie, the change in formant frequencies over time) to understand dynamic articulatory behavior. The interpretation of the formant frequencies should follow from the rules discussed above.

Figure 4–6 shows F1–F2 plots (see Fig. 4–3) for the corner vowels (/i/, /u/, /a/, /ae/) produced by five neurologically normal speakers (top) and five patients with amyotrophic lateral sclerosis (ALS; bottom). The plotted values are means based on five repetitions for each speaker. Note the "compression" of the vowel space in the /i/ and /u/ regions for three of the speakers with ALS, and the apparent expansion of the vowel space in the /a/ region for three of the patients (compare to the plot for normal speakers). One possible articulatory interpretation of these data is that some of these patients have restricted anteroposterior movements of the tongue (hence the compressed F1–F2 plot, especially along the F2 axis) and excessive opening of the jaw for low vowels (inferred from the very high F1 values for /a/). The excessive opening of the jaw could be a compensation for the poor tongue control that appears to be a prominent feature in ALS (Depaul & Brooks, 1993). Taken together, these acoustic characteristics are likely to explain some components of distorted vowels in these patients, and could serve as a basis for evaluation of treatment

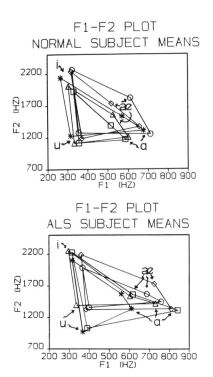

Figure 4–6. Vowel quadrilaterals from five neurologically normal speakers (top) and five speakers with ALS (bottom). Each speaker within a group is represented by a different symbol. Note the compression of the F2 range for some of the ALS speakers, as evidenced by decreased spacing of F2 for /i/ and /u/.

effects or of change in speech production deficits due to disease progression.

On the spectrogram shown in Figure 4–7, the formant trajectories (formant frequencies as a function of time) are traced by white lines for F1, F2, and F3 throughout the vowel nucleus. These trajectories are composed of the formant frequencies at consecutive instants in time projected throughout the duration of the vowel. Formant trajectories provide information on the changing configuration of the vocal tract, rather than the single "position" measurement associated with a set of formant frequencies at one point in time. The trajectories for different formants may change by different amounts and at different times, and parts of any one trajectory may change dramatically over some interval and then remain at the same frequency

for some subsequent interval. The parts of any trajectory associated with large frequency change, reflecting relatively large changes in vocal tract configuration, are often referred to as transitions.

Figure 4–8 shows schematic F1 and F2 formant trajectories for the diphthong /aI/, together with measurements derived from the transitional segment. The transition extent (TE) is the range of frequencies covered by a transition and reflects the relative amount of change in vocal tract configuration; larger TEs are associated with greater amounts of change in vocal tract configuration. The transition duration (TD) is the time taken to complete the transitional segment. Both TE and TD depend on an operational definition of the onset and offset of a formant transition, which is discussed in greater detail in Weismer, Kent, Martin, and Hodge (1988), Weismer, Martin, Kent, and Kent (1992), and Weismer and Martin (1992). When TE and TD are known, the derived measure transition rate (TR) can be computed by dividing TE by TD. This measure is an index of the slope of the formant transition, which can be interpreted in articulatory terms as the speed of change in vocal tract configuration. Small values of TE and TR, and small or large values of TD, may all be associated with the perceptual dimension of distorted vowels. The small values of TE indicate some limitation on changing vocal tract configuration for a given articulatory gesture, perhaps reflecting a failure to reach a "target" configuration for a vowel or a general restriction on the range of articulatory movements. Small values of TR reflect slow articulatory gestures, a common problem in motor speech disorders (see Weismer & Martin, 1992, Table 2, p 86). Small or large values of TD suggest abbreviated or elongated articulatory transitions, both of which are seen in various forms of motor speech disorders. Care must be taken in the interpretation of these measures, because TE, TD, and TR are not independent. For example, TE seems to depend a great deal on TD, with greater TDs resulting in greater TEs (Weismer et al, 1992). Thus the patient who has abnormally

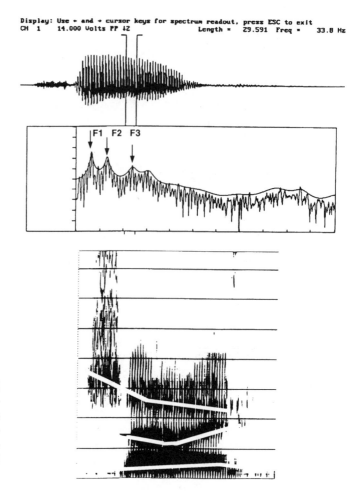

Figure 4–7. Computer-generated waveform, LPC spectrum, and spectrogram that provides easy access to acoustic analysis. Formant trajectories, the instantaneous formant frequencies, are marked with a solid white line.

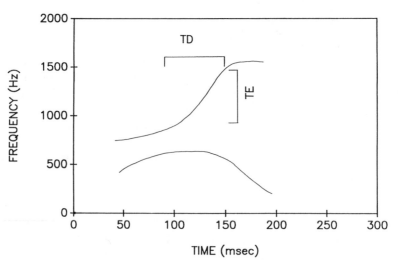

Figure 4–8. Schematic representation of first and second formants. TD = Transition duration, the time taken to complete the part of the F2 transition associated with movement in the vocal tract. TE = Transition extent, the frequency excursion of the F2 transition, a measure that corresponds to the amount change in the vocal tract shape.

long TDs may also have relatively large TEs. In this situation, the TR (TE/TD) will usually be less than normal, indicating long and extensive changes in vocal tract configuration, which are made quite slowly.

Figure 4–9 shows formant trajectories for the word "sigh" for a group of men with ALS and poor speech intelligibility, and a group of neurologically normal male speakers (Weismer et al, 1992). Note that the ALS trajectories are relatively long as compared to normal. In addition, the transitional portion of the ALS trajectories are much more shallow than the normal trajectories, especially for F2. These extended and slow formant transitions may be another component of the perceptual dimension "distorted vowels."

Imprecise Consonants

The perceptual impression of imprecise consonants is common in all types of motor

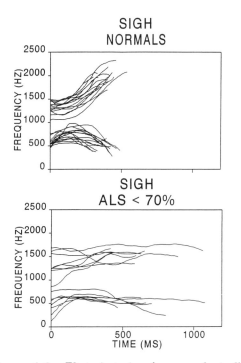

Figure 4–9. F2 trajectories for neurologically normal males (top) and male speakers with ALS (bottom). Notice the difference in the slopes and durations of the trajectories for these two groups of speakers.

speech disorders, and presumably is influenced by a range of consonant misarticulations (eg, distortions, omissions, and substitutions). We will assume for this discussion that consonant distortions contribute heavily to the impression of imprecise consonants, and consider the relevant temporal and spectral measures.

Consonant Durations

As in the case of vowel durations, the temporal measures for consonants are quite straightforward and in most cases easily obtained from either waveform or spectrographic displays (see Fig. 4–1). Typically, stop closure durations, the time during which the vocal tract is completely occluded for the buildup of intraoral air pressure, are measured from the final, full glottal pulse of the preceding vowel to the subsequent stop burst. The burst is the acoustic manifestation of the sudden release of the impounded air pressure. Stop closure durations are usually on the order of 70–120 msec and rarely exceed 150 msec (Stathopoulos & Weismer, 1985).

The commonly measured interval voice onset time (VOT) is measured from the burst to the first full glottal pulse of the following vowel. VOTs are usually in excess of 35 msec for voiceless stops, and less than 20 msec for voiced stops. The closure interval and VOT are measured in a similar way for affricates, which have VOTs greater than those observed in stops of the same voicing status. The duration of voiced and voiceless fricatives is measured from the final full glottal pulse preceding the frication energy to the first full glottal pulse following the frication.

Consonant durations in dysarthric speech are often abnormal, and may be either too long or too short. The influence of abnormal consonant durations on the perception of imprecise consonants is unknown, nor is it clear why such abnormalities would affect a percept of "precision." VOT abnormalities, especially those in a region of ambiguity (ie, between about 20 and 40 msec) could possibly be a component of imprecise consonants. The unusually long durations often seen in apraxia of speech and spastic dysarthria

(Kent & Rosenbek, 1983; Weismer, 1984) are not unexpected in a disorder where slow rate is often encountered. The very brief closure durations seen for the speaker with Parkinson's disease are likely to contribute to the impression of distorted consonants, probably because the contrasts between the consonant and adjacent vowels are "blurred" (Kent & Rosenbek, 1983; Weismer, 1984) by the brief consonant duration.

Consonant Spectra
The spectra of stop bursts and fricative noises would seem to be a valuable source of information concerning articulatory configurations for consonants. There is a fairly well developed literature concerning the normally articulated, acoustic characteristics of consonants (see reviews and data in Stevens & Blumstein, 1978; Forrest, Weismer, Milenkovic, & Dougall, 1988; Kent & Read, 1992; Olive et al, 1994), and in many cases theory relates acoustic characteristics to articulatory configuration in a fairly straightforward way (Fant, 1960). It may therefore seem surprising to encounter so few data in the literature concerning spectral analysis of consonant production in motor speech disorders.

The lack of these data can be explained by considering the measurement issues in quantifying consonant spectra. As discussed above, consonant spectra are typically multi-peaked with energy spread widely throughout the frequency range, and investigators have long felt that some index of the shape of consonant spectra was important (see above). Several investigators have used a categorical system to "measure" spectral shape, wherein spectral templates related to place of articulation are used to categorize consonant spectra (Stevens & Blumstein, 1978; Kewley-Port, 1983). Shinn and Blumstein (1983) have demonstrated the use of the Stevens and Blumstein template system in understanding stop consonant production in aphasia, but little other work has been done in this area. The application of the template system to persons with motor speech disorders is very time consuming, requiring a human observer to generate and classify the spectra on an individual basis. This is an unlikely scenario for the clinician who wishes to use spectral analysis of consonants in a work setting.

Forrest et al (1988) developed a simple quantitative, observer-free approach to the measurement of consonant spectra. The approach treats the spectrum as a statistical distribution that can be described by values for the mean, skewness, and kurtosis. The mean quantifies the central tendency of the energy in the spectrum (see also the "centroid" measure of Harmes, Daniloff, Hoffman, Lewis, Kramer, & Absher, 1984), the skewness the degree to which the spectral energy is tilted toward the low or high frequencies, and the kurtosis the degree to which the spectrum has sharp peaks or is relatively flat. These numerical indices of spectral shape can be generated very quickly with a computer program.

Figure 4–10 shows some sample spectra of stop bursts and frication noises produced by both neurologically normal and dysarthric speakers, along with the values of the mean and coefficients of skewness and kurtosis. It is known that the combination of the three values can uniquely classify place of articulation for stop consonants and some fricatives (Forrest et al, 1988), but the relationship of the values to judgments of dimensions such as "imprecise consonants" or speech intelligibility is unknown. However, initial attempts to categorize different dysarthrias on the basis of spectral moments from the onset spectra of stops, are promising (Thompson, McClean, & Summers, 1992). Values of the mean and the coefficients of skewness and kurtosis for normal speakers can be found in Molis (1992).

Hypernasality

Hypernasality is a prominent perceptual dimension in several of the disorders studied by Darley et al (1969a,b), including flaccid, spastic, and forms of mixed dysarthria, such as that seen in ALS. The underlying articulatory problem in hypernasality is a chronically open velopharyngeal port due to

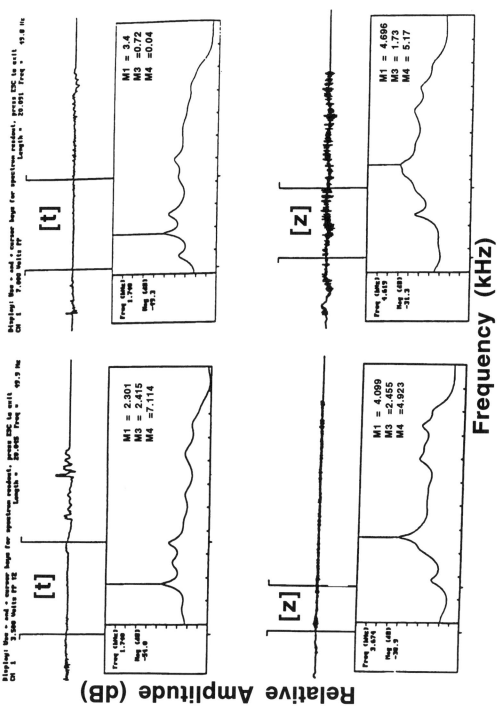

Frequency (kHz)

Relative Amplitude (dB)

Figure 4–10. Spectra and corresponding moments for neurologically normal speaker (left) and a speaker with ALS (right). The top panel presents the waveforms and spectra for /t/ in "tile," and the bottom panel shows spectra for /z/ in "ease." M1 is the first moment, or centroid, of the spectrum; M3 is the coefficient of skewness, a measure of the tilt of the spectrum; and M4 is the coefficient of kurtosis, an index that captures the "peakedness" of the spectrum.

paralysis or paresis of the relevant musculature (ie, the levator veli palatini and superior constrictor muscles of the pharynx) or inappropriately timed closure and opening of the port. The typical acoustic correlates of nasal articulation are (1) an intense, low-frequency F1 around 250–300 Hz, (2) a series of low-intensity formants roughly at 1000 Hz, 2000 Hz, 3000 Hz, and 4000 Hz, (3) regions of the spectrum showing little or no energy, and (4) a relatively low overall intensity compared to vowel intensities. When a nasal is articulated between two vowels (see arrows in Fig. 4–11 for location of nasals), as shown for the utterance (/anə manə piyə/) in the top of Figure 4–11, these features can appear quite clearly. The low-frequency F1 is a resonance of the nasal cavities and the pharynx, and the low intensity of the higher formants is a result of antiresonances and large amounts of sound energy absorption in the nasal cavities (see Kent & Read, 1992, for an explanation of antiresonances). These qualitative features are often fairly easy to spot in a spectrographic display, but it is difficult to quantify degrees of nasality using acoustic techniques. Thus the best use of waveform or spectrographic techniques to detect nasality may, at this time, take the form of qualitative observations. In certain patients with chronic hypernasality, as in selected cases of flaccid dysarthria, the presence of the acoustic markers of nasality described above can actually prevent meaningful analysis of any part of the signal. This is because the chronic presence of antiresonances and absorption of sound energy in the nasal cavities obscures vocalic formant structures and consonantal landmarks, as shown in the bottom part of Figure 4–11, where the sequence "onomanopia," has been spoken with excessive nasality. Note the very dark F1 that extends throughout the entire utterance, and the loss of the boundaries between and vowels and consonants, as compared to the spectrogram in the top of Figure 4–11.

Voice Dimensions

Various voice dimensions figured prominently in Darley et al's (1975) description of the motor speech disorders. Some of these dimensions, such as harsh voice, breathy voice, and strained-strangled voice, are perceptual impressions of voice quality. To a first approximation, voice quality can be said to be determined by the shape of the glottal spectrum and the relative amount of periodic and aperiodic energy in that spectrum. Physiologically, these two acoustic components of voice quality are likely to be interdependent, so we will discuss the acoustic measures of voice quality without differentiating their relationship to different aspects of the glottal spectrum. As we will suggest, this is one of the weaknesses of these measures. Much has been written about the influence of cycle-to-cycle variability of glottal periods on voice quality. The term "jitter" is used to describe variability occurring in time, where successive glottal periods differ from cycle to cycle. Variability in the amplitude of succes-

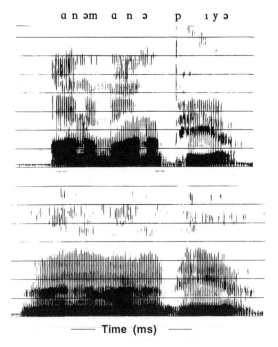

a n ə m e   a n ə   p   ı y ə

Time (ms)

Figure 4–11. Spectrograms of a normal production of the sequence /anə manə piyə/ (top) and the same utterance produced with excessive nasality (bottom). Note the ambiguity of vowel formants in the hypernasal production and the continuous low-frequency energy, typical of nasalization.

sive cycles is referred to as "shimmer." Normal voices are characterized by a certain amount of jitter and shimmer, but too much variability in the period and/or amplitude of successive glottal cycles will typically result in the perception of a "noisy" voice quality.

Figure 4–12 shows time and amplitude variation indicated on a waveform of a normal voice, and a waveform of a voice perceived to be harsh. Note that in the top waveform, there is minimal time and amplitude variation from cycle to cycle of this sustained /a/. In contrast, the waveform for the harsh /a/, shown at the bottom, clearly contains time and amplitude variation. As described in detail by Baken (1987, pp 113-119, 166-188), there are many ways to measure jitter and shimmer, and little agreement on which ways should be preferred (see also Pinto & Titze, 1990; Titze, 1991). We will not review these different approaches to making these measurements, but will note that many speech analysis programs include some form of jitter and shimmer analysis. Generally, the voice quality abnormality, as judged perceptually, will seem increasingly severe as the jitter and/or shimmer values become more

different from normal values. In this sense, the jitter and shimmer measures may serve as useful "hard copy" indices of perceptual events. A major limitation of these measures, however, is the lack of a straightforward relationship between the specific values and the underlying physiological behavior (see Titze, 1991). Thus jitter and shimmer values cannot help differentiate between, for example, a neurologically versus mechanically based problem in the larynx.

The signal-to-noise ratio, sometimes called the harmonic-to-inharmonic ratio, can also be considered as an acoustic counterpart of voice quality. This acoustic index is designed to capture the balance between periodic energy, generated by the cyclic vocal fold vibration, and aperiodic energy, resulting largely from turbulent flows generated in the vicinity of the glottis. High signal-to-noise ratios are typically associated with vocal fold vibration that involves good closure and symmetric action of the two folds; low signal-to-noise ratios will be associated with poor closure (ie, the kind of vocal fold vibration often resulting in the perception of a breathy or hoarse voice). Signal-to-noise values are likely to covary with jitter and shimmer values, so the measures may be somewhat redundant with respect to each other. Like jitter and shimmer values, signal-to-noise ratios may covary with perceptual judgments, but are difficult to interpret in terms of underlying mechanisms.

Finally, Darley et al (1975) employed several voice dimensions designed to reflect insufficient or excessive variability in the output of the larynx. Monopitch, monoloudness, and excess and equal stress are three of these dimensions, and each has acoustic counterparts. The acoustic counterpart of monopitch requires an analysis of a fundamental frequency (F0) contour of a sentence, such as the one shown in the top part of Figure 4–13, where the speech waveform and F0 contour are shown for the utterance, "A yellow lion roared." In this sentence the F0 varies by as much as 50 Hz, which is not unusual for simple declarative utterances spoken by neurologically normal individuals; this variation is shown by the up-and-

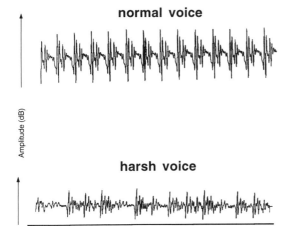

Figure 4–12. Waveform of the vowel /a/ showing the cycle-to-cycle variation found in a normal voice (top) and a voice that is perceived to be harsh (bottom). Notice the temporal and amplitude variation across cycles in the harsh voice.

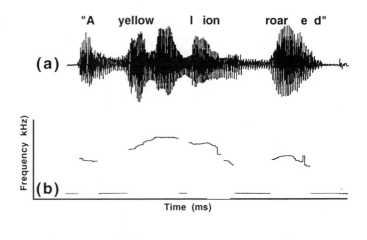

Figure 4–13. Waveforms (a) and fundamental frequency traces (b) for the sentence, "A yellow lion roared," spoken normally (top) and by a male who was perceived to speak with monopitch (bottom). The fundamental frequency traces are plotted with time on the abscissa and frequency along the ordinate.

down movement of the F0 trace in the top figure. In contrast, the relatively flat F0 contour shown in the bottom half of Figure 4–13 is the result of an aberrant production of "A yellow lion roared." The F0 contour for this speaker would almost certainly be scaled as more severe on the monopitch scale than the F0 contour for the normal speaker, but the precise relationship between features of F0 contours and the perceptual scale monopitch is unknown. Studies have shown reduced fundamental frequency range for dysarthric speakers with Parkinson's disease (King, Ramig, Lemke, & Horii, 1993) and ALS (Ramig, Scherer, Klasner, Titze, & Horii, 1990). These reductions in F0 range certainly would contribute to the "mono-" perceptions discussed above. Similarly, computer programs like CSpeech can display a sound-pressure-level trace for an utterance that should correspond at some level to the perceptual dimension "monoloudness." When either the F0 or sound-pressure level trace indicates flatness, one can interpret the underlying mechanism as lacking flexibility, but the reasons for this are not revealed by the acoustic analysis.

The perceptual dimension "excess and equal stress" has already been mentioned in the context of duration measures of vowels, but it is also relevant here because of the effect of F0 and sound pressure level on stress judgments. Stress contrasts in words or at the sentence level are typically characterized by higher F0 and sound pressure level on stressed, as compared to unstressed, syllables. A succession of syllables having roughly equivalent and extreme values of peak F0 and sound pressure levels is likely to promote the perceptual impression of equal and excess stress. The kind of acoustic analysis of sentence-level prosodic events presented here could be used to track progress associated with a naturalness training program (see Yorkston, Beukelman, & Bell, 1988).

Summary

The application of acoustic analysis as a clinical tool in motor speech disorder is a relatively new use for this powerful procedure. A combination of greater understanding of acoustic characteristics of disordered speech, paired with the call for greater explanatory power in the analysis of motor speech disorders (Kent, Weismer G, Kent JF, Rosenbek, 1989) provides motivation for the clinician to gain facility with acoustic analysis. Last, the advent of computer algorithms that are "user-friendly" and relatively inexpensive makes it likely that acoustic analysis will find increasing acceptance in the diagnosis and management of motor-speech-disordered clients.

References

Baken R. (1987). *Clinical Measurement of Speech and Voice*. Boston: Little, Brown.

Crystal TH, House AS. (1982). Segmental durations in connected-speech signals: preliminary results. *J Acoust Soc Am* 72:705–716.

Crystal TH, House AS. (1988a). Segmental durations in connected-speech signals: current results. *J Acoust Soc Am* 83:1553–1573.

Crystal TH, House AS. (1988b). Segmental durations in connected-speech signals: syllabic stress. *J Acoust Soc Am* 83:1574–1585.

Crystal TH, House AS. (1988c). The duration of American English stop consonants: an overview. *J Phonet*.

Crystal TH, House AS. (1988d). A note on the duration of fricatives in American English. *J Acoust Soc Am* 84:1932–1935.

Darley F, Aronson A, Brown J. (1969a). Differential diagnostic patterns of dysarthria. *J Speech Hear Res* 12:246–269.

Darley F, Aronson A, Brown J. (1969b). Clusters of deviant speech dimensions in the dysarthrias. *J Speech Hear Res* 12:462–496.

Darley F, Aronson A, Brown J. (1975). *Motor Speech Disorders*. Philadelphia, PA: WB Saunders.

DePaul R, Brooks BR. (1993). Multiple orofacial indices in amyotrophic lateral sclerosis. *J Speech Hear Res* 36:1158–1167.

Fant G. (1960). *Acoustic Theory of Speech Production*. The Hague: Mouton.

Forrest K, Weismer G, Milenkovic P, Dougall RN. (1988). Statistical analysis of word-initial voiceless obstruents: preliminary data. *J Acoust Soc Am* 84:115–123.

Harmes S, Daniloff R, Hoffman P, Lewis J, Kramer M, Absher R. (1984). Temporal and articulatory control of fricative articulation by speakers with Broca's aphasia. *J Phonet* 12:367–385.

Hillenbrand J, Gayvert RT. (1993). Vowel classification based on fundamental frequency and format frequencies. *J Speech Hear Res* 36:694–700

Kent RD, Read C. (1992). *The Acoustic Analysis of Speech*. San Diego: Singular Publishing Group.

Kent RD, Rosenbek JC. (1983). Acoustic patterns of apraxia of speech. *J Speech Hear Res* 26:231–249.

Kent RD, Kent JF, Weismer G, Sufit RL, Brooks BR, Rosenbek JC. (1989). Relationships between speech intelligibility and the slope of second-formant transitions in dysarthric subjects. *Clin Linguistics Phonet* 3:347–358.

Kent RD, Netsell R, Abbs JH. (1979). Acoustic characteristics of dysarthria associated with cerebellar disease. *J Speech Hear Res* 22:627–648.

Kent RD, Weismer G, Kent JF, Rosenbek JC. (1989). Toward phonetic intelligibility testing in dysarthria. *J Speech Hear Res* 54:482–499.

Kewley-Port D. (1983). Time-varying features as correlates of place of articulation in stop consonants. *J Acoust Soc Am* 73:322–335.

King JB, Ramig LO, Lemke JH, Horii Y. (1993). Parkinson's disease: longitudinal changes in acoustic parameters of phonation. *NCVS Status and Progress Report* 4:135–149.

Klatt DH. (1987). Review of text-to-speech conversion for English. *J Acoust Soc Am* 82:737–793.

Makhoul J. (1975). Linear predication: a tutorial review. *Proc IEEE* 63:561–580.

Milenkovic P. (1992). *Cspeech, Version 4*. Madison, WI.

Miller JL, Grosjean F, Lomanto C. (1984). Articulation rate and its variability in spontaneous speech: a reanalysis and some implications. *Phonetica* 41:215–225.

Molis MR. (1992). Effect of speech material manipulation on the statistical classification of stop burst spectra. Unpublished M.S. thesis, University of Wisconsin-Madison.

Olive JP, Greenwood A, Coleman JS. (1994). *Acoustics of American English Speech: A Dynamic Approach.* New York: Springer-Verlag.

Peterson GE, Barney HE. (1952). Control methods used in a study of vowels. *J Acoust Soc Am* 24:175–184.

Pinto N, Titze IR. (1990). Unification of perturbation measures in speech analysis. *J Acoust Soc Am* 87:1278–1289.

Ramig LO, Scherer RC, Klasner ER, Titze IR, Horii Y. (1990). Acoustic analysis of voice in amyotrophic lateral sclerosis: a longitudinal case study. *J Speech Hear Disord* 55:2–14.

Schiavetti N, Metz DE, Sitler RW. (1981). Construct validity of direct magnitude estimation and interval scaling of speech intelligibility: evidence from a study of the hearing impaired. *J Speech Hear Res* 24:441–445.

Shinn P, Blumstein SE. (1983). Phonetic disintegration in aphasia: acoustic analysis of spectral characteristics for place of articulation. *Brain Lang* 20:90–114.

Shriberg LD, Kwiatkowski J. (1982). Phonological disorders III: a procedure for assessing severity of involvement. *J Speech Hear Disord* 47:256–270.

Stathopoulos ET, Weismer G. (1985). Oral air flow and intraoral air pressure: a comparative study of children, youths, and adults. *Folia Phoniatric* 37:152–159.

Stevens KN, House AS. (1955). Development of a quantitative description of vowel articulation. *J Acoust Soc Am* 27:484–493.

Stevens KN, House AS. (1961). An acoustical theory of vowel production and some of its implications. *J Speech Hear Res* 4:303–320.

Stevens KN, Blumstein SE. (1978). Invariant cues for place of articulation in stop consonants. *J Acoust Soc Am* 64:1358–1368.

Thompson PF, McLean MD, Summers WV. (1992). Discriminant analysis of stop consonant spectra in dysarthria. Poster presented at the American Speech, Language, and Hearing Association Convention. San Antonio, TX.

Titze IR. (1991). A model for neurologic sources of aperiodicity. *J Speech Hear Res* 34:460–472.

Tomiak G. (1990). An acoustic and perceptual analysis of the spectral moments invariant with voiceless fricative obstruents. Unpublished Ph.D. dissertation, State University of New York, Buffalo.

Umeda N. (1977a). Vowel duration in American English. *J Acoust Soc Am* 58:434–445.

Umeda N. (1977b). Consonant duration in American English. *J Acoust Soc Am* 61:846–858.

Weismer G. (In press). Motor speech disorders. In: Hardcastle WJ, Laver J, eds. *A Handbook of Phonetic Science.* London: Blackwell.

Weismer G. (1984). Articulatory characteristics of Parkinsonian dysarthria: segmental and phase-level timing, spirantization, and glottal-supraglottal coordination. In McNeil MR, Rosenbek JC, Aronson AE. (eds). *The Dysarthrias: Physiology, Acoustics, Perception, Management.* San Diego, CA: College-Hill Press.

Weismer G, Martin R. (1992). Acoustic and perceptual approaches to the study of intelligibility. In Kent RD, ed. *Intelligibility in Speech Disorders.* Philadelphia: John Benjamins, pp 67–118.

Weismer G, Martin R, Kent RD, Kent JF. (1992). Formant trajectory characteristics of males with amyotrophic lateral sclerosis. *J Acoust Soc Am* 91:1085–1098.

Weismer G, Kent RD, Hodge M, Martin R. (1988). The acoustic signature for intelligibility test words. *J Acoust Soc Am* 84:1281–1291.

Yorkston KM, Beukelman DR, Bell KR. (1988). *Clinical Management of Dysarthric Speakers.* Austin, TX: Pro-Ed.

Ziegler W, von Cramon D. (1986). Disturbed coarticulation in apraxia of speech: acoustic evidence. *Brain Lang* 29:34–47.

Chapter *5*

Aerodynamics

Donald W. Warren, Anne Putnam Rochet,
and Virginia A. Hinton

Introduction

Events that impact upon the sensorimotor components of the central or peripheral nervous system, such as cerebral vascular accidents, closed head injuries, progressive neurological diseases, and neoplasms, often result in deficits that adversely affect speech performance. Specifically, neurological or neuromuscular damage causing paralysis, paresis, or incoordination in the bulbar or spinal sensorimotor systems can affect the range, velocity, force, or timing of speech movements as well as the respiratory processes that support speech production. Possible deficits in several areas such as respiration, phonation, articulation, and resonation present a significant challenge to clinicians responsible for the assessment and treatment of the resulting speech disorder.

Patients with sensorimotor damage may have difficulty maintaining adequate respiratory support for speech (Hixon, Putnam, & Sharpe, 1983); Hunker, Bless, & Weismer, 1981; Putnam & Hixon, 1981). Generally, this is the result of weakness in the respiratory muscles or in control of muscles that maintain subglottal pressure (Yorkston, Beukelman, & Bell, 1988). Weakness or loss of efficient control of the chest wall muscles may occur during inspiration, expiration, or both.

Laryngeal dysfunction may also occur in individuals with central or peripheral nervous system lesions. In some cases, difficulty with laryngeal control may represent the first signs of a neuromotor disease such as the bulbar form of ALS or indicate further degeneration of a previously diagnosed medical condition (Barlow, Netsel, & Hunker, 1986; Netsell & Kent, 1976; Portney, 1979; Twomey & Espir, 1980). Inappropriate timing of vocal fold closure, inconsistencies in fundamental frequency, and disorders of voice quality such as breathiness, harshness, or hoarseness may be associated with upper or lower motor neuron lesions (Yorkston et al, 1988). The presence of the perceptual characteristics may be the result of specific damage to the processes responsible for the fine motor control of the larynx. However, they may also represent inappropriate interactions between the laryngeal and respiratory systems. The ability to determine the nature of the underlying sensorimotor deficit is crucial for developing an optimal treatment plan for these patients.

Another functional component of speech production frequently impaired by neuromotor disease processes is the mechanism of velopharyngeal closure. Researchers and clinicians have reported the presence of velopharyngeal dysfunction (as indicated by hypernasality and nasal emission) in patients with a variety of nervous system disorders that may be congenital (Barlow & Abbs, 1984; Hardy, 1983; Yorkston, Beukelman, & Honsinger, 1989), acquired but nonprogressive (Aten, McDonald, & Simpson, 1984; Kent & Rosenbeck, 1982; LaVelle & Hardy, 1979), or degenerative (Dworkin & Hartman, 1979; Hoodin & Gilbert, 1989; Ludlow & Bassitch, 1983). Velopharyngeal dysfunction in patients with sensorimotor disorders appears related to reduced velar movement during speech, as well as inappropriate timing of the movement of the velum relative to other structures (Gracco & Muller, 1981; Netsell, 1969; Yorkston et al, 1989). Velopharyngeal dysfunction can range from inconsistent borderline closure to gross inadequacy, and may result in the inability to generate adequate intraoral pressures necessary for obstruent consonant production, as well as problems with oral-nasal resonance balance.

The respiratory, phonatory, and velopharyngeal components of speech production are often dealt with separately when describing the physiologic deficits of patients with CNS lesions (Abbs, Hunker, & Barlow, 1983). However, in reality, these systems interact constantly to produce perceptually adequate speech. For example, maintenance of intraoral air pressure during consonant production requires a constant subglottal pressure, adequate velopharyngeal closure, and sufficient bilabial or lingual-palatal obstruction. Deficits in any of these areas may yield reduced intraoral pressure and serve to decrease overall speech intelligibility. Therefore, clinical assessment and treatment of patients with sensorimotor impairments should include procedures that deal with the integration and coordination of these complex systems.

As noted above and from other sources (Berry, 1983; McNeil, Rosenbeck, & Aronson, 1984; Putnam, 1988; Yorkston et al, 1988), a fairly extensive body of literature has been reported describing the effects of nervous system lesions on the physiologic components of speech. The literature contains some important references to the use of intraoral air pressure and nasal airflow recordings in biofeedback tasks (Netsell & Daniel, 1979; Netsell & Hixon, 1978; Rubow, 1984), and to the use of aerodynamic techniques for the purpose of assessing the progress of surgical or prosthodontic management of velopharyngeal inadequacy (Dworkin & Johns, 1980; Shaughnessy, Netsell, & Farrage, 1983).

More accurate descriptions of the underlying sensorimotor disorder, as well as more quantifiable information concerning the nature of the speech production deficits, are possible with the technology available today (Abbs et al, 1983; Barlow & Abbs, 1984; Moore & Scudder, 1989; Netsell, Lotz, & Barlow, 1989; Weismer, 1989). However, despite their availability, the use of multipurpose instruments for assessment and management of individuals with these speech disorders has been limited (Till & Alp, 1991).

The purpose of this chapter is to describe how aerodynamic techniques can be used for evaluating patients with sensorimotor impairments. Specifically, the use of such procedures should allow clinicians to describe more accurately the nature of a patient's speech production deficits (Dworkin & Johns, 1980; Murry, 1983). Furthermore, these techniques and procedures may be useful in developing new treatment approaches that focus on demonstrating quantifiable changes in physiologic responses rather than judgments of speech performance alone.

Three approaches for assessment of sensorimotor deficits will be described in this chapter. The first involves aerodynamic assessment techniques that are used routinely in evaluation of patients with structural deficits such as velopharyngeal impairment. This approach measures a patient's ability to perform certain activities that are essential for the proper production of consonant sounds: (1) the ability to separate the nose from the mouth during velopharyngeal closure; (2) the ability to bring the tongue, alveolar ridge, and teeth into correct approximation for frication; and (3) the ability to adduct the vocal folds for voicing. The second approach assesses motor activity in terms of the ability of structures to perform tasks within periods of time associated with normal speech motor activities. An example would be how long it takes to effect velopharyngeal closure. The third approach, which is still in the early stage of development in our laboratory, deals with assessment of the sensory side of sensorimotor performance. This is an area that has been essentially neglected except for evaluation of two-point discrimination, assessments of touch recognition, and stereognostic testing (Essick, 1992).

The techniques dealing with sensory evaluation that are described in this chapter represent new methodologies that have not been reported previously. Our experience with normal subjects indicates that aerodynamic sensory testing should be useful in quantifying sensory deficits. However, it should be noted that the authors are just now utilizing this approach in subjects with sensorimotor disorders, and the information provided in this chapter is admittedly anecdotal. Hopefully, the introduction of aerodynamic sensory testing procedures will stimulate others to utilize this approach and ultimately determine its value for this particular group of patients.

Assessing Aerodynamic Performance

During the past decade, the development of instruments capable of measuring aerodynamic variables associated with speech has led to improved, more objective methods for assessing the performance of phonatory structures. These tools range from simple sensing devices to elaborate combinations of pressure transducers and airflow meters (Warren, 1976). While the former are only capable of gross determinations of function, the latter provide acceptable estimates of the performance of discrete activities.

In the past, clinicians have used a number of devices to provide a gross indication of such variables as nasal emission of air, which reflects, to some extent, palatal function. In most instances, the measurements obtained with simple devices related more to respiratory effort than to palatal function. Also, response times were extremely slow, and errors in measurement often occurred. In addition, these measurements were usually made during nonspeech activities such as blowing.

The deficiencies associated with simple manometric instruments led to the development of more elaborate tools for objective evaluation of the structures involved in speech. The basic components of these aerodynamic measuring systems are pressure transducers which record airway pressures within the vocal tract and flowmeters which record volume rates of airflow.

Air Pressure Devices

The pressure transducers currently in use are either variable resistance, variable capacitance, or variable inductance gauges. Resistance wire strain gauges respond to changes in pressure with a change in resistance when the strain-sensitive wire is exposed to stretch. Compression of bellows within the chamber results in a resistance imbalance in a Wheatstone bridge that is proportional to the applied pressure. The resulting output voltage from the bridge is amplified and recorded.

The electrical capacitance transducer is a condenser formed by an electrode separated from a stiff metal membrane by a carefully adjusted air gap. Movements of the membrane in relation to the electrode vary the capacitance, which can be measured by a radio frequency circuit. Membrane displacement is extremely small, and the frequency response is therefore excellent. However, this device is more temperature-sensitive than the strain-gauge manometer. The capacitance-type pressure transducer is distinguishable from other types by its exceptional accuracy, high level outputs, and built-in signal conditioning. Typically, these transducers do not require additional signal conditioning.

The variable inductance pressure gauge utilizes a soft iron slug placed within two coils of wire and fastened to the center of an elastic membrane. Pressure moves the iron slug, and this movement results in a change in magnetic flux. The change in inductance of the coils is then recorded through an appropriate bridge circuit. The advantage of this type of transducer is that it can be made so small that it can be placed directly on the site to be measured.

It is common practice to amplify the signal

from transducers, and usually a carrier-wave amplifier is used. An oscillator supplies an alternating current, and the amplitude is continuously affected by the varying resistance. The output of the transducer enters the capacitance-coupled amplifier, which amplifies the modulated carrier wave. The signals are then rectified, and the carrier wave is filtered out, leaving a DC voltage which powers the recording instrument.

Pressure Measurements

Pressure devices have been used in a variety of ways to measure the aerodynamics of speech production. Usually, measurements are made of oral pressures, nasal pressures, or both. Intraoral pressure can be recorded by placing a catheter in the mouth and attaching it to a pressure transducer and recorder. Pressures in the oral cavity vary from 3 to 8 cm H_2O for nonnasal consonants in normal conversational speech. Voiceless consonants usually are produced with pressures about 20% higher than their voiced cognates (Warren, 1964; Warren & Hall, 1973). This may relate to the need for greater aerodynamic energy for voiceless sounds since there is no accompanying acoustic energy from the vocal folds. Additionally, there is a difference in energy loss across the glottis between the two consonant types (Warren & Hall, 1973).

Consonantal intraoral pressures generally remain above 3.0 cm H_2O even in individuals with impaired palatal function (Warren, 1986). Table 5–1 lists mean intraoral pressures according to degree of velopharyngeal closure for the plosive /p/ in the word

"hamper." A number of factors are involved in maintaining intraoral pressures above 3.0 cm H_2O. Perhaps the most important factor is that the nasal airway provides approximately two-thirds of the total resistance of the respiratory system. Approximately 60–70% of intraoral pressure can be maintained by nasal airway resistance alone even in the presence of velopharyngeal impairment. Since intraoral pressures are usually maintained at levels above 3 cm H_2O, regardless of the degree of palatal dysfunction, it should be obvious that measurements of intraoral pressures alone do not provide an accurate estimate of palatal function.

Nasal pressures have also been used as an index of velopharyngeal function (Hess & McDonald, 1960). This has usually involved the placement of a nasal olive against the more patent nostril while having the subject produce nonnasal consonants within test sounds or phrases. This approach will provide a gross estimate of impairment since nasal pressure should be negligible or zero for adequate closure and in the 1–6 cm H_2O range for inadequacy.

If only pressure measurements are to be made, a more valid approach to screening palatal function involves measuring oral and nasal pressure simultaneously. Warren (1979) described a technique that measures the pressure difference across the velopharyngeal port for rating palatal competency. Closure of the velopharyngeal orifice creates a pressure difference between the nose and mouth. When complete closure occurs, as during production of the consonant /p/, pressure in the mouth is determined by respiratory effort and will vary

Table 5–1. Intraoral pressures and standard deviations according to competency of velopharyngeal closure.

	Adequate	Adequate/ Borderline	Borderline/ Inadequate	Inadequate
AREA	0–.049 cm²	.05–.099 cm²	.10–.19 cm²	>.2 cm²
	6.4 cm H_2O	5.0 cm H_2O	4.3 cm H_2O	3.7 cm H_2O
PRESSURE	±2.2	±1.9	±1.8	±1.9

from about 3 cm H_2O to 8 cm H_2O (Warren, 1964, 1976). Pressure in the nose will be atmospheric or zero since no air leaks into the nasal chamber. However, if there is a velopharyngeal opening, the difference in pressure will vary with the size of the opening. Since a difference in oral and nasal pressures is used, the effect of respiratory effort is canceled out when the velopharyngeal mechanism is not completely closed.

When using differential pressures as an index of velopharyngeal closure, the speech sample should include voiceless plosive consonants in such contexts as "papa" and "hamper." The voiceless plosive /p/ is used because this sound provides an aerodynamic state which varies directly with the degree of velopharyngeal closure. The /p/ is produced by closing the lips and velopharyngeal orifice and stopping airflow for a period of time. If closure is complete at the lips and velopharynx, the pressure measured is equal to intraoral pressure. Any opening results in airflow into the nose which reduces the pressure difference between the nose and mouth. The result is a lower differential pressure. Also, when airflow is stopped in the oral cavity, placement of the tongue does not affect pressure within the stagnant air column. Improper tongue placement is therefore eliminated as a potential problem. This is not true for other sounds. For example, fricative sounds are produced with oral airflow. If tongue-palatal contacts occur, an additional pressure drop would result. This could result in spurious values. Voiced sounds are not preferred because they often have lower, more inconsistent pressure patterns (Warren, 1979).

The nasal-plosive combination, as in the word "hamper," is often used because it stresses the palatal mechanism. Pressure-flow studies have demonstrated that some individuals can close the velopharyngeal port adequately for plosives in nonnasal contexts but cannot do so when the sounds are adjacent to nasal consonants (Warren, 1979). Individuals who have such difficulties tend to experience velopharyngeal inadequacy during continuous speech. Therefore, the nasal-plosive combination is used as a test of velopharyngeal closure ability during ongoing speech. Based upon studies of more than 500 patients with palatal dysfunction, we have found that velopharyngeal closure is usually adequate when differential pressure is greater than 3 cm H_2O. When differential pressure is between 1 and 2.9 cm H_2O, closure is usually borderline. When differential pressure is below 1 cm H_2O, velopharyngeal closure is always inadequate for normal speech.

Airflow Devices

The most accepted airflow device is the heated pneumotachograph which consists of a flowmeter and a differential pressure transducer (Lubker, 1970). This device utilizes the principle that as air flows across a resistance, the pressure drop that results is linearly related to the volume rate of airflow. In most cases, the resistance is a wire mesh screen that is heated to prevent condensation. A pressure tap is situated on each side of the screen, and both are connected to a very sensitive differential pressure transducer. The pressure drop is converted to an electrical voltage that is amplified and recorded. Pneumotachographs are valid, reliable, linear devices for measuring ingressive and egressive airflow rates. In addition, they are easily calibrated with a rotometer.

Airflow Measurement

Measurements of nasal emission frequently have been used to assess velopharyngeal competency (Lubker & Moll, 1965; Machida, 1967; Subtelny, Worth, & Sakuda, 1966). Since there should be little or no nasal emission on any English sounds except /m/, /n/, and /ng/, nasal emission during the production of other sounds usually denotes palatal inadequacy. While nasal emission of air generally increases with increased inadequacy, a number of factors influence the outcome enough to result in a low correlation between the two variables (Laine, Warren, & Dalston, 1988; Warren, 1967). Respiratory effort and nasal airway resistance are factors that influence nasal airflow during speech when tight velopharyngeal closure cannot be attained. For example, an individual with high nasal resistance to airflow will generate sufficient intraoral pressure for nonnasal consonants with less respiratory effort than another individual with the same degree of inadequacy but lower nasal resistance. Thus, the former individual will require less airflow from the lungs and will have less nasal emission as well.

At best, measurements of nasal emission or nasal airflow should be limited to gross estimations of velopharyngeal function. That is, it is safe to consider peak nasal airflow rates above 150 cc/sec during nonnasal consonant productions to be indicative of inadequate closure. However, the converse may not always be true. That is, rates of less than 150 cc/sec may occur despite velopharyngeal inadequacy if there is nasal obstruction or decreased respiratory effort.

The Use of Aerodynamic Principles for Assessing Structural Performance

In general, measurements of pressure and airflow alone have not provided the definitive diagnostic information required by most clinicians. These deficiencies have led to the development of more elaborate approaches for evaluating structural performance (Barlow, 1989; Warren & DuBois, 1964). The techniques involve the application of hydrokinetic principles. Upper airway structures such as the tongue, teeth, lips, and palate form numerous constrictions, which influence airflow and pressure. Hydraulic equations are used to estimate the resistance or size of these constrictions.

There is a self-contained software and related hardware package (PERCI-SARS, Microtronics Corporation, Box 16665, Chapel Hill NC, 27517) available for aerodynamic assessment of speech. This system is used to collect pressure-flow data, and the software provides analysis modes for measuring pressures, airflows, volumes, constriction areas, resistances, conductances, and

timing variables associated with structural movements, as well as acoustic performance.

Area Measurements

Constrictions that form along the vocal tract produce an orifice type of airflow pattern. The pressure drop that results is expressed as

$$\Delta P = \frac{d}{2k^2}\left(\frac{\overset{\circ}{V}}{A}\right)^2$$

where d is the density of air, P is pressure, V is airflow, and k is the discharge coefficient, which depends upon the sharpness of the edge of the orifice and on Reynolds number. The discharge coefficient has a value of 0.6–0.7 in the speech airflow range (Warren & DuBois, 1964).

The relationship of pressure to airflow across vocal tract constrictions has led to the application of hydrokinetic principles to estimate the size of the constrictions formed during speech. The basis for this measurement can be explained in terms of airflow through simple pipes. The size of a constriction in a pipe can be calculated by measuring the airflow through the pipe (V) and the pressure drop across the constriction (P1–P2). The area of the constriction is then calculated from the equation

$$A = \frac{\overset{\circ}{V}}{k\sqrt{\dfrac{2\Delta P}{d}}}$$

where k equals 0.65. Since nearly 80% of patients with sensorimotor deficits are unable to achieve adequate velopharyngeal closure (Netsell et al, 1989), an accurate assessment of velopharyngeal orifice size is particularly important. Figure 5–1 illustrates catheter placement and instrumentation for estimating velopharyngeal orifice area.

Briefly, the pressure drop across the velopharyngeal orifice (oral pressure minus nasal pressure) is measured by placing one catheter in the left nostril and another in the oropharynx. The nasal catheter is secured by a cork which blocks the nostril, creating a stagnant column of air. Both catheters

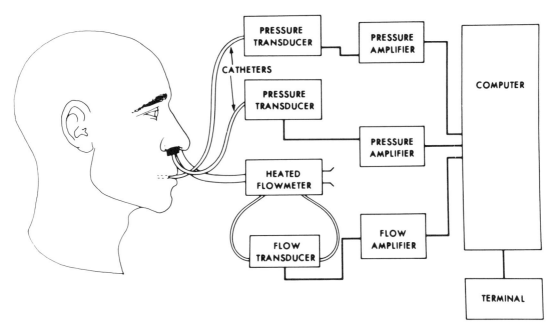

Figure 5–1. Diagrammatic representation of pressure-flow instrumentation for estimating velopharyngeal orifice size. Transducers connected to a nostril and the mouth measure the pressure drop across the velopharyngeal orifice. Airflow is measured by the flow meter and transducer connected to the other nostril. (With permission from Warren et al, 1993.)

measure static air pressures and transmit these pressures to a pressure transducer. Nasal airflow is measured by a heated pneumotachograph connected by plastic tubing to the subject's other nostril. As discussed previously, voiceless plosive sounds should be used in the speech sample. Figure 5–2 is a pressure-flow record from a normal subject producing two series of the word "papa." The first series demonstrates adequate velopharyngeal closure with negligible nasal airflow or nasal pressure. In the second series, the subject is simulating velopharyngeal inadequacy be dropping the velum. Nasal airflow is about 500 cc/sec, and nasal pressures are equivalent to oral pressures. The velopharyngeal opening is in the 2–3 cm² range, which represents a simulation of gross inadequacy.

The rating of velopharyngeal function is based upon data generated from pressure airflow studies of individuals with velopharyngeal impairment associated with cleft palate and from normal subjects (Warren, 1979). An opening greater than

0.2 cm² during nonnasal consonant productions is inadequate for normal speech. Intraoral pressure is usually low (2.5–3.5 cm H₂O range) in these individuals unless the nasal cavity is grossly obstructed. Similarly, nasal emission of air is excessive and audible, and resonance is hypernasal. Figure 5–3 is a pressure-flow record for a patient who received a traumatic brain injury. The velopharyngeal mechanism is grossly inadequate with an area greater than 2.0 cm². Oral pressures are on the low side of normal, but nasal emission of air is excessive with a mean of 341 cc/sec. Normally, the airflow rate at the peak of pressure should be less than 50 cc/sec.

Except in extremely rare instances, oral-nasal resonance balance is within normal limits when the opening is less than 0.05 cm² and any nasal emission present is inaudible. Speech performance is determined by accuracy of articulation rather than palatal closure. Openings between 0.05 and 0.10 cm² are in the adequate-borderline range and are usually small enough not to interfere with an

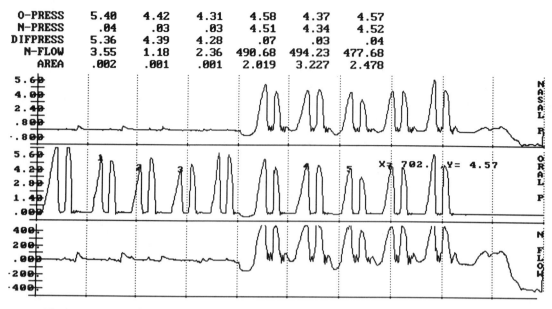

O-PRESS	5.40	4.42	4.31	4.58	4.37	4.57
N-PRESS	.04	.03	.03	4.51	4.34	4.52
DIFPRESS	5.36	4.39	4.28	.07	.03	.04
N-FLOW	3.55	1.18	2.36	490.68	494.23	477.68
AREA	.002	.001	.001	2.019	3.227	2.478

Figure 5–2. Hard copy printout of a subject producing a series of five utterances of the word "papa" normally, and then five utterances in which the velum was lowered to simulate VP inadequacy. Note the lack of nasal airflow and nasal pressure for the normal utterances and high airflow rates and high nasal pressures for the utterances produced with the open orifice. Data for pressures, airflows, and orifice areas are shown above.

individual's ability to impound intraoral pressure. However, nasal emission will occur, and under certain circumstances, it may be audible. If the nasal airway is obstructed, turbulence will produce airflow that will be most audible during fricative and affricate productions since respiratory effort is increased during production of these speech sounds. Otherwise, resonance will be within normal limits or only slightly hypernasal if articulatory performance is normal. If articulatory performance is abnormal, as in the case of many individuals with dysarthrias, then even openings this small may be associated with a speech signal that is perceived by listeners as hypernasal. Again, the indices discussed above are not based on data from individuals with sensorimotor deficits. Additional studies dealing with the effects of more generalized motor dysfunction are needed to determine whether these criteria are valid for populations other than those with cleft palate.

The same instrumental approach can be used for measuring oral port size during fricative productions. This port represents the space between the tongue, teeth, and palate and is approximately $0.06\,cm^2$ during the production of /s/ (Smith, Allen, Warren, & Hall, 1978; Warren, Hall, & Davis, 1981). Values less than $0.02\,cm^2$ or greater than $0.15\,cm^2$ indicate an inability to achieve a proper constriction for frication. This may mean a deficiency in labial or lingual neuromotor activity. Figure 5–4 illustrates catheter placements. One catheter is placed within the oral cavity, and the other within a well-fitting face mask. This measures the pressure drop across the oral port. Oral airflow is measured by a pneumotachograph attached to the oral mask.

Resistance Measurements

Resistance to airflow is opposition to air motion caused by friction (viscous drag). Friction dissipates mechanical energy in the form of heat as air moves through the vocal tract. This energy is supplied by the respiratory muscles, which require more forceful con-

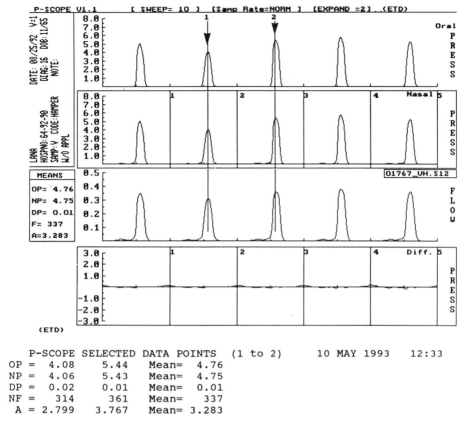

P-SCOPE SELECTED DATA POINTS (1 to 2)   10 MAY 1993   12:33

OP =	4.08	5.44	Mean=	4.76
NP =	4.06	5.43	Mean=	4.75
DP =	0.02	0.01	Mean=	0.01
NF =	314	361	Mean=	337
A =	2.799	3.767	Mean=	3.283

Figure 5–3. Record obtained from a patient with a history of a traumatic head injury. The utterance is the word "hamper." Selected data points show VP orifice areas are between 2.8 and 3.8 cm² of opening during the production of the plosive /p/. Oral and nasal pressures are about equal and differential pressure is close to 0.0.

tractions as airway resistance increases. The measurement of resistance involves the simultaneous recording of the rate of airflow and the pressure drop across the structures involved. The resistance to airflow is explained by an analogy to Ohm's law for electrical currents where

$$R = \frac{\Delta P}{\overset{\circ}{V}}$$

where R is resistance, ΔP is the pressure drop across the constriction, and $\overset{\circ}{V}$ is airflow. Resistance measurements can be made wherever constrictions in the vocal tract occur. Airway resistance is an important factor in maintaining stable speech pressures since the drop in pressure resulting from air moving across a structure is proportional to the recip-

rocal of the fourth power of the radius. Reducing the radius of an airway by one half increases the pressure drop 16-fold (Warren, Hairfield, & Seaton, 1987). Figure 5–5 illustrates that the relationship between area of constriction and resistance is inverse and nonlinear.

Laryngeal Resistance Measurements

Laryngeal resistance can be estimated using an approach suggested by Smitherin and Hixon (1981). Figure 5–6 illustrates the position of the catheter and the mask. Pressure drop across the glottis and glottal airflow are obtained by having the patient repeat the syllable /pi/ several times on one expiration at normal loudness levels. Subglottal pressure is inferred from intraoral pressure obtained

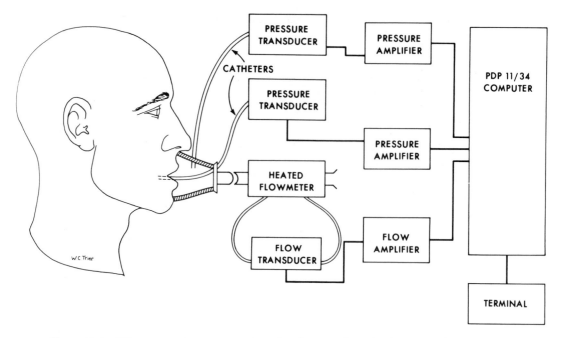

Figure 5–4. Diagrammatic representation of catheter and mask placements for estimating oral port constriction area during sibilant productions. In this case, the pressure drop across the oral port is measured simultaneously with airflow through the oral port. (With permision from Claypoole et al, 1974.)

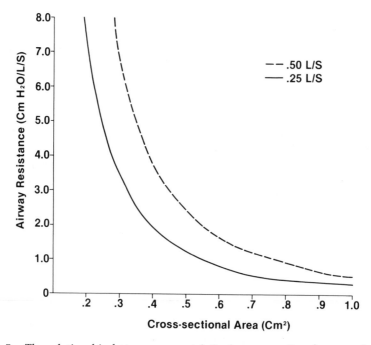

Figure 5–5. The relationship between a constriction's cross-sectional area and resistance across the constriction. As the area increases in size, airway resistance decreases in magnitude. Resistance is also affected by the volume rate of airflow.

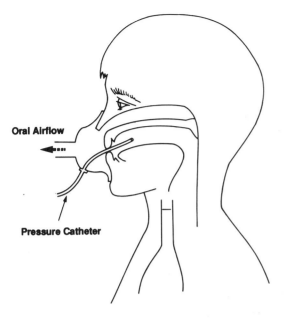

LARYNGEAL RESISTANCE CONFIGURATION

Figure 5–6. Diagrammatic representation of pressure-flow instrumentation for estimating laryngeal resistance. Oral pressure during the stop consonant /p/ is used to estimate subglottic pressure, and airflow during the vowel is used to calculate the value of resistance.

during the production of the stop consonant /p/. Airflow is measured at the midpoint to flow for the vowel /i/. Instrumentation is available to perform these calculations automatically (PERCI-SARS). Figure 5–7 illustrates a printout of pressure-flow data for calculation of laryngeal resistance for three productions of /pi/. Normal resistance values for vowels are in the 30–80 cm H_2O/L/sec range. At normal pitch and conversational loudness levels, very low resistance values may indicate an inability to effect adequate vocal fold adduction for voicing, and voice quality may be perceived as breathy. The combination of a breathy voice quality and low laryngeal airway resistance during voicing in a person with a sensorimotor disorder following CNS damage should also cue the clinician to question the adequacy

of the patient's laryngeal valve for airway protection during swallowing. On the other hand, very high laryngeal airway resistance values at habitual pitch and conversational loudness levels may indicate that vocal fold closure is too effortful during attempts at phonation. For example, in Figure 5–8, laryngeal resistance is estimated at 284 cm H_2O/L/sec, which is approximately 10 times the normal value. This record was obtained from a 10-year-old boy 18 months following a brainstem stroke. His laryngeal aeromechanical characteristics include extraordinarily high respiratory driving pressures and abnormally low translaryngeal flows despite voluntary weakness of the respiratory system and other signs of reduced respiratory capabilities, such as short breath groups and limited loudness during attempts at connected utterance.

Timing Studies

Aerodynamic assessment techniques can also be used to evaluate timing patterns associated with structural movements (Warren, Dalston, & Morr, 1989; Warren, Dalston, & Trier, 1985). For example, individuals with palatal dysfunction can be differentiated on the basis of specific timing parameters such as the onset, peak and end of pressure, and airflow pulses. Patients who present with differing degrees of velopharyngeal inadequacy manifest different patterns of pressure-flow pulsing over time. Figure 5–9 illustrates the pressure-flow patterns of an individual with adequate velopharyngeal function producing the word "hamper." Airflow for the /m/ ends (3) prior to pressure peak (5) for /p/. Figure 5–10 illustrates the change that occurs with palatal inadequacy. The entire airflow record shifts to the right. In fact, the peak of airflow (2) coincides with the peak of pressure (5).

Timing studies also discriminate between individuals who exhibit hypernasality associated with delayed, but adequate, velopharyngeal closure on obstruent segments and those who exhibit hypernasality associated with inadequate closure on

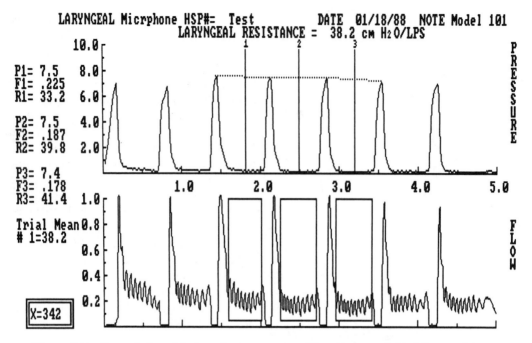

Figure 5–7. Record of a subject producing a series of the utterance /pi/. Mean resistance in this subject is 38.2 cm H₂O/L/sec.

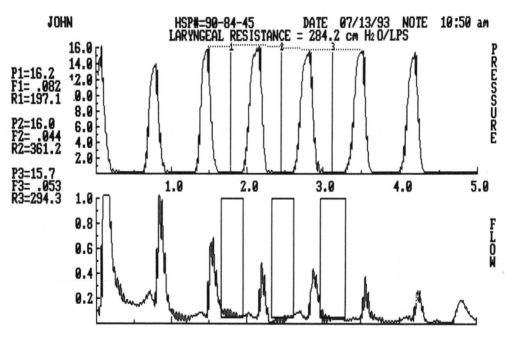

Figure 5–8. High laryngeal resistance resulting from glottal fry secondary to insufficient respiratory support. The precipitating factor in this instance was a brainstem stroke.

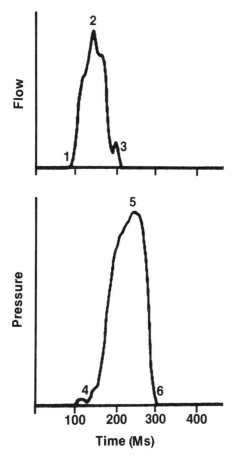

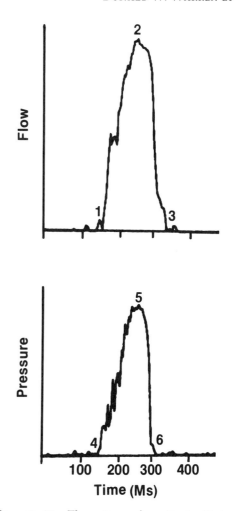

Figure 5–9. Pressure-flow pattern of a patient with competent velopharyngeal closure phonating the nasal-plosive blend /mp/ in "hamper." Note the flow peak (2) is approximately at the beginning of the pressure rise (4) point. End of flow (3) occurs before the pressure peak (5). (With permission from Warren et al, 1985.)

Figure 5–10. The pattern of a patient with inadequate velopharyngeal closure. Note that the flow peak (2) is near the pressure peak (5). End of flow (3) is near the end of pressure (6).

obstruent productions. Figure 5–11 illustrates an individual with a lag in closure. Nasal airflow for the /p/ in "pa" is shown to occur during the pressure-rise phase. There is no airflow at the pressure peak. This suggests the presence of excessive assimilative nasality since, in conversational speech, the delay in closure for the plosive would imply that the subject nasalized the preceding vowels.

Problems associated with timing are frequently observed in patients with sensorimotor deficits. Figure 5–12 illustrates the increase in duration of the airflow pulse (1–3)

in a patient with a traumatic head injury. Normally the duration would be about 140 msec (Warren, Dalston, & Mayo, 1993). Individuals with hypernasal speech are usually in the 200-msec range. On the other hand, this subject, when producing the word "hamper," had a normal time interval for the period that includes the beginning of airflow for /m/ at (1) to the end of the pressure pulse at (6). The mean duration of 190 msec compares favorably to the norm of 184 msec. This suggests that innervation of the muscles associated with velopharyngeal closure was affected (1–3) but that innervation of muscles

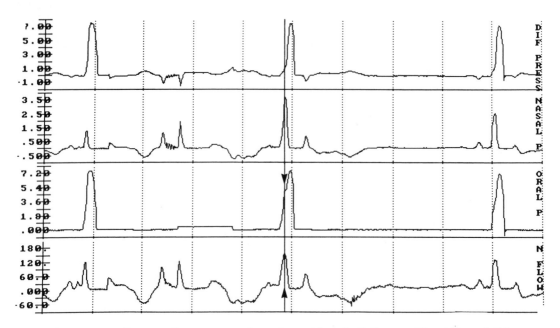

Figure 5–11. Pressure-flow patterns of a patient with assimilative nasality. Although this patient achieves adequate velopharyngeal closure, it is late, thereby nasalizing the preceding vowel. The lower arrow points to the presence of nasal airflow during the pressure buildup phase of consonant production (upper arrow).

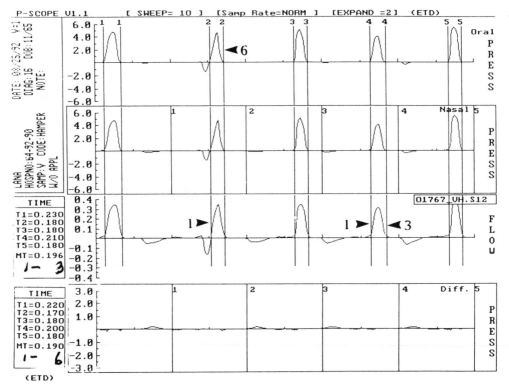

Figure 5–12. A record obtained from a patient who suffered a traumatic head injury. The mean duration of the flow pulse was 0.196 msec, which is substantially longer than normal. However, the entire interval for the /mp/ blend was 0.190 msec, which compares favorably with the norm. This would occur when labial closure is not affected.

associated with labial closure was not. That is, the duration (1–6) measurement more strongly reflects labial movements while the duration (1–3) primarily reflects velopharyngeal movements.

In comparison (Fig. 5–13), another patient, diagnosed as being dysarthric since childhood, shows a duration of 237 msec for the period (1–6). Interestingly, this patient also has two distinct peaks—one for /m/ and the other for /p/. Usually, the two phoneme pulses blend into one when there is velopharyngeal inadequacy. In this case, there appears to be an unsuccessful attempt to separate the /m/ from the /p/. The longer (1–6) duration suggests that there is impairment of the labial musculature as well.

Practical Considerations for Aerodynamic Assessment

Posture/Respiratory Effort

Individuals with speech disorders due to neurological injury or disease also may have problems with body posture control that affect their ability to participate in a speech aerodynamics evaluation. They may slump or list when seated upright, making it difficult for them to reach or stay coupled to pressure-flow data sampling apparatus. Additional time and personnel may be required to ensure that the dysarthric subject is and remains coupled adequately to flow collecting devices and pressure sensors.

The reduced trunk muscle control that compromises a subject's upright posture also

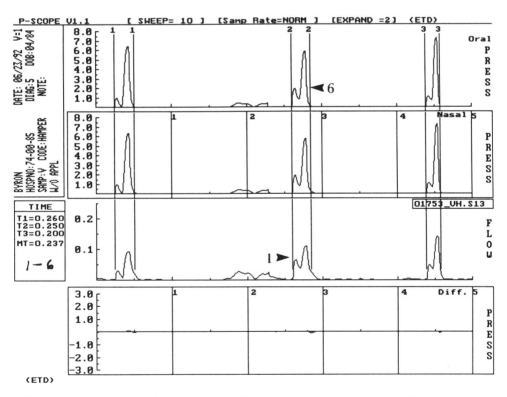

Figure 5–13. A record from a patient diagnosed as dysarthric since childhood. The duration of the /mp/ blend is 237 msec for the period (1–6). The record also shows a twin pulse for the blend, which is unusual. When there is velopharyngeal inadequacy, the two peaks would become one peak, so this indicates an attempt to separate the /m/ from the /p/, although the attempt was not entirely successful.

may reduce or render unreliable that subject's respiratory driving pressure capabilities. When this fluctuating competence is coupled with possible velopharyngeal inadequacy, the subject may not be able to generate enough intraoral pressure to trigger data sampling. It may be advantageous to make the trigger thresholds of pressure and flow transducer systems more sensitive in anticipation of this phenomenon. In automated systems, this can often be done during the calibration procedure. Or, trigger thresholds may be reset as needed by means of software options.

Limited Degrees of Freedom for Compensation, Active Participation, or Assistance

Behavioral signs suggest that subjects with injured nervous systems may be limited in

their on-line compensatory abilities. The neurologically normal subject is usually able to cooperate fully with the assessor during pressure-flow testing—to swallow on command, adjust the head or trunk posture as required to approach the sampling apparatus, hold the catheter, the nasal flow-collecting tube, or both, in place, and accommodate a number of different catheter placements. The dysarthric subject, on the other hand, may be willing to cooperate in these ways but be unable to perform or adjust his performance with such facility. As a general rule, examiners should allow extra time for the assessment of such patients to ensure that adequate, valid, and reliable data are obtained.

As well, some dysarthric subjects appear to be unable to accommodate the presence of the intraoral pressure catheter without adopting articulatory postures that may in-

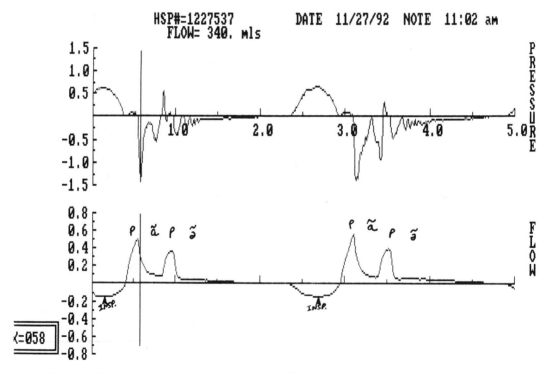

Figure 5–14. A record from a man recovering from brainstem stroke with a long history of alcohol-related cerebral dysfunction. The pressure record indicated differential pressure which is negative because of improper tongue placement during the production of the plosive /p/. The flow record indicates velopharyngeal inadequacy with airflow through the entire word "papa."

troduce artifacts in the pressure-flow data records like those shown in Figures 5–14 and 5–15. The utterance is "papa" in Figure 5–14 spoken twice by a man recovering from a brainstem stroke with a long history of alcohol-related cerebellar dysfunction. He was dysarthric and quadriparetic. His spontaneous connected speech was only 10% intelligible and characterized by imprecise articulation, nasal emission, hypernasal resonance, and short breath groups. The utterance is "hamper" in Figure 5–15 spoken several times by a 7-year-old girl with tetralogy of Fallot. She exhibited mild signs of cerebellar dysarthria including dysprosody and inconsistent, perceptible evidence of nasal emission and hypernasal resonance. Her spontaneous connected speech was 80% intelligible; developmental articulatory errors contributed to this score. Although there is evidence of inappropriate transnasal flow during the bilabial plosives in each figure,

note the instances when the associated pressure pulse is negative. In each of these cases, a single pressure transducer was being used to sense oral and nasal pressures and display their differential pressure (O > N). The negative-going pulse indicates that the pressure sensed by the nasal pressure probe was higher than that sensed by the intraoral probe (ie, N > O). One possible interpretation of this pattern is that the subject's tongue carriage was high and back with velar contact such that the oral catheter was sampling pressure in an oral cul de sac isolated from the "real" pressure of the oropharynx during utterance. Thus, while the transnasal flow suggests that the velopharyngeal sphincter likely is patent to some extent, the differential pressure system is assessing the pressure drop across the lingua-velar contact rather than across the velopharynx. Note also in the records for both subjects and utterances that there is evidence of transnasal flow during

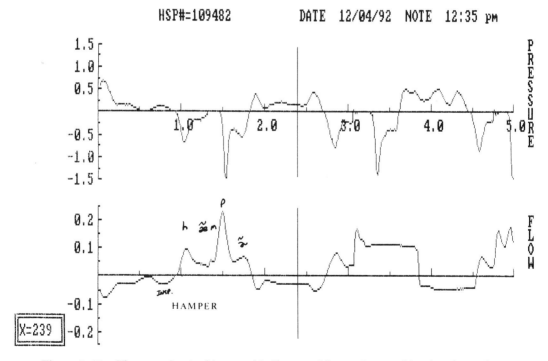

Figure 5–15. The utterance in this record is "hamper" from a 7-year-old girl with tetralogy of Fallot. She also has mild signs of cerebral dysarthria and evidence of nasal emission and hypernasal resonance. Differential pressure of less than zero indicates improper tongue placement, and airflow during production of the plosive /p/ indicates velopharyngeal inadequacy. Nasal air emission is apparent throughout the utterance.

97

the interconsonantal vowel /a/ in Figure 5–14 and throughout the production of "hamper" in Figure 5–15. Furthermore, that the intraoral pressure catheter is somehow trapped in an unusual pressure is confirmed by the positive-going pulse recorded during the subjects' nasal inspiratory gestures in both records. It is not unusual to encounter artifacts of this nature during the pressure-flow assessment of individuals with moderate-severe dysarthria associated with sensorimotor disorders. Assessors must undertake repeated samples, repositioning the intraoral pressure catheter and coaching subjects to alter their tongue positions in an attempt to find a placement that the subject can accommodate and that is legitimate for the measurement of the oropharyngeal pressure in the oral cavity. Examiners should be aware that, although the subject may be willing to cooperate, he or she may be unable to make the necessary intraoral structure placement adjustments to accommodate the catheter or may tire of repeated efforts to obtain measurable data.

Bilabial Incompetence/Closure

Mandibular weakness, labial weakness, or both may make it difficult for some dysarthric subjects to generate valid or reliable pressure-flow records if they are unable to achieve or maintain competent bilabial closure during assessment of velopharyngeal function or laryngeal airway resistance. During the testing of velopharyngeal competence, when a subject is weak and fatiguable but able to achieve bilabial closure with assistance, the assessor may choose to help the subject attain lip closure by means of a digital assist to the mandible for the bilabial plosive in "papa" and "hamper." For a subject in whom aeromechanically competent bilabial closure may be impossible (eg, someone with severe expression of Moebius syndrome), the assessor may experiment with changing the sample utterance for assessment of velopharyngeal competence to "tata" or "hanter," and for laryngeal airway resistance to /ti/, and place the intraoral pressure sensor far-

ther into the mouth to sample pressure behind the lingua-alveolar place of occlusion for /t/ or /n/.

Laryngeal airway resistance assessment may be precluded if neither labial nor lingual competence prevails, because the subject cannot produce a bilabial or lingua-alveolar stop. If only the subject's velopharyngeal closure is not competent, or competence is questionable, data for laryngeal airway resistance estimation can be collected with a mask over the oral airway only and a nose clip managing the nasal airway.

When the subject is troubled by discoordination such that the presence of the intraoral catheter is too disruptive altogether, an estimate of velopharyngeal adequacy can be obtained with measurement of nasal pressure and nasal flow only, preferably along with a voice signal so that interpretation of the aerodynamic data records is as unambiguous as possible.

Drooling

The presence of the intraoral catheter for aerodynamic testing normally stimulates salivation. Hence, clogging of the catheter is a pervasive operational hazard in pressure-flow measurements during speech. Dysarthric subjects who may be dysphagic or have trouble clearing and swallowing their saliva regularly or efficiently are especially at risk for catheter clogging during pressure-flow testing. Assessors must monitor the intraoral pressure signal on line and be alert for baseline shifts in the signal caused by collection of saliva in the pressure-sensing catheter. An example of such a shift is shown in the oral pressure trace in the upper portion of Figure 5–16. When such baseline shifts are observed, the procedure must be stopped, the sensor removed from the subject's mouth, the saliva cleared from the catheter, and the instruments reset to regain true baseline. Under these circumstances, it is important to clear the catheter without undue stress on the differential pressure transducer; to avoid damaging the transducer, the operator should disconnect

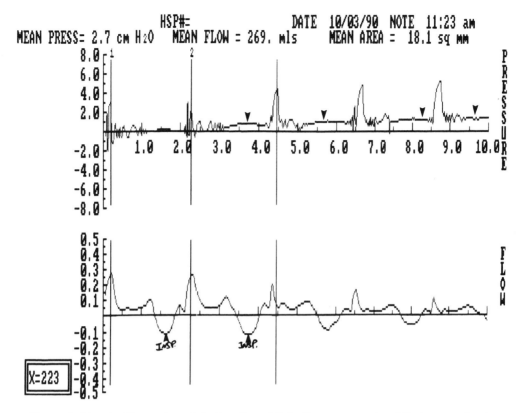

Figure 5–16. An illustration of the baseline shift in the pressure signal that occurs due to saliva in the catheter. Utterance is "hamper." The subject is a dysarthric male 4 years post brainstem stroke.

the catheter from it, especially if suction or positive pressure is to be used to remove the saliva. Coaching subjects to swallow just prior to the placement of the catheter may help to reduce the opportunity for this problem to occur.

Reliability

Clinical and anecdotal evidence suggests that subjects who have suffered central nervous system (CNS) damage may exhibit remarkable performance variability for complex tasks such as pressure-flow measurement due to variations in medication effects, arousal levels, fatigue, and a number of other behavioral or physiological phenomena. Higher performance variability means poorer sample-to-sample and day-to-day sampling reliability after CNS injury. This has implications for aerodynamic data collec-

tion in the assessment of laryngeal and velopharyngeal competence. For best estimates, multiple baseline samples across several recording opportunities should be obtained to make as honest an assessment of respiratory, laryngeal, or velopharyngeal competence as possible.

Assessing Sensory Sensitivity

Speech is primarily a modified breathing behavior with the respiratory system providing the energy source for sound production. Physiologists have long observed that the human body maintains a degree of constancy, or "homeostasis," for its many systems. Respiration is but one example of a highly regulated system (Warren, 1986). The essential characteristics of a regulating system include (1) regulation for the purpose of stability, and (2) control mechanisms to achieve relatively steady-state conditions (Brobeck, 1965). A system is said to be regulated if structures respond to change and, by their activity, preserve some level of constancy. That is, the purpose of a regulating system is to maintain a certain parameter at a generally steady level. For speech production, subglottal pressure appears to be maintained by providing a sufficient level of vocal tract resistance. The control process is the means by which this is accomplished. This implies that the brain receives information, processes it, and then directs control responses such as the movement of articulatory structures and respiratory muscle activity.

Since the production of speech is an overlaid function of breathing, it is not surprising that certain speech activities are similar to respiratory behaviors. Specifically, in breathing, the mechanics of respiration tend to maintain an optimal level of airway resistance in the range of 1.0–3.0 cm H_2O/L/sec (Cole, 1985; Warren, Duany, & Fischer, 1969). This level of resistance, which is maintained primarily by the nasal airway and vocal fold placement, allows sufficient time for alveolar gas exchange. Similarly, in speech, subglottal pressure is maintained at a fairly constant level by controlling airway resistance through movement of such vocal tract structures as the velum, tongue, vocal folds, lips, and respiratory muscles (Warren, 1982). The speech regulating system provides flexible, local energy sources throughout the vocal tract while maintaining a fairly constant subglottal pressure. The point to be emphasized is that, in any regulating system, there must be a relationship among sensory input, central processing, and motor output. Mechanisms to detect or identify changes in such aerodynamic variables as pressure, airflow, or resistance are necessary if responses to modify changes in the vocal tract environment are required (Warren, 1982).

Receptors that respond to pressure, airflow, volume, and resistance have been found in the trachea (Sant'Ambrogio, 1982), the larynx (Sant'Ambrogio, Matthew, Fisher, & Sant'Ambrogio, 1983), and the nasopharynx (McBride & Whitelaw, 1981). Laryngeal receptors sensing pressure, airflow, and muscle contractions have also been described (Sant'Ambrogio, 1982). Studies by England and Bartlett (1982) demonstrate that the larynx controls respiratory flow during breathing by varying the degree of glottal adduction. There is also evidence that muscles in the upper airway play a functional role in instantaneous control of airflow and compensation for changes in airway resistance (Brouillette & Thach, 1980; Cohen, 1975). Remmers and Bartlett (1977) observed a "tracking" behavior involving extrathoracic stretch receptors in which the respiratory muscles compensated for changes in upper airway resistance.

There is evidence that individuals with an intact sensorimotor system can detect imposed changes in the airway environment of approximately 20–40% (Elice & Warren, 1991). For example, an added resistance of less than 2.0 cm H_2O/L/sec during breathing is enough for most young adults to become aware of a change in the airway environment. Although the experimental conditions involved breathing in those studies, there is also evidence that individuals can detect similar changes in the aerodynamic environment during speech as well. Malecot (1966, 1970), Muller and Brown (1980), Wyke (1981), and Williams, Brown, and Turner (1987) have suggested that aerodynamic monitoring may be used to direct the movement of speech structures. They observed that pressure changes as low as 1.0 cm H_2O can be detected.

Methods of Assessment

The simplest approach to testing aerodynamic sensitivity involves using a diaphragm that has an adjustable iris. Opening or closing the aperture changes the resistance load (Fig. 5–17). Data from our studies indicate that normal adults are able to detect changes in resistance that are less than 2.0 cm H_2O/L/sec (Elice & Warren, 1991).

The procedure is simple to perform since it merely involves breathing through a calibrated diaphragm. Determination of thresh-

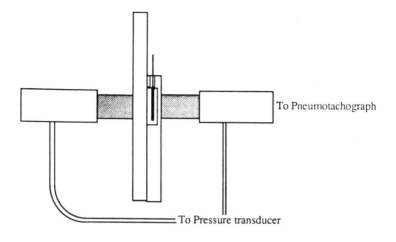

To Pneumotachograph

To Pressure transducer

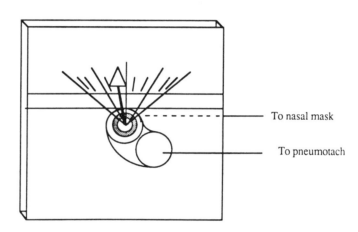

To nasal mask

To pneumotach

Figure 5–17. Diagrammatic representation of the diaphragm used to create a resistance load. The calibrated diaphragm can be opened or closed to change the value of resistance.

olds provides an indication of a patient's ability to detect a change in airway resistance or pressure. Such information should be useful in determining the ability of the patient to sense changes in the aerodynamic environment.

A more dynamic approach is currently undergoing laboratory testing, and preliminary results indicate that this new methodology not only provides an assessment of an individual's ability to sense pressure and resistance changes, but also reveals how fast an individual can respond to such changes. The computer-controlled device, which is considerably faster than a solenoid valve, can alter the aerodynamic environment at any speci-

fied time during phonation in about 20–40 msec, depending upon the magnitude of change desired. This instrument should provide important clinical information on thresholds and response times to dynamic perturbations during speech. For example, in normal subjects, recognition of a change in airway resistance following sudden perturbation during the production of /pi/ occurs at valve openings above $0.10\,\text{cm}^2$. Intraoral pressures fall only slightly even when the valve openings are as large as $0.70\,\text{cm}^2$. Normal individuals are able to compensate almost immediately for the change in airway resistance and maintain an adequate level of intraoral pressure. Under test conditions, the ability to respond to a change in the airway environment depends, to a large extent, on having an intact sensorimotor system. In patients with sensorimotor deficits, large drops in intraoral pressure during and after perturbation may occur, although the loss in pressure does not specifically mean that there is a sensory deficit. That is, the patient may sense the difference but, because of a motor deficiency, may not be able to respond quickly enough to modulate the loss of pressure. On the other hand, a higher threshold for detection of a change in resistance would be indicative of a sensory deficiency. Thus, aerodynamic sensory testing appears to be a feasible way to determine an individual's ability to monitor variables that are associated with the generation of speech. Again, it must be emphasized that there are very few supporting data demonstrating the value of such testing in patients with sensorimotor deficits. However, studies of normal subjects have encouraged us to pursue this line of inquiry.

Although thresholds have often been used as a criterion for judgments of sensory acuity, the ability of the sensory system to monitor changes in the environment must also be assessed at subthreshold levels. That is, a homeostatic system, such as in respiration, utilizes brainstem monitoring mechanisms based on sensory feedback at levels below cognition. In fact, individuals have been found to respond to imposed changes in the airway environment during breathing even before they are cognitively aware of such changes (Laine & Warren, 1995). Table 5–2 presents data that demonstrate this outcome. Various resistances were randomly added to the upper airway during breathing in a group of normal adults. The particular point to be noted is that changes in respiratory behavior occurred in response to the added resistances well before the subjects were cognitively aware that changes in resistance load had occurred. This subliminal monitoring of physiologic events is an essential feature of all human homeostatic sensory systems, and the instrumental approach using experimental resistance loads provides a way to assess this attribute in patients who are suspected of having sensory deficits.

Although the technology used to assess sensory performance is currently available, its use among patients with sensorimotor deficits is infrequent. Obviously, this special group of patients may experience a great degree of difficulty performing some of the

Table 5–2. Effects on inspiratory breathing when adding resistance loads to the nasal airway.

		Difference compared to "unloaded" p-value	Difference compared to loaded prior detection p-value
RESISTANCE (cm $H_2O/l/s$) mean (SD)			
"Unloaded"	1.75 (0.35)		
Load just prior to detection	4.13 (1.98)	0.000	
Load at detection	4.56 (2.30)	0.000	N.S.
AIRFLOW (ml/s) "Unloaded"	352 (82)		
Load just prior to detection	308 (82)	0.000	
Load at detection	303 (84)	0.000	N.S.

The "unloaded" condition is when the diaphragm is open to an extent that no subject can detect a resistance. Load just prior to detection is the highest value that was not perceived by the subject. Load at detection is the threshold value.

tasks, but preliminary experience indicates that the assessment procedures are feasible and that reliable information can be obtained. We are hopeful that, by presenting our ideas on aerodynamic sensory assessments, others will become interested in pursuing these approaches, refine the techniques and, ultimately, determine their validity.

Conclusions

Aerodynamic assessment techniques can be useful for evaluating the motor and sensory abilities of patients with sensorimotor deficits. Motor assessments include measurements of velopharyngeal orifice size, oral port size, and laryngeal resistance. These techniques can also be used to assess timing behaviors associated with the movement of speech structures such as the velopharyngeal port or the anterior oral port constriction. Such information is useful in localizing specific areas of deficiency.

Aerodynamic measurements can also be utilized in combination with apparatus that provides resistance loads to assess the sensory components of a disturbed speech system. Although sensory testing of aerodynamic performance is relatively new, data from normal subjects indicate that valuable diagnostic information can be obtained using relatively simple procedures.

Testing of patients with sensorimotor deficits is often difficult because of the limitations associated with motor problems. However, reliable measurements can be obtained on most patients when the assessor is willing to provide the time and effort necessary to obtain meaningful results.

References

Abbs JH, Hunker CL, Barlow SM. (1983). Differential speech motor subsystem impairments with suprabulbar lesions: neurophysiological framework and supporting data. In: Berry WR, ed. *Clinical Dysarthria.* San Diego: College Hill Press.

Aten JL, McDonald A, Simpson M, et al. (1984). Efficacy of modified palatal lifts for improving resonance. In: McNeil M, Rosenbeck J, Aronson A, eds. *The Dysarthris.* San Diego: College Hill Press.

Barlow SM, Abbs JA. (1984). Orofacial fine motor control impairments in congenital spasticity: evidence against hypertonus related performance deficits. *Neurology* 34:145–150.

Barlow SM, Netsel R, Hunker CJ. (1986). Phonatory disorders associated with CNS lesions. In: *Otolaryngology—Head and Neck Surgery.* St. Louis: CV Mosby.

Barlow SM. (1989). A high-speed data acquisition system for clinical speech physiology. In: Yorkston KM, Beukelman DR, eds. *Recent Advances in Clinical Dysarthria.* Boston: College-Hill/Little, Brown, pp 39–52.

Berry WR, ed. (1983). *Clinical Dysarthria.* San Diego: College-Hill.

Brobeck JR. (1965). Exchange, control and regulation. In: Brobeck JR, Yamamoto WS, eds. *Physiological Controls and Regulations.* Philadelphia: W.B. Saunders.

Brouillette RT, Thach BT. (1980). Control of genioglossus muscle inspiratory activity. *J Appl Physiol* 49:801–808.

Caliguri MP, Murry T. (1983). The use of visual feedback to enhance prosodic control in dysarthria. In: Berry WR, ed. *Clinical Dysarthria.* San Diego: College Hill Press.

Cohen MI. (1975). Phrenic and recurrent laryngeal discharge patterns and the Hering-Breuer reflex. *Am J Appl Physiol* 228:1489–1496.

Cole P. (1982). Upper respiratory airflow. In: Proctor DF, Anderson I, eds. *The Nose–Upper Airway Physiology and the Atmospheric Environment.* Amsterdam: Elsevier, pp 163–189.

Dworkin JD, Hartman DE. (1979). Progressive speech deterioration and dysphagia in ALS: case report. *Arch Physical Med Rehabil* 60:423–425.

Dworkin JD, Johns DF. (1980). Management of velopharyngeal incompetence in dysarthria: a historical review. *Clin Otolaryngol* 5:61–74.

Elice CE, Warren DW. (1991). Perception of nasal airway resistance. *J Dent Res* 70:341.

England SJ, Bartlett D Jr. (1982). Changes in respiratory movements of human vocal cords during hypernea. *J Appl Physiol* 51:780–785.

Essick GK. (1992). Comprehensive clinical evaluation of perioral sensory function. *Oral Maxillofac Clin* 4:503–526.

Gracco V, Muller EM. (1981). Analysis of

supraglottal air pressure variations in spastic dysarthria. Paper presented at the annual convention of the American Speech-Language-Hearing Association, Los Angeles.

Hardy JC. (1983). *Cerebral Palsy*. Englewood Cliffs, NJ: Prentice-Hall.

Hess DA, McDonald ET. (1960). Consonantal nasal pressure in cleft palate speakers. *J Speech Hear Res* 3:201–211.

Hixon TJ, Putnam A, Sharpe J. (1983). Speech production with flaccid paralysis of the rib cage, diaphragm and abdomen. *J Speech Hear Disord* 19:297–356.

Hoodin RB, Gilbert HR. (1989). Parkinsonian dysarthria: an aerodynamic and perceptual description of velopharyngeal closure for speech. *Folia Phoniatr* 41:249–258.

Hunker C, Bless D, Weismer G. (1981). Respiratory inductive plethysmography: a clinical technique for assessing respiratory function for speech. Paper presented at the annual convention of the American Speech-Language-Hearing Association, Los Angeles, CA.

Kent RD, Rosenbeck JC. (1982). Prosodic disturbance and neurologic lesion. *Brain Language* 15:259–291.

Laine T, Warren DW, Dalston RM, et al. (1988). Screening of velopharyngeal closure based on nasal airflow rate measurements. *Cleft Palate J* 25:220–225.

Laine T, Warren DW. (1995). Perceptual and respiratory responses to added nasal airway resistance loads in older adults. *Laryngoscope* 105:425–428.

LaVelle WE, Hardy JC. (1979). Palatal lift prosthesis for treatment of palatopharyngeal incompetence. *J Prosthet Dent* 42:308–315.

Lubker JF, Moll KL. (1965). Simultaneous oral-nasal airflow measurements and cineflurorgraphic observations during speech production. *Cleft Palate J* 2:257–272.

Lubker JF. (1970). Aerodynamic and ultrasonic assessment techniques in speech-dentofacial research. *Am Speech Hear Assoc Rep* 5:203–223.

Ludlow CL, Bassitch CJ. (1983). The results of acoustic and perceptual assessments of two types of dysarthria. In: Berry WR, ed. *Clinical Dysarthria*. San Diego: College Hill Press.

Machida J. (1967). Airflow rate and articulatory movement during speech. *Cleft Palate J* 4:240–248.

Malécot A. (1966). The effectiveness of intraoral air pressure pulse parameters in distinguish-ing between stop cognates. *Phonetica* 14:65–81.

Malécot A. (1970). The lens-fortis opposition: its physiological parameters. *J Acoust Soc Am* 47:1588–1592.

McBride B, Whitelaw WA. (1981). A physiological stimulus to upper airway receptors in humans. *J Appl Physiol* 51:1189–1197.

McNeil M, Rosenbeck J, Aronson A, eds. (1984). *The Dysarthris*. San Diego: College Hill Press.

Moore CA, Scudder RR. (1989). Coordination of jaw muscle activity in parkinsonian movement: description and response to traditional treatment. In: Yorkston KM, Beukelman DR, eds. *Recent Advances in Clinical Dysarthria*. Boston: College-Hill Press.

Muller EM, Brown WS Jr. (1980). Variations in the suproglottal air pressure waveform and their articulatory interpretation. In: Lass N, ed. *Speech and Language: Advances in Basic Research and Practice*, Vol 4. New York: Academic Press, pp 317–389.

Murry T. (1983). The production of stress in three types of dysarthric speakers. In: Berry WR, ed. *Clinical Dysarthria*. San Diego: College-Hill Press.

Netsell R, Daniel B. (1979). Dysarthria in adults: physiologic approach to rehabilitation. *Arch Physical Med Rehabil* 60:502–508.

Netsell R, Hixon T. (1978). A noninvasive method for clinically estimating subglottal air pressure. *J Speech Hear Disord* 43:326–330.

Netsell R, Kent RD. (1976). Paroxysmal ataxia in dysarthria. *J Speech Hear Disord* 41:93–109.

Netsell R, Lotz WK, Barlow SM. (1989). A speech physiology examination for individuals with dysarthria. In: Yorkston KM, Beukelman DR, eds. *Recent Advances in Clinical Dysarthria*. Boston: College-Hill Press.

Netsell R. (1969). Evaluation of velopharyngeal dysfunction in dysarthria. *J Speech Hear Disord* 34:113–122.

Portney RA. (1979). Hyperkinetic dysarthria as an early indicator of tardive dyskinesia. *J Speech Hear Res* 44:214–219.

Putnam A, Hixon TJ. (1981). Respiratory kinematics in speakers with motor neuron disease. In: McNeil M, Rosenbeck J, Aronson A, eds. *The Dysarthrias*. San Diego: College-Hill Press.

Putnam AHB. (1988). Review of research in dysarthria. In: Winitz H, ed. *Human Communication and Its Disorders, A Review*. Norwood, NJ: Apex Publishing Corp.

Remmers JE, Bartlett D Jr. (1977). Reflex control of

expiratory airflow and duration. *J Appl Physiol* 42:80–87.

Rubow R. (1984). Role of feedback, reinforcement, and compliance on training and transfer in biofeedback-based rehabilitation of motor speech and disorders. In: McNeil M, Rosenbeck J, Aronson A, eds. *The Dysarthrias*. San Diego: College-Hill Press.

Sant'Ambrogio G, Matthew OP, Fisher JT, Sant'Ambrogio FB. (1983). Laryngeal receptors responding to transmural pressure, airflow and local muscle activity. *Respir Physiol* 54:317–330.

Sant'Ambrogio G. (1982). Information arising from the tracheobronchial tree in mammals. *Physiol Rev* 62:531–569.

Shaughnessy AL, Netsell R, Farrage J. (1983). Treatment of a four-year-old with a palatal prosthesis. In: Berry WR, ed. *Clinical Dysarthria*. San Diego: College-Hill Press.

Smith ZH, Allen G, Warren DW, Hall DJ. (1978). The consistency of the pressure-flow technique for assessing oral port size. *J Acoust Soc Am* 64:1203–1206.

Smitherin R, Hixon TJ. (1981). A clinical method for estimating laryngeal airway resistance during vowel production. *J Speech Hear Disord* 46:138–146.

Subtelny JD, Worth JH, Sakuda M. (1966). Intraoral pressure and rate of flow during speech. *J Speech Hear Res* 9:498–518.

Till JA, Alp LA. (1991). Aerodynamic and temporal measures of continuous speech in dysarthric speakers. In Moore CA, Yorkston KM, Beukelman DR, eds. *Dysarthria and Apraxia of Speech: Perspectives on Management*. Baltimore: Brookes Publishing Co.

Twomey JA, Espir MLE. (1980). Paroxysmal symptoms as the first manifestations of multiple sclerosis. *J Neurol Neurosurg Psychiatry* 43:296–304.

Warren DW, Dalston RM, Mayo R. (1993). Hypernasality in the presence of "adequate" velopharyngeal closure. *Cleft Palate J* 30:150–154.

Warren DW, Dalston RM, Morr KE, et al. (1989). The speech regulating system: temporal and aerodynamic responses to velopharyngeal inadequacy. *J Speech Hear Res* 32:566–575.

Warren DW, Dalston RM, Trier WC, et al. (1985). A pressure-flow technique for quantifying temporal patterns of palatopharyngeal closure. *Cleft Palate J* 22:11–19.

Warren DW, Duany LF, Fischer ND. (1969). Nasal pathway resistance in normal and cleft lip and palate subjects. *Cleft Palate J* 6:134–140.

Warren DW, DuBois AB. (1964). A pressure-flow technique for measuring velopharyngeal orifice area during continuous speech. *Cleft Palate J* 1:52–71.

Warren DW, Hairfield WM, Seaton D, et al. (1987). The relationship between nasal airway size and nasal airway resistance. *Am J Orthod Dentofacial Orthop* 92:390–395.

Warren DW, Hall D. (1973). Glottal activity and intraoral pressures during stop consonant productions. *Folia Phoniatr* 25:121–129.

Warren DW, Hall DJ, Davis J. (1981). Oral port constriction and pressure airflow relationships during sibilant productions. *Folia Phoniatr* 33:380–394.

Warren DW. (1964). Velopharyngeal orifice size and upper pharyngeal pressure-flow patterns in normal speech. *Plast Reconstr Surg* 33:148–161.

Warren DW. (1967). Nasal emission of air and velopharyngeal function. *Cleft Palate J* 4:148–165.

Warren DW. (1976). Aerodynamics of sound production. In: Lass N, ed. *Contemporary Issues in Experimental Phonetics*. Springfield, IL: Thomas.

Warren DW. (1979). Perci: a method for rating palatal efficiency. *Cleft Palate J* 16:279–285.

Warren DW. (1982). Aerodynamics of speech. In: Lass NJ, McReynolds LV, Northern JL, Yoder DE, eds. *Speech, Language and Hearing*. Philadelphia: Saunders.

Warren DW. (1986). Compensatory speech behaviors in cleft palate: a regulation/control phenomenon? *Cleft Palate J* 23:251–280.

Warren DW. (1986). The velopharyngeal sphincter: a control factor in the speech regulating system. *ASHA* 28:103.

Weismer G. (1989). Articulatory characteristics of parkinsonian dysarthria: segmental and phrase-level timing, spirantization and glottal-supraglottal coordination. In: McNeil M, Rosenbeck J, Aronson A, eds. *The Dysarthrias*. San Diego: College-Hill Press.

Williams WN, Brown WS, Turner GE. (1987). Intraoral air pressure discrimination by normal-speaking subjects. *Folia Phoniatr* 39:196–203.

Wyke B. (1981). Neuromuscular control systems in voice production. In: Bless D, Abbs J, eds. *Vocal Fold Physiology: Contemporary Research and Clinical Issues*. San Diego: College-Hill Press, pp 71–76.

Yorkston KM, Beukelman DR, Bell KB. (1988).

Clinical Management of Dysarthric Speakers, San Diego, College-Hill Press.

Yorkston KM, Beukelman DR, Honsinger MJ. (1989). Perceived articulatory adequacy and velopharyngeal function in dysarthric speakers. *Arch Physical Med Rehabil* 70:313–331.

Acknowledgments

Supported in part by grants DE07105 and DE06957, NIDR. We thank the Voice and Resonance Clinic, Glenrose Rehabilitation Hospital, Edmonton, Alberta, for providing some of the clinical material.

Chapter *6*

Kinematic Measurement of the Human Vocal Tract

Steven M. Barlow, Donald S. Finan,
Richard D. Andreatta, and L. Ashley Paseman

Introduction

The human vocal tract, including the abdomen and rib cage, larynx, velopharynx, tongue, jaw, and lips, represents an anatomically and neurophysiologically diverse collection of tissue-muscle subsystems. An issue of special importance is the relation between orofacial motor control and speech production. It is well known that damage to brain structures important to the selection, sequencing, and activation of vocal tract muscles will degrade the motor control of speech and reduce intelligibility. Measurement of muscle performance variables in these subsystems, however, has been limited for the most part to descriptive kinematics and nonspeech force control. The development and implementation of a dynamic systems approach for the study of speech movements is needed. Limitations in transduction technology, motor task, and motor reorganization continue to present significant problems for *in vivo* studies of vocal tract structures. These problems are compounded by the complexity of brain structures that innervate scores of muscles involved in generating speech. As Larson (1988, p 309) summarized in a recent review of the neural control of vocalization, "We know almost nothing about those aspects of vocalization related to human speech and singing. We cannot even be sure about exactly where in the brain such functions are controlled—whether it is in the neocortex, supplementary cortex, anterior cingulate gyrus, or in subcortical structures."

Neural Substrate for Speech Movements

The nervous system, consisting of both central and peripheral representations of the vocal tract, is at the heart of the speech production process. The activity of the human brain in the programming, selection, and sequencing of vocal tract muscles for speech is considered by many to represent the pinnacle of phylogenetic elaboration (see review in Barlow & Farley, 1989). Numerous signal transformations are hypothesized to occur between neuronal firing (involving premotor and motor areas of central nervous system) and intelligible speech including program selection, specification of appropriate neural networks and relays (ie, corticomotoneurons), controlled inhibition, gating of appropriate sensory mechanisms, enabling of feedback and predictive neural mechanisms, outputs directed along final common pathways to selected effector muscle groups, and generation of active forces and subsequent movements to accurately modify the acoustic tuning properties of the vocal tract. Since there are many structures and dozens of muscle groups along the vocal tract, timing becomes an important factor to maintain coordination between structures (ie, larynx and velopharynx). While these elements of neuromotor control are widely recognized in the neuroscience literature in the context of movement generation, it remains a conundrum as to exactly where in the brain some of these functions may occur, and the relative timing of such operations for speech. The following summary represents a very brief overview of some of the major brain structures involved in the sensorimotor control of speech movements. The interested reader is encouraged to pursue additional sources for a more detailed consideration of the neural substrate underlying speech (Barlow & Farley, 1989; Kandel, Schwartz, & Jessell, 1991).

Implications for Neuromotor Control of the Vocal Tract

Damage to the motor cortices can seriously disrupt vocal tract movement control since the cells of origin for both pyramidal and extrapyramidal inputs are involved. Decreases in the rate of force change and movement velocity of orofacial structures characterizes the articulatory dynamics of individuals with congenital forms of the Upper Motor Neuron (UMN) syndrome (Barlow & Abbs, 1986). The fact that co-ordination among multiple structures may also be disrupted is consistent with the hypothesis that the overlapping representation of laryngeal and supralaryngeal structures in sensorimotor cortex probably serves to co-ordinate articulatory and phonatory activity in speech.

Orofacial muscle systems contain a variety of specialized mechanoreceptors and muscle afferents. Sensory information generated as a result of orofacial force and movement generation is hypothesized to play an important role in the development and maintenance of speech motor control (Bosma, 1970; Barlow et al, 1993). Bosma (1970, p 550) stated, "The mouth's sensory experiences are generated principally by its own actions, and its actions are responsive to its sensory experiences." This supposition seems equally applicable to the domain of the vocal tract and appropriate to a text dedicated to the study of sensorimotor speech disorders.

Certain "premotor" areas that have bilateral and direct access to the primary motor cortex are thought to contribute to the organization of skilled movement and the programming of motor cortex output (Matsumura & Kubota, 1979; Muakkassa & Strick, 1979; Pandya & Vignolo, 1971). Tract tracing techniques (horseradish peroxidase) in primates have led to the identification of at least four spatially separate and somatotopically organized premotor areas with projections to the primary motor cortex, including (1) the inferior limb of the arcuate sulcus (caudal bank), (2) rostrally in the supplemental motor area, (3) rostrally in the ventral bank of the cingulate sulcus, and (4) the lateral bank of the inferior precentral sulcus (Muakkassa & Strick, 1979). The densest projections originate from the premotor cortex and the supplementary motor area. Collectively, these premotor areas represent important elements in parallel pathways that influence motor cortex output and motor behavior. Of special note is the fact that the supplementary motor area contains a somatotopic representation of orofacial structures and is generally considered to function in programming motor sequences, including preparatory states for forthcoming movements (Brickman & Porter, 1978). The supplementary motor area appears to be directly involved in the planning of propositional speech (see review in Barlow, Netsell, & Hunker, 1986). In fact, small lesions limited to this area of the brain have been associated with a disorder of speech initiation. Therefore, lesions of the supplementary motor area could significantly alter orofacial muscle performance and contribute to delays in the time course of force generation. These features combined with its strategic position as one of the primary premotor inputs to the primary motor cortex is one reason to hypothesize a special role for the supplementary motor area in programming and ongoing motor control for speech.

Subcortical-Thalamo-Cortical Relations

Cerebral premotor centers reciprocate information and also receive highly segregated inputs via the ventrolateral thalamus from at least two major subcortical motor structures including the cerebellum and the basal ganglia. Outputs from the cerebellum and basal ganglia form three parallel systems of subcortical efferents to the ventrolateral thalamus that project, in a segregated fashion, to motor and premotor areas of the cerebrum (Schell & Strick, 1984). One parallel pathway originates in the caudal portions of the deep cerebellar nuclei and most directly influences the premotor cortex. A second pathway originates in the substantia nigra pars reticulata and the internal segment of the globus pallidus with direct access to the supplementary motor area. The third pathway originates in rostral portions of the deep cerebellar nuclei and most directly influences the primary motor cortex. These important motor centers form parallel pathways to motor and premotor cortical areas and are hypothesized to contribute to the programming of skilled movement and the sequencing of motor tasks. Interruption and/or progressive disease of the substantia nigra is associated with Parkinsonian dysarthria. Physiologic studies of orofacial and respiratory structures in Parkinson's disease patients generally indicate that aberrations in voluntary movement control and speech intelligibility may result from (1) involuntary tremor, 2) voluntary movement initiation delays related to the synchronizations of voluntary muscle activity with the excitatory phase of the tremor cycle, 3) labial hypertonus as inferred from electromyography (EMG) or increased muscle stiffness, and 4) impaired mechanisms of sensorimotor integration.

Anatomical evidence in monkeys indicates that the somatotopic organization of the pallidonigral and cerebellar systems are maintained in their thalamic projections. For example, the "face" representation in the substantia nigra pars reticulata projects to a "face" representation in the medial division of the ventrolateral nucleus of the thalamus which in turn projects to the "face" representations in the supplementary motor area (Schell & Strick, 1984). In a similar fashion, "face" efferents from caudal regions of the deep cerebellar nuclei projecting to area X of the thalamus have access to neurons in the face representation of the motor cortex (Asanuma et al, 1983; Brooks & Thach, 1981).

In addition to its important role in postural control and the initiation, coordination, learning, and execution of voluntary movements, the cerebellum also plays a vital role in speech motor control. Lesions of the cerebellum and/or its connections via the cerebellar peduncles result in a very distinct sounding dysarthria called "ataxic dysarthria." The voice of ataxic speakers is characterized by excessive variations in fundamental frequency (f_o) and intensity. This is accompanied by significant reductions in displacement velocity of the lips and jaw during speech production. Although the gross features of speech coordination are preserved, significant timing errors between labial-mandibular, lingual, velopharyngeal, laryngeal, and respiratory subsystems contribute to the distorted, inebriated sound associated with ataxic dysarthria.

Dynamics Encoding by the Central Nervous System

One question of special significance concerning the control of vocal tract muscles is the encoding of force and displacement by the brain. Much of what is known about movement dynamics is the result of animal experiments designed to quantify the relations between limb force/movement control and neural firing patterns in primate motor cortex. In general, firing patterns of neurons in primary motor cortex appear to be more highly correlated with select parameters of force, especially the rate of force change, than with other movement parameters (Smith, Hepp-Reymond, & Wyss, 1975; Humphrey, Schmidt, & Thompson, 1970). A large proportion of pyramidal tract neurons recorded from MI manifest a stronger relation to the rate of force change than to static force (Fetz,

Cheney, & German, 1976). Another important feature of the motor cortex is that the activity level of MI is increased when the force levels and increments are small and occurring within the physiologic operating range for skilled motor behavior (Hepp-Reymond, Wyss, & Anner, 1978). This feature of MI may be especially important for the large number of muscles among the major vocal tract systems involved in generating relatively low levels of force necessary for speech.

Vocal Tract Dynamics

Generating the source-excitation and shaping the anterior portion of the vocal tract to achieve a sequence of acoustic targets involves coordinated muscle actions and movements of the chest wall, larynx, velopharynx, tongue, jaw, and lips. The integrity of the underlying performance anatomy, including contractile elements, connective tissue, bone, and the neural substrate, is central to a discussion of motor proficiency during speech. In some instances, the accurate positioning of one structure (ie, the lower lip) may be dependent upon another structure (ie, the mandible). Motor goal acquisition often involves reorganization of motor patterns for individual structures during the course of speech production. Kinematic studies of speech often involve recording from multiple structures in an attempt to understand the trading relations between structures, patterns of organization, and reorganization following brain injury or disease. Feedback and predictive or "forward looking" neural mechanisms are hypothesized to play an important role in the acquisition of speech movements, and in the maintenance of this behavior. Knowledge about the biomechanics of some of the more prominent structures along the vocal tract such as the lips, tongue, jaw, velopharynx, larynx, and chest wall is useful when attempting to define the kinematic variables and operating ranges important in assessing speech motor control in normal and disordered systems.

Why Assess Kinematic Performance Among Individual Structures of the Vocal Tract?

The need to assess individual muscle systems of the vocal tract in individuals with neuromotor disease is motivated by the fact that (1) these structures often manifest differential degrees of motor impairment, (2) the neural plasticity for an impaired articulatory system may vary according to location in the vocal tract, and (3) the patterns of reorganization among intact structures may be dependent upon premorbid motor control. There are numerous examples in the literature of differential motor impairment following CNS lesions. For example, lower lip muscles were found to have significantly higher stiffness coefficients than upper lip muscles in a group of dysarthric individuals with Parkinson's disease (PD) (Hunker, Abbs, & Barlow, 1982). Large differences in force control and tremor amplitude were found for the upper lip and lower lip of PD and traumatically brain-injured adults. Differences in force control between the upper lip and lower lip have been quantified in adult subjects with a congenital form of the upper motor neuron syndrome during the production of steady state, and ramp-and-hold activations (Barlow & Abbs, 1986). Interestingly, the impairments in nonspeech force dynamics were found to be highly predictive of nonspeech kinematics.

Performance Anatomy of the Vocal Tract

Perioral System

Most limb muscles are characterized by relatively well defined origins and insertions, segregated by fascial sheaths, and organized about skeletal joints. Perioral muscles on the other hand lack fascia and tendons. Most labial muscles originate from the bony surfaces of the maxilla and mandible with insertion into the integument surrounding the mouth. The lips are composed of several different muscles, varying greatly in plane and orientation. Even the simplest lip gestures involves the coordination and activation of multiple muscle groups. One perioral muscle group that is especially distinct from the muscles of the limbs is the orbicularis oris (OOm). It consists of two parts, the external and internal layers. The external part of the OOm originates in the periosteum of the mandible and maxilla in the region of the frontal teeth. The internal part of OOm has been described as a sphincterlike muscle with fibers generally coursing from one corner of the mouth to the other. Neither its origin nor insertion lies in the bony substrate. Action of the OOm results in rounding and compression at the oral commissure and is considered important for speech.

The complex arrangement of interdigitating muscle fibers in the lower face makes the lips rather difficult structures to study during force generation. Although accessibility is good, establishing the biomechanical properties of the lips is further complicated by other factors including lip-jaw relations, dentition, facial asymmetry, and muscle length. Therefore, it is important to consider these factors when attempting to study the dynamics of the perioral system.

The Tongue
The tongue is an important speech articulator capable of three-dimensional conformation through multivectorial muscle activation of intrinsic and extrinsic muscles. There are four intrinsic lingual muscles including the superior longitudinal (superior lingualis), the inferior longitudinal (inferior lingualis), the transverse (transverse lingualis), and verticalis (vertical lingualis). The superior longitudinal muscle is confined to the middle portion of the tongue with fibers coursing from the root and from the median fibrous septum to the anterior edges of the tongue and terminate in the fibrous membrane. Activation of this muscle tends to shorten the tongue and elevate the tip. Muscle fibers of the inferior longitudinal course from the root to the apex of the tongue along the under surface of the tongue. Activation of this muscle tends to shorten the tongue or depress the tip. The

transverse muscle fibers originate from the median fibrous septum and course laterally to insert in the submucous fibrous tissue distributed along the lateral margins of the tongue. Activation of this muscle results in narrowing and elongation of the tongue. The vertical muscle fibers extend between the dorsum of the tongue and the inferior and lateral margins of the tongue. Activation of the vertical muscle flattens the tongue. Articulatory movement velocities during speech range from 5 to 20 cm/sec.

There are also several important extrinsic lingual muscles, including the genioglossus, styloglossus, palatoglossus, and hyoglossus, that generally act to position the whole of the tongue in the anterior-posterior and inferior-superior dimensions. For example, posterior fibers of the genioglossus act to draw the tongue anteriorly to protrude the tip from the mouth, whereas the styloglossus provides antagonistic muscle action to draw the tongue upward and backward.

The Mandibular System
The muscle systems of the jaw share many features of muscle systems in the limbs. The striated muscles of the jaw originate from several bones of the skull, including the maxilla, sphenoid, pterygoid, and palatine. The muscles of the jaw are heavily sheathed with fascia and organized into three to five compartmentalized planes about the temporomandibular joint. Mandibular depressors include the digastricus, mylohyoid, geniohyoid, and lateral (external) pterygoid muscles. The mandibular levators include the masseter, temporalis, and medial (internal) pterygoid muscles. Jaw velocities during speech range from 2 to 10 cm/sec and are usually slower than those of the lips and tongue. The presence of muscle spindles, joint receptors, and tendon organs are well established in the jaw. Muscle spindle afferents from jaw closers project directly to the trigeminal mesencephalic nucleus en route to the motor nucleus of the trigeminal nerve thereby forming a monosynaptic stretch reflex pathway.

The Velopharynx

The role of the velopharyngeal mechanism for speech is to vary the degree of acoustic coupling between the nasal and oral cavities. Adequacy of velopharyngeal closure and appropriate timing of the valving action are two important parameters of articulation. Closure is achieved by retraction and elevation of the soft palate in conjunction with constriction of the nasopharynx. The posterior pharyngeal wall may move anteriorly to approximate with the soft palate. Quite often, one observes a combination of movements involving both the lateral and posterior pharyngeal wall to achieve velopharyngeal closure during the production of pressure consonants such as /p/ and /b/. The palatopharyngeus and palatoglossus are velar depressors. The levator veli palatini is the prime levator. Contraction of the musculus uvulus results in an increase in the cross-sectional area of the velum. This effectively increases the bulk of the velum at the point of approximation with the posterior pharyngeal wall. Activity of the superior pharyngeal constrictor muscles assists in achieving the sphincterlike closure pattern frequently observed during speech.

The Laryngeal System

The course of laryngeal engagement following burst-release (ie, /pa/) involves a sequence of interrelated articulatory adjustments along the length of the vocal tract. For plosive production, the lips are compressed together to form a tight seal, the velopharynx is closed, the glottis is open, and the chest wall is under nervous system control to generate the desired level of subglottal air pressure, usually on the order of 6 to 8 cm H_2O. During production of the syllable /pa/, at least two valving adjustments occur during the plosion segment. The first adjustment finds the lips and velopharynx closed and the vocal folds abducted. The abducted position of the vocal folds is largely due to the activity of the posterior cricoarytenoid muscles (PCA). The second adjustment, known as burst-release phase, is associated with an abrupt opening of the lips. At the beginning of this adjustment, the open glottal configuration moves rapidly toward adduction. Vocal fold adduction results from inhibition of the PCA and activation of the interarytenoids (IA) and lateral cricoarytenoid muscles (LCA). The primary laryngeal adductors contract to create a tight seal along the vocal fold margin. Normally, the posterior cricoarytenoids remain quiescent during vocal fold adduction. It is this very transition from plosive burst-release to voice onset that we operationally define as laryngeal engagement. Extrinsic laryngeal muscles are secondarily involved in laryngeal engagement, serving primarily to stabilize the laryngeal apparatus, allowing the intrinsic muscles to act. The cricothyroid muscle is located on the superior border of the anterior cricoarytenoid, and inserts into the inferior margin of the thyroid. The function of this muscle is to rock or adduct the thyroid cartilage ventrally. This mechanical action serves to elongate the thyroarytenoid muscle, thereby elevating the vocal fundamental frequency.

As stated above, during steady-state voice production, the arytenoids must translate to bring the vocal processes midline. Activity of the IA and LCA muscles is regulated in concert with chest wall dynamics during steady-state voice production to maintain subglottal pressure on the order of 6 to 8 cm H_2O. The adducted laryngeal configuration is associated with a relatively small cross-sectional area that presents a load or resistance to the flow of air from the lungs. If the subglottal pressure is great enough to overcome the active forces associated with vocal fold adduction, periodic bursts of high velocity airflow will occur with each open phase of the glottal cycle. Shortly after each transient burst of flow, a short phase of negative air pressure over the medial surfaces of the vocal folds is apparent. Described as the Bernoulli effect, this aeromechanical phenomenon provides the restoring force to move the folds towards another closed phase. The dynamics of vocal fold vibration is maintained through an alternating balance between subglottal air pressure that drives the vocal folds apart and muscular, elastic and Bernoulli restoring forces that draw them together (Holmberg, Hillman, & Perkell, 1988).

The Chest Wall

Under normal conditions, the movements and forces generated by the chest wall provide the pressure-flow source for speech. From a kinematic standpoint, the human chest wall is an exquisitely complex machine (Hixon, 1987a,b,c; Hixon, Goldman, & Mead, 1973; Hixon, Mead, & Goldman, 1987; Hixon & Putnam, 1987; Putnam & Hixon, 1987; Hixon, Putnam, & Sharp, 1987). The body trunk or torso is divided into the upper and lower cavities by a dome-shaped muscle called the diaphragm. The upper cavity is known as the throrax or chest and is filled with the lungs and heart. The thorax is bounded by an elaborate skeletal framework that includes the pectoral girdle, vertebrae, ribs, sternum, and associated cartilage. Muscle and nonmuscular tissues fill the spaces between the ribs and line the inner and outer surfaces of the ribcage (Hixon, 1987a). The contiguous architecture of this lining is necessary for the hydrostatic coupling of the lungs to the inner surface of the ribcage by way of two pleural membranes and the intrapleural fluid. Inspiratory movements of the ribs above tidal volume translates to expansion of the lungs against a force of elastic recoil and is used by kinesiologists to make inferences concerning changes in lung volume. The lower cavity is known as the abdomen and contains most of the digestive system among other organs and glands. It is essentially a fluid filled cavity that is hydrostatically coupled to the abdominal surface of the diaphragm. The lower portion of the vertebral column and the pelvic girdle provide provide a relatively stable base of support for the contents of the abdomen. Movements of the abdominal belly are closely coupled to inferior-superior displacements of the diaphragm. For instance, when the diaphragm is "domed" or in the up position near the end of expiration, the belly appears to be inward. During inspiration, the diaphragm is flattened and the belly of the abdomen moves anteriorly.

Normal speakers are quite proficient at regulating the balance between active and passive forces in the thorax and abdomen, compensate for changes in gravitational load due to posture (prone or supine) or body movement (running), and rapidly effect adjustments in flow/pressure outputs in a changing mechanical environment to satisfy the demands (speaking louder) of speech. All of this is done to achieve a relatively uniform driving pressure (5–10 cm H_2O) through the "valves" or upper airway of the vocal tract. The formidable task of speech respiration actually encompasses the coordination between the chestwall and the upper airway including the larynx, velopharynx, tongue, jaw and lips. Obviously, the controller is the brain. The activation and timing of scores of muscle and nerve systems among the various levels of the neuraxis for speech is accomplished in nearly automatic fashion by the neurologically intact adult speaker. Luckily, as normal speakers, we pay little attention to our chest walls and upper airway structures during speech. On the other hand, patients with sensorimotor speech disorders due to brain injury or disease can manifest tremendous difficulty generating speech. Patients with CNS involvement affecting chest wall control may exhibit an inability to generate the necessary levels of subglottal air pressures required for vocalization and pressure consonant production. Furthermore, these patients may show impairments in the ability to sustain adequate breath pressures and flows for speech. Patients suffering from damage to the cerebellum may manifest problems in coordination and timing of muscle events in the chest wall contributing to changes in the pattern of speech output. Therefore, injury or disease to certain nuclei and/or fiber tracts within the CNS may produce qualitatively different kinematic patterns of chestwall impairment.

For this reason, it is very important to view the chestwall as more than a flow source. It is a dynamic articulatory apparatus. The chestwall produces movements and forces, is influenced by gravitational and inertial forces and by the intrinsic biomechanical properties of the connective tissues (elasticity and viscosity) that bind the thorax and abdomen as a functional unit.

Measures of Muscle Output

Activation of muscle yields a number of measurable outputs including force, displacement, heat, vibration, and electrical activity. Contractile force and displacement have been studied in the context of assessing orofacial muscle performance in normal and disordered speakers. In a limited number of experiments, select parameters of force control have been examined in relation to movement and quantitative measures of speech intelligibility in individuals with dysarthria. Force as a controlled variable is central to theories of motor control. The elaborate neural representation of sensorimotor systems subserving the static and dynamic parameters for movement and force supports this theoretical framework. Active displacement is dependent upon the action(s) of the force generators (muscles) organized about joints or within soft tissues. Kinematic variables typically studied include the amplitude of displacement, velocity, acceleration, phase and relative timing among multiple articulatory structures, phase relations to EMG muscle patterns, and spectral properties of movement (frequency domain) (Smith, 1992).

Instrumental Methods of Movement Transduction

The technical aspects of a variety of movement transduction methods will be considered including the response properties, usable displacement range, bandwidth, calibration, linearity, hysteresis, subject preparation, supporting instrumentation, 2D and 3D dimensions, and cost.

Tracking Orofacial Movements

Labial-Mandibular Strain Gage Transduction

Over 10 years ago, strain gage movement transducers similar to those described by Abbs and Gilbert (1973) and Muller and Abbs (1979) were redesigned and incorporated into a system that allowed two-dimensional measurement of upper lip, lower lip, and jaw movements in individuals with dysarthria. The transducers were coupled to a specially designed headmount that allowed subjects to generate speech without the discomfort of head restraint (Barlow, Cole, & Abbs, 1983). As shown in Figure 6–1, the headmount consists of a low-mass tubular frame assembly, which can be adjusted in three dimensions to accomodate variations in head size and asymmetry of the skull. The basic idea was to build a device that could be clamped to five amuscular/bony contact sites on the human head using double adhesive tape collars. The frame was designed with a counterbalance to offset the mass of the three-beam transducer array. Slippage of this instrument relative to the head was quantified under a wide range of head accelerations. For head acceleration in the inferior/superior dimension on the order of 500 degrees/sec^2, movement transduction artifact was 0.1 mm or less. Relative to lip or jaw displacements of 1 cm, the resulting transduction error is approximately 1%. It is usually the case that head accelerations during actual recording of speech is considerably less than the inertial test condition of 500 degrees/sec^2.

Since its design, the headmounted lip-jaw movement transduction system has been in wide use in the United States, Canada, and Europe. It offers the user with a low-cost solution for sampling inferior-superior (I-S) and anterior-posterior (A-P) movements of the lips and jaw during speech and oromotor control. Calibration of the movement cantilevers can be done statically using a micrometer-controlled linear translation stage (~$50) or dynamically with an electromechanical oscillator. The beams and

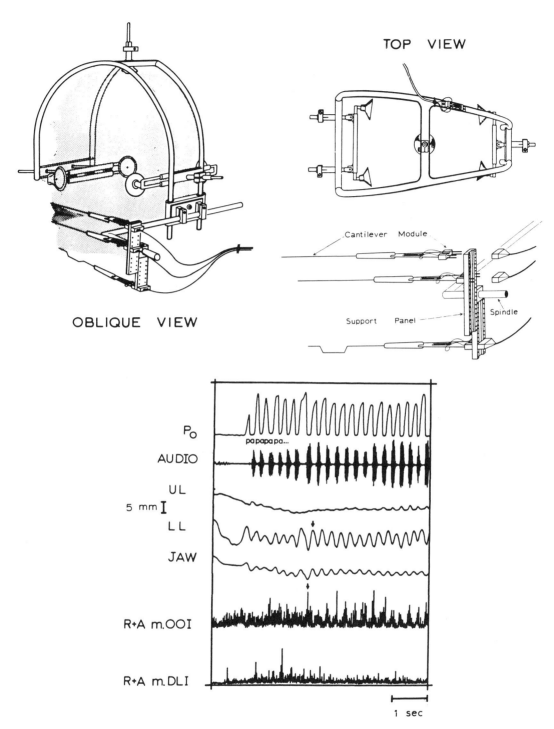

Figure 6–1. A line illustration of the headmount superstructure and the lip and jaw movement transducers shown in two profiles (top figures). Intraoral air pressure (Po), audio, movements (upper lip = UL, lower lip = LL, jaw = J) and IEMG from m. orbicularis oris inferior (OOI) and m. depressor labii inferior (DLI) from a 21-year-old man with a congenital spastic form of the UMN syndrome. The speaker was instructed to repeat the syllable /pa/ at a rate of 4 per second (Barlow, Cole, & Abbs, 1983).

headmount can be safely cold sterilized. The cantilevers are linear over a 30-mm range and have a stable frequency response from DC to 18 Hz with negligible time delay. Use of the headmounted system has made it possible to unobtrusively sample speech movements simultaneously with other signals such as EMG, aerodynamic, and acoustic outputs from many neurologic populations. Some multichannel kinematic data are shown in the lower panel of Figure 6–1 obtained from an adult with a congential form of the UMN syndrome who was instructed to repeat the syllable /pa/. In this example, intraoral air pressure (Po), audio (voice), I-S displacements of the upper lip (UL), lower lip (LL), and jaw (JAW) are shown in relation to the IEMG firing patterns sampled from electrodes positioned over the orbicularis oris inferior and depressor labii inferioris muscles.

Strain gage systems have been used widely in studies of speech kinematics in normal adults (DeNil & Abbs, 1991; Folkins, 1981; Folkins & Canty, 1986; Gracco, 1988, 1994; Moon, Zembrowski, Robin, & Folkins, 1993; Moore, 1993; Moore, Smith, & Ringel, 1988; Nelson, Perkell, & Westbury, 1984; Perkell & Matthies, 1992; Shaiman, 1989; Shaiman & Porter, 1991; Sussman & Westbury, 1981), hearing-impaired speakers (Tye-Murray & Folkins, 1990), children (Sharkey & Folkins, 1985; Smith & Gartenberg, 1984; Smith & McLean-Muse, 1986, 1987a,b), geriatric adults (Forrest, Weismer, & Adams, 1990), stutterers (McClean, Goldsmith &, Cerf, 1984; McClean, Kroll, & Loftus, 1990), Parkinson patients (Forrest, Weismer, & Turner, 1989), and a variety of apraxic, aphasic and dysarthric subjects (Abbs, Hunker, & Barlow, 1983; Barlow & Abbs, 1983, 1986; Hunker, Abbs, & Barlow, 1982; McClean, Beukelman, & Yorkston, 1987; McNeil, Weismer, Adams,, & Mulligan, 1990). This technology remains popular and is in widespread use due to its low initial cost, ease of maintenance and operation, and noninvasive application. The most obvious limitation with strain gage cantilevers is that they are not well suited for tracking the tongue. Therefore, most published work to date on speech production using strain gage technology has focussed on lip-jaw kinematics.

Orofacial Tracking Using X-ray Microbeam

The X-ray microbeam is a computer-controlled system that uses a narrow beam of X-rays to localize and track the two-dimensional movements of small gold pellets attached to the various speech structures (Abbs, Nadler, & Fujimura, 1988).

A report by Kiritani, Itoh, and Fujimura (1975) includes a description of one of the first X-ray microbeam systems in existence. The X-ray microbeam principle was developed in the early 1960s, and a prototype system was constructed and evaluated at the University of Tokyo by 1966. The spatial resolution of the X-ray microbeam system was adjustable, depending on the size of the pinhole and the distance between the tungsten target and the pinhole. With a target to pinhole distance of 15 cm, a pinhole diameter of 250 μm, and the object plane 52 cm from the pinhole, the useful field on the image plane was a 14 cm square, and the object plane spatial resolution was approximately 1 mm. The X-rays produced in this system were rated at 150 kV voltage, with a current of 1 mA. Although the amount of radiation the subject receives is minimal compared to cineradiographic methods, the X-ray beam may be programmed to exclude particular radiosensitive organs from scanning.

The X-ray microbeam system at the University of Wisconsin (Madison) was designed to record the trajectories (Fig. 6–2) of small (2–3 mm in diameter) radiodense markers (gold pellets) which may be attached to various articulators (Abbs, Nadler, & Fujimura, 1988; Westbury, 1991). A typical application may include a total of 10 pellets that are cemented in a midsagittal plane to the tip, body, and dorsum of the tongue, the lower lip, a mandibular incisor, and in a lateral sagittal plane to a mandibular molar. The remaining two pellets are attached to the

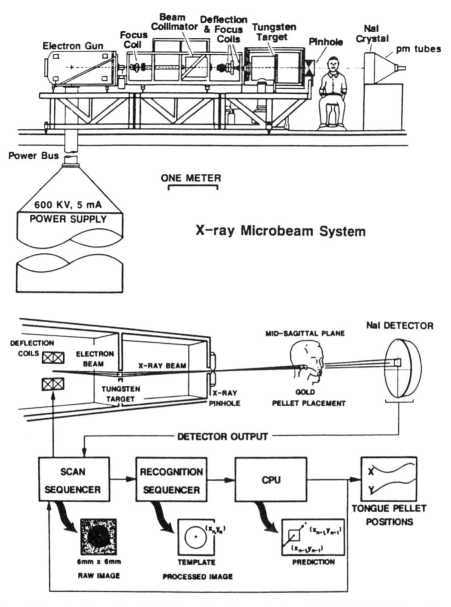

Figure 6–2. A schematic of the X-ray Microbeam System located at the University of Wisconsin (Abbs, Nadler, & Fujimura, 1988).

bridge of the nose and a maxillary incisor to serve as reference points that are immobile relative to the skull.

The X-ray microbeam system was originally implemented at the University of Tokyo (Fujimura, Kiritani, & Ishida, 1973; Kiritani, Itoh, & Fujimura, 1975). The system generates an electron beam accelerated by a voltage source of up to 600kV at a 5mA current. The system produces a narrow beam (approximately 0.4mm in diameter) of X-rays which are generated by channeling the electron beam toward a tungsten target. The resulting X-rays pass through a pinhole aperature (approximately 300μm in diameter) and are focused at the various pellets. As the X-ray beam is scanned across a pellet, a recognizeable "shadow" is registered on a

117

NaI (sodium iodide) crystal detector. The path of the X-ray beam toward a pellet is determined by predictions of the position of the pellet generated by current and previous locations. At periodic intervals, the location of each pellet (defined as the centroid of its shadow) is assigned rectangular coordinates relative to axes specified by the reference pellets. The sequence of scanning, recognition, prediction, and calculation of location for up to 10 pellets may be completed with an aggregate cycling rate of up to 700 Hz. Each pellet may be assigned its own cycle rate in the range of 40–180 Hz (Westbury, 1991).

Error in the evaluated positions of pellets may arise as a result of translation (along the Z axis) or rotation of the head. Translation error relates to the proportion of the distance between the pinhole and the image plane (NaI detector) that the head moves. For example, for a pinhole to image plane distance of 500 mm, movement of the head along the z axis +/−10 mm will generate a maximum error of +/−2%. Thus, two pellets known to be 20 mm apart may intermittently appear to be spread by 20.4 or 19.6 mm. Furthermore, head rotation of +/−10% results in +/−5% error. Measurements of head rotation and translation in a group of six speakers indicate high intratrial stability but somewhat variable intertrial accuracy (Westbury, 1991). Also, measurement error due to head translation or rotation appeared to be within +/−5%.

The X-ray microbeam system has been used successfully in the study of speaking rate by examining the velocity profiles of movements of the lower lip and tongue tip during the production of stop consonants in five young normal adults (Adams, Weismer & Kent, 1993). They found that changes in speaking rate were associated with changes in the topology of the speech movement velocity-time function. Fast speaking rates yielded symmetrical, single-peaked velocity functions whereas slow speech produced asymmetrical, multipeaked velocity profiles. These authors suggested that motor control strategies differ across speaking rate conditions. It was suggested that speech produced

at fast rates appears to involve unitary movements that may be preprogrammed and executed with little or no dependence on sensorimotor integration, whereas articulatory gestures produced at slow speaking rates may be influenced by feedback mechanisms. In another study, real acoustic and X-ray microbeam data from three subjects were utilized to train a neural network designed to infer movements of the vocal tract (Papcun, Hochberg, Thomas, Laroche, Zachs, & Levy, 1992). The use of real articulatory information is in sharp contrast to previous research that utilized synthesized articulatory data. Speech samples consisted of English stop consonants. Three articulators, which were considered the most critical for the production of English stop consonants, were chosen to form a rudimentary vocal tract from which the neural network would infer articulatory trajectories and gestures. These three articulators were the lower lip, tongue tip and tongue dorsum. A neural network was created for each individual articulator, subsequently combined to form a composite neural network. After initial training of the neural network on the entire data set, the network was trained on a portion of the training set to investigate generalization. Three primary results were identified in this study. The neural network, trained on stop consonants, learned the critical components of each articulation and was able to infer trajectories of the critical articulator and noncritical articulators. In other words the network learned the relationship between acoustics and articulation (derived from the X-ray microbeam data). After secondary training on a portion of the initial training set, the neural network was able to generalize to consonants absent from the training set as well as to consonants from the training set. Secondly, 75% of articulatory gestures (defined as the dynamic patterns of articulation across the three primary articulators) were correctly identified from the inferred trajectories when compared to templates created from the real data set. Finally, consistent differences were noted between critical and noncritical articulators. Critical articulators (articulator most importantly involved in the production of a consonant) had a greater operating range yet less variability. Reduction in variability of the critical articulator is perhaps the result of an increase in necessary constraint, considering the responsibility of the critical articulator to production of the consonant. Stable patterns of movement for the critical articulator were identified from the real data set as well as from the inferred trajectories of the neural network.

X-ray microbeam data have been combined with cinefluorography to examine the displacement of the tongue body during opening articulatory gestures in three deaf and two hearing subjects (Tye-Murray, 1991). Speech samples consisted of CVC syllables embedded within a carrier phrase. Displacement patterns in deaf and hearing subjects were examined for variation in vocalic contexts between subjects. Measures of jaw displacement were also analyzed. Deaf subjects were observed to have displacements of the tongue body during an open gesture, in contrast to previous research. Hearing subjects were found to have dissimilar tongue displacement trajectories across different vowels, whereas deaf subjects demonstrated similar tongue displacement trajectories across the different vowels examined. The authors indicated that deaf speakers had less flexible tongue bodies as a result of compensatory and incorrectly learned principles for constraining tongue movement during speech. The authors present suggestions for better quantifying lingual behaviors.

de Jong (1991) used the X-ray microbeam system to obtain trajectories of the articulators during the production of target words in sentences in order to determine the effects of consonants on the duration of the preceding vowel. Tracking pellets were placed in a midsagittal plane on the tongue tip, blade, and dorsum; upper and lower lips; and a mandible incisor. Also, a pellet was placed on a molar of the mandible. Articulatory trajectories and acoustic information were simultaneously recorded to provide measures of phoneme and syllable timing, articulatory positions, velocities, and accelerations.

X-ray microbeam and electromyographic recording techniques were used to assess velar movement and eustachian tube opening during swallowing and speech activities (Hamlet & Momiyama, 1992) For the X-ray microbeam, a 2.5-mm-diameter gold pellet was sutured in a midsagittal plane to the lingual surface of the velum at the level of the apex of the palatoglossal arch. Other pellets were fixed to the bridge of the nose and to a maxillary incisor and molar to be used as reference points. Electromyographic potentials were simultaneously recorded by hookwire electrodes inserted into the tensor and levator veli palatini muscles. Pellet tracking was completed using a sampling rate of 120 Hz, and EMG signals were sampled at 5 kHz. Spatial resolution of the pellet tracing was 0.5 mm. To detect the initiation of swallows, an audio signal and a throat accelerometer signal were also recorded. Subjects performed a series of dry swallows, swallows of 10 mL water, and the utterance "that's nonsense." Microbeam data were postprocessed to obtain positional measurements of the velum, and velar pellet velocity in the direction of motion. EMG data was high-pass filtered at 150 Hz and half-wave rectified. Results indicated that swallowing was composed of a superior/posterior movement, with a rapid anterior motion component following. The burst of EMG activity signaling levator and tensor veli palatini activity was associated with the rapid anterior component of the movement. Velar movement during speech, however, was primarily vertical in trajectory. Furthermore, large intersubject differences were observed.

Orofacial Magnetometry

Alternating magnetic field devices have been used in the past to track orofacial movements, including the jaw (Hixon, 1971) and lips (Van der Giet, 1977). These systems did not have a provision for correcting for rotational misalignment between the magnetic field transmitters and the transducers. Since then, a more elaborate system has been developed and extensively tested over the past 12 years at the Massachusetts Institute of Technology. Known as the Electro-Magnetic Midsagittal Articulometer (EMMA), this system offers up to 10 channels of high-resolution kinematic recordings of intraoral structures such as the tongue and velum during speech, swallowing, and chewing. Signals are corrected for rotational misalignment. With the EMMA system, it is possible to record movements of multiple midline points on vocal-tract structures. A 10-channel EMMA system costs approximately $90,000. The EMMA system can provide the needed quantities of accurate articulatory data with minimal risk to experimental subjects. Figure 6–3 illustrates the EMMA system that was developed at M.I.T. (Perkell, Cohen, Svirsky, Matthies, Garabieta, & Jackson, 1992; Perkell, Svirsky, Matthies, & Manzella, 1993). It includes three transmitter coils, labeled **T**, which are held in a transmitter assembly, with the coil axes perpendicular to the midline plane. The transmitter assembly is positioned so its midline coincides with the subject's midsagittal plane. Each transmitter coil is excited by a sinusoidal signal at a different frequency, between 60 and 80 KHz. This generates an alternating magnetic field having a strength that decreases approximately in proportion to the cube of the distance from the transmitter.

The alternating magnetic fields from the transmitters induce alternating voltages in the transducers, which are then conditioned by receiver electronics. The electronics convert the induced high frequency signals to three slowly varying output signals from each transducer which are digitized simultaneously with the speech acoustic signal. Special signal processing software is used to convert the digitized signals to X and Y coordinates in the midline plane.

As the articulators move, the transducer axes can vary in their alignment "rotational misalignment" with the transmitter axes, causing measurement error. Signal process-

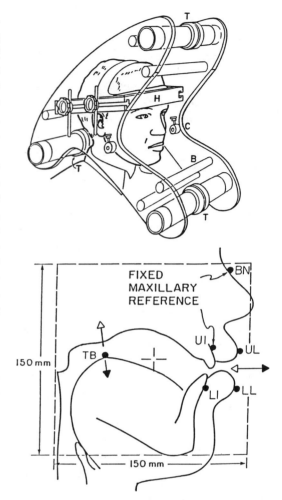

Figure 6–3. The electromagnetic midsagittal articulometer (EMMA) system that was developed at MIT is shown in the top figurine. It includes three transmitter coils, labeled **T**, which are held in a transmitter assembly, with the coil axes perpendicular to the midline plane. The transmitter assembly is positioned so that its midline coincides with the subject's midsagittal plane. Each transmitter coil is excited by a sinusoidal signal at a different frequency, between 60 and 80 KHz. This generates an alternating magnetic field having a strength that decreases approximately in proportion to the cube of the distance from the transmitter. Small, encased transducer coils are mounted on the subject's articulators, including the tongue blade, tongue body, lower incisors, lips and possibly the velum using a special biomedical adhesive (bottom panel). Special care is given to mount the transducers as close as possible to the midline, with their axes parallel to the transmitter axes. (Perkell, Cohen, Svirsky, Matthies, Garabieta, & Jackson, 1992; Perkell, Svirsky, Matthies, & Manzella, 1993).

ing software includes a calculation that corrects for this rotational misalignment.

Small, encased transducer coils are mounted on the subject's articulators, including the tongue blade, tongue body, lower incisors, lips, and possibly the velum using a special biomedical adhesive. As shown in bottom panel of Figure 6–3, transducers are also mounted on the bridge of the nose and upper central incisors for a maxillary frame of reference. Special care is given to mount the transducers as close as possible to the midline, with their axes parallel to the transmitter axes.

The EMMA system is well suited for the study of speech production. Large quantities of kinematic data can be acquired to help reveal the underlying principles of speech motor control. Risk to experimental subjects is deemed minimal.

Tracking Tongue Movements

From the late 1940s through the mid-1970s, our understanding of tongue movements relied heavily on studies using X-ray and cineradiography (Potter, Kopp, & Green, 1947; Chiba & Kajiyama, 1958; House, 1967; Perkell, 1969; Kiritani, Itoh, Fujisaki, & Sawashima, 1976). Tongue contact patterns were studied with the popular dynamic palatometer (Kuzmin, 1962; Kydd & Belt, 1964; Shibata, 1968; Harley, 1972; Palmer, 1973; Fletcher, McCutcheon, & Wolf, 1975). Since then, technological advances have been made in optics, magnetometry, ultrasound, and X-ray microbeam for real-time tracking of the lingual surface during speech and swallowing. Some of these technologies are reviewed in the following sections.

Glossometry—Optical Tracking

Nearly 20 years ago, work was under way to develop an optical distance detection system to track the superior surface of the tongue in real time for studies of speech motor control (Chuang & Wang, 1978). As shown in the upper left panels of Figure 6–4, this system was composed of an array of four LED and photosensor modules positioned adjacent to each other and mounted on a thin acrylic psuedo-palate that was molded from a stone cast of the subjects' hard palate. LED and photosensor pairs may be placed sagittally and/or in the coronal plane to obtain two- or three-dimensional representations of tongue configurations. In this system, the need for an artificial object to be placed on the surface of the tongue is eliminated.

Light is reflected directly off of the tongue and received by a photosensor. The underlying principle of optical distance detection is based upon the premise that the lumen (brightness) of an area illuminated by a light source is proportional to the inverse square of the distance. At distances ranging between zero and 20 mm, the precision of distance measurement was better than 0.5 mm. The precision of distance measurement deteriorates as distance is increased beyond 20 mm. For example, error of estimation increases from 0.5 mm to 4 mm at 40 mm distance. Fortunately, according to Chuang and Wang (1978), the distance between the tongue and palate usually does not exceed 25 mm in continuous speech. The effects of tongue rotation (rotation of the reflecting plane) in relation to the LED-sensor pair are discussed. Tongue surface rarely maintains a perpendicular relationship with the sagittal aspect of the hard palate during speech. Error with spatial resolution of the optical track increases as the tongue is repositioned with regard to the pseudo-palate. In summary, the optical tongue tracking system described above offers real-time signal display, and temporal and spatial resolution comparable to that of currently available magnetic, ultrasonic, and X-ray systems.

Fletcher and colleagues (1989, 1991) described an optoelectronic system very similar to the previously described instrument to measure tongue height, shape, and movements within the oral cavity during speech. As shown in Figure 6–5, the glossometer consists of paired infrared light emitting diodes and phototransistors embedded in a

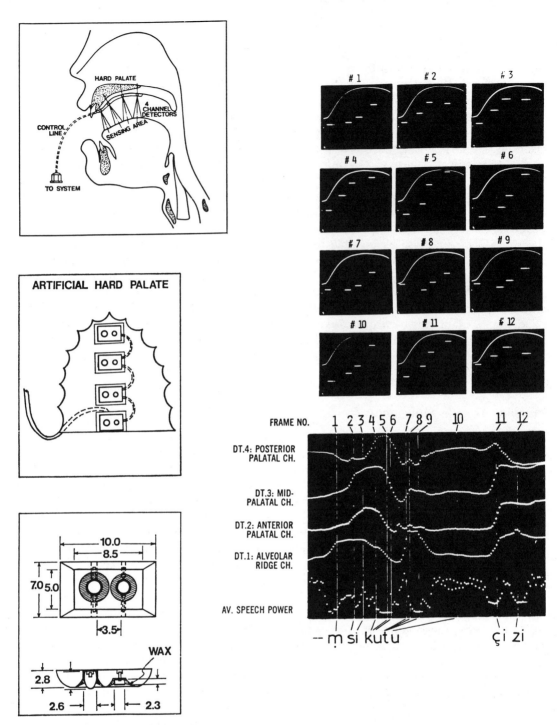

Figure 6–4. Schematic representations of the optical tongue tracking system, the arrangement of the four optical detection units, and the mounting structure of the basic unit of light-source-sensor pairs are shown in successive panels on the left. Successive displays of discrete tongue configurations and the associated time functions of the four optical detector pairs are shown in the upper right with the associated time domain display of tongue trajectories shown below. Total 12-frame time span: 1.5 sec; sampling span, 12 msec (Chuang & Wang, 1978).

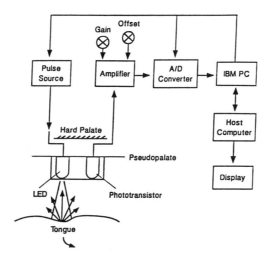

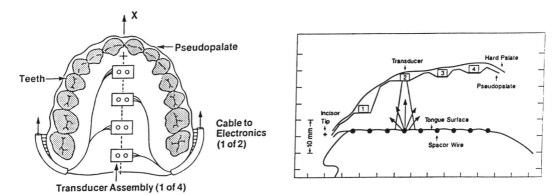

Figure 6–5. The glossometer consists of four pairs of infrared light emitting diodes and phototransistors embedded in a 0.3 mm thick heat pressure molded acrylic pseudopalate. A schematic of the conditioning electronics and recording system is shown (Fletcher, 1989b).

0.3-mm-thick heat pressure-molded acrylic pseudopalate. These authors claim a number of improvements over previous designs including a software-based linearization function, and computer-controlled activation of the LEDs for real-time sampling of tongue displacements at 100 samples per second. Each channel is calibrated in situ from zero to approximately 22 mm using intraoral spacers placed between the tongue and palate. Measurement resolution is reported to be 0.5 mm. It is important to note that discrete points on the tongue are not identified using this method, and that actions of individual muscles can only be inferred from relative changes in position.

Palatometry—Tongue and Palate Contact Patterns

Palatometry (Fletcher, Hasegawa, McCutcheon, & Gilliom, 1980; Fletcher, McCutcheon, & Wolf, 1975; Johnson, 1969; Michi, Suzuki, Yamashita, & Imai, 1986) is used to study and modify the place of linguapalatal contact in both consonant and vowel articulation. As described by Fletcher (1989a), the palatometer employs 96 tiny (0.5-mm) bead electrodes embedded on the oral surface of an acrylic pseudo-palate to sense the pattern of tongue contact during speech production (see Figure 6–6). An AC carrier signal at 27.8 kHz is delivered to the palatal

123

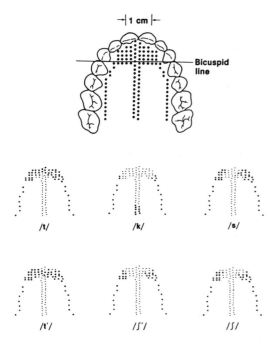

Figure 6–6. The distribution of 96 sensors (configurable) on a pseudopalate (top). Palatograms showing linguapalatal contact for /t,k,s,t',ʃ,ʃ'/ produced in CV (V = /i/) syllables by a normal 14-year old male subject. The squares represent sensors contacted in 80% of the tokens. Uncontacted sensors are indicated by dots (Fletcher, 1989a).

electrode array (current limited to 100 µamp) and referenced to the wrist. The system described by Michi et al (1986) employs a palatal reference electrode and uses considerably less current at just 8 µamp. Tongue contact on any electrode in the array completes the circuit and is registered as a sensor location in a palatometric display on a videoscreen. According to Fletcher, each vowel in English is associated with a unique stationary linguapalatal contact map. For example, during the stable contact portion of /i/, the tongue is in contact with sensors extending from the cuspid-bicuspid region of the palate to the posterior border of the alveolar ridge. During the /ae/ the contact is against the most posterior-lateral sensors. Diphthongs are characterized by movements between two stable monophthong positions.

The glosssometer (optical tracking) and palatometer (lingua-palatal contact) have been used extensively in training or retraining vowel space and consonant production in hearing impaired (Fletcher, 1989b; Fletcher, Dagenais, & Critz-Crosby, 1991) and cleft palate patients (Michi, Suzuki, Yamashita, & Imai, 1986). An example of improved tongue placement using the glossometer is shown in Figure 6–7 for a profoundly hearing-impaired subject during repeated production of /i/ (dashed lines) and /I/ before and after a 3-week training program (Fletcher, 1989b).

Ultrasonic Imaging of the Tongue

The measurement of tongue movement, during speech may be accomplished by a variety

PRE-TRAINING

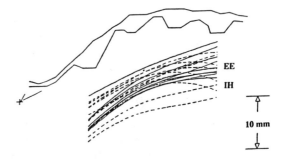

POST-TRAINING

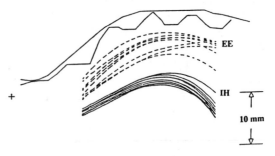

Figure 6–7. An example of improved tongue placement using the glossometer is shown for a profoundly hearing-impaired subject during repeated production of /i/ (dashed lines) and /I/ before (top panel) and after a 3-week training program (bottom panel) (Fletcher, 1989b).

of ultrasonic techniques. Keller and Ostry (1983) described a computerized system for the measurement of tongue dorsum movements with pulsed-echo ultrasound using the A-scan method.

A-scan methods consist of mounting the ultrasound transducer below the chin and measuring the reflected ultrasonic pulses. Ultrasound pulses are reflected according to changes in the acoustic impedance of tissues in their path. The transition between the tongue dorsum and the air in the air cavity produces such a change in acoustic impedance. Therefore, A-scan techniques provide measurements of the distance between the transducer and the surface of the tongue. Averaging and curve fitting procedures are used to reduce artifact in the recorded ultrasound signal. The A-scan ultrasound technique affords the recording of tongue dorsum placement, velocity, and acceleration. The transducer is placed under the chin at an axis perpendicular to the Frankfort line (imaginary line connecting the inferior margin of the orbit with the upper margin of the external auditory meatus) and is held in place by a headband. The orientation of the transducer is modified so that maximum tongue movements for the production of /k/ to /a/ is imaged. The ultrasound technique allows calculation of displacement and velocity relations for posterior vowels, speech rates, and stress levels as well as temporal events of speech production. The system produces approximately 0.39-mm error in spatial resolution, which amounts to approximately 1.5% of the total displacement seen in the production of /ga/ by adult speakers. The authors report that ultrasound techniques allow for greater intermeasure consistency as compared to conventional cineradiographic methods.

The report by Shawker, Stone, and Sonies (1985) described the development of a method to accurately track a fixed point on the tongue surface using localized reverberation artifact from ultrasound imaging. A sector ultrasound transducer with a rotating head was used in this study. The scanner consisted of three 3MHz transducers mounted to a central axis, with 120° separation between the individual transducers. Video frame rate ranged between 34Hz and 44Hz, with an axial distance resolution of 1mm and 1.9mm laterally. Various substances were tested to derive the best substance with the most clearly evident reverberation artifact. Lead, aluminum, copper, and stainless steel all generated sufficient artifact to be visualized on recorded ultrasonic images.

Stainless steel was chosen as the material of choice due to its inert qualities. Periodicity of the reverberation pattern was directly related to pellet size (diameter). Reverberation artifacts are produced from reflection of the sound waves from the anterior and posterior surface of the pellet. The authors suggest the possibility of using stainless steel pellets for both ultrasound and X-ray microbeam tracking, due to the pellets high reverberation and radio-opaque quality, respectively. The authors discuss several potential drawbacks to utilizing X-ray imaging techniques. These include difficulty in visualizing the tongue due to the interference of radiodense structures such as bone and teeth, the use of barium paste or liquid to highlight the image, and exposure of delicate structures to X-ray emissions. X-ray microbeam imaging presents lower doses of radiation exposure than cineradiography and is capable of tracking pellets without the need for barium pastes. However, the X-ray microbeam system is unable to visualize the surface of the tongue and is prohibitively expensive. The ability to use ultrasound and reverberation artifact for pellet tracking permits localized configuration changes in tongue with regard to a reference point. Recent advances in ultrasound technology, such as the ability to scan and display images in real time with better resolution than older forms of X-ray imaging, may provide a cost-effective and accurate system for describing tongue kinematics in three dimensions.

Stone, Shawker, Talbot, and Rich (1988) described a newly designed ultrasound transducer holder and head restraint system for accurately imaging cross-sectional tongue movement during speech. Speech samples consisted of 10 English vowels embedded within two contexts, /pVp/ and /sVs/. Primary goals of the study were to assess A/P coronal tongue shape, determine coarticulatory effects of /s/ on cross-sectional tongue shape of neighboring vowels, and third, to compare cross-sectional data with models of tongue shape based on sagittal and lateral data. Subjects were seated in a dental chair with their heads stabilized by means of a Velcro strap placed over the forehead and upper skull. The strap did allow for a small amount of mobility by the subject. The transducer was suspended via a cantilever submentally in relation to the subject. The transducer cantilever allowed 90° rotation in the vertical plane, 180° translation in a horizontal plane, and only allowed superior/inferior movement. A dual goniometer, a device used to measure joint angles, was utilized to align the ultrasound transducer with the mandible. The transducer cantilever foundation was attached to a constant force spring that acted in opposition to the load created by the transducer. The ultrasound transducer was capable of tracking all movements of the jaw during execution of the speech samples while maintaining contact submentally. Hysteresis measures of the transducer with relation to the jaw were performed using strain gages. These data confirm that the transducer cantilever is capable of accurately tracking the movements of the mandible during speech. Two distinct scanning angles demonstrating oral and pharyngeal constriction points were performed during the protocol. Video frames were digitized and analyzed by hand using a graphics cursor to identify surface points along the tongue dorsum. Results indicate that cross-sectional tongue shape is directly related to the position of the tongue, and the lateral and sagittal shape of the tongue. In general, midsagittal grooving was evident for all vowel types, with posterior grooves being deeper than anterior grooves. In the /p/ context, posterior grooving was greater than in the /s/ context. Grooving for vowels in the /p/ context demonstrated a continuum, whereas in the anterior /s/ context two groups of vowels were identified (high group/shallower grooves, and back group with deeper grooves). In the anterior /s/ context, tongue shape for /i/ and /u/ was convex.

These authors outline the benefits of using real-time ultrasound data with regard to advancements in the imaging technology (ie, motion during speech and swallowing, tracking of a single point via localized reverberation artifact, analysis of tongue shape and surface). They also discuss the drawbacks of other imaging techniques such as MRI and CT scan with regard to vocal tract analysis. In general, MRI and CT scanning utilize static postures in order to image the shape of the vocal tract and necessitate prolonged acquisition times. Maintaining a static posture for a phoneme eliminates the possibility of any dynamic and coarticulatory description of vocal tract structures during speech and introduces artifact into the resultant image due primarily to the subjects potential inability to reliably maintain the shape of the vocal tract over lengthy acquisition periods.

Ultrasound technology has been combined with X-ray microbeam data to develop a 3D model of tongue movement in one female subject (Stone, 1990). Speech materials consisted of VCVC utterances using the consonants /s/ and /l/, and vowels /i/, /a/, and /o/. Ultrasound technology was utilized to obtain coronal views of the tongue in three locations; anteriorly, dorsally, and posteriorly. The X-ray microbeam tracked radiodense pellets that were attached to the superior surface of the tongue, midsagittally. These two distinct forms of data were combined to conclude that the tongue may be divided into a sagittal and coronal segment, with quasi-independent movements of these segments resulting in local displacements and rotation of the tongue. These two major segments were further subdivided into four functionally based sagittal sections (anterior, middle, dorsal, and posterior) and three bilateral coronal segments (medial, lateral, most lateral). Segment boundaries were

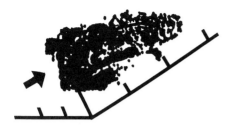

Figure 6–8. An example of a reconstructed 3D image of the tongue from the posterior-superior oblique view is shown. The arrow is positioned at the tongue root (Watkin, *personal communication*, 1993).

variable. Movement of these segments in different combinations accounted for the total movement and rotation of the tongue during speech. Sagittal segment movements reflect local contractions and displacements as well as anterior/posterior changes. Coronal segment movements produced midsagittal grooving and left-right asymmetries in surface structure. A three-tiered nested organizational scheme is offered as an hypothesis for tongue movement. The first level consists of coronal segments, whose movements would result in local displacements at level 2, the sagittal segments. Jaw movement is considered the third level, due to the effect jaw movement has on relative tongue positioning, which in turn affects the sagittal segments at level 2.

Watkin and colleagues have been closely involved in the development of high-speed 3D reconstruction of ultrasonic images. They described the development of a method whereby three-dimensional tongue surface could be reconstructed from ultrasound scans (Watkin & Rubin, 1989). An example of a reconstructed 3D image of the tongue from the posterior-superior oblique view is shown in Figure 6–8. The arrow in the figure is positioned at the tongue root (Watkin, 1993). A sweep or series of cross-sectional scans of the tongue were required to reconstruct the tongue surface. The subject was required to sustain an /s/ during scanning with the ultrasound transducer. Variables such as pressure of the transducer on skin, angle, and position of the device were not

controlled in this study. Algorithms were developed and written to code for rapid analysis and three-dimensional reconstruction. Five measurement parameters were extracted from the two-dimensional image in order to develop the 3D composite. Image scans of the tongue were examined on a frame-by-frame basis. X-Y coordinates were established for each video frame of the tongue. Tongue surface asymmetries were noticed during /s/ production from the reconstructed 3-D image.

According to Watkin et al (1993), three-dimensional ultrasonic imaging techniques have the potential to provide important information on the morphology of complex structures, such as the tongue, as well as provide developmental data. Current efforts are aimed at the development of 3D reconstruction techniques of freehand ultrasonic images using advanced graphic workstations. A standard ultrasound device and a 6-DF multichannel tracking system were used to localize the freehand position and orientation of the ultrasound transducer in 3D space. Data are digitized and stored in real time for image processing, surface mapping, and volume rendering.

The diagnostic advantages of freehand image acquisition and associated computer-based projection include: (1) increased sampling range compared to the limited range of mechanical and electronic techniques; (2) operator control of the 3D viewing point; (3) rapid reconstruction, enhancement, and volume rendering; (4) oblique slicing of the reconstructed 3D image; and (5) volume estimation of imaged objects.

Tracking Velar and Laryngeal Movements

As one proceeds beyond the lips and tongue and ventures into the depths of the vocal tract, the task of recording movements generated by the "invisible valves" of speech, such as the velopharynx and larynx, becomes technologically more challenging. Acceptable sampling methods in humans usually reflect a concession between the invasiveness of the instrument and the quality of the acquired signals. The small size and inaccessibility of both the velopharynx and larynx present real problems for the bioengineer attempting to transduce these articulatory elements. Measurement error, common to all forms of transduction, becomes an even bigger concern in measures of velopharyngeal and laryngeal output. While it is acceptable to attach small sensors to the lips and jaw in the form of pellets or cantilevers, or magnetic coils to the rib cage or abdomen, no such mechanical device is acceptable to the delicate tissue boundary of the human vocal fold for this maneuver would disrupt the behavior and health of the organism. Instead, techniques have evolved that rely on imaging, acoustics, and/or fluid mechanics. These procedures are described in the following sections.

Velopharynx

The velopharynx, strategically situated to divert acoustic and aerodynamic energy through the oral and nasal cavities, constitutes a very complex anatomical region of the vocal tract. The size of the velar port determines the oral or nasal nature of speech sounds. Movements of the velum, lateral pharyngeal walls, and the posterior pharyngeal wall collectively determine the size of the velar port.

Methods aimed at measuring the size and/or movements of select components of this port roughly fall into one of two categories: direct and indirect. Direct methods include a number of imaging techniques such as cineradiography (Moll, 1962; Moll & Daniloff, 1971), video nasendoscopy (Bell-Berti & Hirose, 1975), electromechanical (Christiansen & Moller, 1971; Moller & Christiansen, 1969; Moller, Martin, & Christiansen, 1971), optomechanical transduction (Horiguchi & Bell-Berti, 1987; Bell-Berti & Krakow, 1991) of velar displacement, and others. Line drawings of strain gage, optomechanical, and phototransistor devices to track velar movements are shown in Figures 6–9, 6–10, and 6–11, respectively. These

transducers for measuring velar activity and radiographic imaging techniques share a common limitation in only resolving movement in a single plane. In most radiographic studies, discrete points are tracked on a frame-by-frame basis which is useful in resolving velocity and displacement profiles. However, since the radiographic methods are limited to one plane or slice through the velopharynx, one is never quite sure if closure has actually occurred. It is quite possible that velar apertures may exist at locations opposite the lateral pharyngeal walls on one or both sides. It is well known that the patterns of velopharyngeal closure are highly variable both within and across speakers.

It is well known from radiography (Moll, 1962; Moll & Daniloff, 1971), nasendoscopy (Bell-Berti & Hirose, 1975), direct observation (Bloomer, 1953; Calnan, 1953; Harrington, 1944), photodetection (Dalston, 1982, 1989; Keefe & Dalston, 1989; Moon & Lagu, 1987) and acoustic analysis (House & Fairbanks, 1953) that complete velopharyngeal closure is not always obtained during vowel production. Moll's (1962) pioneering work was aimed at characterizing normal patterns of velopharyngeal closure using cinefluorographic techniques. The main results of this

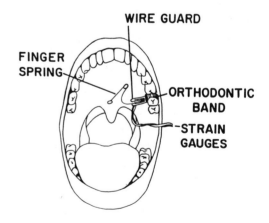

Figure 6–9. Strain gage instrumented velar displacement transducer (Hixon, 1987b; adapted from Christiansen & Moller, 1971; Moller & Christiansen, 1969; Moller, Martin, & Christiansen, 1971).

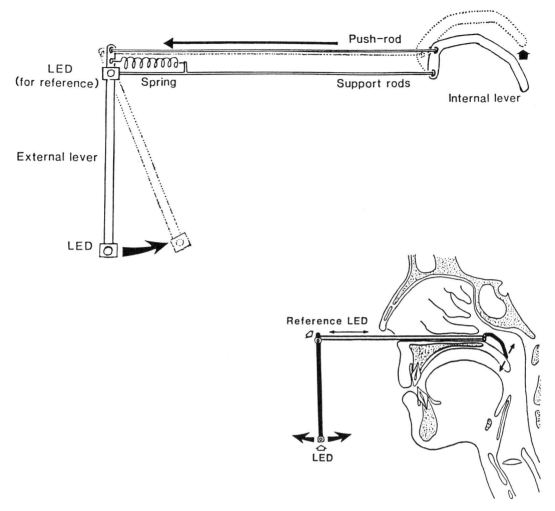

Figure 6–10. Optomechanical transducer for measuring velar movements known as the Velotrace (top). A midsagittal schematic drawing of the Velotrace in position with the internal lever resting on the velum (bottom) (Horiguchi & Bell-Berti, 1987).

study indicated that high vowels exhibit greater velopharyngeal closure than low vowels, regardless of consonant context. Moll also observed that complete closure of the velopharynx was not always present during production of the low vowels. Moll also reported that velopharyngeal closure is not attained on vowels adjacent to a nasal consonant. In fact, under these conditions, the velum does not return to its rest position, but assumes what has been referred to as the "ready" position (Graber, Bzoch, & Aoba, 1959; Moll, 1962). One of the limitations of the early cinefluorographic studies was temporal resolution in that the dwell time between frames was too long to provide detailed information on the dynamics of the velopharyngeal mechanism during speech. For example, in the Moll (1962) study, lateral images of the velopharynx were sampled every 41.66 msec. This relatively low sampling rate would be inadequate to capture the dynamics of velopharyngeal movement during speech. Later on, introduction of high-speed imaging have made it possible to sample lateral cinefluorographic images

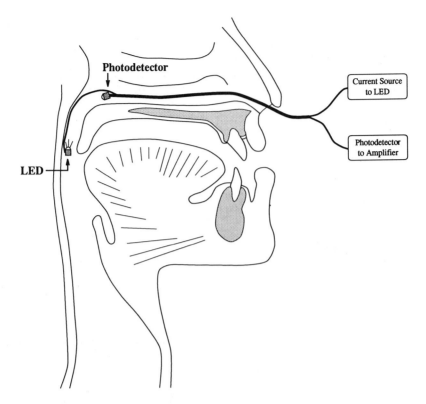

Figure 6–11. Phototransistor and light emitting diode assembly used for tracking changes in the size of the velopharyngeal orifice. Photodetector (100° acceptance cone) is positioned over the superior surface of the velum, and a wide-dispersion (180° dispersion cone) LED is suspended below the velopharyngeal port. The current input to the LED is modulated at 10 kHz. The cable assembly is reported to be less than 3 mm in diameter. (Redrawn from Moon & Lagu, 1987.)

every 6.66 msec (see Moll & Daniloff, 1971). Although this greatly improved temporal resolution, radiographic measures were still limited to two-dimensional planar images of the port (ie, lateral, basal, or anteroposterior). The spatial resolution was also limited in radiographic studies due to blurred or "fuzzy" boundaries making it difficult to identify the relative positions of the velum and posterior pharyngeal wall during closure. Measurement error was reported to be 0.91 mm for velar movement towards the posterior pharyngeal wall and 0.45 mm for estimating the velopharyngeal opening. Based on area calculations of the velopharyngeal orifice, Warren and colleagues (Laine, Warren, Dalston, Hairfield, & Morr, 1988; Laine, Warren, Dalston, & Morr, 1989; Warren, 1967,

1982) have clearly demonstrated that openings of this magnitude can yield significant airflows through the nasal cavity.

Flexible fiber optic nasoendoscopy has the potential of becoming a powerful quantitative tool to resolve some of this uncertainty regarding the dynamics of the velopharyngeal port. The camera, fiber optic, and recording technology has evolved to the point where very good images of the velopharynx can be acquired in real time. It should be possible to develop high-speed graphics-imaging software to identify edges and features of the port in real time, including computation of portal area and edge velocity, range of displacement, and calibration schemes for determining absolute distance. Not only would data be available on the size of the port, but the added information on the kinematics would be useful for studies of motor control in patients with sensorimotor disorders affecting this important speech valve.

Indirect measures of velopharyngeal port function offer some unique perspectives on the actual behavior of this valve during speech. Compared to nasendoscopy or cineradiography, aerodynamic methods can reveal the pressure-flow dynamics of the port over a wide range of speech behaviors. Contemporary aerodynamic protocols provide reasonably accurate estimates of the aeromechanical inputs and outputs of the velopharynx during speech in fluid mechanics terms without the biohazards of cineradiography, or the invasiveness of placing a 3- or 4-mm fiber optic bundle deep into the nasal cavity. Area functions (Warren & Dubois, 1964; Warren, 1982, 1988; see Chapter 5 of this volume), resistance estimates (Barlow & Suing, 1991; Barlow, Suing, & Andreatta, 1994; Netsell, Lotz, & Barlow, 1989), and temporal pattern studies (Warren, Dalston, Trier & Holder, 1985; Samlan & Barlow, 1996; Barlow, Suing, & Andreatta, 1994) have been used effectively to characterize the activity of the velopharynx during speech.

Many features of velopharyngeal and upper airway coarticulatory dynamics remain to be studied in normal speakers and explored in patients with sensorimotor speech disorders. Information gained from these experiments, involving relatively noninvasive aeromechanical measures, should prove to be of considerable value to clinicians responsible for the diagnosis and management of individuals with velopharyngeal dysfunction due to musculoskelatal abnormalities and/or neuromotor disease.

Recent reports have described some of the temporal relations between pressure-flow variables during nasal-plosive blends in the hopes of stressing the velopharyngeal mechanism to reveal the coarticulatory dynamics between velopharynx and other upper airway structures in normal and cleft palate speakers (Dalston, Warren, & Smith, 1990; Samlan & Barlow, 1994; Warren,

Dalston, Trier, & Holder, 1985). For example, Dalston et al (1990) used the pressure-flow technique previously described (Warren & DuBois, 1964; Warren, 1975) to study velopharyngeal aerodynamics in repaired cleft palate adults and normal controls instructed to produce five repetitions of the nasal-plosive blend /mp/ within the carrier word "hamper." Measures of nasal air flow rate, intraoral air pressure, and timing differences between the pressure and airflow curves were obtained from the five /mp/ productions for each subject. Compared to normals, the magnitude of the average intraoral air pressure was slightly less and the average nasal airflow rate was significantly less in the repaired cleft speakers. Dalston et al (1990) also found that the nasal airflow pulse overlapped into the rising phase and peak of the pressure pulse associated with /p/ in the word "hamper." Dalston et al (1990) argued that a decrease in respiratory effort may have been a compensatory strategy used by patients with repaired cleft palates to achieve adequate velopharyngeal closure and minimize shunting through the velopharyngeal port. This conclusion was based on careful study of the temporal relations between the airflow and pressure curves associated with production of the nasal-plosive blend. This line of investigation is important in demonstrating the utility of indirect measurement techniques such as aerodynamics in formulating inferences about the underlying articulatory dynamics of the velopharyngeal mechanism. It is clear from this work that much remains to be learned about the factors that influence articulatory dynamics of this "invisible" speech valve.

Larynx

The deepest of the "invisible" speech valves is the larynx. Laryngeal function during speech involves more than simply providing a sound source to excite the dynamically changing cavities of the vocal tract. The larynx is a microcosm of the entire speech mechanism in that it provides a sound source in coordination with the respiratory system, acts as a dynamic "articulator", capable of rapid adductor and abductor adjustments, generates frequency modulation or intonation, and conveys emotion and personal identity (Barlow, Netsell, & Hunker, 1986).

During the past 20 years, endoscopy has become a very important clinical tool in the assessment of laryngeal movement disorders affecting speech in adults (Paseman, Barlow, & Philippbar, 1994; Chait, D'Antonio, Lotz, & Netsell, 1984; D'Antonio, 1985; D'Antonio, Chait, & Lotz, 1986; D'Antonio, Chait, Lotz, & Netsell, 1987). Endoscopy is best applied in conjunction with other assessment methods and has demonstrated application in infants and children (D'Antonio et al, 1986). A detailed case history is followed by an ENT exam and an auditory-perceptual evaluation of speech/voice function. Chait et al (1984) advocated the use of aerodynamics in order to provide inferential and quantitative information concerning laryngeal and chest wall function; however, the analyses are limited to the vocal phase only and do not include a consideration of the articulatory dynamics associated with laryngeal engagement. Somewhat more invasive, fiber optic evaluations of the nasopharynx, hypopharynx, and larynx are obtained and recorded on videotape along with an audiotape recording of the speech. Use of fiber optic nasopharyngoscopy and laryngoscopy in conjunction with low-light cinematography allows observation of the dynamic processes of speech production. This technique allows the clinician to visualize the overall articulatory dynamics of the larynx during speech and other behaviors such as swallowing, coughing, and respiration. Information obtained during the nasendoscopic examination has proven useful for biofeedback in the remediation of select laryngeal and velopharyngeal impairments affecting speech. To date, observation has been limited primarily to visual impressions of the video image, relative medialization of one vocal process versus another, or hyperconstriction of the ventricular folds, etc. Videofluoroscopy offers additional information for evaluation of gross

muscle activity over a large expanse of the upper airway, from the larynx to the velopharynx, pharynx, and the hypopharynx. It is most useful for evaluation of gross movement patterns and coordination of movements of the upper articulators. The combination of perceptual-physiologic methods appears to have considerable value in cases where there are multiple factors involved with the speech/voice disorders, the diagnosis is elusive, or therapy has not produced adequate results.

An emerging technology that is finding wider application in voice clinics and laboratories is electroglottography. This instrument consists of a flexible neck collar supporting an array of electrodes and a signal conditioning unit. In electroglottography, a small DC bias current is fed through the tissues of the neck and the conditioning unit senses changes in the electrical resistance in the region of the larynx. Essentially, the electroglottogram (EGG) signal correlates with vocal fold contact area (Childers & Krishnamurthy, 1985). It is regarded as a useful assessment technique in drawing inferences about vocal fold vibration during speech.

Some of the electroglottographic measures that have been used clinically include timing measures between voiced segments, and an analysis of the cycle-by-cycle dynamics of voicing (Baken, 1992; Childers & Krishnamurthy, 1985; Titze, 1990). These dynamic measures are usually obtained in combination with inverse filtered flow signals (AC flow) for the purpose of detailing the organization and timing of the open and closed phases of the glottis during voice production. Since information derived from EGGs is based on the vocal segment and subtle changes in vocal fold contact area, it would offer limited potential for drawing inferences about the aeromechanical events underlying vocal fold engagement. Furthermore, the reliability and validity of the EGG signal associated with the early phases of laryngeal engagement are questionable. The beginning phases of arytenoid rotation are associated with displacement of the vocal folds in free space. During this interval, one would not expect appreciable increases in vocal fold contact area until arytenoid advancement results in actual tissue approximation. Therefore, the EGG output during this phase of engagement may yield little or no output signal even though significant displacements of the vocal folds have occurred.

The value of considering aerodynamic testing for collecting information on the dynamic and phonatory aspects of voice production is underscored in neurogenic patients. Netsell, Lotz, and Barlow (1989) illustrated the differences in pressure-flow patterns during consonant-vowel production in a normal and dysarthric patient. As shown in Figure 6–12, the sharp flow peaks associated with burst-release in the normal waveform are not as obvious in the dysarthric data. These peaks are presumed to correspond to the vocal fold position of maximum abduction during plosion of the /p/ consonant. The rapid decrease from peak flow in the normal subject reflects the rapid articulatory phase of vocal fold adduction toward midline for phonation. Also, the declination of flow throughout the vowel segments indicates that the folds were not abducting for the upcoming /p/ segment

to the extent that they do in normal productions. Therefore, it appears that this dysarthric subject had at least two different problems with laryngeal control, including difficulties with rapid abduction/adduction of the folds as well as inefficient midline compression during vowel production.

Patients with sensorimotor voice disorders frequently exhibit impairments in the ability to efficiently make the transition from the plosive environment to the subsequent voiced segment. This results in air being wasted when the speaker attempts to engage (adduct) the vocal folds for voice production. Patients with adductor spasmodic dysphonia manifest exaggerated medial compression of the vocal processes of the arytenoids. Often, this pattern of adduction includes the ventricular or false folds and results in a sudden interruption of the breath stream during voicing. Therefore, it appears that a comprehensive evaluation of the vocal apparatus should include a physiologic assessment of how the vocal folds/arytenoids are engaged for voicing in addition to the usual battery of tests aimed at determining glottal efficiency during phonation. Disruption of this important articulatory adjustment due to neural and/or biomechanical factors can dramatically influence the man-

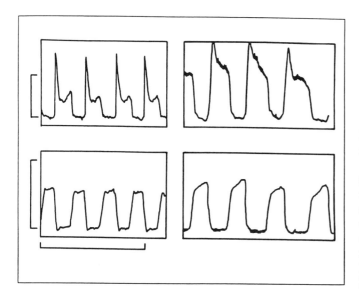

Figure 6–12. Laryngeal aerodynamic data from a normal subject (left) and a dysarthric subject (right). Subjects were asked to produce a series of [pa] syllables at a rate of four syllables per second. Total air flow (top traces) and intraoral air pressure (bottom traces). Calibration: flow = 500 cc/sec; pressure = 10 cm H$_2$O; time = 1 sec (Netsell, Lotz, & Barlow, 1989).

ner in which the vital capacity is used for speech. In cases of slow or mechanically limited engagement, it seems likely that significant portions of the lung vital capacity may be wasted by a defective laryngeal articulatory apparatus independently from the pressure-flow dynamics associated with voice production.

A new aerodynamic analysis method (Paseman, Barlow, & Philippbar, 1994) was designed to inferentially assess the articulatory proficiency of laryngeal engagement. The transducer configuration for sampling intraoral air pressure and translaryngeal flow using the MS Windows based AEROWIN (version 1.3) data acquisition and analysis program (Barlow, Suing, & Andreatta, 1994) is shown in Figure 6–13. Unlike most systems, the instrumentation is very compact. The flow transduction (pneumotach/differential pressure transducer/tubing/orofacial mask), signal conditioning, and control of analog-to-digital conversion (A/D) has been integrated into a single lightweight hand-held instrument. An example of the burst-release flow dynamics analysis of laryngeal engagement is shown in Figure 6–14 for a dysarthric patient with an advanced form of ALS. The audio (voice), translaryngeal air flow, intraoral air pressure, and derived laryngeal resistance (L_R) are displayed in sequence on the right side of

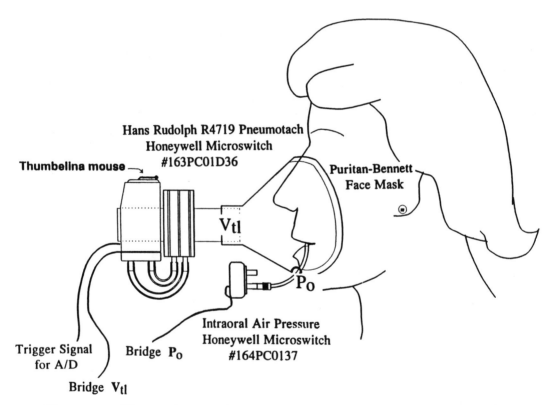

Figure 6–13. The transducer configuration for sampling laryngeal airway resistance is shown. The system includes a speech pneumotach and associated differential pressure transducer to sample the pressure drop correlated with air volume velocity. A PE 260 tube is passed through a full face mask and positioned behind the lips to sample intraoral air pressure. Finally, a miniature Thumbelina serial mouse, attached to the superior surface of the pneumotach assembly, is used to trigger the computer to begin analog-to-digital conversion and control all AEROWIN program functions. Components are cold-sterilized (Paseman, Barlow, & Philippbar, 1994).

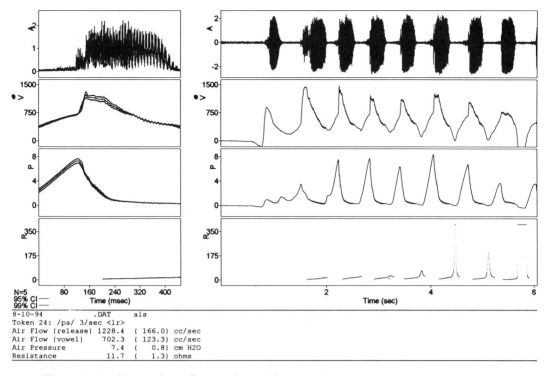

Figure 6–14. Burst-release flow analysis of laryngeal engagement in a dysarthric patient with ALS. Patient was instructed to produce the syllable /pa/ at a rate of 3/sec. A 450-msec window, referenced to the peak of translaryngeal flow, was ensemble-averaged for several syllable productions (Paseman, Barlow, & Philippbar, 1994; Barlow & Suing, 1994).

this figure. The patient was instructed to repeat the syllable /pa/ at a rate of 3 per second and given a tape recorded model of the desired utterance. Several features of the time domain displays pressure and flow reveal gross abnormalities in vocal tract function. First, the pressure peaks are very brief and do not show the characteristic plateau shape characteristic of a normal speaker (see Figure 6–15). Second, the magnitude of the burst-release flow is excessive, approaching an average of 1240 cc/sec. The control subject produced burst flows of 526 cc/sec on the average. Third, the ALS patient voiced before plosive release. Fourth, the normal pattern of rapid decline in the air flow following burst-release to steady-state phonation levels is much different for the ALS patient. The time course of flow declination is much longer than expected, taking some 300 msec. The control subject stabilizes flow following

burst-release in less than 40 msec. In fact, the translaryngeal flows in this ALS patient never really reached steady state before the next bilabial was produced. In looking at these records, one gets the impression that the arytenoid movements underlying medialization of the vocal folds for this ALS patient are very slow. Likewise, the forces associated with medial compression are less than normal since the midvocalic laryngeal resistance for this ALS patient is only 11.7 cm H_2O/LPS. The control subject manifests L_R of 38.6 cm H_2O/LPS. The laryngeal dysfunction for this ALS patient is compound in nature. There is clearly a decrease in medial compression which partially explains the breathy voice. The second problem centers around the articulatory dynamics of the arytenoid/vocal fold machinery. The digital signal processing scheme also includes an analysis of the composite translaryngeal air

135

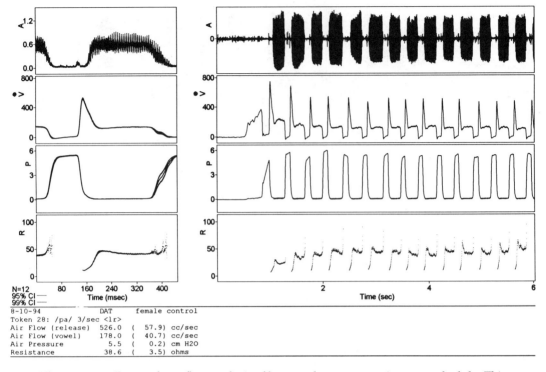

N=12
95% CI —
99% CI —

8-10-94   DAT   female control
Token 28: /pa/ 3/sec <lr>
Air Flow (release)   526.0 (57.9) cc/sec
Air Flow (vowel)   178.0 (40.7) cc/sec
Air Pressure   5.5 (0.2) cm H2O
Resistance   38.6 (3.5) ohms

Figure 6–15. Burst-release flow analysis of laryngeal engagement in a normal adult. This subject was instructed to produce the syllable /pa/ at a rate of 3/sec. A 450-msec window, referenced to the peak of translaryngeal flow, was ensemble-averaged for several syllable productions (Paseman et al, 1994; Barlow & Suing, 1994).

flow ensemble averaged around the peak flow associated with burst-release for syllable repetitions. These plots are shown on the left side of Figures 6–14 and 6–15. The protracted nature of the flow declination function, indicative of a slowly adducting laryngeal apparatus, is evident in this ALS patient. The magnitude and time course of translaryngeal flow, described mathematically as air volume and flow rate declination functions, are presumed to reflect the underlying kinematics of vocal fold adduction toward the phonatory phase. Well established measures of pressure-flow dynamics can also be determined for the phonatory phase of syllable production to provide for a comprehensive evaluation of the articulatory dynamics of laryngeal behavior (Smitheran & Hixon, 1981; Holmberg, Hillman, & Perkell, 1988, 1989). The net result of an impaired adductory mechanism is that lung volume is

wasted during the articulatory gymnastics of rotating the arytenoids for vocal fold approximation. The lung volume available for speech is depleted and overall utterance length is decreased. Therefore, the evaluation of laryngeal function in patients with sensorimotor speech disorders would benefit from an analysis of the kinematic properties of transitory (engagement-disengagement) and phonatory (voice efficiency) phases.

The few reports that exist in the dysarthria literature clearly suggest that the dynamics underlying flow-source utilization can be quite different for these two laryngeal behaviors, and that disruption in one or both aspects of laryngeal control may degrade the overall efficiency of the vocal output. Obviously, in the case of patients with slow moving arytenoids but adequate medial compression (hypokinetic dysarthria), the time course of laryngeal engagement may be protracted considerably in time when compared to the normal system. Under these conditions, it is predicted that an excessive volume of air would be forced through the glottis en route to engagement, but, once the folds reach approximation, it is entirely possible for the system to yield near normal laryngeal airway resistance values.

In Parkinson's disease the rapid positioning of the vocal folds for alternating between phonatory onset and offset during connected speech is particularly impaired (Ludlow, 1976, 1981; Ludlow & Bassich, 1981). According to Ludlow (1981), procedures for measuring adduction and abduction during speech and vocalization would be useful for assessing laryngeal neuromotor disorders.

In summary, the larynx is a dynamic articulator. The repetition of consonant-vowel syllables requires dynamic articulations from the larynx in the form of rapid alternating movements. For the most part, "these rapid muscular contractions and movements and their contributions to laryngeal dysfunction have been overlooked in examinations restricted to sustained vowel productions" (Netsell & Lotz, in preparation, p 4). As previously reviewed, AC flow studies of vibratory cycle dynamics focus on the phonatory aspects of voice production and do not provide measures of the articulatory dynamics of laryngeal adduction/abduction. An individual's voice problem need not be restricted to difficulty with phonation (Netsell & Lotz, in preparation) but may include problems in abduction/adduction (Ludlow, 1976, 1981; Ludlow & Bassich, 1981; Paseman, Barlow, & Philippbar, 1994) for consonant production and variable amounts of constriction during vowel production.

Tracking Chest Wall Movements

Chest Wall Magnetometry

As described by Hixon (1987a), the chest wall includes, except for the lungs and airways, all parts of the respiratory apparatus including the rib cage, diaphragm, the abdomen and its contents. The rib cage and diaphragm constitute the thoracic cavity. The abdominal cavity is defined by the diaphragm and abdominal wall bounding an incompressible mass of liquid. According to Hixon, Goldman, & Mead (1987), the chest wall is reduced to a two-structure model consisting of the rib cage and "diaphragm-abdomen." One of the central assumptions in chest wall kinematics during speech is that "the extent each of the two parts of the chest wall exhibits a fixed shape at a given volume of the part, all motions of points within a part must bear fixed relationships to the volumes that part displaces. It follows that volume displacements can be estimated from measurements of motions of a single point within the part in question, after, of course, the relationship between volume displacement and linear motion of that point is determined" (Hixon, Goldman, & Mead, 1987, pp 96–97). Isovolume maneuvers involve equal and opposite volume displacement by the surfaces of the abdomen and rib cage.

The transduction method preferred by Hixon and colleagues involves the use of magnetometers. A schematic of the magnetometers in situ, and the recording system are shown in Figure 6–16. Changes in the anterior-posterior diameters of the rib cage and abdomen are transduced with electromagnetic devices consisting of small coils ($2\,cm \times 0.5\,cm$) set up in pairs, one for signal generation and the other for sensing changes in inductance due to displacement. Typically, two generator-sensor pairs are used. The generator coils are attached midline on the anterior surface of the chest wall. The first is glued to the skin at the level of the nipples, and the second coil is attached to the abdomen immediately above the umbilicus. The sensor coil mates are attached to the dorsal surface of the body on midline at the same axial level as their respective generator mate coils. As shown in Figure 6–16, all four coils are oriented with their long axes perpendicular to the sagittal plane. Subjects are usually placed on a tilt table to allow for recordings of chest wall movements in the supine and prone positions. Each generator coil is driven sinusoidally at its resonant frequency

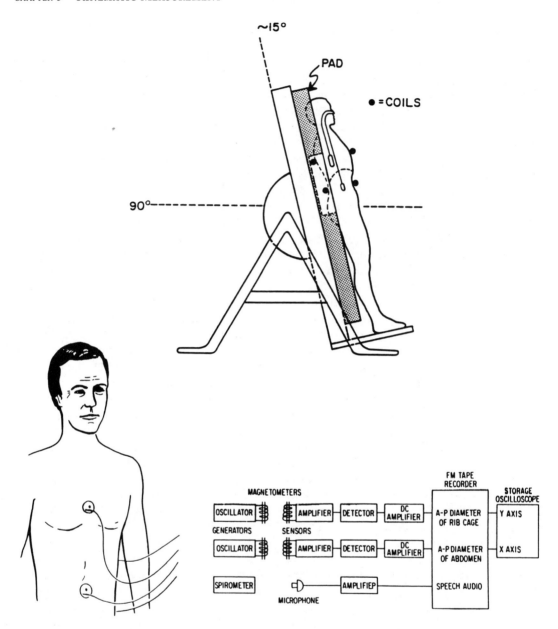

Figure 6–16. Orientation of the generator and sensor coils for chest wall magnetometry is shown for the rib cage and abdomen (top) (Hixon, Goldman, & Mead, 1987, adapted from Hixon, Goldman, & Mead, 1973). A block diagram of the electronic equipment used is shown at the bottom (Putnam & Hixon, 1987).

which turns out to be 1.53 kHz for the rib cage and 0.69 kHz for the abdomen. Signal conditioning involves coil excitation, amplification of sensor coil output, half-wave rectification, filtering, DC-coupled amplification, and output to recording and/or display devices. The usable frequency response for inductive systems is approximately one-tenth of the coil excitation frequency. A conservative estimate for the system used by Hixon and colleagues indicates a usable bandwidth from DC to 70 Hz. This is more than adequate to faithfully capture the relatively low-frequency displacements of the rib cage and abdomen.

Calibrating the chest wall is straightforward. As shown in Figure 6–17, the idea is to perform a series of isovolume maneuvers at several known lung volumes in order to reveal the functional relation between the relative motion of the abdomen and rib cage. With knowledge of the relative motion relations determined during isovolume maneuvers with lung volume constrained, it then becomes possible to estimate the component volume contributions of the abdomen and

rib cage during an unconstrained task such as speech. Examples of A-P diameter changes by rib cage and abdomen during conversation, soft reading, normal reading, loud reading and singing are shown graphically in Figure 6–18.

Speech breathing kinematics using magnetometers has been studied in individuals with profound hearing impairments (Forner & Hixon, 1987), voice disorders (Hixon & Putnam, 1987), motor neuron disease (Putnam & Hixon, 1987), flaccid paralysis (Hixon, Putnam, & Sharp, 1987), Parkinsonian dysarthria (Solomon & Hixon, 1993),

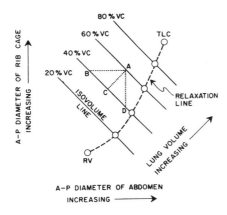

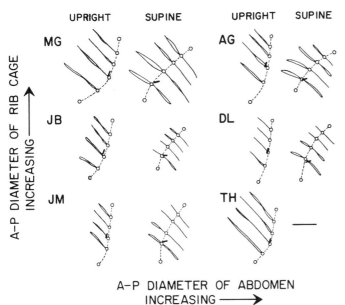

Figure 6–17. Schematic drawing of a relative motion chart (rib cage versus abdomen—upper panel) similar to those used for actual subject data in the upright and supine positions shown in the lower panels. Dashed lines depict relaxation characteristics; thin solid lines, configurations assumed during isovolume maneuvers; and short thick lines, resting breathing patterns (Hixon, Goldman, & Mead, 1987, adapted from Hixon, Goldman, & Mead, 1973).

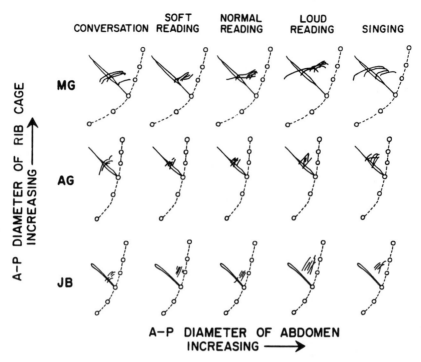

Figure 6–18. Relative volume charts for normal subjects in the upright position, showing data obtained during conversation, reading, and singing. Relaxation curves and 40% vital capacity isopleths are shown for each subject (Hixon, Goldman, & Mead, 1987, adapted from Hixon, Goldman, & Mead, 1973).

spinal cord injury (Hoit, Banzett, Brown, & Loring, 1990), and in a variety of normal subgroups where factors such as age (Hoit & Hixon, 1987), body type (Hoit & Hixon, 1986), and sex (Hodge & Rochet, 1989) are the dependent variables.

Another transducer system that has been used to measure chest wall kinematics is the strain gage belt pneumograph. This setup is quite simple and involves a clip gage attached to a circumferential belt with velcro (see Figure 6–19). A bridge amplifier provides DC excitation and conditioning for each belt. Signals are typically low-pass filtered (LP @ 50 Hz) and routed to a digital computer or instrumentation recorder. Murdoch and colleagues have utilized this method to study respiratory function in subjects with Parkinson's disease (Murdoch, Chenery, Bowler, & Ingram, 1989), cerebellar degeneration (Murdoch, Chenery, Stokes, & Hardcastle, 1991), pseudobulbar palsy (Murdoch, Noble, Chenery, & Ingram, 1989),

closed head injury (Murdoch, Theodoros, Stokes, & Chenery, 1993), and normal subjects (Manifold & Murdoch, 1993). Use of the strain gage belt pneumographs by Murdoch and colleagues has come under strong criticism recently (Hoit, 1994; Solomon & Hixon, 1993). Much of the debate centers on the exact placement of the abdominal belt. Murdoch, Chenery, Bowler, and Ingram (1989) stated that the abdominal belt was placed above the umbilicus. According to Hoit (1994), this placement is considered appropriate for A-P measurements, but not for circumferential measurements because the lower ribs contribute to movement of the abdominal belt.

Summary

Many new and exciting methods are available to researchers and clinicians interested in the kinematics and motor control of the human vocal tract. With most transducer systems it is possible to simultaneously acquire physiologic outputs from several articulatory flesh points and even combine with electromyographic, aerodynamic, acoustic, and electrical impedance measures of vocal tract function. High-speed microprocessors, especially graphics workstations, now make it possible to reduce many channels of information, including signal processing transformations, in real time. As the

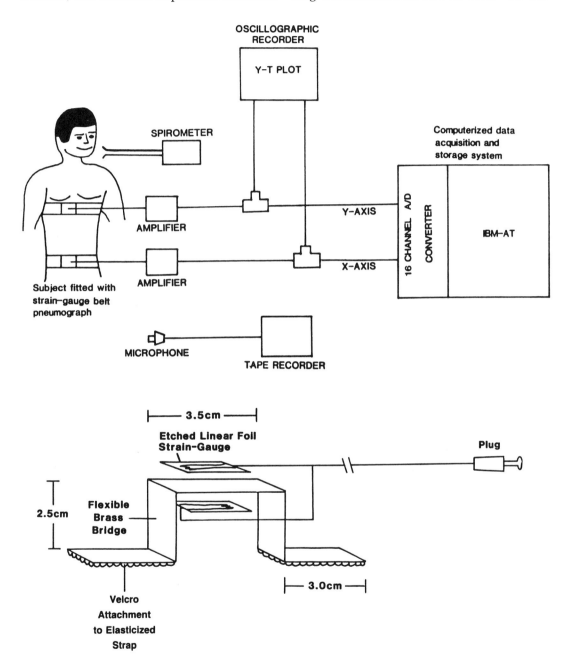

Figure 6–19. The strain gage belt pneumograph and block diagram of electronics for sampling circumferential changes in ribcage and abdomen during speech breathing (top) (Manifold & Murdoch, 1993). The structure of the clip gage and Velcro mounting pads (bottom) (adapted from Murdoch, Chenery, Bowler. & Ingram, 1989).

technologies and scientific underpinnings of speech motor control continue to advance, so will the depth of inquiry into sensorimotor speech movement disorders. Purely descriptive experiments will be superseded with studies addressing the mechanisms underlying sensorimotor impaired speech. Improved instrumentation also means that the complexity of task dynamics will be increased, using more subjects and external agents to induce reorganization and change in motor programming. Exciting dividends are being realized in the clinical setting as well. Many of the technologies reviewed in this report have been applied toward improved diagnostic methods of respiratory, laryngeal, velopharyngeal, and orofacial function in patients suffering from neurologically based speech disorders. The speed of processing data and higher resolution graphics has resulted in the emergence of new biofeedback tools that await clinical trial. Continued cooperation among the disciplines of speech science, physiology, neuroscience, bioengineering, and computer science will undoubtedly have a dramatic impact on the study of vocal tract kinematics.

REFERENCES

Abbs JH, Gilbert BW. (1973). A strain gage transducer system for lip and jaw motion in two dimensions. *J Speech Hearing Res* 16:248–256.

Abbs JH, Hunker CJ, Barlow SM. (1983). Differential speech motor subsystem impairments with suprabulbar lesions: neurophysiological framework and supporting data. In: Berry WR, ed. *Clinical Dysarthria*. San Diego: College-Hill Press, pp 21–56.

Abbs JH, Nadler RD, Fujimura O. (1988). X-ray microbeams track the shape of speech. *SOMA* 2:29–34.

Adams SG, Weismer G, Kent RD. (1993). Speaking rate and speech movement velocity profiles. *J Speech Hear Res* 36:41–54.

Asanuma C, Thach WT, Jones EG. (1983). Cytoarchitectonic delineation of the ventral lateral thalamic region in the monkey. *Brain Res Rev* 5:219.

Baken RJ. (1992). Electroglottography. *J Voice* 6:98–110.

Barlow SM, Abbs JH. (1983). Force transducers for the evaluation of labial, lingual, and mandibular function in dysarthria. *J Speech Hear Res* 26:616–621.

Barlow SM, Abbs JH. (1986). Fine force and position control of select orofacial structures in the upper motor neuron syndrome. *Exp Neurol* 94:699–713.

Barlow SM, Cole KJ, Abbs JH. (1983). A new headmounted lip-jaw movement transduction system for the study of motor speech disorders. *J Speech Hearing Res* 26: 283–288.

Barlow SM, Farley GR. (1989). Neurophysiology of speech. In: Kuehn DP, Lemme ML, Baumgartner JM, eds. *Neural Bases of Speech, Hearing, and Language*. Boston: College-Hill Press, pp 146–200.

Barlow SM, Finan DS, Bradford PT, Andreatta RD. (1993). Transitional properties of the mechanically evoked perioral reflex from infancy through adulthood. *Brain Res* 623:181–188.

Barlow SM, Netsell R, Hunker CJ. (1986). Phonatory disorders associated with CNS lesions. In: Cummings CW, ed. *Otolaryngology—Head and Neck Surgery*. St. Louis: C.V. Mosby, pp 2087–2093.

Barlow SM, Suing G. (1991). AEROSPEECH: Automated digital signal analysis of speech aerodynamics. *J Comput Users Speech Hear* 7(2):211–227.

Barlow SM, Suing G, Andreatta RD. (1994). AEROWIN: Windows-based automated speech aerodynamics aquisition and analysis program. In: *Technical Report*. Bloomington: Neuro Logic Inc. and Indiana University Speech-Orofacial Physiology and Biomechanics Laboratory.

Bell-Berti F, Hirose H. (1975). Palatal activity in voicing distinctions: a simultaneous fiberoptic and electromyographic study. *J Phonet* 3:69–74.

Bell-Berti F, Krakow RA. (1991). Anticipatory velar lowering: a coproduction account. *J Acoust Soc Am* 90(1):112–123.

Bloomer, H. (1953). Observations on palatopharyngeal movements in speech and deglutition. *J Speech Hear Disord* 19:230–246.

Bosma JF. (1970). Summarizing and perspective comments. Part V. In: Bosma JF, ed. *Second Symposium on Oral Sensation and Perception*. Springfield, IL: Charles C. Thomas, pp 550–555.

Brooks VB, Thach WT. (1981). Cerebellar control of posture and movement. In: Brooks VB, ed. *Handbook of Physiology. Section I: The Nervous System. Vol. II: Motor Control.* Bethesda, MD: American Physiological Society, 1981.

Brinkman C, Porter R. (1978). Supplementary motor area in the monkey: activity of neurons during performance of a learned motor task. *J Neurophysiol* 42:681.

Calnan JS. (1953). Movements of the soft palate. *Br J Plast Surg* 5:286–296.

Chait D, D'Antonio LD, Lotz W, Netsell RW. (1984). Physiologic evaluation of speech disorders. *Neb Med J* 69:294–298.

Chiba T, Kajiyama M. (1958). *The Vowel, Its Nature and Structure.* Chiyoda Press, 1958.

Childers DG, Krishnamurthy AK. (1985). A critical review of electroglottography. *CRC Crit Rev Biomed Eng* 12:131–161.

Christiansen R, Moller K. (1971). Instrumentation for recording velar movement. *Am J Orthodont* 59:448–455.

Chuang CK, Wang WSy. (1978). Use of optical distance sensing to track tongue motion. *J Speech Hear Res* 21:482–496.

Dalston RM. (1982). Photodetector assessment of velopharyngeal activity. *Cleft Palate J* 19:1–8.

Dalston RM. (1989). Using simultaneous photodetection and nasometry to monitor velopharyngeal behavior during speech. *J Speech Hear Res* 32:195–202.

Dalston RM, Warren DW, Smith LR. (1990). The aerodynamic characteristics of speech produced by normal speakers and cleft palate speakers with adequate velopharyngeal function. *Cleft Palate J* 27(4):393–399.

D'Antonio L. (1985). Clinical aerodynamics for the evaluation and management of voice disorders. *Ear Nose Throat J*.

D'Antonio L, Chait D, Lotz W. (1986). Pediatric videonasendoscopy for speech and voice evaluation. *Otolaryngol Head Neck Surg* 94:578–583.

D'Antonio L, Chait D, Lotz W, Netsell R. (1987). Perceptual-physiologic approach to evaluation and treatment of dysphonia. *Ann Otol Rhinol Laryngol* 2:182–190.

de Jong K. (1991). An articulatory study of consonant-induced vowel duration changes in English. *Phonetica* 48:1–17.

DeNil LF, Abbs JH. (1991). Influence of speaking rate on the upper lip, lower lip, and jaw peak velocity sequencing during bilabial closing movements. *J Acoust Soc Am* 89(2):845–849.

Fetz EE, Cheney PD, German DC. (1976). Corticomotoneuronal connections of precentral cells detected by postspike averages of EMG activity in behaving monkeys. *Brain Res* 114:505.

Fletcher SG. (1989a). Palatometric specification of stop, affricate, and sibilant sounds. *J Speech Hear Res* 32:736–748.

Fletcher SG. (1989b). Visual articulatory training through dynamic orometry. *Volta Rev* 91(5):47–64.

Fletcher SG, Dagenais PA, Critz-Crosby P. (1991). Teaching vowels to profoundly hearing-impaired speakers using glossometry. *J Speech Hear Res* 34:943–956.

Fletcher SG, Hasegawa A, McCutcheon MJ, Gilliom J. (1980). Use of linguapalatal contact patterns to modify articulation in a deaf adult. In: McPherson DL, ed. *Advances in Prosthetic Devices for the Deaf: A Technical Workshop.* Rochester, NY: National Technical Institute for the Deaf.

Fletcher SG, McCutcheon J, Smith SC, Wilson HS. (1989). Glossometric measurements in vowel production and modification. *Clin Linguist Phonet* 3:359–375.

Fletcher SG, McCutcheon MJ, Wolf MB. (1975). Dynamic palatometry. *J Speech Hear Res* 18:812–819.

Folkins JW. (1981). Muscle activity for jaw closing during speech. *J Speech Hear Res* 24(4):601–615.

Folkins JW, Canty JL. (1986). Movements of the upper and lower lips during speech: interactions between lips with the jaw fixed at different positions. *J Speech Hear Res* 29(3):348–356.

Forner LL, Hixon TJ. (1987). Respiratory kinematics in profoundly hearing-impaired speakers. In: Hixon TJ, ed. *Respiratory Function in Speech and Song.* Boston: Little, Brown, pp 199–236.

Forrest K, Weismer G, Adams S. (1990). Statistical comparison of movement amplitudes from groupings of normal geriatric speakers. *J Speech Hear Res* 33(2):386–389.

Forrest K, Weismer G, Turner GS. (1989). Kinematic, acoustic, and perceptual analyses of connected speech produced by Parkinsonian and normal geriatric adults. *J Acoust Soc Am* 85(6):2608–2622.

Fujimura O, Kiritani S, Ishida H. (1973). Computer controlled radiography for observation of articulatory and other human organs. *Comput Biol Med* 3:371–384.

Graber TM, Bzoch KR, Aoba T. (1959). A functional study of the palatal and pharyngeal structures. *Angle Orthodont* 29:30–40.

Gracco VL. (1988). Timing factors in the coordination of speech movements. *J Neurosci* 8:4628–4639.

Gracco VL. (1994). Some organizational characteristics of speech movement control. *J Speech Hear Res* 37(1):4–27.

Hamlet SL, Momiyama Y. (1992). Velar activity and timing of eustachian tube function in swallowing. *Dysphagia* 7:226–233.

Harley WT. (1972). Dynamic palatography — A study of linguapalatal contacts during the production of selected consonant sounds. *J Prosthet Dent* 27:364–376.

Harrington R. (1944). A study of the mechanism of velopharyngeal closure. *J Speech Dis* 9:325–345.

Hepp-Reymond M-C, Wyss UR, Anner R. (1978). Neuronal coding of static force in the primate motor cortex. *J Physiol (Paris)* 74:287–291.

Hixon TJ. (1971). An electromagnetic method for transducing jaw movements during speech. *J Acoust Soc Am* 49:603–606.

Hixon TJ. (1987a). Respiratory function in speech. In: Hixon TJ, ed. *Respiratory Function in Speech and Song.* Boston: Little, Brown, pp 1–54.

Hixon TJ. (1987b). Some new techniques for measuring the biomechanical events of speech production: one laboratory's experiences. In: Hixon TJ, ed. *Respiratory Function in Speech and Song.* Boston: Little, Brown, pp 55–91.

Hixon TJ. (1987c). Speech breathing kinematics and mechanism inferences. In: Hixon TJ, ed. *Respiratory Function in Speech and Song.* Boston: Little, Brown, pp 237–257.

Hixon TJ, Goldman MD, Mead J. (1973). Kinematics of the chest wall during speech production: volume displacements of the rib cage, abdomen, and lung. *J Speech Hear Res* 16:78–115.

Hixon TJ, Goldman MD, Mead J. (1987). Kinematics of the chest wall during speech production: volume displacements of the rib cage, abdomen, and lung. In: Hixon TJ, ed. *Respiratory Function in Speech and Song.* Boston: Little, Brown, 1987, pp 93–133.

Hixon TJ, Mead J, Goldman MD. (1987). Dynamics of the chest wall during speech production: function of the thorax, rib cage, diaphragm, and abdomen. In: Hixon TJ, ed.

Respiratory Function in Speech and Song. Boston: Little, Brown, pp 135–197.

Hixon TJ, Putnam AHB. (1987). Voice abnormalities in relation to respiratory kinematics. In: Hixon TJ, ed. *Respiratory Function in Speech and Song.* Boston. Little, pp 259–280.

Hixon TJ, Putnam AHB, Sharp JT. (1987). Speech production with flaccid paralysis of the rib cage, diaphragm, and abdomen. In: Hixon TJ, ed. *Respiratory Function in Speech and Song.* Boston: Little, Brown, pp 311–336.

Hodge M, Rochet A. (1989). Characteristics of speech breathing in young women. *J Speech Hear Res* 32:466–480.

Hoit JD. (1994). A critical analysis of speech breathing data from the University of Queensland (letter). *J Speech Hear Res* 37(3):572–580.

Hoit JD, Banzett R, Brown R, Loring S. (1990). Speech breathing in individuals with cervical spinal cord injury. *J Speech Hear Res* 33:798–807.

Hoit JD, Hixon TJ. (1986). Body type and speech breathing. *J Speech Hear Res* 29:313–324.

Hoit JD, Hixon TJ. (1987). Age and speech breathing. *J Speech Hear Res* 30:351–366.

Holmberg EB, Hillman RE, Perkell JS. (1988). Glottal airflow and transglottal air pressure measurements for male and female speakers in soft, normal, and loud voice. *J Acoust Soc Am* 84:511–529.

Holmberg EB, Hillman RE, Perkell JS. (1989). Glottal airlflow and transglottal air pressure measurements for male and female speakers in low, normal, and high pitch. *J Voice* 3:294–305.

Horiguchi S, Bell-Berti F. (1987). The velotrace: a device for monitoring velar position. *Cleft Palate J* 24(2):104–111.

House AS, Fairbanks G. (1953). The influence of consonant environment upon the secondary acoustical characteristics of vowels. *J Acoust Soc Am* 25:105–113.

House RA. (1967). A study of tongue body motion during selected speech sounds. Doctoral dissertation, Univ. of Michigan.

Humphrey DR, Schmidt EM, Thompson WD. (1970). Predicting measures of motor performance from multiple cortical spike trains. *Science* 179:758.

Hunker CJ, Abbs JH, Barlow SM. (1982). The relationship between parkinsonian rigidity and hypokinesia in the orofacial system: a quantitative analysis. *Neurology* 32:755–761.

Johnson K. (1969). Mapping the movements of the human tongue. *Atom* 6:12–16.

Kandel ER, Schwartz JH, Jessell TM, eds. (1991). *Principles of Neural Science*, 3rd ed. New York: Elsevier Science.

Keefe MJ, Dalston RM. (1989). An analysis of velopharyngeal timing in normal adult speakers using a microcomputer based photodetector system. *J Speech Hear Res* 32:39–48.

Keller E, Ostry DJ. (1983). Computerized measurement of tongue dorsum movements with pulsed-echo ultrasound. *J Acoust Soc Am* 73(4):1309–1315.

Kiritani S, Itoh K, Fujimura O. (1975). Tongue-pellet trackig by a computer-controlled x-ray microbeam system. *J Acoust Soc Am* 57(6): 1516–1520.

Kiritani S, Itoh K, Fujisaki H, Sawashima M. (1976). Tongue pellet movement for the Japanese CV syllables—observations using the X-ray microbeam system. *Annl Bull Res Inst Logoped Phoniat* (Tokyo) 10:19–27.

Kuzmin YI. (1962). Mobile palatography as a tool for acoustic study of speech sounds. Report of Fourth International Congress on Acoustics, Copenhagen, paper G35.

Kydd W, Belt DA. (1964). Continuous palatography. *J Speech Hear Dis* 29:489–492.

Laine T, Warren DW, Dalston RM, Morr KE. (1989). Effects of velar resistance on speech aerodynamics. *Eur J Orthodont* 11:52–58.

Laine T, Warren DW, Dalston RM, Hairfield WM, Morr KE. (1988). Intraoral pressure, nasal pressure and airflow rate in cleft palate speech. *J Speech Hear Res* 31:432–437.

Larson CR. (1988). Brain mechanisms involved in the control of vocalization. *J Voice* 2:301–311.

Ludlow CL. (1976). Acoustic study of speech in Parkinson's disease. Paper presented at the Acoustical Soceity of America, San Diego.

Ludlow CL. (1981). Research needs for the assessment of phonatory function. *Proc Conf Assessment Vocal Pathol* 11:3.

Ludlow CL, Bassich CB. (1981). The differential diagnosis of syndromes of dysarthria using measures of speech production. In: *Speech and Language: Advances in Basic Research and Practice*. New York: Academic Press.

Manifold J, Murdoch B. (1993). Speech breathing in young adults: effect of body type. *J Speech Hear Res* 36:657–671.

Matsumura M, Kubota K. (1979). Cortical projection to hand-arm motor area from post-arcuate in macaque monkeys: a histological study

of retrograde transport of horseradish peroxidase. *Neurosci Lett* 11:241.

McClean MD, Beukelman DR, Yorkston KM. (1987). Speech-muscle visuomotor tracking in dysarthric and non-impaired speakers. *J Speech Hear Res* 30(2):276–282.

McClean MD, Goldsmith H, Cerf A. (1984). Lower lip EMG and displacement during bilabial disfluencies in adult stutterers. *J Speech Hear Res* 27(3):342–349.

McClean MD, Kroll RM, Loftus NS. (1990). Kinematic analysis of lip closure in stutterer's fluent speech. *J Speech Hear Res* 33(4):755–760.

McNeil MR, Weismer G, Adams S, Mulligan M. (1990). Oral structure non-speech motor control in normal, dysarthric, aphasic, and apraxic speakers: isometric force and static position control. *J Speech Hear Res* 33(2):255–268.

Michi K-I, Suzuki N, Yamashita Y, Imai S. (1986). Visual training and correction of articulation disorders by use of dynamic palatography: serial observation in a case of cleft palate. *J Speech Hear Dis* 51:226–238.

Moll KL. (1962). Velopharyngeal closure on vowels. *J Speech Hearing Res* 5:30–37.

Moll KL, Daniloff RG. (1971). Investigation of the timing of velar movements during speech. *J Acoust Soc Am* 50:673–684.

Moller K, Christiansen R. (1969). Instrumentation for recording velar movement. Paper presented at the Annual Convention of the American Speech and Hearing Association, Chicago.

Moller K, Martin R, Christiansen R. (1971). A technique for recording velar movement. *Cleft Palate J* 8:263–276.

Moon JB, Lagu RK. (1987). Development of a second-generation phototransducer for the assessment of velopharyngeal activity. *Cleft Palate J* 24(3):240–243.

Moon JB, Zembrowski P, Robin DA, Folkins JW. (1993). Visuomotor tracking ability of young adult speakers. *J Speech Hear Res* 36(4):672–682.

Moore CA. (1993). Symmetry of mandibular muscle activity as an index of coordinative strategy. *J Speech Hear Res* 36(6):1145–1157.

Moore CA, Smith A, Ringel RL. (1988). Task-specific organization of activity in human jaw muscles. *J Speech Hear Res* 31(4):670–680.

Muakkassa KF, Strick PL. (1979). Frontal lobe inputs to primate motor cortex: evidence for four somatotopically organized "premotor" areas. *Brain Res* 177:176–182.

Müller EM, Abbs JH. (1979). Strain gage transduction of lip and jaw motion in the midsagittal plane: Refinement of a prototype system. *J Acoust Soc Am* 65:481–486.

Murdoch B, Chenery H, Bowler S, Ingram J. (1989). Respiratory function in Parkinson's subjects exhibiting a perceptible speech defect: a kinematic and spirometric analysis. *J Speech Hear Dis* 54:610–626.

Murdoch B, Chenery H, Stokes P, Hardcastle W. (1991). Respiratory kinematics in speakers with cerebellar disease. *J Speech Hear Res* 34:768–780.

Murdoch B, Noble J, Chenery H, Ingram J. (1989). A spirometric and kinematic analysis of respiratory function in pseudobulbar palsy. *Aust J Hum Commun* 17:21–35.

Murdoch B, Theodoros D, Stokes P, Chenery H. (1993). Abnormal patterns of speech breathing in dysarthric speakers following severe closed head injury. *Brain Injury* 7(4):295–308.

Nelson WL, Perkell JS, Westbury JR. (1984). Mandible movements during increasingly rapid articulations of single syllables: preliminary observations. *J Acoust Soc Am* 75(3):945–951.

Netsell R, Lotz WK. (1994). Aerodynamic abnormalities and dysphonia (Personal communication).

Netsell R, Lotz WK, Barlow SM. (1989). A speech physiology examination for individuals with dysarthria. In Yorkston KM, Beukelman DR, eds. *Recent Advances In Clinical Dysarthria.* Boston: Little, Brown, pp 3–39.

Palmer JM. (1973). Dynamic palatography—general implications of locus and sequencing patterns. *Phonetica* 28:76–85.

Pandya DN, Vignolo LA. (1971). Intra- and interhemispheric projections of the precentral, premotor, and arcuate areas in the rhesus monkey. *Brain Res* 26:217.

Papcun G, Hochberg J, Thomas TR, Laroche F, Zacks J, Levy S. (1992). Inferring articulation and recognizing gestures from acoustics with a neural network trained on x-ray microbeam data. *J Acoust Soc Am* 92(2):688–700.

Paseman LA, Barlow SM, Philippbar S. (1994). The aerodynamics of laryngeal engagement in voice disorders. Convention Abstracts for the American Speech-Language-Hearing Association.

Perkell JS. (1969). Physiology of speech production: results and implications of a quantitative cineradiographic analysis. *Res Monogr* No. 53. Cambridge MA: MIT Press.

Perkell JS, Cohen MH, Svirsky MA, Matthies ML, Garabieta I, Jackson MTT. (1992). Electromagnetic midsagittal articulometer systems for transducing speech articulatory movements. *J Acoust Soc Am* 92:3078–3096.

Perkell JS, Matthies ML. (1992). Temporal measures of anticipatory labial coarticulation for the vowel /u/: within- and cross-subject variability. *J Acoust Soc Am* 91(5):2911–2925.

Perkell JS, Svirsky MA, Matthies ML, Manzella J. (1993). On the use of electro-magnetic midsagittal articulometer (EMMA) systems. *Forshungsberichte des Instituts für Phonetic und Sprachliche Kommunikation der Universität München (FIPKM)* 31:29–42.

Potter RK, Kopp GA, Green HC:. (1947). *Visible Speech.* New York: Van Nostrand.

Putnam AHB, Hixon TJ. (1987). Respiratory kinematics in speakers with motor neuron disease. In: Hixon TJ, ed. *Respiratory Function in Speech and Song.* Boston: Little, Brown, pp 281–309.

Samlan R, Barlow SM. (1996). The effects of transition rate and vowel height on velopharyngeal airway resistance. *Cleft Palate J* (in press).

Schell GR, Strick PL. (1984). The origin of thalamic inputs to the arcuate premotor and supplementary motor areas. *J Neurosci* 4:539.

Shaiman S. (1989). Kinematic and electromyographic responses to perturbation of the jaw. *J Acoust Soc Am* 86(1):78–88.

Shaiman S, Porter RJ Jr. (1991). Different phase-stable relationships of the upper lip and jaw for production of vowels and diphthongs. *J Acoust Soc Am* 90(6):3000–3007.

Sharkey SG, Folkins JW. (1985). Variability of lip and jaw movements in children and adults: Implications for the development of speech motor control. *J Speech Hear Res* 28(1):8–15.

Shawker TH, Stone M, Sonies BC. (1985). Tongue pellet tracking by ultrasound: Development of a reverberation pellet. *J Phonet* 13:135–146.

Shibata S. (1968). A study of dynamic palatography. *Annu Bull Res Inst Logoped Phoniat (Univ Tokyo)* 2:28–36.

Smith A. (1992). The control of orofacial movements in speech. *Crit Rev Oral Biol Med* 3(3):233–267.

Smith AM, Hepp-Reymond M-C, Wyss UR. (1975). Relation of activity in precentral cortical neurons to force and rate of force change during isometric contractions of finger muscles. *Exp Brain Res* 23:315–332.

Smith BL, Gartenberg TE. (1984). Initial observations concerning developmental characteristics of labio-mandibular kinematics. *J Acoust Soc Am* 75(5):1599–1605.

Smith BL, McLean-Muse A. (1986). Articulatory movement characteristics of labial consonant productions by children and adults. *J Acoust Soc Am* 80(5):1321–1328.

Smith BL, McLean-Muse A. (1987a). An investigation of motor equivalence in the speech of children and adults. *J Acoust Soc Am* 82(3):837–842.

Smith BL, McLean-Muse A. (1987b). Effects of rate and bite block manipulations on kinematic characteristics of children's speech. *J Acoust Soc Am* 81(3):747–754.

Smitheran J, Hixon TJ. (1981). Clinical method for estimating laryngeal airway resistance during vowel production. *J Speech Hear Dis* 46:138–146.

Solomon NP, Hixon TJ. (1993). Speech breathing in Parkinson's disease. *J Speech Hear Res* 36:294–310.

Stone M. (1990). A three dimensional model of tongue movement based on ultrasound and x-ray microbeam data. *J Acoust Soc Am* 87(5):2207–2217.

Stone M, Shawker TH, Talbot TL, Rich H. (1988). Cross sectional tongue shape during the production of vowels. *J Acoust Soc Am* 83(4):1586–1596.

Sussman HM, Westbury JR. (1981). The effects of antagonistic gestures on temporal and amplitude parameters of anticipatory labial co-articulation. *J Speech Hear Res* 24(1):16–24.

Titze IR. (1990). Interpretation of the electroglottographic signal. *J Voice* 4:1–9.

Tye-Murray N. (1991). The establishment of open articulatory postures by deaf and hearing talkers. *J Speech Hear Res* 34:453–459.

Tye-Murray N, Folkins JW. (1990). Jaw and lip movements of deaf talkers producing utterances with known stress patterns. *J Acoust Soc Am* 87(6):2675–2683.

Warren DW. (1967). Nasal emission of air and velopharyngeal function. *Cleft Palate J* 4:148–156.

Warren DW. (1975). The determination of velopharyngeal incompetence by aerodynamic and acoustical techniques. *Clin in Plast Surg* 2(2):299–304.

Warren DW. (1988). Aerodynamics of speech. In: Lass NJ, ed. *Handbook of Speech-Language Pathology and Audiology*. Toronto: Decker.

Warren DW. (1982). Aerodynamics of speech. In: Lass NJ, McReynolds LV, Northern JL, Yoder DE, eds. *Speech, Language, and Hearing*. Philadelphia: W.B. Saunders, pp 219–245.

Warren DW, Dalston RM, Trier WC, Holder MB. (1985). A pressure-flow technique for quantifying temporal patterns of palatopharyngeal closure. *Cleft Palate J* 22:11–19.

Warren DW, DuBois A. (1964). A pressure-flow technique for measuring velopharyngeal orifice area during continuous speech. *Cleft Palate J* 1:52–71.

Van der Giet G. (1977). Computer-controlled method for measuring articulatory activities. *J Acoust Soc Am* 61(4):1072–1076.

Watkin KL. (1993). Personal communication. Ultrasonic Imaging Laboratory. McGill University, Montreal, Quebec, Canada, 1993.

Watkin KL, Baer LH, Mathur S, Jones R, Hakim S, Diouf I, Nuwayhid B, Khalife S. (1993). Three-dimensional reconstruction and enhancement of freely acquired 2D medical ultrasonic images. Canadian Conference on Electrical and Computer Engineering.

Watkin KL, Rubin JM. (1989). Pseudo-three-dimensional reconstruction of ultrasonic images of the tongue. *J Acoust Soc Am* 85(1):496–499.

Westbury JR. (1991). The significance and measurement of head position during speech production experiments using the x-ray microbeam system. *J Acoust Soc Am* 89(4):1782–1791.

Acknowledgment

This work was supported in part by a grant from the National Institutes of Health (DC-00365-08) and Neuro Logic, Incorporated, Bloomington, Indiana.

Chapter 7

Electromyographic Techniques for the Assessment of Motor Speech Disorders

Erich S. Luschei and Eileen M. Finnegan

Introduction

Scientists discovered, during the mid-19th century, that very small electrical currents were generated by contracting muscles. By 1912 (Piper, 1912), instruments used for detecting these "action currents" had become sensitive enough to record voluntary muscle activity in humans. Limitations in the photographic recording devices available at that time provided records that were only a second or 2 in duration, but these records were sufficient to provide our first insights into the control of muscle by the nervous system. The signal recorded by this method was called the "electromyogram," and is still known by that name today. It is often abbreviated to "EMG." Although the study of the EMG signal has been widely used as a research tool for studying muscle and the general principles of motor control in the body, it has also evolved into a medical procedure that is used in hospitals and clinics throughout the world.

The primary purpose of this chapter is to help the reader better understand EMG procedures: where the signal comes from, the instrumentation used to record it, and how the signals may be processed and interpreted. Before considering those topics, however, it may be of interest to consider a few examples of how EMG recording is used in modern medical settings.

Diagnosis of Systemic Neurological Diseases

Suppose a patient comes to clinic complaining of very significant weakness. This could result from diseases at several sites in the peripheral or central nervous system. One site is the neuromuscular junction, where action potentials in motor nerve fibers cause action potentials in muscle cells. Failure of the neuromuscular junction is the cause of diseases such as myasthenia gravis, or the result of poisoning by toxins (botulinum toxin for example). Another potential cause is failure of conduction in peripheral nerves (peripheral neuropathy). Another chilling possibility is amyotropic lateral sclerosis (ALS), in which motoneurons slowly die. In considering this problem, it should be emphasized that an experienced clinician would probably have a good idea about which of these possibilities was the most likely cause of the weakness without using an EMG exam, based upon the history and a physical exam. The prognosis and treatment of the weakness would be very different, however, for the different possible causes, so any responsible clinician would want to have as much reliable information as possible before informing the patient and/or starting treatment. In this case, as in all others, EMG recordings yield additional information that has to be interpreted within the context of all other medical information. It is likely, in this hypothetical case of weakness, that a neurologist would order an EMG exam from a special diagnostic lab. Peripheral nerves in the forearm containing motor nerves to muscles in the hand may be percutaneously stimulated while recording the EMG of the hand muscles. The synchrony of the electrical nerve stimulation produces a large evoked EMG potential that can document the viability of the neuromuscular junction and also measure the conduction velocity of the action potentials in the peripheral nerves. The types of activity and waveforms of EMG potentials, recorded with needle electrodes inserted into the muscles, may definitively diagnose the disease of ALS.

Generally speaking, the diagnosis of motor disorders in neurological clinics is currently the main well-established clinical use of EMG recording and analysis. Texts such as that by Kimura (1989) cover the substantive issues in detail, so will not be repeated in the current chapter. The types of electrodes used in neurological EMG analysis will be covered later, however, since the terminology can be a matter of significant confusion.

Evaluation of Paralyzed or Spastic Muscles

When a person cannot move a limb or articulator, it can be surprisingly difficult to know the exact cause. Damage to a particular nerve, either as the result of trauma, a surgical procedure, or simply as a "spontaneous" event can produce what appears to be "paralysis." One such problem that is familiar to speech-language pathologists who work in the field of voice and their colleagues in the medical field of otolaryngology, is unilateral vocal fold paralysis. The condition is given this name because one of the vocal folds does not appear to move. The presumptive cause is damage to or cutting of the recurrent laryngeal nerve. One of the pioneers in the use of electromyography of laryngeal muscles, Faaborg-Andersen (1957), studied EMG signals from "paralyzed" laryngeal muscles of patients with a presumptive diagnosis of unilateral vocal

fold paralysis, and observed that many of them in fact exhibit EMG activity. Other otolaryngology studies have confirmed this observation (Blair, Berry, & Briant, 1978; Haglund, Knutsson, & Martensson, 1972; Hirano, Nozoe, Shin, & Maeyama, 1987; Hiroto, Hirano, & Tomita, 1968; Min, Finnegan, Hoffman, Luschei, & McCulloch, 1994; Parnes & Satya, 1985; Thumfart, 1981). Failure of a limb or articulator to move, or exhibit a normal range of motion, can have several causes: damage to motoneurons or motor nerves, mechanical changes in joints, cocontraction of antagonist muscle groups, or inappropriate reinnervation of muscles following nerve damage. Laryngeal muscle EMG recording is beginning to be used to help resolve some of these possibilities as they relate to unilateral vocal fold paralysis (Berry & Blair, 1980; Crumley, 1989; Hoffman, Brunberg, Winter, Sullivan, & Kileny, 1991; Kokesh, Flint, Robinson, & Cummings, 1993; Lewis, Crumley, Blanks, & Pitcock, 1991; Mu & Yang, 1991), but the procedure is far less widespread and "mature" than the procedures used in neurological diagnostic EMG labs.

Many readers may wonder, at this point, "Why don't the voice specialists with a patient with an immobile vocal fold just send the patient to the neurology EMG lab?" This could very well be done. The premise of this chapter is, however, that the interests of patients with dysarthrias will be best served by speech-language pathologists who are directly involved in EMG procedures. An appreciation of the anatomy and physiology of the articulators, the characteristics of speech and swallowing, and certain technical aspects of doing EMG recordings from inaccessible muscles that move vigorously during function will greatly improve any EMG procedures that are done. A speech-language pathologist may have more knowledge in these areas than a neurologist who has not specialized in the study of the articulators. Thus the speech-language pathologist has much to offer even if an EMG recording were conducted in a neurology EMG lab.

Many dysarthrias result from central nervous system disorders that produce abnormally high levels of activity (spasticity) in groups of muscles of the limbs and articulators. In some cases the ability of patients to walk, for instance, can be improved by surgically cutting the tendon of certain spastic muscles that are causing the most interference with the function. It may be difficult to know, ahead of time, which muscle is the "culprit" just using physical examination. In these cases, surgeons can use EMG recording to help make their decision about which muscle to tenotomize (Cahan, Adams, Perry, & Beeler, 1990; Keenan, 1988; Sutherland, Larsen, & Mann, 1975). Although surgery of this type is not used to treat the dysarthrias, a related procedure, reversible paralysis of muscles by injection of botulinum toxin has been widely used to treat certain dystonias (Brin et al, 1987; Cohen & Thompson, 1987; Cohen, Hallett, Geller, & Hochberg, 1989; Jankovic & Orman, 1987; Mauriello, 1985; Scott, 1980; Stager & Ludlow, 1994; Tsui, Eisen, Mak, Caruthers, Scott, & Calne, 1985). In this procedure, EMG recording can be used as an aid to verify the injection site (Blitzer, Brin, Fahn, & Lovelace, 1988; Ludlow, Hallett, Sedory, Fujita, & Naunton, 1990; Ludlow, Naunton, Sedory, Schulz, & Hallett, 1988; Ludlow, Naunton, Terada, & Anderson, 1991; Miller, Woodson, & Jankovic, 1987; Min, Luschei, Finnegan, McCullough, & Hoffman, 1994).

The goal of this chapter is provide a resource for anyone who wishes to use or better understand how to record and interpret the EMG. It seems likely that it has many uses in addition to the examples given above, including the study and treatment of motor speech disorders. It is appreciated by the authors that technical procedures of this type are somewhat foreign to many clinical speech pathologists, not only because they appear to interfere with the person-to-person relationship, which is the heart and soul of the profession, but also because the instrumentation has too many knobs and wires. On the first point, it may be helpful to consider the fact that EMG recording is merely a way of extending the clinician's senses to obtain information that we can't ordinarily

sense. As for the second point, it seems likely that the problems of "too many knobs and wires" will be eased a great deal in the future by EMG instrumentation designed for clinical use rather than for research. In addition, however, most clinicians will find the knobs and wires relatively simple once they are understood.

Principles of EMG Recording

Source of the EMG Signal

An action potential must sweep along muscles cells in order for a muscle to contract. These action potentials create, as they move along, minute electrical currents flowing outside the muscle cells (Fig. 7–1). These tiny currents don't really do anything. They are just there as a part of the process, like the bow wave on a ship going through the water.

The nervous system activates muscles in terms of motor units, defined as "a motoneuron and all the muscle cells it innervates."

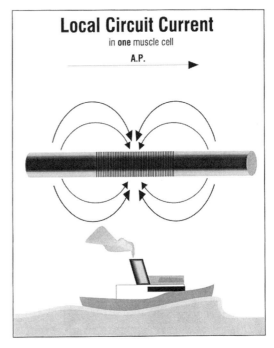

Figure 7–1. The extracellular current caused by an action potential sweeping along the muscle cell is analogous to the bow and stern wave caused by a ship going through the water.

Because all the muscle cells in one motor unit "fire" (have action potentials) at the same time, the tiny extracellular currents from individual muscle cells add up to produce a current which is rather easily detected by recording electrodes. Since these currents are going in the same direction at the same time, the total waveform is stereotyped. Such a potential is called a "single motor unit potential" (Fig. 7–2). This potential is equivalent to a group of ships going through the water in precise synchrony; their bow waves would add up and produce quite a wave!

Because the firing of the motoneurons of a naturally activated muscle is not synchronized, the single motor unit potentials interact with one another in a complex manner, and produce an interference pattern. Referring to our earlier analogy, one may imagine hundreds of groups of ships racing up and down the waterway. Their bow waves would interact and produce a "chop," which is just an hydraulic interference pattern. One may intuitively sense that the size of the "chop" will be related to the number of groups of ships that are traveling about. Obviously the more ships, the higher the "chop." The EMG interference pattern is no different; the more motor units that are active, the "higher" the EMG signal. (Typical records showing such an interference pattern are illustrated in Fig. 7–7a.) The metric to be used for describing the "height" of the EMG is a complicated matter, however, which will be considered later. For the moment, it can be taken as a fact that the size of the EMG signal bears a monotonic relationship to the degree to which the muscle has been activated.

Electrode Configuration in EMG Recording

The EMG signal is almost always recorded with a differential amplifier, which creates an output that is proportional (and much larger) than the difference in the voltage of its two inputs. How these two inputs are spaced with respect to the active muscle has a large effect on the nature of the EMG signal and the interpretation one can apply to it. Let's go back to the hydraulic analogy. Suppose we wanted to measure the "chop" on the water created by the ships dashing about. The use of a differential amplifier is equivalent to measuring the height of the water between two points. Suppose these two points are close together, say a foot apart. If a bunch of ships were steaming around miles away from our two recording points, the size of the chop would be much attenuated by the time it got to us. Also, all the little peaky white caps would be gone; we would just see small slow "rollers" going by. So our signal would be small, and it would be composed of low frequencies. However if we had our two recording points right out in the midst of all those ships, we would detect large water height differences, And many of the waves would have sharp peaks. In this case, our signal would be large and be composed of much higher frequencies than when the recording points were distant from "the action."

When the electrodes are far apart, they are able to "survey" activity over large areas. This has some advantages in some circumstances, but in this case the source of the activity is not known with precision. This can

Single Motor Unit Response
From **many** muscle cells

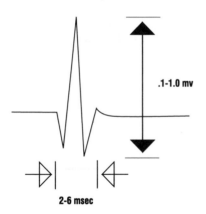

.1-1.0 mv

2-6 msec

Figure 7–2. Drawing of a typical "single motor unit potential" caused by synchronous firing of muscle action potentials in all the muscle fibers innervated by a single motor unit.

be a major diagnostic problem. Suppose your electrodes are far apart in a paralyzed muscle. Adjacent muscles that are active may produce a sizable EMG signal. Such "distant" activity would be relatively small compared to what one would expect of a normally active muscle, and would be composed of low frequency waveforms. Thus one would suspect (hopefully) that the activity was not from the muscle under study. Close-spaced electrodes tend to "reject" muscle activity from distant active muscles, however, and would be preferable, therefore, in assessing a muscle suspected of being paralyzed.

Four generalizations about amplification and electrodes spacing may be offered at this points:

1. Differential amplifiers are essential.
2. Close electrode spacing is the best in the majority of cases.
3. Muscle activity close to the electrodes is represented by a signal having high frequencies, often showing characteristic single motor unit waveforms. Such signals sound "crisp" in the audio monitor (see below).
4. Signals from distant active muscles may be picked up even by electrodes that are very close together. These signals are composed predominantly of low frequencies, however, and sound "dull" and "muffled" compared to the signals of nearby muscle fibers.

For readers desiring a more rigorous treatment of this topic, an excellent review article is that by De Luca (1986). Another excellent source, covering myoelectric theory and many very pragmatic issues in EMG recording, is that by Loeb and Gans (1986).

Instrumentation

Overview

The scheme represented in Figure 7–3 identifies some of the major aspects of an overall instrumentation system. Three electrodes

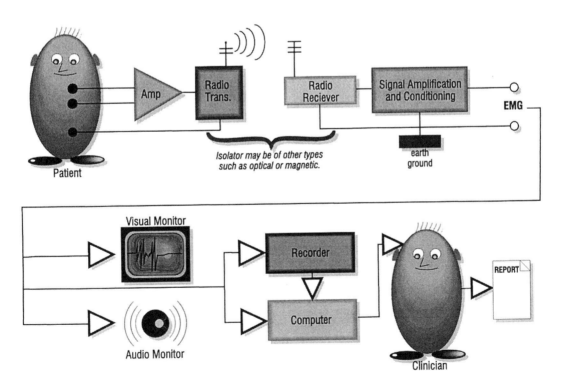

Figure 7–3. Major components of an EMG instrumentation system.

are attached to the patient. One of these, the "reference" lead, is attached to the skin with a conductive gel electrode, and serves to hold the subject's body, as a whole, to the electrical reference voltage of the EMG amplifier and input stage of the isolator. The other two electrodes are the inputs to the differential amplifier, and their difference in voltage is amplified by the gain of the amplifier. This amplified voltage difference is applied to the input stage of the isolator. The input stage of the isolator modulates a very low power radio transmitter as a simple linear function of the signal. It should be realized, however, that radio transmission is only one of several ways of sending the information in the signal across an insulating gap. The output stage of the isolator is a radio receiver that demodulates the radio signal to recover an exact replica of the EMG signal which now can be safely referenced to earth ground. The rationale for use of the isolator stage will be discussed in detail below.

The EMG signal may be further amplified and processed, such as being bandpass filtered, before it is presented to the eye and/or ear of the clinician. On-line monitors are very useful to make sure the recordings are proceeding appropriately, but documentation and objective analysis requires that the signal be permanently recorded. This can be done by tape recorders, which then may be played back off-line to a computer for analysis. Alternatively, state-of-the-art computers may now be used as the data acquisition recording device, as well as serve for data analysis. The last stage of this "system," perhaps the most essential, is the experience and intelligence of the clinician in interpreting the EMG signal.

The instrumentation system just described may be usefully regarded as being like a "chain" insofar as it is only as strong as its weakest link. Inappropriate electrodes, amplifiers, or recorders that are noisy or lacking in fidelity, or lack of experience by the clinician in recognizing artifactual signals, for example, can all defeat an otherwise adequate system. It will, therefore, be useful to

consider these various parts of the system in detail.

Electrodes

There are basically three types of electrodes that have been widely used in EMG recording: skin electrodes, intramuscular fine-wire (hooked-wire) electrodes, and intramuscular rigid needle electrodes. The latter two types are schematically illustrated, along with their usual connections to a differential amplifier, in Figure 7–4.

Skin Electrodes

Muscle activity from large muscles directly under the skin may be easily detected and quantified by simply attaching metal disk electrodes to the skin surface. This approach often seems most desirable because it is noninvasive. No one seems to like needles! The fact of the matter is, however, that there are major limitations to the use of skin electrodes by speech-language pathologists; most of the muscles involved in speech and oral functions such as swallowing are not directly under the skin. These muscles are also relatively small and complex in their anatomy, so records obtained with skin electrodes provide only a limited measure of how these muscle systems are operating. The lips are an exception, however. Lip EMG during speech may be easily recorded with skin electrodes (Cole, Konopacki, & Abbs, 1983; McClean, 1991; Smith, 1989; Smith, McFarland, Weber, & Moore, 1987). The surface lip EMG signal can sometimes be misleading, however, because it may reflect the activity of different muscles or functionally different motor units within what is anatomically one muscle (Blair & Smith, 1986). Surface electrodes placed over the masseter muscles can record an EMG signal related to vigorous jaw motion or relatively forcible biting. These electrodes may detect some low-level activity during speech tasks (Moore, Smith, & Ringel, 1988), but the exact source of this activity is uncertain. It could be from remote jaw muscles or from small facial muscles located under the skin close to

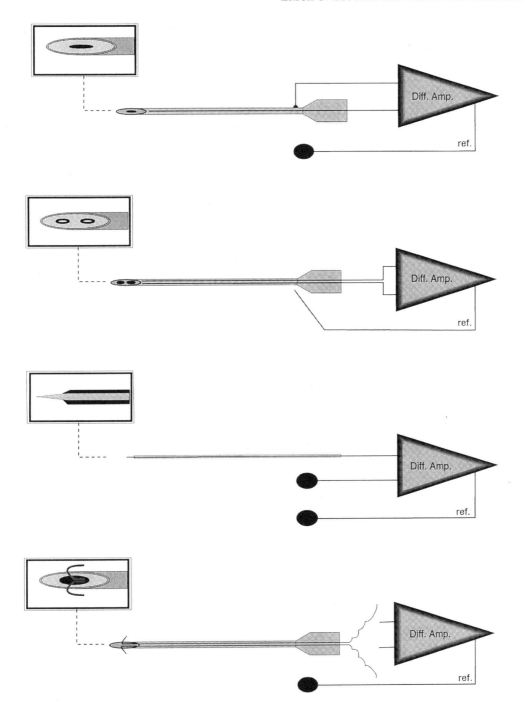

Figure 7–4. Four types of needle electrodes, numbered from top down, respectively: (1) concentric needle electrode; (2) bipolar concentric needle electrode; (3) monopolar needle electrode; and (4) bipolar hooked-wire electrodes.

or overlying the masseter muscle—ie, buccinator or platysma.

One skin electrode that is common to all of the recording schemes to be discussed is the electrode attached to the reference (common) input to the differential amplifier. This is a very important electrode because a stable low-resistance contact between the skin and metal wire carrying the signal to the amplifier is critical to good noise-free recording conditions. This is facilitated by carefully cleaning the skin before the electrode is secured in place by an adhesive collar. After cleaning the skin, a conductive electrode gel is then applied to the "cup" of the electrode containing the metal surface, and the electrode attached to the skin. The metal inside the electrode "cup" is a complicated material generally made of compressed silver powder and "special ingredients" known only to the manufacturer. In the experience of the author, some commercial skin electrodes are better than others, and all of the good ones are surprisingly expensive (but well worth the cost). Large commercial disposable electrodes made for hospital recording of the electrocardiogram (ECG) are too large for placing over most muscles, but make excellent skin electrodes for the reference electrode. They come with the gel and adhesive collar in place, and because of their large size, provide an excellent electrical contact without excessive skin preparation.

Rigid Needle Electrodes
Needle electrodes for recording the EMG are basically a long thin hypodermic needle with one or two insulated wires in the lumen. If there is one wire, the needle is usually called a "concentric" EMG electrode. If there are two wires, then it is called a "concentric bipolar" electrode. When using a concentric electrode, one input of the differential amplifier is connected to the center wire of the electrode, and the shaft of the hypodermic needle (which is uninsulated) is connected to the other amplifier input. The signal that is picked up by this electrode is any voltage difference that exists between the exposed center wire at the tip and the shaft, which is

essentially held at a neutral "reference" voltage by its large uninsulated area. This electrode can be quite "selective" in recording single motor units. The third wire of the electrode is connected to the reference point on the patient (the skin of the forehead is often convenient when studying cranial muscles).

When using concentric bipolar electrodes, the inputs to the differential amplifier are connected to the two wires in the lumen of the needle. The shaft of the needle may be connected to the reference input of the amplifier, but this is not necessary. The reference input may be connected to a distant point on the skin. The concentric bipolar electrode is more "selective" than the concentric electrode, particularly if the needle can be rotated when in place. This can change the alignment of the two exposed wire tips at the lumen of the needle with respect to the direction of the muscle fibers; such alignment can have a dramatic effect on the degree to which a particular muscle fiber action potential is picked up. From a practical standpoint, concentric bipolar electrodes are more expensive than concentric electrodes, and thus used mainly for research or specialized studies.

Monopolar EMG electrodes are insulated solid needles whose tip has been bared of the insulating material. The wire from the needle is connected to one input of the differential amplifier, and the other input of the amplifier is connected to a second skin electrode (in addition to the electrode connected to the reference input to the amplifier). One might suppose it would be simpler to connect the second input of the amplifier directly to the reference input. If this is done, however, the resistance to ground of the two inputs will be greatly unbalanced. This condition increases the response of the system to external noise. Monopolar electrodes record muscle activity just as well as the other types, but they are also more responsive to activity generated in muscles distant to the one being studied, i.e. they are less selective. The monopolar arrangement is, in effect, the type of recording configuration used when one records from the tip of an insulated hypodermic needle used to inject botulinum toxin in a laryngeal muscle.

Rigid needle electrodes are used almost exclusively in most EMG diagnostic clinics, such as those found in departments of neurology. This is because the waveform and firing patterns of single motor units are of primary interest in diagnosing most neurological diseases that affect muscle activity. These electrodes can be advanced and withdrawn by the clinician to isolate particular units. When used in muscles directly under the skin during isometric contraction, in which there is relatively little actual movement of the muscle tissue, these electrodes are relatively painless to the patient, and do little damage to the muscle. When used to record from small and/or thin muscles, particularly during functions that involve significant movements, this type of electrode has serious problems. First of all, an EMG interference pattern, as distinct from single motor unit activity, is useful for determining if and how much a muscle can be activated. Concentric bipolar electrodes are very selective for single motor units, so one might see little, if any, evidence of activity in a normal muscle, even at fairly high levels of activation. Another serious problem is that movement of a muscle with a rigid needle in it can be quite painful. Pain from this source may have large effects on the motoneuron pool that one is attempting to study, as well as hurt the patient. If the larynx, pharynx, or other oral structure remained very still, this probably wouldn't be a significant factor, but large, vigorous, movements occur during speaking and swallowing. Movements of the very sharp tip of a rigid needle electrode within a small muscle could cause damage. Furthermore, these movements could cause the population of motor units under observation to change each time they occur. This would make it difficult to quantitatively compare a current EMG record with one taken before the movement occurred. There are currently no empirical studies to show that these possible problems actually occur, although this is the subject of an ongoing study in one of the authors' laboratory. To start with, however, it is worth keeping in mind that rigid EMG electrodes are not the only or necessarily the best electrodes when one is attempting to study natural movements, particularly of the articulators.

The main advantage of rigid needle electrodes is that they may be advanced and withdrawn in the muscle to explore various parts of a muscle, or to be redirected to other muscles. The potentials they record during short periods of relative immobility of muscles can provide valuable information. Such information has to do with the shape of action potentials. These potentials can confirm diagnoses of diseases such as ALS, or indicate whether a muscle is being reinnervated. When these are the main diagnostic questions, the EMG recording and interpretation is obviously best done by an experienced neurologist.

Bipolar Hooked-Wire Electrodes

Hooked wire electrodes were first used by Basmajian and Stecko (1962), who, in collaboration with several colleagues, described the activity of many muscles of the body during natural movements. These observations are summarized in a classic book *Muscles Alive* (Basmajian & De Luca, 1985). This type of intramuscular electrode has also been used for study and assessment of laryngeal muscles (Freeman & Ushijima, 1978; Gartlan, Peterson, Luschei, Hoffman, & Smith, 1993; Hirano & Ohala, 1969; Hirose, 1987; Koda & Ludlow, 1992; Thumfart, 1988; Woo and Arandia, 1992), tongue (Borden & Gay, 1978; Hrycyshyn & Basmajian, 1972; Mowrey & McKay, 1990; Palmer, Rudin, Lara, & Crompton, 1992; Sauerland & Mitchell, 1975), velum (Basmajian & Dutta, 1961; Bell-Berti, 1976; Benguerel, Hirose, Sawashima, & Ushijima, 1975; Cooper & Folkins, 1985; Fritzell, 1969; Fritzell & Kotby, 1976; Hairston & Sauerland, 1981; Kiritani, Hirose, & Sawashima, 1980; Kuehn, Folkins, & Cutting, 1982; Kuehn, Folkins, & Linville, 1988; Seaver & Kuehn, 1980; Ushijima & Hirose, 1974), and pharynx (Hairston & Sauerland, 1981; Palmer, Tanaka, & Siebens, 1989; Perlman, Luschei, & DuMond, 1989; Rowe,

Miller, Chierici, & Clendenning, 1984) as well as some combinations of these muscles (Hunker & Abbs, 1990; Neilson & O'Dwyer, 1984; O'Dwyer, Neilson, Guitar, Quinn, & Andrews, 1983; Palmer, Tippett, & Wolf, 1991; Schaefer et al, 1992). They are made with two very fine, flexible, insulated wires. For recording gross EMG, about 1 mm of insulation is removed from each wire. These two wires are placed in the lumen of a suitable hypodermic needle so that the bared portions extend just beyond the tip, and then the ends of the wire are bent over to form a "hook." When the needle is placed into the muscle and then withdrawn, the hooks catch in the muscle and the wires are left behind in the muscle. Because of the flexibility of the wires, the muscle may make large movements without causing pain. Most people find these electrodes quite comfortable. They may be left in place during repeated measures of speech and swallowing.

While there are several good reasons for using hook-wire electrodes, they have the major disadvantage of not permitting adjustments of the electrode position once the hypodermic needle has been withdrawn. Obviously the electrode cannot be pushed further into the muscle. One could imagine (naively) that one could gently tug on the wires and pull them along the route of the wires through the muscle. To do this, however, the hooks have to be straightened out, and once this is done, the wires do not generally remain in the muscle. For all practical purposes, one gets one attempt per needle. When recording from laryngeal muscles, it is advisable to have extra electrode assemblies to try a second or third time to get the wires into the desired muscle.

Choosing the wire for these electrodes is a compromise between using wires that are too ductile and wires that are too stiff. Very ductile wires can be inserted with very fine needles, and cause no sensation in the muscle. But their hooks are very weak, and they often do not "hook" into the muscle, and get pulled out with the needle. On the other hand, their weak hooks probably do minimal damage when these wires have to

be pulled out after the recording is over. Stainless steel wire with an uninsulated diameter of 50 or 75 μm (0.002 or 0.003 inch) are the most widely used types of wire. They generally hold the "hook," and produce only a slight "funny feeling" in the muscle. They probably damage some muscle cells when the hook is pulled out, but there is no pain associated with this event, so the damage is quite limited. Single-strand 75-μm stainless steel wire with various types of insulation is available in small quantities from several vendors in the United States. Some companies will fabricate special configurations of fine wire (usually for a minimum order of 1000 ft). One such configuration, "bifiler," where two strands of wire are bonded together along their entire length, has two advantages to using two wires that are not bonded together. First of all, the bared ends of bonded wire remain in a fixed relationship, and in particular cannot "short together" in the muscle as it moves. Second, the fact that the two wires have to move together greatly reduces their tendency to produce movement artifacts and microphonics when they are mechanically disturbed. An explanation of this property is offered later in the chapter.

Once the wire is chosen, one has to select a needle size. A 25-gauge hypodermic needle is suitable for a pair of 75-μm diameter wires. In some cases, one can choose a smaller needle that will accept the wires, but the fit is so close that the wires often "hang up" when the needle is withdrawn, so the wires get pulled out; the wires have to have enough room in the lumen of the needle to accommodate slight bends in the wire. A single strand of insulated 75-μm wire can be inserted with a 30-gauge needle, but this requires two needle insertions for differential recording. The larger electrode spacing obtained in this case may be advantageous, however, if the goal is to sample a large area of a muscle.

When placing the electrode in a package for sterilization, it is important to use a relatively large package so the wires may be loosely looped in a way that allows them to be straightened out without forming kinks when the package is opened. Once formed, these kinks are impossible to remove. Because the hypodermic needle cannot be pulled passed a kink in the wire, such an electrode might as well be discarded before the electrode is inserted into the muscle.

Connecting the amplifier to fine wires can be more troublesome than one might suppose. If one uses very long pieces of fine wire, then these leads may be taken directly to the inputs to the amplifier and put under a screw-type terminal (gold-plated surfaces are a very good idea). However, these long wires have a tendency to become tangled and form kinks when removed from the sterilization packages. The wires may be kept much shorter if the amplifier has a preamplifier stage in a small box that can be placed close to the patient. Such a preamplifier stage may have screw-type terminals as well, but spacing usually makes it desirable to have a wire "grabber" that requires less manipulation than a screw terminal. One may use spring-loaded commercial "grabbers," but keep in mind that the very small size of the wire requires a close-tolerance fit of the "jaws," and that an oxide coating on either the wires or the grabber surfaces can cause electrical "noises" that can interfere with recording. Grabbers with gold-plated surfaces are, for this reason, much to be preferred. We currently use gold-plated extension springs to make contact with the fine wires. The

springs are bent to open a few loops, the wire inserted between them, and the spring allowed to straighten out. They seem to be a vast improvement over other methods we have used previously.

Amplifiers

To detect and study the activity of muscles requires one or more differential amplifiers that have a selection of gains between about 1000 and 50,000 (60 dB to 94 dB) with a bandpass between 30 Hz and 5 kHz. These characteristics are easily obtained with modern electronics. In a clinical situation, it is often difficult to control external sources of 60-cycle interference, so a 60-Hz notch filter in the amplifier can be quite helpful. A very important feature of the amplifier is its "common mode rejection ratio" (CMRR). When used with the proper electrode configuration, an amplifier with a high CMRR is the most effective way to prevent amplification of the 60 cycle electrical fields. There are companies that manufacture amplifiers that are marketed specifically for recording EMG activity. One pays a premium for such equipment, however, and the fact of the matter is that the electronic requirements are easily met by devices made from a few integrated circuits, resistors, and capacitors. Whatever amplifier is purchased or fabricated, it is crucial that it include an isolation

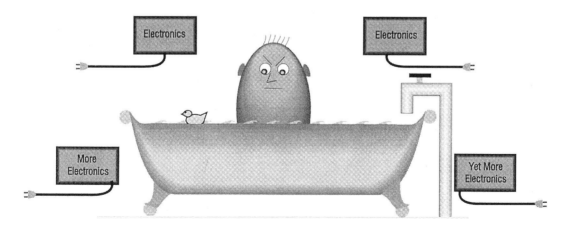

Figure 7–5. Earth-grounding a person is like putting them in a bath tub, from the standpoint of electrical safety.

stage. The function of an isolation stage is to avoid having the patient connected to earth ground. Connecting a subject to earth ground with a low resistance electrode (the large skin electrode) is essentially like standing the patient in a bathtub (Fig. 7–5). In this condition, the patient could be electrocuted by coming into contact with any equipment that is electrically "hot."

In the scheme illustrated earlier, such isolation is represented by using radio signals to transmit the output of the first stage of amplification to the earth-grounded part of the system. In this case, the patient could possibly be on the moon! *It is impossible to accidentally electrocute anyone who has no electrical connection to earth ground!* Use of the proper equipment eliminates this danger, but it is possible for a person to unwittingly defeat this safety feature by connecting the reference (indifferent) electrode to earth ground, or, for example, by having the patient sitting on a grounded chair. It should be noted that radio transmission is certainly not the most common way of achieving isolation. It was chosen for illustration because it is intuitively easy to understand. The same effect can be achieved by using modulated light or magnetic fields to couple the signal across a "gap" that keeps the patient totally isolated from earth ground.

Setting the appropriate gain of an amplifier is a matter of some judgment. Usually, the gain is set so the largest potentials observed stay within the input range of the recording instrument. If one suspects muscle paralysis, or is seeking evidence of low-level activity, one should not hesitate to try the highest gains on the amplifier, even if some other events and/or noise go outside the range. Some motor unit activity in a muscle is very small, and can "hide" within the noise of the baseline if gains of 1K–5K are the only ones used. Unless higher gains are used, the "failure to observe activity" in a muscle is questionable.

Monitors

A type of monitor that has traditionally been used with the EMG is an audio amplifier connected to a loudspeaker. This type of monitor has several advantages. It is inexpensive, you don't have to watch it, and the human can, with some experience, use his or her "ears" to perform an acoustic analysis that can provide critical on-line information. For example, the sound of muscle activity that is close to an intramuscular electrode sounds "crisp" because it has mainly high-frequency components. EMG from muscles located at greater distance has a "dull" sound. This is because the tissue that intervenes between the EMG source and the electrodes acts like a low-pass filter (DeLuca, 1979). Single motor unit "spikes", which are produced by the near-simultaneous action potentials in the muscle cells innervated by the same motoneuron, produce a "crack" or "pop," which has a unitary sound. The ear can quickly detect the pattern and rate of firing of a single motor unit. In fact, a subject who can control his or her muscles can quickly learn to turn a unit on and off by listening to its discharges. An inexpensive receiver amplifier, which can be purchased from a commercial electronics store for a little over $100, is quite adequate for this purpose.

The limitation of an audio monitor is that it provides no permanent record, and the amplitude of the EMG cannot be determined with any precision. It also cannot reveal the presence of some problems such as high frequency interference (as from a near-by video monitor) and large low-frequency movement artifacts. Another problem with audio monitors is that they produce a terrible 60-cycle din when the electrode is removed or a wire becomes detached. A very good idea is to have an audio monitor with a handy volume control, or an assistant who can anticipate the "blast" and turn the volume down before it happens.

A visual monitor such as an oscilloscope or a computer capable of providing on-line display of waveforms is very useful. They can be used to reveal the many types of artifacts that interfere with EMG recording, and by knowing the gain of the amplifier which is being used, it can be used to estimate the actual amplitude of the signals. Waveforms that can't be discriminated by the audio monitor carry potentially important information. If an oscilloscope were to be purchased for this use, then a very basic digital oscilloscope, costing about $1000, would be quite adequate. A digital oscilloscope can "freeze" a picture on-line, and thus the EMG signal can be studied in order to make a decision during the procedure. Older analog oscilloscopes are still quite useful, however, for verification of the signal's basic characteristics. There are also computer hardware/software systems (see below) that are very useful for on-line monitoring.

Recorders/Data Acquisition and Storage Devices

It will be very important for any person or group of people making decisions based upon EMG recordings to be able to directly compare records from different patients. Historically, polygraph records or tape recorders have been used for permanent storage of EMG records. Both of these instruments have serious problems, both for storing data and for its subsequent display and analysis. Another approach, made possible by the recent development of powerful but inexpensive computer systems, is direct digitization of EMG records and "streaming" of these data to computer disk. Commercial software systems operating on personal computers are currently capable of continuously acquiring and storing 80,000 samples per second. This would make it possible, for example, to acquire data on four channels of EMG at a sampling rate of 20,000 samples per second, quite fast enough to resolve the finest details of the waveform of a motor unit response. Some software/hardware data acquisition systems provide a continuous display of the EMG traces, whether or not data are actually being stored to disk, so they provide a very good visual monitor of the records as well as a means of data storage. These same computer programs can also provide a method of

quantitatively analyzing the EMG records. The use of one such data acquisition and analysis system, that developed by DATAQ Instruments, Inc., Akron, Ohio, will be illustrated later in conjunction with the section on data analysis.

Direct digitization and storage of EMG records will unquestionably produce very large data files. Consider, for example, the need to store 10 minutes of data at 80,000 samples per second. Remember each sample needs two bytes of storage (assuming 12-bit A/D conversion). This would produce a record of almost 100 MB. If this record were left on a computer's "hard disk," it would be a major problem. Such a record could be moved, off-line, however, to another storage medium such as a magneto-optical disk. Currently, each removable magneto-optical disk stores 230 MB of data, so the recording sessions would require less than half of such a disk for storage. The storage cost would thus be less than $25, and it is very likely that this cost will go down over time.

Although it is natural to look at data storage systems in terms of technical problems and costs, the most important factors, in the long run, are those related to ease of access. Simply put, stored data that don't get looked at and analyzed are absolutely worthless. If data are stored in a way that requires a great deal of human time for it to be accessed and/or analyzed, they may never be used, and if they are, wages provided to assistants for this process may easily wipe out any savings associated with a less expensive storage system or storage medium. In this respect, directly digitized and archived EMG recordings have great advantages. The fact that we do not already have well-established norms for using EMG for diagnostic purposes is probably a result of the prodigious task of analyzing EMG with the instruments that have previously been available for storing and analyzing these records. The development of digital data acquisition systems, which are currently just in their formative stage, will change this situation dramatically.

161

Source and Recognition of Artifactual Signals (Noise)

The 60-Cycle Beast

As most people know, the power supplied to homes, hospitals, and labs by the Electric Company comes out of the wall (in the United States) as a 60-Hz sinewave at a root-mean-square voltage of about 115 volts. This power line signal often contaminates EMG records. In dealing with 60-cycle interference, there are three important steps to take:

1. Minimize the electrode impedance, including the impedance of the reference electrode.
2. Remove the sources of the interference.
3. Shield against the interference, and/or selectively filter it out of the amplification process.

Reducing Source Impedance
Other factors being the same, the amount of 60-cycle problems one encounters can be related to the "source" resistance of the electrodes, which in this case is the sum of the resistances from each electrode to the reference electrode. Consider the extreme: Suppose you directly connect both input electrodes directly to the reference electrode with a piece of wire. You could put that "electrode" configuration in the middle of a generator and you wouldn't have a problem! At the opposite extreme, suppose the electrodes are "open," i.e. there is nothing but air between the electrodes and the reference electrode. The source impedance is now the input impedance of the amplifier, which is extremely high. In this condition, very small 60-cycle fields will be able to create comparatively large voltages (but see comment below on "blocking" of amplifiers). There is really little that one can do about the resistance of the electrode contact with the body fluids. One has a small area of bared stainless steel wire on the end of each wire, and that it that. The thing that one CAN do something about is the resistance between the reference electrode and skin of the patient. Good skin

preparation and/or use of large gel electrodes, such as those for ECG recording in intensive care units, will be helpful. Appreciation of the effect of having a high source impedance will help you understand a frequent problem in EMG recording: the mysterious appearance of high level of 60-cycle noise where it was absent earlier in the recording, or where exactly the same conditions were used in a previous recording session. The best guess is that either a connection is "open" somewhere in the circuit, or you have an air bubble between the gel in the skin electrode and the metallic part of the electrode.

Eliminating the Source of the 60-Cycle Field
Interference from 60-cycle sources comes from two types of "fields." The easy problem (usually) to solve is caused by inductive fields from transformers or wires carrying large AC currents that are physically close to the electrodes. The 60-cycle interference from inductive sources usually has a characteristic waveform, which does not contain "spikes" (Fig. 7–6). You cannot shield against this type of field, but physically moving the source of the magnetic field away from the recording site is usually sufficient to solve the problem. Moving just a few feet sometimes helps a great deal. The other type of 60-cycle interference comes from electrostatic influences. Any two conductors separated by an insulator form a capacitor. If a capacitor has a significant capacitance (a number that indicates how much charge can be stored at a given voltage difference between the conductors), then an AC voltage impressed upon one of the conductors can "couple" some fraction of that AC voltage to the other conductor. Large currents do not have to flow to cause this type of interference. Equipment that is plugged into the wall socket, but which is not turned on, can still cause problems. The power cord to the equipment, and the wires running internally to the power switch, can form a conductor having peak voltages of +/−160 volts with respect to ground. Any other conductor in the area, in particular the leads to the ampli-

Typical 60-cycle noise waveforms

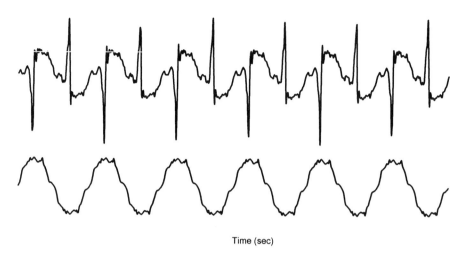

Time (sec)

Figure 7–6. Typical waveforms of 60-cycle noise from florescent lights (top trace) and from power cord inductive field (botton trace). Traces are 0.1 sec in duration, and therefore show exactly 6 cycles.

fier, can have a large AC voltage coupled to it if the resistance to ground is large (see above re source impedance). In this case, the insulator between the "plates" of this capacitor is the air in the room. One strategy for finding the source of a 60-cycle interference problem is to systematically unplug any unnecessary equipment in the vicinity of the recording site. If the equipment has to be plugged in, then sometimes moving the offending equipment to another location is helpful.

Florescent light can be a terrible problem. They all have a "ballast" in them, which increases the voltage across the florescent tube to about 750 volts. The waveform of this type of interference typically has large "spikes" in it (Fig. 7–6). The waveforms seen can vary a great deal, but they will always have a period of 16.667 msec. Keep in mind that a 60-cycle notch filter will not attenuate these "spikes" at all, so one should check the period of regular "spikes" of any type, even if there is no evidence of a sinusoidal waveform at a frequency of 60 Hz. Turning off florescent lights close to the recording site usually gets rid of the problem, but if one has to use high amplifier gains, then one may have to turn off all the florescent lights. Incandescent lights,

which use only 115 volts, cause far less interference. Sometimes florescent lights are not the source of the problem, however. You can answer this question by turning off the lights to see if the problem goes away.

One factor that seems to greatly increase 60-cycle interference is the presence of large ungrounded metal structures of any type close to the patient or amplifier. For example, we have found it very helpful, to eliminate 60-cycle noise problems in a minor surgery room used for EMG recording, to earth-ground the metal frame holding the patient's bed. It is important to note that the patient was not in contact with this frame, so this arrangement did not ground the patient.

Shielding and Filtering

After the source of the 60-cycle noise has been minimized, there are two additional strategies to reduce 60-cycle interference: shielding and filtering. If one is working in a normal environment, having an electrically shielded room to do the recording in is generally not practical. Some people shield the leads going from the subject to the amplifier, but this makes the leads rather stiff and

163

much heavier than is desirable. A much more common strategy, that accomplishes the same thing, is to use a small input stage on the amplifier (a first-stage amplifier in a small box) that is held close to the patient. Thus the leads can be kept fairly short. If these leads are only a few feet long, then putting them in a cable with a braided "shield" really doesn't help much. Shielded input leads can also be a major source of movement artifact (discussed later), so we recommend short unshielded leads to the amplifier. Although the primary attempt to control 60-cycle noise should be to get rid of the source, some environments, such as a surgical facility, make this very difficult. In this case, 60-cycle notch filters can be very helpful. They will help by reducing the 60-cycle component of the noise 10-fold, compared to what it would be without the filter. They will also produce corresponding amplitude and phase distortions of the biological signals in this frequency range, but that should not be a problem for diagnostic EMG recording.

Besides 60-cycle noise, one can encounter other forms of extraneous noise signals, such as high frequency fields from TV or computer monitors. Interference from a TV monitor will be seen on an oscilloscope as a broad band of "fuzz" around the recorded signal. You can't hear it on the audio monitor, because most audio amplifiers can't reproduce it and/or most of the "seniors" can't hear that high (about 16 kHz). Generally it isn't a serious problem, but if it is too large, it can "block" the input stage of the amplifier and thus affect amplification of the EMG signal. The easiest solution is to move the TV monitor as far away from the patient as possible. A few feet of movement can often totally eliminate the problem.

Movement Artifacts

Another type of artifact one has to recognize is related to movement of the electrode leads between the patient and the amplifier inputs. In most cases, these electrode lead movements cause large low-frequency excursions

of the recording baseline. A "tap," or high-frequency vibration, of the leads may also cause artifactual signals whose frequency components are high enough to be in the pass band of the amplifier. In fact, they sound like someone tapping on the bottom of a metal can when heard over the audio monitor. An important source of movement artifact is the electrochemical system at the interface of the electrode, which is a metallic conductor in a salt solution. There is usually a significant DC junction potential at each electrode. In effect, each electrode acts like a miniature "battery." The voltage from this battery charges the distributed capacitance of the electrode lead with respect to ground. Movements of the electrode leads cause changes in the distributed capacitances, and changes in these "capacitors" cause charging and discharging currents to flow back and forth across the electrode resistance, thus producing voltage changes. If the changes in the capacitance of both electrode leads are exactly the same, the voltage changes produced across each electrode will be identical, and thus will not be amplified by a differential amplifier; ie, they will be a "common-mode signal." This conceptual model of movement artifact would explain why the use of bifiler wires, where both electrode leads have to move together, dramatically reduces problems with movement artifact.

Sometimes one sees a sinusoidal signal at the frequency of phonation when recording from laryngeal muscles. Don't suppose you are observing phase-locking of the EMG. This is another version of the movement artifact discussed above; the wires going to the amplifier are probably vibrating at the frequency of phonation. Another type of movement artifact may be observed when using hooked-wire electrodes: rather large "spikes" associated with the start of movements. They look somewhat like large single motor units, except for two things. They are usually monophasic (go in only one direction from the baseline), and they typically have much longer durations than motor units responses. While they may occur several times in each burst, they don't exhibit a repetitive pattern at a respectable rate—ie, something on the order of 10–50 spikes per second. One possible cause of these large spikes would be intermittent contact of the two wires of the electrode within the muscle. Such contact would discharge the "standing" electrochemical junction potential (see above).

Even with bipolar hooked-wire electrodes having large tip exposures, it is fairly common to observe single motor unit activity in most muscles. One has to separate these potentials from artifacts that can produce spike-like potentials in the record. Real single motor unit potentials are distinguished by several features: (1) they are almost always biphasic; (2) they usually fire at least several times in a row at rather regular intervals; (3) they generally correlate with some aspect of motor activity; (4) they do not correspond to external events like someone switching a piece of electronic equipment on and off; and (5) they do not fire at a steady interval of 16.667 msec (the interval of 60-cycle interference). Another thing to look for, when recording from two or more muscles, are potentials occurring simultaneously in two or more channels. Such events are very unlikely to be biological in their origin. They can result from irregular powerline transients, sometimes caused by someone in another part of the building turning on or off large motors. We have seen "strange" potentials of this variety quite often when recording in a surgical suite.

"Blocking" of Amplifiers

If the lead to the reference electrode or to either of the inputs electrodes is "open," ie, has an extremely high resistance, the output of many (if not most) modern EMG amplifiers will show a perplexing behavior that can be quite confusing to the novice. The amplifier output may be very quiet for extended periods of time, as if there were absolutely no muscle activity, and even noise signals will be absent. Then one may observe brief periods of high amplitude 60-cycle noise and/or large movements artifacts that gradually die out, leaving a quiet baseline once again.

These periods of "noise" recording can usually be produced at will by moving the leads to the electrodes, or by any movements of the preamplifier or the patient/subject. This is the behavior of a "blocked" amplifier, and it can only be corrected by establishing a reasonable resistance from each electrode to the reference electrode and making sure the reference electrode is connected to the reference input of the amplifier. "Blocking" in an amplifier is caused by the very small currents that have to flow from the inputs. These currents are, in modern amplifiers, in the picoampere range, and so are ordinarily of no consequence. However, if they have no path back to the reference input of amplifier, they will create a relatively large DC differential signal at the inputs. This will cause the first-stage amplifier to "saturate" it's output at the plus or minus power supply voltage. Subsequent high-pass amplifier circuits, always present in an EMG amplifier system, will make this steady DC voltage into a steady zero-voltage output. Any movements of the wires or electrodes will momentarily allow this input current to redistribute itself, and thereby amplify the noise signals that one ordinarily sees when the electrodes have a very high resistance. Pragmatically, the main lesson is this: if you observe a VERY quiet baseline, interrupted by "funny" episodes of recording, check to see that you have intact electrode wires and good connections to the amplifier.

Analysis of EMG Records

Qualitative Analysis: Using the Calibrated Eyeball

Although it is natural, from a scientific standpoint, to gravitate toward numerical comparisons when using physical measurements for diagnostic purposes, the fact remains that probably one of the most sophisticated analyzers available to us is our own senses. Therefore it is very useful, in using EMG records to understand and/or diagnose dysarthrias, to be able to locate regions of interest in the record and then observe them in detail. In doing this, however, certain simple transformations of the original waveforms may improve our ability to observe relationships in the recordings. The best way to make such observations is to use a computer program specifically designed for display and analysis of physiological recordings. Figure 7–7 illustrates an example of how this may be done, using a program such as Windaq (DATAQ Instruments Inc., Akron, OH). It is the result of an analysis of laryngeal EMG obtained from a normal subject during three repetitions of the phrase, "Pop took his socks off." Keep in mind that this presentation is not intended as a definitive statement of how laryngeal muscles are used during speech, nor as a "sales pitch" for a particular commercial computer program. What is intended is to convey to the reader at least one approach to finding information in an EMG recording of some of the muscles involved in speech.

The recording to be presented below was obtained from a healthy, normal adult female speaker. She repeated the phrase at normal pitch and somewhat increased loudness, using normal prosody and emphasis. Recordings were made from the cricothyroid (CT) and thyroarytenoid (TA) muscles respectively using bipolar hooked-wire electrodes. Amplifier gain was 2000, and the band pass of the amplifiers was 30 Hz to 5 kHz. Before being digitized on-line at a sampling rate of 5 kHz, all channels were filtered at 2.5 kHz for purposes of antialiasing. Figure 7–7A illustrates a "compressed" portion of the recording. Compression of the record is accomplished by having the computer display a vertical line representing the maximum and minimum value of data found in each compressed "block" of data (in this case, 80 data points) at each horizontal pixel of the screen. This algorithm is much preferable to other types of "compression," such as just displaying every 80th data point or displaying the average of the 80 data points; it preserves the occurrence of transient responses whose duration is shorter than the duration represented by each pixel, in particular single motor unit responses. The ability to

display a compressed record is very useful in locating a region in which some activity of interest is occurring.

In a long record, where the subject perhaps speaks several phrases, one may wonder how you can be sure what the subject is saying at a particular point of the record. The computer program has the capability of outputting the data from a selected channel (in this case the microphone channel) to the digital-to-analog converter (DAC). The data to be output are selected using the cursor, and at a keystroke, they are played back and one hears the spoken phrase. Because of the relatively low sampling rate, such speech is not suitable for acoustic analysis, but it is clearly intelligible. We can thus be sure that this portion of the record is of interest.

The details of the muscle activity are obscured by this degree of compression. This problem is easily solved by having the computer decrease the compression of the record corresponding to the location of the cursor. In effect, we want to "magnify" the record around the cursor. The decompressed record, displaying all data samples around the position of the cursor in Figure 7–7A, is shown in Figure 7–7B.

Even though the speaker is perfectly normal, an initial reaction to inspection of the EMG recordings of these laryngeal muscles is, "What a bunch of junk!" There is clearly modulation of activity, but the pattern is uncertain. It might be supposed that the electrodes are not actually in the intended muscles, a possibility that always has to be considered when attempting to record from laryngeal muscles. However, certain transformation of the "raw" EMG records makes it easier to recognize patterns of modulation (Fig. 7–7C). The "raw" EMG is first rectified (the sign bit of each data point is simply set to be positive). The record is then smoothed with a moving average. In this operation, the computer calculates, for each data point, the average of that data point and all the data points coming X points before and after the data point. In effect, a "window" containing 2X+1 samples is averaged, and the data point at the middle of this window is re-

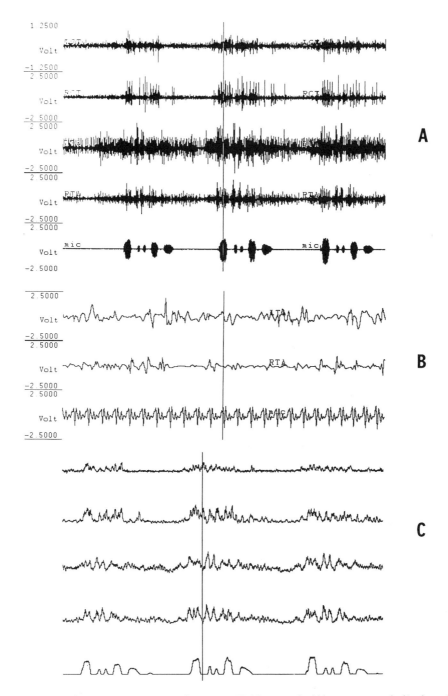

Figure 7–7. Three ways to view the same EMG record: (A) compressed display; (B) decompressed display (bottom three traces from 7a), plotting all data points; and (C) rectified and smoothed (moving average). See text for discussion.

placed with this average. Then the window is moved one data point to the right, etc. In Figure 7–7C, the averaging window is 30 msec. The resulting record shows, with more clarity, the "trend" of EMG amplitude changes. In particular, there appears to be two peaks of activity in both TA muscles preceding the "his socks" portion of the phrase

167

(immediately following the cursor), which correspond to two smaller peaks of activity in the CT that seem out of phase with the TA modulation. Obviously, appreciation of these features would benefit from being able to superimpose these repetitions, lining them up on some point that seems relatively invariant. This can be easily done by "clipping" 2.2-sec portions of the record around each token, where the beginning of each of these subfiles begins exactly 1.1 sec before the peak of the "his" in the microphone record. The computer program allows these subfiles to be saved in a spreadsheet format. When these files are opened in a spreadsheet program, the three tokens may be aligned in time (superimposed), and the values normalized to the highest values found in each channel. The resulting data may then be graphed, resulting in Figure 7–8. In this final form, the modulation of the laryngeal muscle activity, and its repeatability, is very clear.

Even knowing that the subject studied in Figure 8 was a normal speaker, we cannot assert that this pattern of laryngeal muscle activity is "normal." It could in fact be quite atypical: one would only know by applying the analysis to a large number of speakers. Had the health status of the speaker been unknown, however, the results illustrated in Figure 8 would establish important facts:

1. The nerves to the TA and CT muscle are intact bilaterally.
2. The motoneurons to these muscles are activated in a coordinated manner that seems related to speech, and thus corticopontine neural systems controlling laryngeal motoneurons are intact.
3. Absence of long duration or polyphasic single motor unit waveforms would be evidence against previous nerve injury followed by reinnervation.

With additional research, it may eventually be possible to make more detailed interpretations of these records. Asymmetric modulation of pairs of muscles involved in speech, or

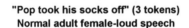

"Pop took his socks off" (3 tokens)
Normal adult female-loud speech

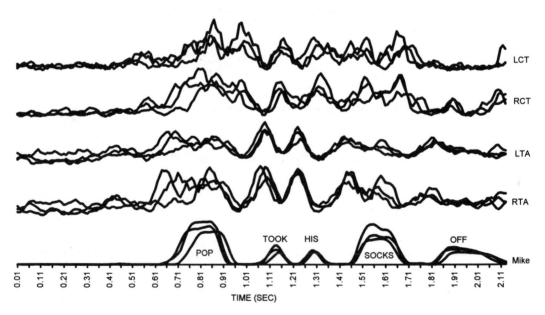

Figure 7–8. Superimposed traces of rectified and smoothed laryngeal EMG generated after importing data into a spreadsheet. Nomal adult female speaker. All trace amplitudes have been normalized to the highest value occurring in the three tokens.

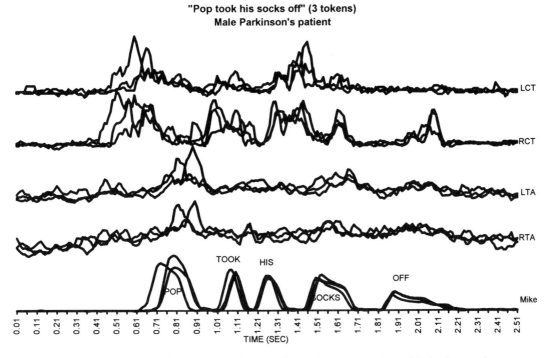

Figure 7–9. Analysis of the laryngeal EMG of a Parkinson's patient. Methods exactly as described for Figure 7–8.

absence of modulation, may be characteristic of some diseases of the nervous system. For example, Figure 7–9 shows an analysis of the recordings from the laryngeal muscles of an elderly male with Parkinson's disease during three repetitions of the phrase, "Pop took his socks off." Methods of analysis were identical to those described for Figure 7–8. The TA muscles in this patient are quite active during the phrase, but there is no modulation of their activity in the central part of the phrase. Cricothyroid muscles are, on the other hand, active and well modulated. This observation could possibly be related to the rather weak and breathy voice of the patient. Warning! This comparison is VERY preliminary, and is only presented here to illustrate the potential use of EMG analysis.

Quantitative Analysis of the EMG

There are two basic features of the EMG signal that can be fairly easily reduced to a constrained set of numbers: its amplitude, and

its temporal properties (when it starts and stops). There are some surprisingly "sticky" problems about making these measurements, however, and our eventual ability to say whether a measure of EMG amplitude is "normal" or "abnormal' will depend upon attention to these details. Let's first consider the problem of measuring the EMG of a muscle in a patient with weakness during a static maximal response. The amplitude of this response, measured in volts, could have diagnostic value. For example, if this measure in this patient were statistically the same as a normal subject, it would suggest that the contractile aspects of muscle, rather than muscle activation, were disordered. In arriving at this conclusion, what factors need to be considered?

Electrode Characteristics

First of all, the electrode type and/or physical configuration, such as interelectrode spacing, that is used to make the measurement has to be the same as that used to gen-

169

erate the normative data. For those interested in muscles of the articulators, intramuscular electrodes are usually required. Rigid needle electrodes, in which tip exposure and electrode spacing are fixed, would have advantages in this regard, but making maximal responses could be painful and thus might interfere with the patient's ability or willingness to "give it all they've got." Hooked-wire electrodes are not painful, even for maximal responses. Historically, their tip exposure and spacing have been treated rather casually, but this could be easily improved, particularly by the use of bifiler wire. Let us suppose we make the measurement with hooked-wire electrodes manufactured with great attention to uniformity of their tip characteristics. We will still have to consider that some degree of variation will occur because of differences in the geometry of the electrode in the muscle or because of its location in a particular part of the muscle. A good example of this problem is illustrated in Figure 7–7A. All EMG channels were amplified at a gain of 2000. Note that the top trace (LCT) is displayed at twice the sensitivity as the other traces (2.5 rather than 5.0 volts full-scale). From this display one may see that a 2:1 difference in the general amplitude of EMGs may be expected in a normal subject, when observing bilateral pairs of muscles (which we are assuming are excited to the same degree). This problem, that of difference of EMG amplitude as a function of "whimsy," could be reduced by repeated measurements in a patient. If several electrode placements in the muscle all yielded low amplitudes, then much more significance could be attached to the observations.

Measures of EMG Amplitude

Periods of relatively steady EMG may be numerically summarized in two ways: (1) rectification (taking the absolute value) and computing the mean amplitude over an established interval or (2) computing the RMS (root-mean-square) value of the unrectified signal over an established interval.

Given the same record, these two methods give somewhat different values. The squaring operation in the RMS method gives greater "weight" in the final value to high-amplitude portions of the record, which are usually single-motor unit responses. Root-mean-square values will obviously be larger than mean rectified EMG values, but how much larger is difficult to predict from a theoretical viewpoint. Figure 7–10 presents an empirical treatment of this problem. Six 200-msec periods representing low, medium, and high levels of EMG were chosen from the "Pop took his socks off" record shown in Figure 7–7A, and the ratio of the RMS value and mean rectified value was determined from each sample. These values are plotted as a function of the mean rectified amplitude of the LTA, the muscle in this record usually having the largest value. One may observe the ratio of RMS/mean rectified EMG ranges between one and two. For three of the muscles, the ratio does not change much as the EMG signal goes from small to large. Nevertheless, it is worth noting that the LTA ratio does decrease as the signal gets larger, and one may also observe that the ratio for LCT is quite a lot smaller than the other muscles. This is just an example, but it makes it clear that there is a complex relationship between RMS and mean rectified EMG "amplitudes." There is no "right" or "wrong" about the use of either measure, but the use of mean rectified EMG seems much more common in current publications than the use of RMS values, even though it requires the additional step of rectification.

Another detail to be considered when attempting to quantify EMG amplitude is the sampling rate used to digitize the signal. Whatever rate is chosen, the signal has to be low-pass filtered at a cutoff frequency of half the sampling rate to avoid the creation of false (aliased) components. Such filters are often called "antialias filters." Thus, all high-frequency components of the EMG signal above the cutoff frequency of the antialias filter will be lost. If the EMG signal contains large high-frequency components, then the

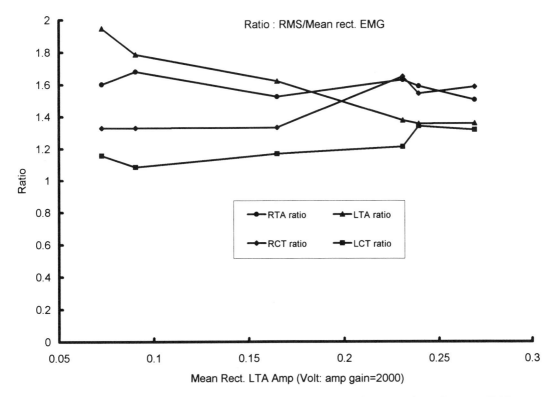

Figure 7–10. Ratio of values obtained for RMS vs mean rectified EMG from the same EMG record as a function of the mean rectified EMG amplitude.

mean rectified or RMS value of this signal will obviously be spuriously low if these high frequencies are removed before they are digitized. One might avoid this problem by using a very high sampling rate, but if this is not necessary, then one would be wasting a great deal of storage space and processing time to work with the resulting large files. One might digitize the same EMG signal, recorded on a tape recorder, with a wide range of sampling rates to empirically determine the lowest sampling rate that would produce an accurate value of EMG amplitude. Spectral analysis of a typical example of EMG signal to be analyzed can also provide this information, however. Figure 7–11 compares the spectra of EMG signals recorded from the wrist extensor muscles of one of the authors using skin electrodes and also an intramuscular bipolar hooked-wire electrode. Signals from both electrode pairs were antialias

filtered at 5 kHz and digitized at 10 kHz. The skin electrodes produced an EMG signal whose high-frequency components (above 300 Hz) are attenuated by 20 dB or more. The dominant frequency components are around 100 Hz. Therefore one can conclude that digitizing EMG from large skin electrodes at rates of 400 to 500 Hz would provide accurate measures of EMG amplitude. The situation would be very different for the intramuscular recording, however. The spectrum of this signal does not fall to an attenuation level of 20 dB until frequencies of 2 kHz are reached. Therefore, we routinely use 5 kHz sampling for our studies of intramuscular EMG.

Measuring the Temporal Characteristics of EMG Activity
The duration and timing of EMG activity of muscles used in speech or swallowing have potential diagnostic value. In most respects,

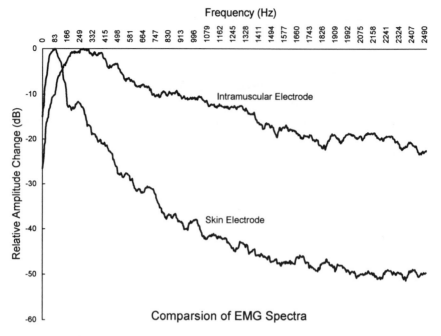

Figure 7–11. Comparison of the spectra of EMG obtained using intramuscular (hooked-wire) vs skin (surface) electrodes.

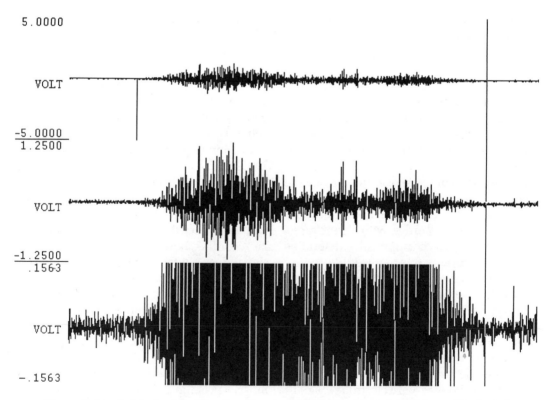

Figure 7–12. Subjective identification of onset of EMG activity can be influenced by "gain" of EMG display.

making these measures is merely a matter of placing the cursor at the beginning, peak, or end of periods of activity (a "burst" of EMG) and having the computer record the time (really the sample number in the record) of the cursor position. While this sounds simple, anyone who has actually done this task has quickly come to discover that the "beginning" or "end" of EMG activity usually is somewhat arbitrary. The usual solution is to try to adopt some systematic rule, such as "the beginning is the first signal clearly larger than the baseline activity that persists and becomes larger." In making these judgments, however, it should be realized that very different values can be obtained by honest and diligent observers if they use the EMG trace displayed at different "gains." If the main body of the EMG burst is kept on the scale of the display, then very often the actual baseline activity cannot be seen with enough detail to know when it actually changes. This situation is illustrated in Figure 7–12, which shows exactly the same burst of submental EMG activity, associated with a swallow, at three different display gains. The bottom trace, which displays the EMG at a very high gain, allows one to detect the true beginning the change in the baseline activity. The cursor position marking the beginning of the burst, as determined by the bottom trace, intersects the top trace at a point on the trace that appears to come about 200 msec before the beginning of the burst, as seen in this low gain display. In the end, people do their best, and check the reliability within and between observers. It is well to keep in mind, however, that very different measurements of EMG burst duration might result from the manner in which the signals to be measured were displayed on the computer.

References

Basmajian JV, De Luca CJ. (1985). *Muscles Alive: Their Functions Revealed by Electromyography.* Baltimore: Williams & Wilkins.

Basmajian JV, Dutta CR. (1961). Electromyography of the pharyngeal constrictors and levator palati in man. *Anat Rec* 139:561–563.

Basmajian JV, Stecko G. (1962). A new bipolar electrode for electromyography. *J Appl Physiol* 17:849.

Bell-Berti F. (1976). An electromyographic study of velopharyngeal function in speech. *J Speech Hear Res* 19:225–240.

Benguerel AP, Hirose H, Sawashima M, Ushijima T. (1975). Electromyographic study of the velum in French. *Ann Bull Res Inst Logoped (Tokyo)* 9:79–90.

Berry H, Blair RL. (1980). Isolated vagus nerve palsy and vagal mononeuritis. *Arch Otolaryngol* 106:333–338.

Blair C, Smith A. (1986). EMG recording in human lip muscles: can single muscles be isolated? *J Speech Hear Res* 29:256–266.

Blair RL, Berry H, Briant TDR. (1978). Laryngeal electromyography: Technique and application. *Otolaryngol Clin North Am* 11:325–346.

Blitzer A, Brin MF, Fahn S, Lovelace RE. (1988). Localized injections of botulinum toxin for the treatment of focal laryngeal dystonia (spastic dysphonia). *Laryngoscope* 98:193–197.

Borden GJ, Gay T. (1978). On the production of low tongue tip /s/: a case report. *J Commun Disord* 11:425–431.

Brin MF, Fahn S, Moskowitz C, Friedman A, Shale HM, Greene PE, Blitzer A, List T, Lange D, Lovelace RE, McMahon D (1987). Localized injections of botulinum toxin for the treatment of focal dystonia and hemifacial spasm. *Movement Disord* 2:237–254.

Cahan LD, Adams JM, Perry J, Beeler LM. (1990). Instrumented gait analysis after selective dorsal rhizotomy. *Dev Med Child Neurol* 32:1037–1043.

Cohen LG, Hallett M, Geller BD, Hochberg F. (1989). Treatment of focal dystonias of the hand with botulinum toxin injections. *J Neurol Neurosurg Psychiatry* 52:355–363.

Cohen SR, Thompson JW. (1987). Use of botulinum toxin to lateralize true vocal cords: a biochemical method to relieve bilateral abductor vocal cord paralysis. *Ann Otol Rhinol Laryngol* 96:534–541.

Cole K, Konopacki R, Abbs J. (1983). A minature electrode for surface electromyography during speech. *J Acoust Soc Am* 74:1362.

Cooper DS, Folkins J. (1985). Comparison of electromyographic signals from different electrode placements in the palatoglossus muscle. *J Acoust Soc Am* 78:1530–1540.

Crumley RL.(1989). Laryngeal synkinesis: its significance to the laryngologist. *Ann Otol Rhinol Laryngol* 98:87–92.

De Luca C. (1979). Physiology and mathematics of myoelectric signals. *IEEE Trabsact Biomed Engin* BME-26:313–325.

Faaborg-Andersen K. (1957). Electromyographic investigation of intrinsic laryngeal muscles in humans. *Acta Physiol Scand* 41:9–148.

Freeman FJ, Ushijima T. (1978). Laryngeal muscle activity during stuttering. *J Speech Hear Res* 21:538–562.

Fritzell B, Kotby MN. (1976). Observations on thryroarytenoid and palatal levator activation for speech. *Folia Phoniatr* 28:1–7.

Fritzell B. (1969). The velopharyngeal muscles in speech: an electromyographic and cineradiographic study. *Acta Oto-Laryngol* (suppl 250)1–81.

Gartlan MG, Peterson KL, Luschei ES, Hoffman HT, Smith RJ. (1993). Bipolar hooked-wire electromyographic technique in the evaluation of pediatric vocal cord paralysis. *Ann Otol Rhinol Laryngol* 102:695–700.

Haglund S, Knutsson E, Martensson A. (1972). An electromyographic investigation of intrinsic laryngeal muscles in humans. *Acta Oto Laryngol* 74:265–270.

Hairston LE, Sauerland EK. (1981). Electromyography of the human palate: discharge patterns of the levator and tensor veli palatini. *Electromyogr Clin Neurophysiol* 21:299–306.

Hairston LE, Sauerland EK. (1981). Electromyography of the human pharynx: discharge patterns of the superior pharyngeal constrictor during respiration. *Electromyogr Clin Neurophysiol* 21:299–306.

Hirano M, Nozoe I, Shin T, Maeyama T. (1987). Electromyography for laryngeal paralysis. In: Hirano M, Kirchner J, Bless D, eds. *Neurolaryngology: Recent Advances.* Boston: College-Hill, pp 232–248.

Hirano M, Ohala J. (1969). Use of hooked-wire electrodes for electromyography of the intrinsic laryngeal muscles. *J Speech Hear Res* 12:362–373.

Hirose H. (1987). Laryngeal articulatory adjustments in terms of EMG. In: Hirano M, Kirchner J, Bless D, eds. *Neurolaryngology: Recent Advances.* Boston: College-Hill, pp 200–208.

Hiroto I, Hirano M, Tomita H. (1968). Electromyographic investigation of human vocal cord paralysis. *Ann Otol Rhinol Laryngol* 77:296–304.

Hoffman HT, Brunberg JA, Winter P, Sullivan MJ, Kileny PR. (1991). Arytenoid subluxation: diagnosis and treatment. *Ann Otol Rhinol Laryngol* 100:1–9.

Hrycyshyn AW, Basmajian JV. (1972). Electromyography of the oral stage of swallowing in man. *Am J Anat* 133:333–340.

Hunker CJ, Abbs JH. (1990). Uniform frequency of parkinsonian resting tremor in the lips, jaw, tongue, and index finger. *Movement Disord* 5:71–77.

Jankovic J, Orman J. (1987). Botulinum A toxin for cranial-cervical dystonia: a double-blind, placebo-controlled study. *Neurology* 37:616–623.

Keenan MA. (1988). Surgical decision making for residual limb deformities following traumatic brain injury. *Orthopaed Rev* 17:1185–1192.

Kimura J. (1989). *Electrodiagnosis in Diseases of Nerve and Muscle: Principles and Practice,* 2nd ed. Philadelphia: F.A. Davis Co.

Kiritani S, Hirose H, Sawashima M. (1980). Simultaneous X-ray microbeam and EMG study of velum movement for Japanese nasal sounds. *Ann Bull Res Inst Logoped Phoniatr* 14:91–100.

Koda J, Ludlow CL. (1992). An evaluation of laryngeal muscle activation in patients with voice tremor. *Otolaryngol Head Neck Surg* 107:684–696.

Kokesh J, Flint PW, Robinson LR, Cummings CW. (1993). Correlation between stroboscopy and electromyography in laryngeal paralysis. *Ann Otol Rhinol Laryngol* 102:852–857.

Kuehn DP, Folkins JW, Cutting CB. (1982). Relationships between muscle activity and velar position. *Cleft Palate J* 19:25–35.

Kuehn DP, Folkins JW, Linville RN. (1988). An electromyographic study of the musculus uvulae. *Cleft Palate J* 25:348–355.

Lewis WS, Crumley RL, Blanks RH, Pitcock JK. (1991). Does intralaryngeal motor nerve sprouting occur following unilateral recurrent laryngeal nerve paralysis? *Laryngoscope* 101:1259–1263.

Loeb GE, Gans C. (1986). *Electromyography for Experimentalists.* Chicago: University of Chicago Press.

Lubker JF, Fritzell B, Lindqvist J. (1970). Velopharyngeal function: an eletromyographic study. *STL-QPSR* 20:9–20.

Ludlow C, Hallett M, Sedory S, Fujita M, Naunton R. (1990). The pathophysiology of spasmodic dysphonia and its modification by botulinum toxin. In: *International Medical Society of Motor Disturbances. Motor Disturbances II.* San Diego. Academic Press, pp 273–288.

Ludlow CL, Naunton RF, Sedory SE, Schulz GM, Hallett M. (1988). Effects of botulinum toxin injections on speech in adductor spasmodic dysphonia. *Neurology* 38:1220–1225.

Ludlow CL, Naunton RF, Terada S, Anderson BJ. (1991). Successful treatment of selected cases of abductor spasmodic dysphonia using botulinum toxin injection. *Otolaryngol Head Neck Surg* 104:849–855.

Mauriello JA. (1985). Blepharospasm, Meige's syndrome, and hemifacial spasm: treatment with botulinum toxin. *Neurology* 35:1499–1500.

McClean MD. (1991). Lip muscle EMG responses to oral pressure stimulation. *J Speech Hear Res* 34:248–251.

Miller RH, Woodson GE, Jankovic J. (1987). Botulinum toxin injection of the vocal fold for spasmodic dysphonia. A preliminary report. *Arch Otolaryngol Head Neck Surg* 113:603–605.

Min YB, Finnegan EM, Hoffman HT, Luschei ES, McCulloch TM. (1994). A preliminary study of the prognostic role of electromyography in laryngeal paralysis. *Otolaryngol Head Neck Surg* 111:70–75.

Min YB, Luschei ES, Finnegan EM, McCullough TM, Hoffman HT. (1994). Portable telemetry system for electromyography. *Otolaryngol Head Neck Surg* 111:849–852.

Moore CA, Smith A, Ringel RL. (1988). Task-specific organization of jaw muscles. *J Speech Hear Res* 31:670–680.

Mowrey RA, McKay IRA. (1990). Phonological primitives: electromyographic speech error evidence. *J Acoust Soc Am* 88:1299–1312.

Mu L, Yang S. (1991). An experimental study on the laryngeal electromyography and visual observations in varying types of surgical injuries to the unilateral recurrent laryngeal nerve in the neck. *Laryngoscope* 101:699–708.

Neilson PD, O'Dwyer NJ. (1984). Reproducibility and variability of speech muscle activity in athetoid dysarthria of cerebral palsy. *J Speech Hear Res* 27:502–517.

O'Dwyer NJ, Neilson PD, Guitar BE, Quinn PT, Andrews G. (1983). Control of upper airway structures during nonspeech tasks in normal and cerebral-palsied subjects: EMG findings. *J Speech Hear Res* 26:162–170.

Palmer JB, Rudin NJ, Lara G, Crompton AW. (1992). Coordination of mastication and swallowing. *Dysphagia* 7:187–200.

Palmer JB, Tanaka E, Siebens AA. Electromyography of the pharyngeal musculature: technical considerations. *Arch Physical Med Rehabil* 70:283–287.

Palmer JB, Tippett DC, Wolf JS. (1991). Synchronous positive and negative myoclonus due to pontine hemorrhage. *Muscle Nerve* 14:124–132.

Parnes SM, Satya MS. (1985). Predictive value of laryngeal electromyography in patients with vocal cord paralysis of neurogenic origin. *Laryngoscope* 95:1323–1326.

Perlman AL, Luschei ES, DuMond CE. (1989). Electrical activity from the superior pharyngeal constrictor during reflexive and nonreflexive tasks. *J Speech Hear Res* 32:749–754.

Piper H. (1912). *Elektrophysiologie menschlicher Muskeln.* Berlin: Springer.

Rowe LD, Miller AJ, Chierici G, Clendenning D. (1984). Adaptation in the function of pharyngeal constrictor muscles. *Otolaryngol Head Neck Surg* 92:392–401.

Sauerland EK, Mitchell SP. (1975). Electromyographic activity of intrinsic and extrinsic muscles of the human tongue. *Tex Rep Biol Med* 33:445–455.

Schaefer SD, Roark RM, Watson BC, Kondraske GV, Freeman FJ, Butsch RW, Pohl J. (1992). Multichannel electromyographic observations in spasmodic dysphonia patients and normal control subjects. *Ann Otol Rhinol Laryngol* 101:67–75.

Scott AB. (1980). Botulinum toxin injection into extraocular muscles as an alternative to strabismus surgery. *J Pediatr Ophthalmol Strabismus* 17:21–25.

Seaver EJ, Kuehn DP. (1980). A cineradiographic and electromyographic investigation of velar positioning in non-nasal speech. *Cleft Palate J* 17:216–226.

Smith A, McFarland DH, Weber CM, Moore CA. (1987). Spatial organization of human perioral reflexes. *Exp Neurol* 98:233–248.

Smith A. (1989). Neural drive to muscles in stuttering. *J Speech Hear Res* 32:252–264.

Stager S, Ludlow C. (1994). Responses of strutterers and vocal tremor patients to treatment with botulinum toxin. In: Janovic J, Hallett M, eds. *Therapy With Botulinum Toxin.* New York: Mercel Dekker.

Sutherland DH, Larsen LJ, Mann R. (1975). Rectus femoris release in selected patients with cerebral palsy: a preliminary report. *Dev Med Child Neurol* 17:26–34.

Thumfart W. (1981). Electromyography of the larynx. In: Samii M, Gannetta PJ, eds. *The Cranial Nerves.* Berlin: Springer-Verlag, pp 597–606.

Thumfart WF. (1988). From larynx to vocal ability. New electro-physiological data. *Acta Oto Laryngologica* 105:425–431.

Tsui J, Eisen A, Mak E, Carruthers J, Scott A, Calne D. (1985). A pilot study on the use of botulimun toxin in spasmodic torticollis. *Can J Neurol Sci* 12:314–316.

Ushijima T, Hirose H. (1974). Electromyographic study of the velum during speech. *J Phonet* 2:315–326.

Woo P, Arandia H. (1992). Intraoperative laryngeal electromyographic assessment of patients with immobile vocal fold. *Ann Otol Rhinol Laryngol* 101:799–806.

Acknowledgments

We would like to acknowledge the support of the National Center for Voice and Speech (grant No. P60 DC00976 from the National Institutes of Deafness and Other Communication Disorders) and extend our thanks to Drs. Lorraine Ramig and Kristin Larson for permission to use the recordings used in Figures 7–7 through 7–10 . A special expression of thanks goes to Dunc for singing his heart out under adverse circumstances.

Chapter *8*

Speech Imaging

Barbara C. Sonies and Maureen Stone

Introduction

Whereas the speech science literature over the last few decades recognizes that there are many unknown parameters in our knowledge of the vocal tract during speech, specialized methods for viewing or imaging these structures have proven to be critical to expand our knowledge base. This is because the motions of the articulators are rapid, highly variable, complex, and not easily visualized. The internal structures of the vocal tract are difficult to measure without impinging upon normal movement patterns. Imaging techniques overcome that difficulty because they capture internal movement without directly contacting the structures. The question of which is the best imaging system for measuring speech articulation during normal and dysarthric production often arises. Although there is no one best technique, this chapter should assist the reader in understanding the uses, limits, and applications of the commonly used imaging techniques.

In recent times, physiological measurements have improved at an extraordinary pace. Imaging techniques have emerged on the scene and revolutionized the way we view the vocal tract by providing recognizable images of structures deep within the oropharynx. Imaging procedures can be used to compare normal and abnormal patterns and to obtain baseline data for both short-term and longitudinal studies. Short-term studies may be used for acquiring normative information and to collect large amounts of data on fewer subjects. Longitudinal studies of speech production are important in determining maturational changes, effectiveness of treatment and impact of disease, surgical intervention or trauma. Regardless of the length of the study, the following considerations are needed in selection of the appropriate imaging system:

1. Completeness and visibility of the image
2. Dynamic acquisition of speech samples, during coarticulation
3. Soft /hard tissue visualization
4. Multiple image planes
5. Repeatability of studies
6. Comfort and safety of subject
7. Type of format for postprocessing of data (Sonies, 1991)

Applications of Imaging Techniques to Dysarthria

Measuring the vocal tract is an exceedingly difficult task because the articulators differ widely in speed of movement, structural composition, dimensionality of movement, degree of complexity, shape, and location. There are large differences in shape and structural composition between soft tissue structures (tongue, lips, velum) and hard tissue structures (jaw, palate). Therefore, these structures differ significantly in movement dimensionality. For example, the fluid deformation of the tongue needs quite different measurement strategies from the rigid body movements of the jaw. Another difficulty is the different speeds and locations of the articulators. An instrument whose frequency response is adequate for the slow-moving jaw will not necessarily be adequate for the fast-moving tongue tip. As with articulator speed, differences in articulator location significantly affect the type of transduction system needed. For example, structures that are visible to superficial inspection, such as the lips, are much easier to record than structures deep within the oral cavity, such as the velum or tongue base.

The most important complication in measuring articulatory movement is the interaction among articulators. Some articulatory behaviors are more highly correlated than others, and distinguishing the contributions of each behavior can be quite difficult. The most dramatic example of this is the tongue-jaw system. It is clear that jaw height is a major factor in tongue tip height. However, this coupling of the two structures becomes progressively weaker as one moves posteriorly, until in the pharynx, tongue movement is not coupled to jaw movement at all. Thus, trying to measure contribution of the jaw to tongue movement becomes increasingly complex. The problem is complicated further in that no single imaging system measures these contributions simultaneously.

There are several major advantages of using speech imaging techniques. There is no need to infer the position or activity of the various anatomical structures during speech, as is necessary with analog or point tracking techniques such as electromyography (EMG) or electroglottography (EGG). An image of the entire oropharynx or oral cavity, rather than a single point on the structure (muscle, bone, cartilage), can be obtained. Imaging techniques can provide real-time pictorial representations of the actual oropharyngeal and laryngeal anatomy during motion (Sonies, 1991). Techniques such as computed tomography (CT) and X-rays are best able to visualize bones and hard tissue structures, whereas soft tissues are best seen on magnetic resonance imaging (MRI) and ultrasound (US). Some imaging techniques easily allow for acquisition of multiple plane images; this provides an advantage for clinical studies and interpretation of oral-motor function. Each procedure has different capabilities and different advantages for viewing the oropharyngeal structures during speech. There is often a trade-off between safety and image quality or among image quality, resolution, and speed of acquisition of an image.

The four imaging techniques that we describe in this chapter are X-ray, CT, MRI, and US. These technologies differ in the ways in which they generate images, in their applications for speech, and in their specificity for viewing motions of the speech anatomy over time. Each technique will be discussed separately, and their advantages and limitations presented.

X-Ray Studies

Until recent years the X-ray was the most commonly used imaging system for speech investigation (Harshman et al, 1977; Kent & Netsell, 1971; Kent, 1972; Maeda, 1989, Tye-Murray, 1991; Wood, 1979). X-ray images are produced when a beam is projected through the head and the internal tissues to a film plate placed on the opposite side of the body. X-ray studies of the oropharynx provide black-and-white images of the head and neck and clearly depict air-filled cavities, bones, and cartilage. Soft tissues such as the tongue and floor of the mouth muscles are often not able to be seen as they are obscured by the mandible. Another disadvantage in using X-rays for speech is that the major articulator, the tongue, is difficult to visualize unless a contrast medium such as barium is used; even then, the midline surface is often not clearly seen. Since the surface of the tongue is grooved and moves in various planes consecutively, it is not seen reliably on X-ray studies. Although most of the earlier studies of speech were done with X-ray, recent concern over cumulative exposure to ionizing radiation may limit its future use.

The individual can, by moving the body within the radiographic plane, be studied in several upright positions (lateral, anterior/posterior) as well as lying down. Because of beam scatter, the investigator or technician in the room is also accumulating radiation exposure if not properly shielded. Therefore, repeated studies must be carefully considered for cumulative risk to both examiner and client (Beck & Gayler, 1991). The National Council on Radiation Protection and Measurements recommends that maximum dose to an examiner not exceed 500 mrem and not more than 50 mrem in a month if a radiation worker is pregnant or considering pregnancy (Beck & Gayler, 1991; NIH Guidelines, 1994). Additional concern is that the tissues of the thyroid, breast, lungs, and olfactory bulb are exposed to ionizing radiation during speech studies.

Images can also be obtained using more rapid X-rays. Focused beams such as X-ray microbeam and high-resolution video produce less radiation exposure than static spot films. Standard static X-rays are limited to four exposures per second, hardly fast enough for speech studies where the changes in the vocal tract occur in hundredths or tenths of a second during continuous speech. It is recommended that there be a clear rationale for using still X-rays for speech studies as the long-term exposure risks may exceed the benefits. Since speech studies using X-ray are able to be recorded on to video tape, images can be collected and stored at a rate of 30 frames (60 video fields) per second. This appears to be rapid enough to evaluate articulation, velar activity, hyolaryngeal motion, and coarticulation. X-ray studies may also be used to determine structural changes or deviations in the bony skeleton which may impair or alter speech production (ie, cleft palate, velar insufficiency, oropharyngeal syndromes). Dysarthric speech can be studied with videofluorography since the entire vocal tract can be visualized to document the various compensations or muscular patterns characterizing a dysarthria. Videofluorographic examination of speech remains the preferred technique for many investigators in spite of radiation exposure since it is readily available.

Tomography

Tomographic images differ from X-ray images in that slices of the organism are constructed by projecting a beam through tissue in a single plane, thus creating a slice of that plane. Images can be captured in four planes—sagittal, coronal, oblique, and transverse (Fig. 8–1). CT is a static procedure and cannot track motion. The midsagittal plane

IMAGING TECHNIQUES

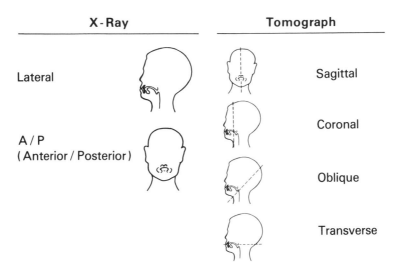

Figure 8–1. Tomographic imaging planes.

is taken longitudinally from top to bottom through the median plane of the body. The parasagittal plane is parallel and lateral to the midsagittal plane and is useful for seeing anatomical changes. The coronal plane is perpendicular to the midline and gives slices from anterior to posterior in the body. The oblique plane is a diagonal between the horizontal and vertical planes and is usually angled from under the chin toward the palate. Transverse images, in the transaxial or axial plane, are taken perpendicular to the long axis of the body. This plane is used to image the posterior tongue, pharynx, and larynx and may show the vocal folds and glottis.

Computed Tomography

CT is an imaging procedure that uses X-radiation to obtain slices or sections of the body. Currently, different thicknesses are used when scanning various structures. The thinnest CT voxel is 1.5 × 1.5 mm used to image the internal auditory canal. A 2 × 3 mm voxel is used for the head and cranium and a 5 × 5 mm voxel for scanning the neck area. All images are based on a 512 × 512 pixel metric scale. The scanner rotates while taking multiple images at different angles of a single section (Fig. 8–2). A composite view is then created from the digitized data that displays structures that were not visible on each plane. A transverse section of the oropharynx at rest is seen on Figure 8–3.

Bone appears as bright white and the air in the vocal tract appears black. The jaw is at the top of the image and a vertebra at the bottom. The hyoid bone is the white horseshoe shaped figure in the center of the image and the epiglottis can also be detected as a gray area beneath the hyoid. Soft tissues such as the tongue (above the hyoid) appear gray and can be visualized more clearly on CT than on X-ray because of digital summing of a series of scans. The typical clinical head/neck CT scan procedure takes approximately 35–40 min to perform. Intravenous nonionic iodine contrast material is used to better visualize vessels and soft tissues.

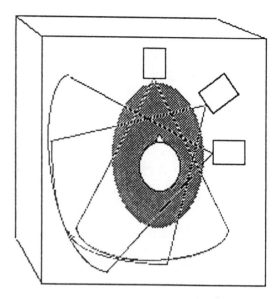

Figure 8–2. Schematic view of the rotation of the CT scanner during image acquisition of a single section. Subject's head is represented by the circle in the center of the block.

The head must be secured and respiration suspended for coronal sections as breathing increases artifacts. To get a clear view of the vocal folds, the neck must be hyperextended to elevate the laryngeal structures out of the way of the shoulders. If this is not done, the shoulders impose streaking artifacts onto the image. However, placement into neck hyperextension posture will inhibit or change articulatory motion.

CT is not typically used for speech imaging because scan rates are too slow for real-time speech production. Dysarthric speech has been examined with CT to evaluate central nervous system abnormalities such as white matter changes (Belli et al, 1993), hydrocephalus (Salvi et al, 1992), and cerebellar atrophy (Demichele et al, 1993). Because of the radiation exposure to the vocal tract and positioning difficulty, very few studies use this technique to evaluate abnormal articulation. Several studies have examined the normal vocal tract with CT (Kiritani et al, 1977; Muraki et al, 1983; Sundberg et al, 1987).

Although the newer, high-speed CT scanners (Imatron) can capture several images

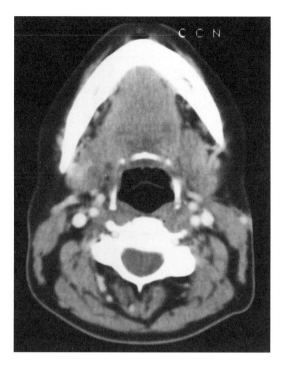

Figure 8–3. Transverse CT section of the resting oropharynx. The following bones appear as bright white structures (from top to bottom of the figure): mandible, hyoid bone, vertebrae. The tongue is a less distinct gray area between the hyoid and mandible. The dark region in the center of the scan is the pharynx.

Table 8–1. Summary of advantages and limits of speech imaging procedures.

X-Ray
1. Ionizing radiation
2. Video format for real-time studies
3. Limited repeatability
4. Poor soft tissue resolution
5. Good resolution of bony skeleton

Computerized Tomography
1. Ionizing radiation
2. Static images
3. Clear definition of structures, especially bone
4. Static images
5. Slow speed of acquisition of images
6. Good ability to detect vascular lesions, and small tumors
7. Positional discomfort during speech acquisition studies

Magnetic Resonance Imaging
1. Nonionizing radiation
2. Easy multiplanar views
3. Excellent tissue definition
4. Slow speed of acquisition of images
5. Image slices too thick
6. Claustrophobic responses
7. Magnetic field problems for metal objects
8. Likely to show continued technological advances

Ultrasound
1. No bioeffects
2. Totally noninvasive
3. Normal acquisition postures for speech
4. No limits on repeatability of studies
5. Real-time imaging
6. Excellent soft tissue definition
7. Bones not imaged
8. 140° sector with variable depth functions
9. Good tongue surface imaging
10. Rapid speech acquisition
11. Video format for playback and analysis

The clinician or investigator who desires to examine speech production in normal or impaired speakers should be able to select from among the various imaging systems which were presented in this chapter. No single existing system is yet that "perfect self-contained" system we need to analyze speech. Therefore knowledge of many advanced technologies is imperative to capture the complexities of human communication.

per second, they are still not fast enough to visualize continuous motions of the tongue and palate during articulation. CT has an advantage in that the images are clear with distinct edges between various surfaces, which allows easy measurement of regions of interest. Composite three-dimensional vocal tract shapes can be reconstructed by combining multiple sections from the 2-mm slices. Although CT has proven to be an excellent means for studying the anatomy and vascular structures, it remains less desirable than MRI because of radiation exposure.

Magnetic Resonance Imaging

MRI and CT provide anatomically equivalent studies in relation to the quality of the images they are capable of producing. MRI relies on relaxation times (T1 and T2) and proton density for contrast between normal and pathologic tissue, while CT relies only on differences in electron density (Mancuso, 1993). MRI uses a magnetic field and radio waves rather than X-radiation to obtain tissue sections.

The MRI system contains electromagnets that create a magnetic field that surrounds the part of the body scanned. Hydrogen atoms occur in abundance in water. MRI detects the presence of hydrogen atoms in human tissues, which are largely composed of water. The following are depicted in Figure 8–4, where A represents a hydrogen proton spinning about an axis which is oriented randomly. Picture B shows what happens when a magnetic field is introduced. The proton's axis aligns along the direction of the poles of the magnetic field. The proton continues to wobble even when aligned. In picture C, a short-lived radio pulse that vibrates at the same frequency as the wobble is introduced. This pulse causes the proton to loose its alignment. In D the proton realigns to the magnetic field and emits a weak radio signal. These radio signals are then assembled from the derived images of the hydrogen density and water content. Thus, MRI is able to differentiate among the various body tissues.

Figure 8–5 shows a coronal MRI image of the head. Although the tongue can be differentiated from the other structures, on this image it is not distinct enough for fine measurements.

Figure 8–6 is a midline sagittal MRI image taken while the tongue was at rest, while

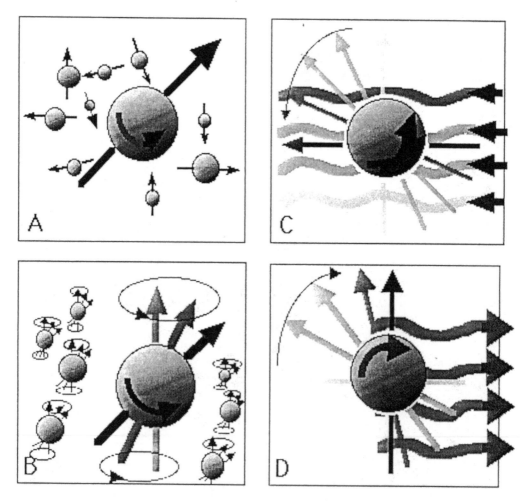

Figure 8–4. Creation of MRI images. (A) Rotation of a hydrogen proton; (B) introduction of a magnetic field; (C) introduction of a short-lived radio pulse; (D) realignment of the proton to the magnetic field and emission of radio signals.

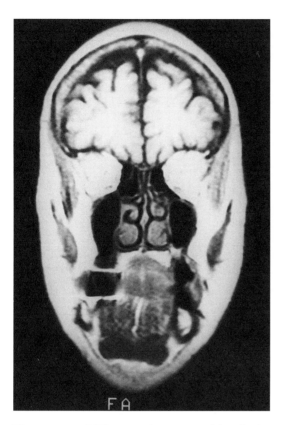

Figure 8–5. MRI coronal section of head, the tongue is the central gray area at the bottom; nasal sinuses, air in oral cavity and teeth are black; cortex seen at top of image; bones are white and nasal turbinates are the curled midline structures.

Figure 8–7 shows a sagittal MRI image of /a/ taken in the nearly identical postalveolar plane. The subject held the /a/ for 45 sec to produce this image. The vocal tract and teeth both appear black because neither contain water. The bone marrow of the palate has high water content. The fat surrounding the head has high hydrogen content. Therefore they both appear bright white. None of the hard tissue structures appear as distinctly as they may on CT.

MRI can depict soft tissue anatomy and therefore has been used to view the vocal tract by various investigators (Christianson et al, 1987; Lufkin et al, 1983; McKenna et al, l990). Several studies used MRI with other imaging techniques such as ultrasound (Takashima et al, 1989; Wein et al, 1990), X-ray (Lakshminarayanan et al, 1990, 1991) and glossometry (McCutcheon et al, 1990). In McCutcheon's work, tongue-palate spacers were used to generate known tongue positions on which to validate both instruments. Several investigators have used MRI to calculate vocal tract volumes (Baer et al, 1987, 1991; Lakshminarayanan et al, 1990, 1991; Moore, 1992). A recent MRI technique reported by Lakshminarayanan, allows for more rapid scan rates of up to 4 seconds per image. This rapid rate was achieved with a specially designed coil to highlight the oral area and a gradient-echo technique. The authors were able to generate formant patterns comparable to actual acoustic data although they found individual formant variations of up to 500 Hz. The authors speculated that these errors could be due to their assumptions of cross-sectional tube area or to the conversion algorithm that they used.

Another new application of MRI is to visualize tongue displacement with rapid tagged magnetization (Kumada et al, 1992; Niitsu et al, 1992, 1994). This tagging snapshot technique has been used to examine tongue position at the beginning and end of a movement to derive the direction of that movement. Tagging stripes were superimposed on a slice of tissue. As the tongue tissue changed its shape and position, the stripes moved and deformed, reflecting the changes in the tissue. The compression and expansion of the body of the tongue was able to be seen. In their most recent study, Niitsu et al (1994) used a "magnetization-prepared gradient-recalled echo imaging sequence" to obtain a midline sagittal section of the tongue and then created additional vertical and/or horizontal tags by added pulses that were superimposed on the resting oropharynx. These appear as high-intensity bands which contrast to the dark tagging stripes produced by the spin-echo techniques. Midline sagittal sections were 10 mm thick, creating 7–10 tags, each 3 mm thick with a 7-mm gap. Tongue displacement was studied on three Japanese speakers during production of /i/.

The positional changes of the tongue have been studied in abnormal populations such

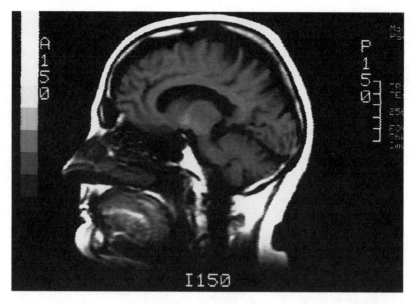

Figure 8–6. MRI resting midline sagittal view of the head showing the tongue and oral structures.

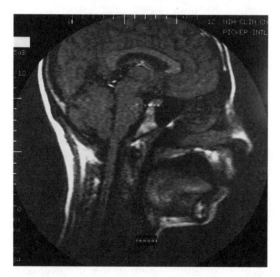

Figure 8–7. Midline sagittal MRI image of /a/. Tongue surface is unclear; vocal tract and teeth appear as black areas above and posterior to tongue tissue.

as ALS (Cha & Patten, 1989). Wein et al (1991) demonstrated the presence of velopharyngeal inadequacy in patients with a variety of pathological conditions. Since cortical tissue changes are visible using MRI, several investigators have examined the cortex of dysarthric speakers with varying eti-

ologies; cerebellar atrophy (Bonni et al, 1993), Gilles-de-la-Tourette syndrome (Leckman et al, 1993), basal ganglia lesions (Krageloh-Mann et al, 1992), and cerebellar infarcts (Barth et al, 1993). Since soft tissues can be clearly visualized, both MRI and CT can be used to see tissue changes, tumors, and cysts.

There are several disadvantages of MRI. Even using the special tagged radio signal, the signal is so weak that is must be summed over time thus reducing the speed of the obtained images. Speed of acquisition thus becomes a major limitation of MRI as imaging time for a picture with good resolution can take up to several minutes (Moore, 1992; Wein et al, 1991). Especially with the newer scanners that take only 50 msec per scan, image resolution is reduced. Since the technology of MRI is rapidly improving and changing, rate of image acquisition might approach real time and be able to assess online speech production.

A second limitation of present MRI systems is the width of the section. Whereas CT sections are 2 mm wide, MRI scans are 5 mm wide or more. The problem with a wide scan is that tomographic scanning compresses 3D space into two dimensions. It essentially represents a cylinder as a circle and therefore, structures that are 5 mm apart in the plane of the image would appear to be in the same plane. The result of this is that the hyoid bone and epiglottis may appear in the same slice even though the hyoid is actually several millimeters below the epiglottis.

Another drawback of MRI is that many subjects (anecdotes indicate about 30%) will experience claustrophobia and cannot tolerate being placed in a narrow enclosed tube for up to the 45 minutes needed to complete a scan. Because of the magnetic field, caution must also be taken to find subjects without dental or steel implants, pacemakers, metal clamps, and any other object that would be affected by the magnet. The MRI signal is stopped when it nears metal and a diffuse dark area appears about the circumference of the object on the MRI.

Another limitation of both CT and MRI is the positioning of the subject within the scanner. Since the individual must lie supine or prone, the forces of gravity affect the opposition of the normal agonist/antagonist muscle relationships as they occur during normal speech output.

In spite of these difficulties, MRI and CT can provide valuable information on the vocal tract as both soft and hard tissues can be visualized in the various planes of the body. These techniques, in their next generation, should allow for three-dimensional reconstruction of the rapid articulatory postures of some of the interesting aspects of speech in both normal and abnormal subjects.

Ultrasound

Ultrasound imaging relies on a completely different principle from the previous imaging technologies in that the images are created by ultra-high-frequency sound waves (20,000 to 20,000,000 Hz) reflected through the tissues. These sounds are well above the range of the human ear and thus the term "ultrasound." The sounds are generated by an electric pulse stimulated by a piezoelectric crystal housed in a transducer which both transmits and receives the reflected sound

wave. When the pulsed sound wave traveling through the tissues reaches an interface with tissue of a different density or elasticity such as bone, fluid, tendons, or air, some (or most) of the sound wave is reflected back to the source. These reflections are converted from acoustic energy to electrical energy and depicted in a computerized gray scale as a video image. Two types of transducers, sector scanner or linear array, can be used to image the oropharynx. Both of these transducers allow the sound reflections to be seen as a section of tissue in a single plane rather than as a single point in time as is obtained using A mode ultrasound. With a sector scanner, a wedge-shaped section of up to 140° is created (Fig. 8–8). With the linear array transducer the crystals fire sequentially and create a rectangular section of tissue (Fig. 8–9).

For speech imaging the transducers are positioned below the chin in the soft tissue depression just posterior to the mandible and superior to the thyroid cartilage (Fig. 8–10). Multiple plane images (sagittal, parasagittal) can be created by changing the transducer angle or moving the transducer from midline off to either side. Coronal images of the tongue are created simply by the rotation of the transducer 90° from the midline sagittal position. Since the tongue is surrounded by air, when the sound waves reach the air/tissue interface at the surface of the tongue, the sound is reflected back to its source, creating a bright white line that represents the tongue surface. The muscles below the tongue surface, the superior and transverse longitudinal muscles, and the genioglossus muscle are clearly visible. All of these muscles, as well as the floor muscles of the mouth, geniohyoid, mylohyoid, and digastric, can be seen in either the sagittal or coronal views (Shawker, Sonies, & Stone, 1984a,b). Closeup details of muscle fibers can be imaged by changing the depth of the image (Fig. 8–11). Since ultrasound is collected with a video format, images are acquired in real time, and detailed muscle activity can be easily studied during speech activity.

185

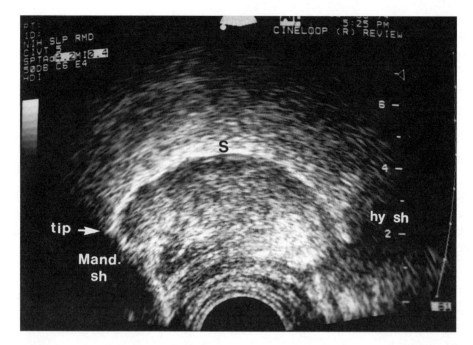

Figure 8–8. Midline sagittal Ultrasound section of tongue showing the various muscle layers and floor muscles. Tongue surface is the bright white curved line, tip is seen at the right with air under the surface as another white line. The point where the muscles insert on the superior cornu of the hyoid bone is the area beneath the dark triangular shadow cast by the hyoid bone. The dark area at the far right is the shadow cast by the mandible.

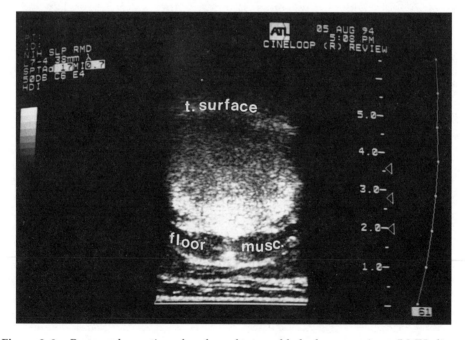

Figure 8–9. Rectangular section of surface of tongue blade dorsum using a 5-MHz linear array transducer (ATL).

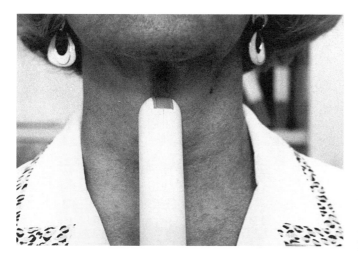

Figure 8–10. Placement of the ultrasound transducer below the chin for imaging the tongue and oropharynx.

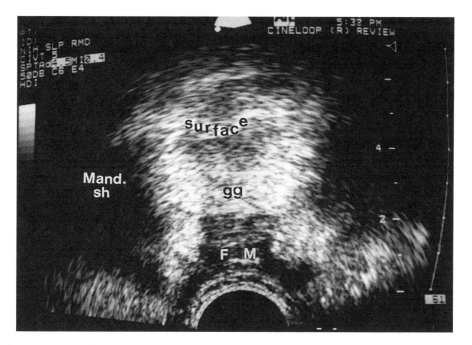

Figure 8–11. Ultrasound coronal view of the tongue. The genioglossus muscle is the center triangular mass, the floor muscles are below, and the surface is the curved white line at the top. The mandible casts a black shadow on both sides of the tongue.

By placing the linear array transducer at the thyroid notch and directing it backwards so the beam is in the transverse plane, the larynx and vocal folds can be seen (Carp & Bundy, 1988; Hamlet, 1980; Raghavendra et al, 1987; Sonies, 1991a,b) (Fig. 8–12). Although the rapid vibrations of the true vocal folds are unable to be captured on ultrasound as it is limited to 60 fields per second by the video capture format, different vocal fold patterns can be visualized (Fig. 8–13). With ultrasound imaging of the larynx, the patterns of adduction/abduction of the folds during repeated or isolated phonation of

187

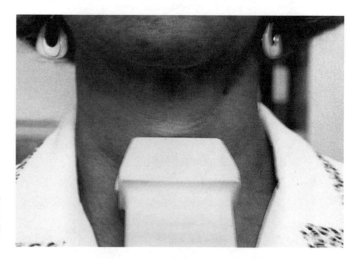

Figure 8–12. Placement of the ultrasound transducer at thyroid notch for transverse view of the larynx.

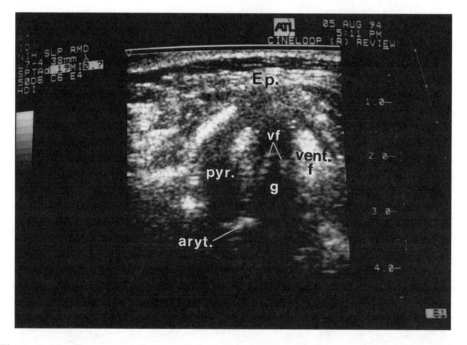

Figure 8–13. Transverse ultrasound view of the larynx. Glottis, ventricular folds, epiglottis, arytenoid cartilages, aryepiglottic ligament, and pyriform sinuses are seen during production of /i/.

consonants and vowels can be examined (Kaneko et al, 1988). If paralysis or abnormal bowing exists, it is readily visible. Polyps, tumors, and other masses that distort vocal fold physiology can also be seen from the transverse view (Fruehwald et al, 1987; Gademann et al, 1986; Gritzman et al, 1989).

Ultrasound has been used to study tongue motions during speech in normal and dysarthric speakers (Shawker & Sonies 1984; Sonies, 1981a,b, 1991; Stone et al, 1987, 1988) and for speech and biofeedback (Shawker & Sonies, 1985). From studying phonation of single vowels and CV and CVC units, it has been discerned that there are several lingual motion patterns such as lateral bracing, inversion, grooving that accompany production (Morrish et al, 1984, 1985; Stone, 1990; Stone et al, 1988).

Among the advantages of using ultrasound for the study of speech is that it is totally noninvasive, uses normal postures and positions, and has no known bioeffects. Because of these features it can be used repeatedly to obtain normative information for longitudinal and short-term studies on subtle tongue configurations that cannot be determined from any other procedure. The real-time and multiple-plane features of ultrasound make it capable of capturing in vivo tongue movements, not static postures, thus allowing for reconstruction of complex movements of the tongue surface needed for three-dimensional studies and modeling of the tongue surface (Stone, 1990; Stone & Lele, 1992; Watkin & Rubin, 1989).

References

Baer T, Gore J, Boyce S, Nye P. (1987). Application of MRI to the analysis of speech production. *Magn Resonance Imaging* 5:1–7.

Baer T, Gore J, Gracco C, Nye P. (19911). Analysis of vocal tract shape and dimensions using magnetic resonance imaging: vowels. *J Acoust Soc Am* 90:799–828.

Barth A, Bogousslavsky J, Regli F. (1993). The clinical and topographic spectrum of cerebellar infarcts—a clinical magnetic resonance imaging correlation study. *Ann Neurol* 33:451–456.

Beck TJ, Gayler BW. (1991). Radiation in video-recorded fluoroscopy. In: Jones B, Donner MW, eds. *Normal and Abnormal Swallowing: Imaging in Diagnosis and Therapy*. New York: Springer-Verlag.

Belli L, Decarlis L, Romani F, et al. (1993). Dysarthria and cerebellar ataxia—late occurrence of severe neurotoxicity in a liver transplant recipient. *Transplant Int* 6:176–178.

Bonni A, Delcarpiooodonovan R, Robitaille Y, Andermann E, Andermann F, Arnold D. (1993). Magnetic resonance imaging in the diagnosis of dominantly inherited cerebello-olivary atrophy. *Can Assoc Radiol J* 44:194–198.

Carp H, Bundy A. (1988). Ultrasound examination of the vocal cords and larynx: a guide to intubation and a diagnostic aid. *Anesthesiology* 60:303.

Cha C, Patten B. (1989). Amyotrophic lateral sclerosis: abnormalities of the tongue on magnetic resonance imaging. *Ann Neurol* 25:468–472.

Christianson R, Lufkin R, Hanafee W. (1987). Normal magnetic resonance imaging anatomy of the tongue, oropharynx, hypopharynx and larynx. *Dysphagia* 1:119–127.

Demichele G, Filla A, Striano S, Rimoldi M, Campanella G (1993). Heterogeneous findings in 4 cases of cerebellar ataxia associated with hypogonadism. *Clin Neurol Neurosurg* 95:23–28.

Fruehwald F, Salomonowitz E, Neuhold A, Pavelka R, Mailath G. (1987). Tongue cancer: sonographic assessment of tumor stage. *J Ultrasound Med* 6:121–137.

Gademann VG et al. (1986). Kernspintomographisches Staging von Tumoren der Mundhohle, des Oro- und Hypopharynx sowie des Larynx: Vergleich mit Computertomographie und Sonographie. [NMR staging of tumors of the oral cavity and oro and hypopharynx as well as the larynx: comparison with CT and sonography.] *Fortschr Rontgenstr* 145(5).

Gritzmann N, Traxler M, Grasl G, Pavelka R. (1989). Advanced laryngeal cancer: sonographic assessment. *Radiology* 171:171–175.

Hamlet S. (1980). Ultrasonic measurement of larynx height and vocal fold vibratory pattern. *J Acoust Soc Am* 68:121–126.

Harshman R, Ladefoged P, Goldstein L. (1977). Factor analysis of tongue shapes. *J Acoust Soc Am* 62:693–707.

Hirose H. (1986). Pathophysiology of motor speech disorders (dysarthria). *Folia Phoniatrica* 38:61–88.

Kaneko T, Numata T, Haruhiko S, Hino T, Komatsu K, Masuda T. (1988). Newly developed ultrasound laryngographic equipment and its clinical application in voice physiology. In: Fujimura O, ed. *Voice Production, Mechanism and Function*. New York: Raven.

Kent R. (1972). Some considerations in the cinefluorographic analysis of tongue movements during speech. *Phonetica* 26:16–32.

Kent R, Netsell R. (1971). Effects of stress contrasts on certain articulatory parameters. *Phonetica* 24:23–44.

Kiritani S, Kakita K, Shibata S. (1977). Dynamic palatography. In: Sawashima M, Cooper F, eds. *Dynamic Aspects of Speech Production.* Tokyo: Tokyo University Press, pp 159–170.

Krageloh-Mann I, Grodd W, Niemann G, Haas G, Ruitenbeek W. (1992). Assessment and therapy monitoring of Leigh disease by MRI and proton spectroscopy. *Pediatr Neurol* 8:60–64.

Kumada M, Niitsu B, Niimi S, Hirose H. (1992). A study on the inner structure of the tongue in the production of the 5 Japanese vowels by Tagging Snapshop MRI. *Res Inst Logoped Phoniatr Annu Bull* 26:1–12.

Lakshminarayanan A, Lee S, McCutcheon M. (1990). Vocal tract shape during vowel production as determined by magnetic resonance imaging. Presented at 13th annual meeting of Society of Computed Body Tomography; Palm Springs, CA.

Lakshminarayanan A, Lee S, McCutcheon M. (1991). MR imaging of the vocal tract during vowel production. *J Magn Resonance Imaging* 1:71–76.

Leckmean J, de Lotbiniere A, Marek K, Gracco C, Scahill L, Cohen D. (1993). Severe disturbances in speech, swallowing, and gait following stereotactic infrathalamic lesions in Gilles de la Tourette's syndrome. *Neurology* 43:890–894.

Lufkin R, Larsson S, Hanafee W. (1983). Work in progress: NMR anatomy of the larynx and tongue base. *Radiology* 148:173–175.

Maeda S. (1989). Compensatory articulation during speech: Evidence from the analysis and synthesis of vocal tract shape using an articulatory model. In: Hardcastle W, Marchal A, eds. *Speech Production and Speech Modeling.* Boston: Kluwer, pp 131–150.

Mancuso A. (1993). CT and MRI of head and neck cancer. University of Florida College of Medicine. Unpublished paper. *Radiol Soc North Am* 1994.

McCutcheon M, Lee S, Lakshminarayanan A, Fletcher S. (1990). A comparison of glossometric measurements of tongue position with magnetic resonance images of the vocal tract. *J Acoust Soc Am* 87:S122. Abstract.

McKenna D, Jabour B, Lufkin R, Hanafee W. (1990). Magnetic resonance imaging of the tongue and oropharynx. *Top Magn Reson Imaging* 2:49–59.

Moore C. (1992). The correspondence of vocal tract resonance with volumes obtained from magnetic resonance images. *J Speech Hearing Res* 35:1009–1023.

Morrish KA, Stone M, Shawker T, Sonies BC. (1985). Distinguishability of tongue shape during vowel production. *J Phonet* 13:189–204.

Morrish KA, Stone M, Shawker T, Sonies BC. (1984). Characterization of tongue shape during normal speech. *J Acoust Soc Am* 75:S23A.

Muraki A, Mancuso A, Harnsberger H, Johnson L, Meads G. (1983). CT and the oropharynx, tongue base and floor of the mouth: normal anatomy and range of variations, and applications in staging carcinoma. *Radiology* 148:725–731.

Niitsu M, Kumada M, Campeau N, Niimi S, Riederer S, Itai Y. (1994). Tongue displacement: Visualization with rapid tagged magnetization-prepared MR imaging. *Radiology* 191:578–580.

Niitsu M, Kumada M, Niimi S, Itai Y. (1992). Tongue movement during phonation: a rapid quantitative visualization using tagging snapshot MR imaging. *Res Inst Logoped Phoniatr Annu Bull* 26.

Raghavendra BN, Horii SC, Reede DL, Rumancik WM, Persky M, Bergeron RT. (1987). Sonographic anatomy of the larynx, with particular reference to the vocal cords. *J Ultrasound Med* 6:225–230.

Salvi F, Michelucci R, Plasmati R, et al. (1992). Slowly progressive familial demential with recurrent strokes and white matter hypodensities on CT scan. *Ital J Neurol Sci* 13:135–140.

Shawker TH, Sonies BC. (1985). Ultrasound biofeedback for speech training. *Invest Radiol* 20:90–93.

Shawker TH, Sonies BC, Stone M. (1984). Sonography of speech and swallowing. In: Saunders RC, Hill M, eds. *Ultrasound Annual.* New York: Raven, pp 237–260.

Shawker TH, Sonies BC, Stone M. (1984). Soft tissue anatomy of the tongue and floor of the mouth: An ultrasound demonstration. *Brain Language* 21:335–50.

Shawker TH, Sonies BC. (1984). Tongue movement during speech: A real-time ultrasound evaluation. *J Clin Ultrasound* 12:125–133.

Sonies BC. (1991a). Instrumental procedures for diagnosis. *Semin Speech Language* 12(3).

Sonies BC: (1991b). Ultrasound imaging and swallowing. In: Jones B, Donner MW, eds. *Normal and Abnormal Swallowing: Imaging in Diagnosis and Therapy.* New York: Springer-Verlag.

Sonies BC, Shawker TH, Gerber L, Leighton S. (1981a). Ultrasonic visualization of motion during speech. *J Acoust Soc Am* 70:693–696.

Sonies B et al. (1981b). Ultrasonic visualization of tongue motion during speech. In: *Working Papers in Biocommunication,* Vol I. College Park, MD: University of Maryland, Department of Hearing and Speech Science.

Stone M, Lele S. (1992). Representing the tongue surface with curve fits. *Proc Int Conf Spoken Language Process* 2:875–878.

Stone M. (1991). Imaging the tongue and vocal tract. *Br J Disord Comm* 26:11–23.

Stone M. (1990). A three-dimensional model of tongue movement based on ultrasound and X-ray microbeam data. *J Acoust Soc Am* 87:2207–2217.

Stone M et al. (1988). Cross-sectional tongue shape during the production of vowels. *J Acoust Soc Am* 34:1586–1596.

Sundberg J, Johansson C, Wilbrand H, Ytterbergh C. (1987). From sagittal distance to area: A study of transverse vocal tract cross-sectional area. *Phonetica* 44:76–90.

Takashima S, Ikezoe J, Harada K, et al. (1989). Tongue cancer: Correlation of MR imaging and sonography with pathology. *Am J Neuroradiol* 10:419–424.

Tye-Murray N. (1991). The establishment of open articulatory postures by deaf and hearing talkers. *J Speech Hearing Res* 34:453–459.

Watkin K, Rubin J. (1989). Pseudo-three-dimensional reconstruction of ultrasonic images of the tongue. *J Acoust Soc Am* 85:496–499.

Wein B, Drobnitzky M, Klajman S, Angerstein W. (1991). Evaluation of functional positions of tongue and soft palate with MR imaging: Initial clinical results. *J Magn Res Imaging* 1:381–383.

Wein B, Bockler R, Huber W, Klajman S, Willmes K. (1990). Computer sonographic presentation of tongue shapes during formation of long German vowels. (In German.) *Ultraschall Med* 11:100–103.

Wood S. (1979). A radiographic examination of constriction location for vowels. *J Phonet* 7:25–43.

Chapter 9

Flaccid Dysarthria

Carlin Hageman

Introduction

Darley, Aronson, and Brown (1975) noted the term dysarthria is a collective name used for a group of speech disorders that arise from disruptions in neuromotor control of the muscular activities necessary for the production of speech. Dysarthria includes motor control disorders of neurologic origin for respiration, phonation, articulation, resonance, and prosody. Darley and his colleagues specifically noted that dysarthria includes speech disorders arising from an isolated injury to a specific cranial nerve affecting even one speech function such as velopharyngeal competence. The purpose of this chapter is to address dysarthria arising from lesions to the cranial and peripheral nerves that support motor speech production.

The peripheral nervous system (PNS) is either the first or final common pathway for all sensorimotor functions. For motor activities, all signals arising in the central nervous system (CNS) which will elicit muscle contractions to produce movements must pass through the final common pathway (FCP), which includes the lower motor neuron (LMN). These LMNs arise from motor nuclei in the brain stem and the spinal cord. Each LMN innervates a specific set of muscle fibers which together comprise a motor unit. Yorkston, Beukelman, and Bell (1988) noted that a variety of speech problems can occur depending upon the location and etiology of the injury to the motor unit. Practical questions concerning the assessment and management of flaccid dysarthria demand that

we take a closer look at the components and neural excitation of the motor unit.

Motor Unit

Darley et al (1975) noted that the motor unit consists of four parts: (1) the neuron cell bodies in the cranial nerve nuclei in the brain stem and the spinal nerve nuclei in the anterior horns of the spinal cord; (2) the axon that leaves the CNS and continues to the muscle; (3) the myoneural junction; and (4) the muscle fibers innervated by the LMN. A full discussion of the motor unit is beyond the scope of this chapter. However, two important points need to be made. First, a breakdown in the function of the lower motor neuron or motor unit can occur at any of these levels. Second, an axon aborizes within a motor unit innervating many muscle fibers and individual muscle fibers from one motor unit may intermingle with fibers from another motor unit. Consequently, Basmajian and Deluca (1985) observed that a single action potential does not characterize a motor unit; rather, a motor unit is distinguished by many action potentials at several sites in the motor unit.

Innervation of Muscle

A skeletal muscle can have thousands of muscle fibers but many fewer motor units. Muscles responsible for large, strong contractions have a relatively larger number of muscle fibers per motor unit whereas muscles responsible for fine, discrete movements have a relatively small number of muscle fibers per motor unit. For example, muscles of the leg or trunk may have a few hundred fibers per motor unit while muscles of a finger or the larynx may have as few as 10 fibers per motor unit. This illustrates the innervation ratio which refers to the ratio of axons to muscle fibers (Larson, 1989). Fewer muscle fibers per motor unit mean that the movements produced by contractions of these muscles can be more finely controlled. In addition, the contractile properties of muscles can be quantified in other ways (see Luschei and Finnegan, Chapter 7).

Contractile Properties of Muscle

Liss, Kuehnz, and Hinkle (1994) described four characteristics of muscle contraction: strength, power, endurance, and fatigue. They defined strength as the maximum force generated by a muscle or group of muscles, regardless of time. Power, on the other hand, also refers to maximum force but it is time-dependent (force generated over a specified time). Endurance was defined as the ability of muscle to maintain a submaximal level of contraction for a specified time period. Finally, they considered fatigue to be exhibited by a muscle when it cannot maintain a specified level of force without increasing neural drive. The threshold for fatigue was defined by Bigland-Ritchie and Woods (1984) as a level of exercise that cannot be sustained indefinitely. Robin, Somodi, and Luschei (1991) reported a technique for measuring tongue strength and fatigue (or endurance). However, they did not distinguish between endurance and fatigue and noted that many variables can affect fatigue (or endurance) including motivation and central recruitment of motor units.

Liss et al. (1994) described the physical correlates of strength, power, and endurance which included muscle fiber type and cross-sectional area of muscle fibers. The type of muscle fiber determines the strength, power, and endurance properties of that muscle. This is because the muscle fiber contractile properties determine contraction speed, fati-

gability, and metabolic characteristics. Chusid (1985) noted that striated muscle in humans can be grossly categorized as red or white. Red, or Type 1, muscle contains more myoglobin and responds slowly (slow contracting or slow twitching) but is fatigue resistant because red muscle has an oxidative mechanism for muscle contraction. These muscles are adapted for long, slow postural control activities. White, or Type 2, muscle typically has fewer muscle fibers per motor unit and short response times, but it fatigues more quickly because white muscle has an anaerobic metabolism specialized for fine skilled movements such as hand, tongue, and eye movements. Liss and colleagues reported that muscle physiologists have further divided Type II muscle to include: (1) Type IIA contract quickly but remain fatigue-resistant; (2) Type IIB contract quickly but are fatigue- sensitive; and (3) Type IIC, found in embryonic, degenerating, and regenerating muscle and have functional contraction properties between those of Type I and Type II muscle fibers.

Breakdown of the Motor Unit

At the level of the motor unit, there are several possibilities for breakdown of neuromuscular function. Darley et al. (1975) provided a useful model for classification of the dysarthrias based on etiology and site of lesion. One could use their model to construct Table 9–1, which summarizes lower motor neuron and motor unit dysarthrias without regard to speech symptoms. Speech problems arise from the specific cranial or spinal nerve affected and the location of the lesion within the peripheral nerve pathways.

Cranial Nerves

A listing of the cranial nerves and their general functions is available from many sources (eg, Larson, 1989) and will not be presented here. However, a summary (Aronson, 1990; Chusid, 1985; Darley et al, 1975; Yorkston et al., 1988) of the speech-related cranial nerves with respect to origin, distribution, etiolo-

Table 9–1. Lower motor neuron and motor unit dysarthria.

Lesion site	Symptoms*
Brainstem or peripheral nerve	Loss of muscle contraction of affected units for reflex and voluntary activity; flaccid muscle; reduced reflexes; hypotonia, muscle atrophy, weakness, paralysis, fasciculation
Myoneural junction	Weakness, increased fatiguability over short time periods
Muscle fibers	Muscle hypertrophy or atrophy, failure to relax; failure to contract, fatty infiltration and fibrosis, hypocontraction

*Chusid (1985).

gies, and symptoms for each is shown in Table 9–2.

Cranial Nerve Syndromes

In addition to those listed in Table 2, there are several syndromes that affect the four most inferior cranial nerves. These include: (1) Avellis' affecting IX and X; (2) Schmidt's affecting X and XI; (3) Jackson's affecting X, XI, and XII; (4) Tapia's affecting X and XII; (5) Babinski-Nageotte Bulbar affecting IX, X, XI, and XII with contralateral hemiplegia; (6) Wallenberg's, similar to Babinski-Nageotte but without hemiplegia; (7) Cestan-Chenais affecting the nuclei of V, X, and XI due to thrombosis of the vertebral artery; (8) Bonnier's affecting VIII, IX, X with Meniere's disease symptoms; (9) Vernet's involving IX, X, and XI often a basilar skull fracture involving the jugular foramen; and (10) Villaret's, Collet's, or Sicard's (retroparotid space injury) with ipsilateral paralysis of IX, X, XI, and XII.

Muscular Weakness and Paralysis

In the previous paragraphs, mention has been made of weakness, paresis, and paralysis. These characteristics were mentioned as potential outcomes of insults to the motor units. For example, what does it mean to have a weak or paretic muscle? Sustained muscle contractions are comprised of a large number of twitches (contractions) of muscles supplied by motor units. A single twitch lasts only a few milliseconds, and it can be repeated but only after a delay. In order to produce a relatively smooth, strong contraction, there is a temporal and spatial summation of motor unit contractions. The process of developing a smooth contraction could be disrupted in several ways. First, signals could be interrupted in the peripheral nerve as it courses to the muscle (eg, trauma or a demyelinating disease). The number of axons in the nerve that were affected or unaffected determines the number of motor units that produce a muscle twitch. Second, if the myoneural junction is disrupted so that the action potential from the neuron does not stimulate a corresponding muscle action potential , then the muscle twitch is stopped in that motor unit. This can occur when the neurotransmitter is depleted either from chronic stimulation (fatigue) or from a disease process that interferes with neurotransmitter uptake (eg, myasthenia gravis). Third, if the muscle is diseased or fatigued, then it may fail to twitch or contract properly (muscular dystrophies). The greater the number of interruptions, the fewer the number of twitches in the motor units that can be summed together to produce a smooth, strong contraction. Titze (1994) described this process in the vocal folds. In his example, maximum forces are generated in two

195

Table 9–2. Nerve, distribution, etiologies, and symptoms resulting from lesions to cranial nerves.

Cranial Nerve V (Trigeminal)

Sensory	Distribution
ophthalmic	forehead, eyes, nose, temples, and nasal mucosa
maxillary	teeth, upper lip, cheeks, hard palate, nasal mucosa
mandibular	teeth, lower lip, buccal mucosa, tongue, auditory meatus
Motor	Distribution
motor root (pons)	masseter, temporal, internal and external pterygoids
otic ganglion	tensor tympani, tensor veli palatini
mylohyoid	mylohyoid, anterior belly of digastric
Etiologies	neuralgias, neuritis, syphilis, tuberculosis, syringobulbia, tumors, basilar meningitis, tic douloureux, para trigeminal
Symptoms	paralysis or weakness of muscles of mastication with mandible deviation to the affected side

Cranial Nerve VII (Facial)

Nerve	Distribution
Sensory	
nervous intermedus	Taste to anterior 2/3 of the tongue
Motor	
temporal	frontalis, orbicularis oculi, dilator naris, nasalis
zygomatic	zygomaticus, quadratis labii superior, orbicularis oris
cervicofacial	risorius, mentalis, quadratis labii inferior, incisivus inferior, buccinator, posterior belly of digastric, stapedius
Etiologies	Bell's palsy, middle ear infections, chilling of the face, tumors
Symptoms	Lesion outside stylomastoid foramen—affected side of mouth droops, buccal stasis of food, no wink, decreased wrinkle of forehead on affected side
	Lesion in facial canal (chorda tympani)—reduced taste and salivation.
	Lesion in internal auditory meatus—deafness and facial weakness.
	Lesion at emergence from pons—facial weakness and other cranial nerve involvement.

Cranial Nerve IX (Glossopharyngeal)

Nerve	Distribution
Sensory	
Fibers from jugular ganglia	pharynx, soft palate, taste posterior 1/3 of tongue, fauces, tonsils, carotid body, and carotid sinus controlling reflexes for respiration, blood pressure, and heart rate.
Motor	stylopharyngeal
Parasympathetic	parotid gland
Etiologies	Bonnier's syndrome, Vernet's syndrome, glossopharyngeal neuralgia (paroxysmal pain)
Symptoms	loss of gag, dysphagia, loss of taste, sensation loss in pharynx and posterior tongue, increased salivation, tachycardia

Cranial Nerve X (Vagus)*

Nerve	Distribution
Sensory	
auricular	external auditory meatus, dura of posterior fossa
ganglion nodosum	pharynx, larynx, trachea, esophageus, abdominal cavity

Table 9–2. *Continued*

internal sup. laryn. Motor (nucleus ambiguous)	internal surface of larynx above vocal folds
pharyngeal	pharyngeal constrictors, levator veli palatini
external sup. laryn.	cricothyroid
recurrent laryngeal	all intrinsic laryngeal muscle except cricothyroid
Etiologies	intramedullary lesions including hemmorrhage, thrombosis, tumors, syphilis, syringobulbia. Peripheral lesions include primary neuritis (alcohol, dipheritic, lead, arsenic), tumors, trauma, surgery, aortic aneurysm
Symptoms	Bilateral recurrent lesions—adductor/abductor paralysis of vocal folds with aphonia, dyspnea, or pseudoasthma, cardiac arrhythmia and death. Unilateral recurrent lesions—unilateral vocal fold paralysis with dysphonia. Unilateral pharyngeal nerve—unilateral velar paralysis with hypernasality with deviation to strong side. Unilateral superior laryngeal nerve—anesthesia of larynx, fatigue, pitch control problems.

Cranial Nerve XI (Spinal accessory)	
Nerve	Distribution
Sensory	None
Motor	
Internal medullary	Via X Cranial Nerve contributes to intrinsic laryngeal muscle
External (spinal)	trapezius, sternocleidomastoid
Etiologies	menningitis, syphilis, trauma, surgery on tuberculoses nodes
Symptoms	
Unilateral	No rotation of head to healthy side; cannot shrug shoulder on affected side, affected shoulder droops
Bilateral	Difficult to rotate head or raise chin, head often drops forward

Cranial Nerve XII (Hypoglossal)	
Nerve	Distribution
Hypoglossal	Intrinsic muscle of tongue, styloglossus, genioglossus, geniohyoid, thyrohyoid, sternohyoid, sternothyroid, omohyoid
Etiologies	Basal skull fractures, dislocation of upper cervical vertebrae, tuberculoses, aneurysm of Circle of Willis, syphilis, and lead, alcohol, arsenic, & carbon monoxide poisonings, brain abscess, syringobulbia

*See Aronson (1990) for detailed examination of the X Cranial Nerve.

muscle groups where the muscle fiber twitch amplitudes are nearly equal. In a muscle group with a 100 motor unit condition, the force is steady, but in the two motor unit condition, the force is unsteady (see Fig. 9–1). This would mean that the strength in that two motor unit muscle would wax and wane producing an unsteady movement. Since the number of motor units is reduced in flaccid weakness, movements would be unsteady, which could lead to vocal variability in flaccid weakness of laryngeal muscles. Vocal variability is actually preferred by listeners, but only to a certain extent. When the vari-

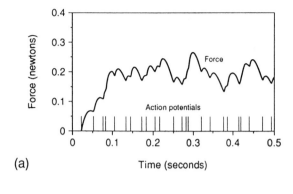

(a)

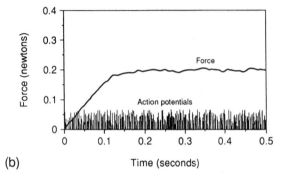

(b)

Figure 9–1. Stimulation of motor unit action potentials and corresponding muscle forces for (a) two motor units with equal twitch amplitudes and (b) 100 motor units with varying twitch amplitudes. (Titze, 1994; with permission.)

ability becomes too great, the voice is heard as rough.

When the entire peripheral nerve is interrupted, the specialized muscle receptors receive no neural input from the CNS. In this condition, no movement is possible and muscle tone is absent. The muscle is ultimately weak or paralyzed. Fasciculation, a spontaneous twitching, may occur within individual muscle fiber bundles. There will also be muscle atrophy. When some of the remaining LMN axons reach the muscle intact, then those muscle fibers are stimulated. Consequently, some degree of muscle tone is maintained, but since fewer motor units are available to contract, the muscle produces weaker and more irregular contractions. Muscle atrophy may occur because some motor units are nonfunctional due to the muscle fibers lack of stimulation from the

CNS. Finally, when the problem is at the myoneural junction, the effect depends upon the amount of neurotransmitter available and released and the amount that can be received by the specialized muscle. Since the muscle does receive input from the CNS, there will be no atrophy or fasciculation. During the course of a sustained contraction(s), neurotransmitter will be used up and motor unit dysfunction will occur, resulting in fewer motor unit twitches. As a result, muscle weakness from LMN involvement is a continuum from complete paralysis to variably reduced muscle contractions.

Neural Adaptation

The previous discussion concerning muscle weakness and motor units leads directly to neural adaptation. Within the realm of muscle strengthening, Liss et al (1994) noted that those "changes within the nervous system that correspond to muscle use and function are referred to as neural adaptation" (p 44). While the mechanisms of neural adaptation are not confined to lower motor neuron activities, the influence of neural adaptation on the functioning of weakened muscle due to LMN injury is potentially quite strong. Sale (1986) reported that strength and power training bring about changes in the nervous system. These changes allow the person to better organize the activation of muscle groups. Liss et al (1991) concluded that the goal of strength training is not to simply make muscles stronger but to make muscle activity more efficient. Increased efficiency in muscle activation could lead to strategies to improve weak speech musculature. Liss et al (1994) noted that muscle physiology research has shown that resistance training at any submaximal force level leads to reduced neural activity, suggesting greater efficiency. Sale (1986) reported data suggesting that early or rapid improved strength performance is likely due to neural adaptation rather than increased muscle size or metabolic capacity. Several investigators have suggested that neural adaptation occurs when one can recruit previously untapped motor units or increase the firing rate of already activated motor units (Kraemer, Deschenes, & Fleck, 1988; Liss et al, 1994; Sale, 1986; Sale, McComas, MacDougall, & Upton, 1982). Speech pathologists have yet to take advantage of the literature in exercise physiology and apply it to muscle retraining in dysarthria.

Muscle Training

Speech pathologists often utilize therapy time to enable the patient to strengthen weak, flaccid muscle. These attempts would seem to be right on target because the hallmark of LMN disease is weakness caused by the failure of muscle to contract properly. The success of these endeavors has been problematic. It may be that our attempts to strengthen weakened speech musculature were not as successful as they could have been because we did not utilize specific muscle training activities.

First, the literature strongly suggests that neural changes in muscle training are task-specific (Kraemer et al, 1988). This means that neural adaptation to increase a specific pattern of motor unit recruitment will occur only when the characteristics of the target movement match the training movement. Kraemer et al (1988) found that type of contraction, joint angle, and proper velocity must be considered. Sale and MacDougall (1981) reported four kinds of training specifics: (1) movement patterns, (2) velocity, (3) contraction type, and (4) contraction force. Liss et al (1994) utilized these concepts to develop a specific training procedure for velopharyngeal musculature. They attempted to exploit the relationship between neural adaptation, which leads to more efficient muscular activity for a task, and muscle training. This could lead to more strength in a muscle that is poorly innervated due to injuries to some number of the motor units innervating that muscle.

Liss et al (1994) summarized the specifics of muscle training and noted that specificity of movement means that the greatest strength increases will occur when the train-

ing occurs in the position(s) that the movement operates through. Thus, if we were to apply that notion to the lip, then strength training for the lip should vary according to the intended target. When the intended target is movement from an open to a closed position and then to open again, the strength training should have the lip moving against resistance from open to closed to open while fixing the mandible. If the target was tight lip closure to prevent leakage during eating, then pushing against resistance in the closed position while allowing the jaw to move might be more appropriate. For the tongue, it will be more difficult to develop movements that operate against resistance yet mimic the movements of speech. Since the tongue is a hydrostat and does not operate around a joint, position angles and movement strategies to attain those angles (positions) during strength training may be quite different for the tongue compared to the arm. Finally, when constructing movement activities one might want to consider compensatory postures/movements that might change the movement requirements and consequently the strength training requirements. Liss and colleagues (1994) concluded that the palliative affect of strength training that is designed around these considerations resulted from neural adaptation rather than muscle change per se. If this is true, then one could expect changes in strength to occur sooner rather than later since neural adaptation seem to occur relatively quickly compared to muscle fiber change.

Second, the training should occur at similar velocities as the target movement. Again, neural adaptation is probably the mechanism responsible. Liss et al (1994) suggested that the CNS may respond differently to slow versus fast movments. This would mean that therapy to improve tongue velocity using slow, protrusion movements against a tongue blade has two strikes against it with respect to the efficiency of muscle training. The movement (or lack of movement) does not approach the velocity of speech and the position of the tongue is clearly incorrect to tongue positions that occur during speech and may be, in fact, deleterious to the learning of natural tongue movements during speech.

Third, Liss et al (1994) noted that the type of contractions should match the intended movment and muscle contraction type. Three forms of contraction against a resistance are possible: (1) concentric—muscle is shortening during the movement; (2) eccentric—the muscle is lengthening during the movement; and (3) isometric—the muscle does not change length against the resistance. Many exercises that have been used by speech pathologists were isometric. Dworkin (1991) has developed some clever strategies for strengthening exercises for the speech mechanism. However, it will be up to the individual speech pathologist to utilize his ideas and others to meet the muscle training requirements noted here. For example, Liss and colleagues (1994) reported a unique application of continuous positive airway pressure (CPAP) to employ air pressure as a resistance for the velum to move against during muscle training exercise.

Measurement, Assessment, and Management

The challenges facing the speech pathologist in treatment of the dysarthric individual are numerous and difficult. Models have been suggested as a way to organize our efforts. Wertz (1985) combined measurement and assessment into appraisal and suggested five objectives: (1) to measure the patient's symptoms and recognize the hierarchical relationship among them to determine the relative contribution to the speech deficit; (2) to determine the speech diagnosis (eg, presence and type of dysarthria); (3) to determine the severity of the disorder; (4) to determine the probability for improvement (prognosis); and (5) to focus the therapy. Rosenbek and LaPointe (1985) also suggested that speech pathologists need to use models to guide their assessments. They proposed using a point-place model (Netsell, 1973) (see Table 9–3) complemented with a process model

Table 9–3. Point-place model adapted by Rosenbek and LaPointe (1985).

Point	Place
1	Muscles & structures of respiration
2	Larynx
3	Velopharyngeal port
4	Tongue blade
5	Tongue tip
6	Lips
7	Jaw

(articulation, resonation, phonation, respiration, and prosody) to appraise speech difficulties of dysarthria.

Models focus one's attention and lead to more systematic appraisal. However, they may lead to a relatively inflexible mental set when the model is not revised. The mental set with which one approaches the measurement and assessment of dysarthria establishes the perceptual and cognitive filters that determine our actions and subsequently our conclusions. Arguments about whether nonspeech measures or only speech measures should be used to measure and assess dysarthria may be the result of perceptual and cognitive filters leading us in one direction or another. For a more in-depth discussion of these issues, readers are referred to Luschei (1991), Weismer and Liss (1991), and Kent (1994). Luschei argued elegantly that just because the extent of the relationship between, for example, tongue strength and articulatory accuracy is not known with certainty, it is not sufficient reason to refrain from investigating the utility of objective nonspeech measures of tongue function. This would seem to be especially true in the case of flaccid dysarthria because it is the execution of motor commands that is disrupted and not the planning, organizing, or ideation of speech. The bottom line is that speech pathologists are trying to minimize the effects of dysarthria on the patient's life and to accomplish that goal in the most efficient and cost effective way possible. With the present state-of-the-art measurement methods and assessment strategies, it is probably possible to achieve that goal in different ways, depending upon the perspective and goals.

Yorkston et al (1988) noted that there are at least three perspectives from which dysarthria is addressed—neurology, speech physiology, and speech pathology (or rehabilitationist). To successfully manage the dysarthric patient, the speech pathologist must be able to change perspectives (mental set or filter) to fit the purpose at hand. One way to remain flexible, yet organized and efficient, might be to utilize a model that fosters measurement and assement from different perspectives. Since dysarthria can be viewed as a chronic disorder, models that could address dysarthria in that way (Frey, 1984; Wood, 1980; Yorkston et al, 1988) might be useful to the speech pathologist to create a perspective (filter set) that is adaptive. Frey's (1984) model included three levels: (1) impairment, "any loss or abnormality of psychological, physiological, or anatomical structure or function" (eg, paralyzed velum); (2) disability, "restriction or lack (resulting from impairment) of the ability to perform an activity in the manner or within the range considered normal for the human being" (eg, reduced intelligibility); and (3) handicap, the "disadvantage for a given individual (resulting from an impairment or disability) that limits or prevents the fulfillment of a role that is normal (depending upon age, sex, social, cultural factors) for that individual" (eg, loss of a teaching position). In the paragraphs that follow, the management of flaccid dysarthria is addressed within the "chronic disorder" model. Since this chapter is devoted to flaccid dysarthria, it will be assumed that the measurement and assessment procedures have been completed and that the sequelae of flaccid dysarthria have been found. Sources with more complete discussions of measurement and assessment are widely available (Dworkin, 1991; Kent, Kent, & Rosenbek, 1987; Linebaugh, 1983; McNeil & Kennedy,

1984; Rosenbek & LaPointe, 1985; Wertz, 1985; Yorkston et al, 1988) and are found in other chapters in this text.

Management

After a diagnosis of flaccid dysarthria has been made, the therapeutic decisions regarding treatment priorities have not. Dworkin (1991) proposed a hierarchical approach to management in which respiration and resonation were first-order (top-priority) subsystems, which meant that they should be treated to their maximum potential first. He suggested that second-order (phonation) and third-order (articulation and prosody) should not be treated until first-order problems are resolved to a criterion established by the clinician. In contrast, Rosenbek and LaPointe (1985) suggested that the management approach should be based on a hierarchy of symptoms. The clinician establishes the hierarchy based on his or her judgment about the causative relationship among symptoms and their contribution to the intelligibility reduction of the dysarthria. Rosenbek & LaPointe's (1985) management strategy suggested eight specific treatment goals. These goals addressed each of the point-place issues in Netsell's (1973) model (eg, modify respiration, modify phonation etc.), targeted process-based issues (eg, modify prosody), sought the remediation of impairments (eg, modify abnormalities of posture, tone and strength), and finally pursued the reduction of handicap (eg, help a person to become a productive client). Since the author of this chapter, cut his therapeutic teeth, so to speak, following Rosenbek and LaPointe's (1985) advice, the discussion that follows borrows heavily from their ideas.

General Principles

Previously, several principles of muscle training gleaned from the exercise physiology literature were discussed. Briefly, the main points were that strength increases after muscle training through neural adaptation and increased contractile properties of the muscle itself. The rapid increases in strength at the early stages of training are believed to occur through neural adaptation. Liss et al (1994) observed that resistance training at any submaximal force level improves neural innervation efficiency by eliciting previously untapped motor units or by increasing neural firing rates. In addition, muscle training activities are task specific for position, velocity, and contraction type. In flaccid dysarthria, the direct management of the impairment caused by the dysarthria must address the weakness caused by the loss or interruption of LMN innervation. It should be recalled that muscle training can improve strength (maximal force), power (force over time), and endurance (sustained submaximal contraction). Strength training for flaccid muscle should attempt to increase neural activation, and improve muscle synergist efficiency. To do this, training must be specific over four variables: (1) movement pattern, (2) velocity, (3) contraction type and (4) contraction force.

If the LMN innervation is completely lost, then activities to strengthen muscle are a waste of time. In these cases, impairment is reduced by physical compensations (eg, surgery), by reinnervating the muscle or through behavioral compensations (eg, using an artificial larynx). In the treatment suggestions offered in the following pages, an attempt will be made to distinguish between therapy strategies that are muscle-strengthening activities and those that are compensatory.

Respiration

Assuming that we have flaccid respiratory muscle, the problem, then, is to decide the contribution to disability and handicap resulting from muscular impairments of the respiratory system. At least four treatment decisions need to be made: (1) Can respiratory drive itself be improved? (2) Is the maximum respiratory drive possible being utilized by the patient? (3) What compensa-

tions can be made to lessen the disability and handicap? (4) What is the prognosis for favorable outcomes at each level? In addition, it would seem prudent to note that the patient's handicap will change as the patient's medical and social expectations change. The very sick (acute) patient may be concerned only with sufficient communication ability to signal for assistance while the more chronic patient may be increasingly concerned with more general communication goals. Thus, management of the dysarthric patient with respiratory impairments is influenced by continuous assessment and must adapt to changing ability levels as well as changing social demands.

The speech-language pathologist's first goal of intervention with a patient experiencing severe respiratory deficiencies should be to establish communication. Many patients fear their inability to speak. If the flaccid respiratory impairment is so severe that breathing for speech purposes is impossible, the immediate goal is to reduce the handicap which, at this point, may be to be able to signal caregivers concerning pain or other needs. A simple switch activating an alerting signal (eg, a light or sound) can be used by the patient to alert them. When prolonged ventilator assistance is required, then the clinician should consider devices which direct airflow into the larynx providing the patient is able to phonate and articulate. As it becomes apparent that the compromised respiratory support is permanent and speech breathing is impossible, then augmentative devices as complicated as the patient's cognitive abilities will support are necessary.

Assuming the person's immediate communication needs are met and that respiration for speech is inadequate, the clinician must turn his or her attention to improving respiratory support for speech (reducing impairment and disability), a first-order problem for Dworkin (1991). For flaccid respiratory problems, there are essentially two possibilities: either improve respiratory muscle dynamic contraction, or compensate for the weakness by making maximum use of phonatory, articulatory, and postural adjustments to improve air stream management.

Strength

Strength training of the respiratory muscle is problematic for speech pathologists. Shelton's (1963) counsel that speech pathologists should leave strength training to physical therapists should lead us to the consideration of this option. Certainly, efforts to improve respiration capacity beyond that needed for speech would seem to be misplaced. On the other hand, speech breathing has dynamic characteristics quite different from resting respiration for which physical therapists would have little working knowledge. Further, since muscle training is task specific, it would seem prudent for speech pathologists to explore this problem more thoroughly. Dworkin (1991) stated that patients with flaccid respiratory muscle may need exercise to improve the strength of inspiratory and expiratory muscle. He prudently warns us that a multidisciplinary approach is required here and that any therapeutic efforts for breathing should be cleared by those professional colleagues who are specifically trained to know the dynamics of respiration for living.

A number of writers have described devices or techniques believed to be useful for improving speech breathing (Dworkin, 1991; Hixon, Hawley, & Wilson, 1982; Netsell & Hixon, 1978; Rosenbek & LaPointe, 1985; Yorkston et al, 1988). The applications range from practicing expiratory breath control using a glass of water 12 cm or greater with a straw inserted to 10 cm (Hixon et al., 1982), using a water manometer with a "leak" tube (Putnam & Hixon, 1984), using the Sea Scape (Dworkin, 1991), and utilizing pressure matching tasks using an oscilloscope (Rosenbek & LaPointe, 1985). Readers are referred to those sources for specific strategies. Of concern here is whether these exercise strategies improve dynamic strength (ie, throughout a full range of motion) or something else. It must be kept in mind that to increase muscle strength, one should move against resistance throughout the entire range of motion and velocities required by the target task. When these exercises employ a "bleed tube," which is an analog to laryngeal resistance, respiratory (expiratory) movements are completed throughout the range of motion and at nearly the same velocity as during speech. The goal of these strategies is usually to establish a level of pressure (5 cm H_2O) for a specific length of time (5 sec), which is considered the minimum necessary for speech breathing.

These exercises used to strengthen respiratory support muscles are problematic. First, only expiratory activity is targeted. Second, lung volumes at which these exercise occur determine which muscles are forced to work. At high lung volumes, inspiratory muscles perform checking action; so to obtain higher expiratory breath pressures, the inspiratory muscles would actually relax rather than contract. At middle to low lung volumes, the expiratory muscles work to increase pressure and to maintain a constant pressure against the column of water while overcoming resistance of the "leak" tube would require extra effort from the expiratory muscle. Consequently, practicing constant air pressures against leaks probably works more on control than strength per se, especially for expiratory muscle. This is not to say that exercises are not helpful; rather it would seem that they are helpful for one aspect of respiratory support for speech, and when they fail, inspiration could be the source of the problem.

Putnam and Hixon (1984) noted that problems of inhalation are frequently found in flaccid dysarthria. The literature is sparse with respect to strengthening inspiratory muscle. Dworkin (1991) described a clever application of the Sea Scape for inspiratory muscle strengthening. His step-by-step approach has several levels of practice designed to increase lung volume and faster breathing. Since he approaches the exercises utilizing both prolonged and rapid inspirations, these exercises would appear to approach two of the components of muscle strengthening exercise; that is, movement through the entire range of motion and at velocity similar to the task requirement (speech breathing). For most of these exercises, inspiratory resistance to the movement is provided by the natural resistance of the chest wall and viscera. Dworkin (1991) developed at least one exercise that provided external resistance in which the clinician resisted abdominal distension during inspiration by applying light pressure with his or her hands. This would appear to be appropriate if the target of muscle strengthening was the diaphragm. However, if the diaphragm was not active in inspiration due to paralysis and the chest wall muscles were carrying the load, then resistance to chest wall expansion would be necessary to increase chest muscle strength.

Compensation
Learning to modify a rather automatic behavior such as speech breathing and articulation is difficult. At first, the new movements have to be highly controlled. This requires a directing of attention to the speech act (Darley et al, 1975). The compensations cannot require continuously high cognitive direction unless the goal is to use the compensations in short bursts in specific situations. To be successful, the compensations must become as automatic as possible. For movements to become automatic, they must be programmed, and feedback about performance is essential. Feedback can take two forms. There can be the knowledge of the results of the behavior (eg, successful or not successful performance), and there can be knowledge concerning the actual performance of the task (feedback) (Schmidt, 1991). Many of the pathologies (not all) that affect the lower motor neuron, certainly can affect the afferent pathways as well. Thus, just as the muscle may not be completely innervated with efferent signals, neither may the sensory pathways from a muscle be completely functional. In order for the speaker with flaccid dysarthria to know what the muscles are doing, external feedbacks may be necessary but not necessarily sufficient. To learn new movements, the person must be able to develop memories of the performance

(feedback concerning movement parameters) to serve as a comparator against which future movements (practice) can be compared (knowledge of results) and then modified. The clinician treating the flaccid dysarthric, regardless of the level of the speech production system being addressed, must ascertain which afferent pathways are available to contribute to the memory of movements. Compensations that make use of unimpaired pathways would seem to make the most sense.

Compensations for deficits imply that more intact mechanisms will take over or supplement muscle activity in the impaired system. For respiration, the compensations can take the form of extra respiratory drive or better management of the respiratory support available. For example, Hixon et al (1983) described a subject with flaccid paralysis of the respiratory muscle who learned to use neck movements to store recoil energy to inspire and used glossopharyngeal pumping to extend breath groups. These strategies represented compensations for respiratory drive. Hixon et al. (1983) recommended that patients with progressive LMN disorders begin to learn these compensatory movements as soon as chest wall paresis is showing moderate levels of dysfunction. The glossopharyngeal pumping during speech utilized by this patient can be taught (Dail, Zumwalt, & Adkins, 1983), but there are medical issues to address. For example, Hixon et al. (1983) noted that glossopharyngeal pumping may be hazardous to individuals without normal vasomotor reflexes. Again, the implementation of this particular strategy highlights the necessity for speech pathologists to consult with expert pulmonary physicians and receive medical clearance before implementing respiratory training.

The report by Hixon et al (1983) points the way for downstream compensations for the respiratory difficulties of flaccid dysarthria. Their subject became efficient using his air supply that relied on only 5% of his predicted vital capacity during speech. He accomplished this by using a tighter laryngeal closure leading to a mild strained quality and by modifying his articulation to become more efficient. He shortened fricatives, used stops instead of fricatives, and interrupted airflow with intrusive glottal stops. Even though this patient learned these compensations without specific training, his success does show that potential compensations utilizing upstream valving modifications can be learned. The challenge for the clinician is to provide the environment where instruction, feedback, and knowledge of results can be provided so that the new behaviors can be learned.

Postural adjustments to improve respiratory drive are valuable for some patients. Patients with predominately inspiratory difficulties may do better in a sitting position because gravity will assist in lowering the diaphragm during inspiration (Putnam & Hixon, 1984). On the other hand, patients with expiratory problems may do better in a supine position. Binders and corsets have been reported to improve expiratory air pressure especially in patients with good diaphragm function but weak expiratory muscles (Duffy, 1995; Rosenbek & LaPointe, 1985; Yorkston et al, 1988). Again, the necessity for medical approval is paramount due to the potential pulmonary complications from binding. Rosenbek and LaPointe (1985) pointed out that leaning into a flat surface during exhalation can assist respiratory drive reducing the complications of binding. However, poor trunk support, poor balance, or general weakness can make this compensation difficult to implement and to time (Yorkston et al, 1988).

Phonation

Flaccid dysphonia has been widely addressed in texts devoted to voice disorders. The voice that results from LMN interruption depends upon which branches of the Vagus nerve have been damaged. Flaccid paralysis of the vocal folds can be unilateral or bilateral. When the external branch of the superior laryngeal nerve is affected, the pitch-changing cricothyroid muscle is af-

fected. When the recurrent branch is affected, all of the intrinsic laryngeal muscles, except for the cricothyroid, are weakened with impairment of laryngeal adduction, abduction, and active tensing.

Within the model of chronic disorders, the flaccid dysarthria of the vocal folds creates impairment of phonation with subsequent disability in speech intelligibility, loudness, and quality. The handicap varies with the vocal requirements of the individual affected and is determined by an analysis of the patient's capability to meet those requirements. Smith and colleagues (1994) reported that a voice disorder is perceived by patients as having a moderate to severe negative impact in numerous important areas including, for example, the workplace, social activities, and interpersonal communication. Treatments targeting impairment involve strengthening in a few instances and compensation in most others.

Strengthening
Two medical approaches to manage flaccid laryngeal muscle address muscle strengthening directly. Pharmacologic management of myasthenia gravis directly affects the ability of muscle to contract by improving neuromuscular synaptic function. Flaccid dysarthria caused by myasthenia gravis can be treated with the anticholinesterase drug pyridostigmine (Mestinon). Dworkin (1991) noted that the long term effects of pyridostigmine on dysarthria are uncertain but that it seems to assist voice return in those patients in the initial stages of the disease is most likely. Surgical interventions have been developed to reestablish neural innervation to the intrinsic laryngeal muscles. Crumley and Izdebski (1986) have reported a procedure which improves voice quality by an ansa hypoglossi transfer. Crumley (1992) stated that the ansa cervicalis/recurrent laryngeal nerve anastomosis usually results in a near-normal voice and attributed the good results to the reinnervation of the four ipsilateral intrinsic muscles innervated by the recurrent nerve. Leddy and Canfield (1991) and Dworkin

(1991) have proposed therapeutic exercise to directly strengthen the laryngeal muscle. Leddy and Canfield's (1992) contribution is a computerized home program which utilizes vowel prolongation at different pitches and pitch ranges to improve vocal fold function. Dworkin's programs are much more complex and target improved strength (or improved vocal closure) through a hierarchical exercise program including exercises at the contextual speech level. These exercises are designed to increase the force with which the vocal folds close during phonation. His exercises make use of nonspeech valving and hard glottal attack. Whether any of these exercises can or actually do strengthen the muscles rather than improve the utilization of existing strength is not readily apparent. However, Dworkin (1991) does provide a valuable, though complex, method of documentation of progress through each level with valuable admonitions to establish objective baselines and criteria for treatment continuation or termination.

Compensation

Compensation for laryngeal paralysis includes behavioral changes and surgical interventions. Most behavioral strategies attempt to improve vocal fold adduction taking advantage of the closure capabilities that occur while protecting the airway (eg, during swallowing) or when providing constriction to increase thoracic pressure during lifting, pushing, and pulling. Surgical interventions improve closure by moving the paralyzed vocal fold closer to midline or by increasing the mass of the paralyzed fold.

Effort closure techniques have been reported to induce phonation while pushing, pulling, or lifting a resistance, or producing a controlled cough to improve adduction and subsequent voice (Aronson, 1990; Duffy, 1995; Rosenbek & LaPointe, 1985; Yorkston et al., 1988). Boone and McFarlane (1994) preferred to use other techniques such as the "half-boom" swallow or a change of head position to facilitate better voice. They claimed that these techniques resulted in a

clearer voice than other effort closure techniques. Rosenbek and LaPointe (1985) pointed out that techniques which create postures that are cosmetically undesirable should be reserved for specific situations. Regardless of which technique is chosen, the clinician has the responsibility to restore the patient's voice as close to "normal" as possible. Careful attention to the integration of closure attempts with good respiratory support without inducing hyperfunctional behavior is a must.

A variety of sources are available for specific step-by-step guidance to implement facilitating techniques. Boone and McFarlane (1994) provide detailed descriptions of 25 techniques for improving voice of which at least six are directly applicable to flaccid weakness of the larynx. These facilitation techniques do not address muscle strengthening; rather they are designed to elicit the most muscle contraction possible with the existing LMN innervation. Dworkin's (1991) systematic approach of charting baselines and progress could easily be combined with any facilitory approach.

Laryngeal framework surgery or phonosurgery is often completed to improve vocal fold closure. Medialization laryngoplasty improves laryngeal closure by introducing a mass between the vocal fold and thyroid cartilage on the affected side (Koufman, 1986), which moves the paralyzed vocal fold closer to midline. Gray et al (1992) have noted that even though improvement in pitch and loudness usually results, breathiness, vocal harshness, and fatigue may continue. Since this procedure is reversible, the mass can be removed if reinnervation occurs.

Arytenoid adduction surgery repositions the paralyzed vocal fold without lateral compression. One advantage is that it can place the vocal process into a position more consistent with the vocal fold position during phonation. However, medialization of the membranous portion of the vocal fold may not occur. In that case, Type I thyroplasty or injection thyroplasty may be necessary (Bauer, Valentino, & Hoffman, 1994).

There are a variety of techniques to augment the bulk of the paralyzed vocal fold to increase mass and reduce the glottis. Boone and McFarlane (1994) observed that the most common surgery for vocal fold paralysis in the open, paramedian position is Teflon injection. Weber, Neumayer, Alford, and Weber (1984) reported 111 patients in whom 85% demonstrated improvement of voice. However, Teflon injection is not removable without damaging the vocal fold structure itself.

Bauer et al (1994) reported the successful use of autogenous fat to augment vocal fold mass. They noted that questions remain concerning the long-term survival of the graft and the amount of over correction needed. A clear advantage to the use of autogenous fat is the increased tolerance of the vocal folds to the graft. In their opinion, this would lead to a more naturally moving vocal fold during phonation.

Injectable collagen has also been used for augmenting the vocal fold bulk (Ford & Blexx, 1986; Ford, Staskowski, & Blexx, 1995; Remacle, Marbaiz, Hamoir, Bertrand, & Van den Eeckhout, 1990). Ford and colleagues observed that FDA concerns about the potential immunologic response to bovine source material which is used in the airway has slowed the approval for the use of collagen. They went on to describe the use of autologous collagen vocal fold injection which produced comparable vocal fold function results to bovine collagen. The large advantage is that the likelihood of a hypersensitivity response is negligible. Other advances accrue during the preparation of the material and should contribute to increased tolerability with longer duration of effectiveness.

Although considerable progress has been made in surgical compensation for vocal fold paralysis, McFarlane et al (1991) concluded that a conservative approach to unilateral vocal fold paralysis (without significant dysphagia), which utilizes behavioral therapy, is the most cost-efficient and risk-free approach to restoring voice. Voice therapy should be considered as a primary treatment to maximize voice production in cases of unilateral vocal fold paralysis because it resulted in superior voice to Teflon injection. An average of 9 hours of voice therapy was required for older and more severely impaired voice patients to be rated as successful as the surgery group and more successful than the Teflon group. McFarlane and colleagues (1991) suggested that most laryngologists agree that a waiting period of at least nine months is recommended before proceeding with surgical interventions but that they may not consider voice therapy during this time. They concluded that voice therapy, utilizing facilitation techniques, can provide a cost-effective treatment during that initial waiting period without the risks of surgery.

New approaches to decision making regarding management of laryngeal paralysis is on the horizon. Min et al (1994) have described electromyographic measures that predict innervation recovery leading to better decisions regarding the type and timing of surgical intervention for laryngeal paralysis. Electromyography completed prior to 6 months but preferably within 6 weeks of onset was successful in predicting recovery outcome at 89%. A positive prognosis for laryngeal recovery was present when the following EMG features were present: (1) normal motor unit waveform morphology; (2) overall EMG activity at an RMS value greater than $40\,\mu V$ in any one task; and (3) no electrical silence during voluntary tasks. These data suggest that it will be possible to predict innervation outcome and assist speech pathologists and laryngologists in the managment of voice disorder secondary to laryngeal paralysis. Recent developments in the use of magnetic resonance imaging (MRI) (see Sonies & Stone, this volume) may lead to better application of vocal fold medialization techniques (Ford, Unger, Zundel, & Bless, 1994). Placement and durability of the medialization medium can be precisely defined by MRI and should lead to better decisions regarding the repair of suboptimal results.

Finally, prosthetic management of voice disorders is possible. Speech amplifiers, such as the SPEECHMAKER Voice Amplifier and the PERSONAL PA (Williams Sound Corp. Eden Prairie, MN) can be used to amplify a weak voice. Personal experience with these systems suggests that careful evaluation of articulatory competence is necessary before recommending these systems. Amplifying unintelligible, soft speech will result in loud, unintelligible speech. In addition, when using FM systems, such as the PERSONAL PA, it is necessary to check for interference from other FM systems being used in the same facility. Consultation with audiologists who are knowledgeable about sound amplification in a classroom was invaluable in the many decisions regarding placement of speakers, desirable sound levels, and measurement of effect. Patients with bilateral vocal fold paralysis without voice, but with good articulation, could make use of an artificial larynx.

Resonance

Even though the term resonance is applied often to the functional outcome of the velopharyngeal port, other parameters of speech are affected by velopharyngeal function. Since speakers with velopharyngeal incompetence (VPI) are unable to impound air for intraoral pressure consonants, nasal emission or articulatory substitutions (eg, glottal stop or pharyngeal fricative) are likely. In addition, the open velopharyngeal port allows acoustic energy to be diverted into the nasal passages, damping the acoustic signal and reducing overall loudness. To complicate matters further, respiratory air wastage makes intelligible speech even more difficult for those speakers with compromised respiratory, phonatory, or articulatory systems. VPI due to flaccid velar musculature can range from mild hypernasality to unintelligible speech. When VPI is severe, management of VPI becomes a necessity so that more intelligible speech can be produced. As with other levels of the point-place model, the handicap brought about by VPI is determined by the communication requirements of the individual patient. The management of the impairment of VPI caused by flaccid muscle can take three forms: behavioral, prosthetic, and surgical.

Behavioral

Several exercises have been put forward as ways to improve velopharyngeal closing including blowing and sucking (Johns, 1985). Johns (1985) also noted facilitation techniques such as pressure, icing, brushing, stroking, and electrical stimulation have been advocated to improve VPI due to flaccid muscle. Johns was pessimistic and wrote that "these exercises are disappointing and generally ineffective" (p 158). Duffy (1995) concluded that further controlled investigations of the effectiveness of palatal stimulation and strengthening may be warranted. Indeed, it could be argued that none of the previous attempts at muscle strengthening addressed any of the known principles of muscle training. Certainly, blowing and sucking exercises require the velum to assume a static position and while sucking can create a negative intraoral pressure that may have acted as a resistance (load) to the closing action of the levator palatini muscle, blowing would not. Consequently, exercises through representative velocities, ranges of movement, or types of muscle contraction would not be possible; hence, neural adaptation as a means to increase velar function would be unlikely. This is not surprising given the inaccessibility of the velum.

Recently, Kuehn and Wachtel (1994) and Liss et al (1994) have reported a creative application of a device which provides continuous positive airway pressure (CPAP). CPAP is used with those who experience sleep apnea due to collapsing of the upper airway. CPAP provides a continuous positive pressure within the nasopharyngeal and pharyngeal spaces keeping them open during sleep. The applications reported above have taken advantage of that positive pressure to provide a resistance against which the velum can operate through a full range of motion, at speech related velocities, with the correct muscle contraction type. Liss et al (1994) have developed a standard protocol and are currently testing the procedure in clinical trials. Variables that continue to require investigation include exercise quantity, intensity, and frequency as well as the role of feedback and fatigue.

Dworkin (1991) described behavioral techniques that he has used with VPI. He suggested that 10 hours of concentrated (undefined) behavioral therapy be completed before alternative methods of repairing VPI are tried. Dworkin (1991) delineated a series of exercises (and charting techniques) to reduce VPI. His techniques center around systematically increasing oral pressure capability into activities that progressively approximate conversational speech. The activities have been designed to use the See-Scape and tape recordings to provide feedback. These exercises would not appear to address strength (power, force, or endurance) directly except in the sense that the patient is taught to make better use of existing strength. Consequently, the 10-hour limit is probably a good one because it provides a window of opportunity for the patient to demonstrate learning but does not provide an unrealistic expectation of strength change.

Prosthetic

A palatal lift prosthesis lifts the velum to approximate the posterior pharyngeal wall. Yorkston et al (1988) reported that this technique has been the most successful strategy to improve VPI in patients with dysarthria. Detailed explanations of the utilization and fitting of palatal lifts have been provided (Aten, McDonald, Simpson, & Gutierrez, 1984; Dworkin, 1991; Johns, 1985; Yorkston et al, 1988). Duffy (1995) observed that the best candidates for palatal lift management are those with minimal deficits throughout the speech production system, static rather than progressive conditions, adequate dentition, and a hypoactive gag reflex. Since the gag reflex is usually diminished or absent in flaccid dysarthria, the palatal lift is well suited for the task of improving VPI in the face of isolated flaccid paralysis of the velum. However, Shaughnessy, Netsell, and Farrage (1983) cautioned that clients may need to be taught to use the palatal lift. The amount of rehabilitation is determined by the degree of successful use of oral pressure during speech.

Surgical

Surgical intervention to improve VPI has not been as successful as prosthetic management. Two general approaches have been tried: pharyngeal flap, and Teflon injection. Noll (1982) remarked that any form of surgical management of VPI due to neuromotor problems is not as successful compared to surgical approaches with structural deficits. Johns (1985) furnished a detailed report delineating approaches to surgical management and their usefulness. He concluded that pharyngeal flap surgery is effective for some patients. Lewy, Cole, and Wepman (1965) reported on the use of Teflon injection in the posterior wall along Passavant's line in one patient who appeared to benefit. Further study and documentation of the effectiveness of this procedure has not been forthcoming.

Articulation

Successful articulation of speech requires the integration of all the points and places represented on Netsell's point-place model. This particular section deals with the anterior and posterior tongue, lips, and mandible. Since these elements are innervated by different cranial nerves, the deficits found will vary widely. The movements of these articulators valve and shape the oral cavity to produce constrictions for consonants and resonances for vowels. To be effective, the articulatory movements must be integrated across places and levels. The movement relationships among respiration, phonation, and articulatory mechanisms necessary to produce linguistic contrasts, such as the voice and voiceless distinction, are complex across space and time. Further, the systems involved are quite disparate in terms of their architecture. For example, the tongue operates as a hydrostat while the muscles of the jaw operate around a joint. The effect of flaccid weakness, especially bilateral, is to slow articulatory movements and reduce the range of motion so that articulatory targets are not reached either in space or time. Management of impairment of articulation due to flaccid weakness can be behavioral, surgical, and pharmaceutical.

Behavioral

At first glance, strengthening of flaccid articulatory muscle would seem to be the correct target of remediation. Many authors (DePaul & Brooks, 1993; Dworkin, 1991; Duffy, 1995; Rosenbek & LaPointe, 1985; Yorkston et al, 1988) have contributed discussions dedicated to strengthening the articulatory musculature. There is no consensus regarding the necessity to strengthen articulatory muscles. For example, it has been reported that only 10% to 30% (jaw only 2%) of maximum forces are utilized during speech and that up to one-third of the motor nerve fibers can be lost before functional impairments are encountered (Duffy, 1995). Indeed, many clinicians have observed dysarthric patients for whom unilateral weakness of the tongue posed no difficulty whatsoever. On the other hand, Dworkin, Aronson, and Mulder (1980) and Robin et al. (1992) have discussed positive relationships between measures of tongue strength and amount of articulatory deficit in speech disordered subjects. For the purposes of this chapter, strength will be considered an important treatment variable. It is likely that much of the difference in opinion regarding lingual, lip, and jaw strength, its importance and potential for remediation stems from dissimilar definitions and methods of increasing and measuring strength.

To improve the muscle strength of the articulators, the challenge is to design exercises which will provide movement at the right velocity, with the right movement pattern, and with sufficient contraction to engender neural adaptation, which is the quickest way to increased strength. Duffy

(1995) noted that the "jaw can be opened, closed or lateralized; the lips can be rounded, spread, puffed, closed isometrically with or without clinician provided resistance; the tongue can be protruded and lateralized against resistance or pushed against the alveolus, cheeks or a tongue blade and so on" (p. 398). We must carefully consider whether these movements of the tongue or lips capture the elements of dynamic strengthening activity necessary to generate neural adaptation for speech movements. For the most part, it would appear that they do not. For example, pushing against the alveolus with the tongue certainly approximates an appropriate target position but utilizing that as a strengthening technique will not elicit the neural adaptation necessary to strengthen the dynamic aspect of tongue activity. To create neural adaptation, the patient should move the articulator against a resistance through a variety of movement velocities, which mimic speech movements. Of course, that is easier said than done, especially for the tongue.

At present we are conducting clinical trials with an 8-year-old-boy (C.T.) who has congenital flaccid dysarthria. We have adapted Dworkin's (1991) creative use of tongue blades to provide resistances against which the tongue can work. Since C.T. can produce two positions with the posterior aspect of his tongue (high and low), we have had him initiate anterior tongue movements toward and from the alveolus with the posterior tongue in elevated and depressed positions. We also have him move the tongue quickly and slowly. At this point, the results are encouraging in that we have proceeded from zero tongue tip articulations to being able to produce a /d/ consistently in single words.

Since this patient also has flaccid lips, we are attempting to strengthen lip movement too. Traditional lip strengthening activities would usually have the lips press together or purse. However, these activities represent only one aspect of strength necessary for successful lip movement during speech. It especially ignores lip retraction, which is an important aspect of anterior oral shaping.

Early exercise with this patient attempted to increase lip strength by having the patient resist the pulling of a button placed behind the lips. This exercise may have led to increased lip closure during chewing because the parent reported less drooling and loss of food during meals. However, there was no change in his ability to produce lip closure for bilabial consonants or anterior oral shaping for vowels. Most recent exercise has been directed toward eliciting a retraction movement from a closed position with light resistance provided by the clinician followed immediately by a closing gesture against resisted. We believe that we have begun to see more movement, but these treatment attempts are in their earliest stages and many more repetitions are needed.

We have found Dworkin's (1991) ideas about exercise to provide quite useful starting points from which we have devised other exercises. His ideas are particularly appealing to the practicing clinician because he has made creative use of routine clinical materials such as tongue blades, buttons, and string. His ideas provide an interesting basis from which it should be possible to develop resistance exercises which more closely resemble speech movements.

Before we jump onto the exercise band wagon too completely, Kent et al (1987) have observed that maximal strength may not be a useful measure to predict speech motor capability. Duffy (1995) admonished us to establish that weakness is clearly related to the speech impairment and subsequent disability. To do this, though, we need improved methods of measuring lingual and labial strength. Typical clinical measures of tongue strength, such as pushing anteriorly against a tongue blade or laterally against the cheek, are inadequate. Not only do these measures fail to approximate any of the natural targets or vectors of speech movement, but they are dependent upon subjective estimates of strength by the clinician. Recent developments in the measurement of tongue strength and movement may provide methods which will allow the creation of standardized measures of tongue, lip, and jaw

strength or movement. In Chapter 5 of this book, Barlow, Finan, Andreatta, and Paseman, detail the use of force transducers to quantify labial, lingual, and mandibular functioning in dysarthria. Also, in Chapter 3, Robin, Solomon, Moon, and Folkins provide an extensive discussion of the relationship between nonspeech measures such as the IOPI and physiologic parameters (eg, strength, endurance).

Interestingly, the supranormal speakers of Robin, Goel, Somodi, and Luschei (1992) had not "lifted" weights with their tongues but they rather had practiced speaking in certain ways (ie, speaking very rapidly while maintaining good intelligibility in the case of debaters). Luschei (1991) argued that the architecture of the tongue requires sufficient strength to overcome its intrinsic viscous load. Consequently, exercise, which elicits rapid tongue movement, may provide sufficient resistance to improve tongue strength. Further, Robin and his colleagues suggested that the minimum strength (eg, 20% of normal) to support sufficient movement for speech is not known. Duffy (1995) also observed that only 20–30% of maximum forces may be required for speech. However, to conclude that some level of strength above these levels is unnecessary may be premature. Robin et al (1992) have pointed out that "sense of effort" plays an important role in task compliance and that speakers who are weak may articulate adequately for short periods of time but not for longer times or in conditions which demand more of the speech mechanism. These notions might be particularly important in trying to reduce the handicap of an individual who articulates well enough in therapy but has trouble at work. For example, DePaul and Brooks (1993) concluded that weakness is not directly related to intelligibility and suggest that the orofacial system can compensate for the lingual weakness. Intelligibility measures in their report were obtained under optimal speaking conditions for a relatively short period of time (2 minutes). While that might be good enough for someone who was homebound, for another who wanted to return to work in a more challenging environment (handicap), it might not be. Without a doubt, the influence of strength upon articulatory performance is far from understood, especially with respect to critical levels of strength and endurance. Finally, the relationship of strength and endurance to articulatory performance in children may be different from that in adults. Certainly, the competency of compensatory strategies would be affected and would likely be directly related to the amount and level of successful articulatory performance that was obtained before the onset of weakness. Clearly, much clinical investigation remains to be done.

Surgical

First, myasthenia gravis is often managed surgically. A thymectomy is often used to change the neurochemistry at the myoneural junction (Aronson, 1990). Two surgical approaches to recovery of nerve function associated with Bell's palsy are occasionally used. Although controversial, decompression of the facial nerve has been advocated for some forms of VII cranial nerve involvement. Fisch (1981) found increased recovery with decompression surgery compared to no surgery when the surgery was performed within 24 hours of onset of the facial palsy. Neural anastomosis has also been used to restore facial nerve innervation. Typically a branch of the XII cranial nerve is connected to the VII cranial nerve (Mingrino & Zuccarello, 1981). These authors pointed out that hypoglossal-facial anastomosis can result in facial synkinesis during speech which could be cosmetically unappealing and affect speech articulation. Yorkston et al. (1988) stated that patients should have intact lingual function to minimize the chance of impaired tongue function after the anastomosis.

Pharmacologic

Pharmacologic management of flaccid dysarthria in patients without myasthenia gravis is primarily limited to pain prevention and lessening of degeneration. Steroids in conjunction with acyclovir are usually prescribed. In patients with myasthenia, pyridostigmine bromide (Mestinon) is prescribed, and speech pathologists encourage conservation of effort to reduce fatigue. A number of treatment approaches for flaccid dysarthria have been discussed in this chapter. There have been attempts to persuade the speech clinician that we should explore the relationship between strength (in all of its manifestations) and articulation more carefully, especially in flaccid dysarthria. The hallmark of flaccid dysarthria is weakness and if we want to treat the bottom line, then we need to find a way to increase strength. This is not to say, that strategies to compensate for the weakness are not appropriate. Indeed, in many cases, that's all there is.

References

Aronson AE. (1990). *Clinical Voice Disorders: An Interdisciplinary Approach* (3rd ed.). New York: Thieme, Inc.

Aten J, McDonald A, Simpson M, Gutierrez B. (1984). Efficacy of modified palatal lifts for improved resonance. In: McNeil M, Rosenbek J, Aronson A, eds. *The Dysarthrias: Physiology, Acoustics, Perception, Management.* San Diego, CA: College-Hill Press, pp 231–242.

Barlow SM, Finan DS, Andreatta RD, Paseman LA. (1997). Kinematic measurement of the human vocal tract. In: McNeil MR, ed. *Clinical Management of Sensorimotor Speech Disorders.* New York: Thieme Medical Publishers Inc.

Basmajian JV, DeLuca CJ. (1985). *Muscles Alive: Their Functions Revealed by Electromyography* (5th ed.). Baltimore: Williams and Wilkins.

Bauer C, Valentino J, Hoffman H. (1994). Long-term result of vocal cord augmentation with autogenous fat. *Natl Center Voice Speech: Status Prog Rep* 6(5):61–66.

Bigland-Ritchie B, Woods JJ. (1984). Changes in muscle contractile properties and neural control during human muscular fatigue. *Muscle & Nerve* 7:691–699.

Boone DR, McFarlane SC. (1994). *The Voice and Voice Therapy* (5th Ed.). Englewood Cliffs, NJ: Prentice Hall.

Chusid JG. (1985). *Correlative Neuroanatomy and Functional Neurology.* Los Altos, CA: LANGE Medical Publications.

Crumley RL, Izdebski K. (1986). Voice quality following laryngeal reinnervation by ansa hypoglossi transfer. *Laryngoscope* 96:611–616.

Crumley RL. (1992). Response to McFarlane & co-authors. *Am J Speech-Language Pathol* 1:65–67.

Dail C, Zumwalt M, Adkins H. (1983). *A Manual of Instruction for Glossopharyngeal Breathing.* New York: National Foundation for Infantile Paralysis.

Darley FL, Aronson AE, Brown JR. (1975). *Motor Speech Disorders.* Philadelphia: W.B. Saunders.

DePaul R, Brooks B. (1993). Multiple orofacial indices in amyotrophic lateral sclerosis. *J Speech Hear Res* 36:1158–1167.

Duffy JR. (1995). *Motor Speech Disorders: Substrates, Differential Diagnosis and Management.* St. Louis: Mosby-Year Book, Inc.

Dworkin JP, Aronson A, Mulder D. (1980). Tongue force in normals and dysarthric patients with amyotrophic lateral sclerosis. *J Speech Hear Res* 23:828–837.

Dworkin JP. (1991). *Motor Speech Disorders: A Treatment Guide.* St. Louis: Mosby–Year Book, Inc.

Fisch U. (1981). Surgery for Bell's palsy. *Arch Otolaryngol* 107(1):1–11.

Ford C, Unger J, Zundel R, Bless D. (1994). Magnetic resonance imaging (MRI) assessment of vocal fold medialization surgery. *Natl Center Voice Speech: Status Prog Rep* 7(Dec.): 23–27.

Ford CN, Bless DM. (1986). A preliminary study of injectable collagen in human vocal fold augmentation. *Otol Head Neck Surg* 94:104.

Ford CN, Staskowski PI, Bless D. (1995). Autologous collagen vocal fold injection: A preliminary clinical study. *Natl Center Voice Speech: Status Prog Rep* 8:75–80.

Frey WD. (1984). Functional assessment in the '80s: A conceptual enigma, a technical challenge. In: Halpern AS, Fuhrer MJ, eds. *Functional Assessment in Rehabilitation.* Baltimore: Paul H. Brookes.

Gray S, Barkmeier J, Druker D, Shive C, Van Denmark D, Jones D, Alder S. (1992). Vocal evaluation of thyroplasty surgery in treatment of unilateral vocal cord paralysis. *Laryngoscope* 102:415–421.

Hixon T, Hawley J, Wilson J. (1982). An around-the-house device for the clinical determination of respiratory driving pressure: a note on making the simple even simpler. *J Speech Hear Disord* 47:413.

Hixon TJ, Putnam A, Sharpe J. (1983). Speech production with flaccid paralysis of the rib cage, diaphragm, and abdomen. *J Speech Hear Disord* 48:315–327.

Johns DF. (1985). Surgical and prosthetic management of neurogenic velopharyngeal incompetency in dysarthria. In: Johns DF, ed. *Clinical Management of Communicative Disorders* (2nd Ed.). Boston: Little, Brown, pp 153–178.

Kent RD, Kent JF, Rosenbek JC. (1987). Maximum performance tests of speech production. *J Speech Hear Disord* 52:367–387.

Kent RD. (1994). The clinical science of motor speech disorders: A personal assessment. In: Till JA, Yorkston KM, Beukelman DR, eds. *Motor Speech Disorders: Advances in Assessment and Treatment.* Baltimore: Paul H. Brookes, pp 3–18.

Koufman JA. (1986). Laryngoplasty for vocal cord medialization: An alternative to Teflon. *Laryngoscope* 96:726.

Kraemer WJ, Deschenes MR, Fleck SJ. (1988). Physiological adaptations to resistance exercise: Implications for athletic conditioning. *J Sports Med* 6:246–256.

Kuehn DP, Wachtel JM. (1994). CPAP therapy for treating hypernasality following closed head injury. In: Till JA, Yorkston KM, Beukelman DR, eds. *Motor Speech Disorders: Advances in Assessment and Treatment.* Baltimore: Paul H. Brookes, pp 207–212.

Larson C. (1989). Basic neurophysiology. In: Kuehn DP, Lemme ML, Baumgartner JM eds. *Neural Basis of Speech, Hearing and Language.* Boston: College-Hill; Little, Brown.

Leddy M, Canfield MR. (1992). Laryngeal muscle strengthening exercises: A computerized home study program. Paper presented at the Annual Convention of the American Speech-Language and Hearing Associatio, San Antonio, TX.

Lewy R, Cole R, Wepman J. (1965). Teflon injection in the correction of velopharyngeal insufficiency. *Ann Otol Rhinol Laryngol* 28: 874.

Linebaugh C. (1983). Treatment of flaccid dysarthria. In: Perkins W, ed. *Dysarthria and Apraxia.* New York: Thieme Stratton.

Liss J, Kuehn D, Hinkel K. (1994). Direct training of velopharyngeal musculature. In: *National Center for Voice and Speech: Status and Progress Report* 6(5):43–52.

Luschei ES, Finnegan EM. (1996). Electromyographic techniques for the assessment of motor speech disorders. In: McNeil MR, ed. *Clinical Management of Sensorimotor Speech Disorders.* New York: Thieme Medical Publishers.

Luschei ES. (1991). Development of objective standards of nonspeech oral strength and performance: An advocate's perspective. In: Moore CA, Yorkston KM, Beukelman DR, eds. *Dysarthria and Apraxia of Speech: Perspectives on Management.* Baltimore: Paul H. Brookes, pp 3–14.

McFarlane SC, Holt-Romeo TL, Lavorato AS, Warner L. (1991). Unilateral vocal fold paralysis: Perceived vocal quality following three methods of treatment. *Am J Speech-Language Pathol* 1:45–48.

McNeil MR, Kennedy JG. (1984). Measuring the effects of treatment for dysarthria: Knowing when to change or terminate. *Semin Speech Lang* 4(4):337–358.

Min YB, Finnegan EM, Hoffman HT, Luschei ES, McCulloch TM. (1994). A preliminary study of the prognostic role of electromyography in laryngeal paralysis. *Natl Center Voice Speech: Status Prog Rep* 6(May):67–72.

Mingrino S, Zuccarello M. (1981). Anastomosis of the facial nerve with accessory or hypoglossal nerves. In: Samii M, Jannetta PJ. eds. *The Cranial Nerves.* New York: Springer-Verlag.

Netsell R, Hixon TJ. (1978). A noninvasive method for clinically estimating subglottal air pressure. *J Speech Hear Dis* 43:326–330.

Netsell R. (1973). Speech physiology. In Minifie FD, Hixon TJ, Williams F, eds. *Normal Aspects of Speech, Hearing, and Language.* Englewood Cliffs, NJ: Prentice-Hall, pp 211–234.

Noll JD. (1982). Remediation of impaired resonance among patients with neuropathologies of speech. In: Lass N, McReynolds L, Northern J, Yoder D, eds. *Speech, Language and Hearing.* Vol. III: *Pathologies of Speech and Language.* Philadelphia: W.B. Saunders.

Putnam A, Hixon TJ. (1984). Respiratory kinematics in speakers with motor neuron disease. In: McNeil M, Rosenbek J, Aronson A, eds. *The Dysarthrias: Physiology, Acoustics, Perception, Management.* San Diego, CA: College-Hill Press, pp 37–67.

Remacle M, Marbaiz E, Hamoir M, Bertrand B, Van den Eeckhaut J. (1990). Correction of glottic insufficiency by collagen injection. *Ann Otol Rhinol Larygol* 99:438–444.

Robin DA, Goel A, Somodi LB, Luschei ES. (1992). Tongue strength and endurance: Relation to highly skilled movments. *J Speech Hear Res* 35:1239–1245.

Robin DA, Somodi LB, Luschei ES. (1991). Measurement of tongue strength and endurance in normal and articulation disordered subjects. In: Moore CA, Yorkston KM, Beukelman DR, eds. *Dysarthria and Apraxia of Speech: Perspectives on Management.* Baltimore: Paul H. Brookes, pp 173–184.

Rosenbek JC, LaPointe LL. (1985). The dysarthrias: Description, diagnosis and treatment. In: Johns DF, ed. *Clinical Management of Communicative Disorders* (2nd Ed.). Boston: Little, Brown, pp 97–152.

Sale D, MacDougall D. (1981). Specificity in strength training: A review for the coach and athlete. *Can J Appl Sports Sci* 6:87–92.

Sale DB. (1986). Neural adaptation in strength and power training. In Jones NL, McCartney N, McComas AJ, eds. *Human Muscle Power.* Champaign, IL: Human Kinetics, pp 281–305.

Sale DG, McComas AJ, MacDougall JD, Upton ARM. (1982). Neuromuscular adaptation in human thenar muscles following strength training and immobilization. *J Appl Physiol Respir Environ Exer Physiol* 53:419–424.

Schmidt RA. (1991). *Motor Learning and Performance: From Principles to Practice.* Champaign, IL: Human Kinetics Books.

Shaughnessy AL, Netsell R, Farrage J. (1983). Treatment of a four-year-old with a palatal lift prosthesis. In: Berry WR, ed. *Clinical Dysarthria.* San Diego: College-Hill Press.

Shelton RL. (1963). Therapeutic exercise and speech pathology. *ASHA* 5:855.

Smith E, Verdolini K, Gray S, Nichols S, Lemke J, Barkmeier J, Dove H, Hoffman HT. (1994). Effect of voice disorders on quality of life. *Natl Center Voice Speech: Status Prog Rep* 7(12):1–17.

Titze IR. (1994). *Principles of Voice Production.* Englewood Cliffs, NJ: Prentice-Hall.

Weber RS, Neumayer L, Alford BR, Weber SC. (1984). Clinical restoration of voice function after loss of the vagus nerve. *Head Neck Surg* 7:448–457.

Weismer G, Liss J. (1991). Reductionism is a dead-end in speech research: Perspectives on a new direction. In: Moore CA, Yorkston KM, Beukelman DR, eds. *Dysarthria and Apraxia of*

Speech: Perspectives on Management. Baltimore: Paul H. Brookes, pp 15–29.

Wertz RT. (1985). Neuropathologies of speech and language: An introduction to patient management. In: Johns DF, ed. *Clinical Management of Communicative Disorders* (2nd Ed.). Boston: MA: Little, Brown, pp 1–96.

Wood PHN. (1980). Appreciating the consequences of disease—the classification of impairment, disability and handicap. *WHO Chron* 43:376–380.

Yorkston KM, Beukelman DR, Bell KR. (1988). *Clinical Management of Dysarthric Speakers.* Boston: College-Hill; Little, Brown.

Chapter 10

Ataxic Dysarthria

Michael P. Cannito and Thomas P. Marquardt

Introduction

Ataxic dysarthria (AD) is a disorder of sensorimotor control for speech production that results from damage to the cerebellum or to its input and output pathways. The dragging and blurred quality of AD speech has sometimes been likened to "drunken speech" (Netsell, 1986), which results from the particular vulnerability of the cerebellum to the immediate effects of alcohol ingestion. Patients with AD suffer not from inebriation, however, but from a dramatic disintegration of fundamental motor processes, termed "ataxia," due to disturbance of the essential role played by the cerebellum in the regulation of movement. The cerebellum or "little brain" is a highly complex structure which, like the cerebrum that overlays it, consists of a convoluted outer cortex replete with gyri and sulci, two hemispheres subdivided into various lobes, subcortical white matter projections and paired deep nuclei, as well as diverse efferent and afferent projections via the cerebellar peduncles which interconnect with other central nervous system structures. Due to its distinct complexity of structure and connectivity, the cerebellum cannot be viewed as subserving any single function: Its duties are manifold and have been described as ranging from the regulation of muscle spindle activity for postural maintenance (Granit, 1977), to ongoing comparison and correction of intended with achieved postural goals (Thach, 1980), to rapid timing generation and ballistic motor programing (Kornhuber, 1975), to sensorimotor learning (Eccles, 1977), to auditory and visual information processing (Mortimer, 1975), and even cognitive linguistic behavior (Leiner, Leiner, & Dow, 1991).

The present discussion will emphasize those aspects of sensorimotor function that are most relevant to the assessment and treatment of the speech deficits associated with AD. For a more comprehensive discussion of cerebellar structure and function, the reader is referred to Ito (1984). In the sections that follow, this chapter will review the pathophysiology of ataxia and its nonspeech symptomatology; discuss existing research findings on the physiological, acoustic, and perceptual characteristics of AD speech; and provide a systematic framework for treatment supported with efficacy data where available.

Pathophysiology of Ataxia

Cerebellar Structure and Function

Gilman (1986) has suggested that it is clinically useful to conceptualize the cerebellar cortex in terms of three saggital subdivisions or zones: a *medial zone* which includes the cerebellar vermis, a "worm-shaped" band of midline cortex that lies between the hemispheres; a *paravermal zone*, which includes the more medial aspects of each cerebellar hemisphere adjacent to the vermis; and a *lateral zone* which includes the more lateral portions of the hemispheres. Each cortical zone projects axonal fibers to the subcortical nuclei, bilaterally paired neuronal masses, deep within the cerebellum. The medial zone comprises only about 5% of the human cerebellum and projects to the fastigial nuclei; the paravermal zone comprises about 7% of the cerebellum and projects to the globose and emboliform nuclei; and the lateral zone, comprising about 88% of the human cerebellum, projects to the dentate nuclei (Eccles, 1977). Major inputs to the medial (vermal) zone include spinal cord and the vestibular, reticular, and trigeminal nuclei of the brainstem, while major outputs (via the fastigial nuclei) include vestibulospinal and reticulospinal projections. The paravermal zone of the cerebellar hemispheres receives input from the cerebral motor cortex, brainstem, and spinal cord, and projects output (via the globose and emboliform nucei) back to these areas. The lateral zone of the cerebellar hemispheres receives major cerebral input relayed via pontine and reticular nuclei of the brainstem, and projects its output (via the dentate nuclei) to brainstem and thalamic stuctures, which in turn relay information to both spinal and cerebral levels.

According to Gilman (1986), the medial zone contributes primarily to locomotion and posture: clinical symptoms associated with damage to this region include abnormalities of stance and gait, truncal titubation, rotated postures of the head, and disturbances of extraocular movement. Gilman suggests that at our present state of knowledge the functions of the paravermal zone are not well understood and for clinical purposes it may be grouped with the lateral zone. Symptoms associated with damage of the cerebellar hemispheres relate primarily to voluntary movement and include hypotonia, dysmetria, dysdiadochokinesis, excessive rebound, impaired check, tremors, decomposition of movement, eye movement disorders, and dysarthria (Gilman, 1986).

It is clear that the cerebellum serves as a component in a number of control loops for sensory motor systems (eg, cortical-pontine-cerebellar-thalamic-cortical) which appear to be involved in movement initiation and specification of muscular activation patterns necessary for coordinated movements

(Alexander & Delong, 1986). The cerebral premotor cortex (which includes Broca's and supplemental motor areas in man) and the primary motor cortex project via brainstem nuclei onto the lateral cerebellum and receive back cerebellar projections, via the ventrolateral thalamus (Leiner et al, 1991; Sasaki, 1984; Schell & Strict, 1984). Studies by Thach (1975, 1978) of neuroelectrical activity in awake monkeys during wrist flexion and extension have demonstrated that neuronal activity in the dentate nucleus precedes activity in the motor cortex, which in turn precedes the appearance of EMG activity in the extremity. In contrast, the interpositus nucleus (analogous to the human globose and emboliform nuclei) is active during movement, or in response to perturbations of static holding positions. These and other, similar studies collectively suggest that contributions of the cerebellum to voluntary movement control include initiation, continuation and termination of movements, regulation of slow ramp, ballistic and compound movements, maintaining static postures and compound postural adjustments (Brookes & Thach, 1981). Although few physiological data of this type are available on the role of the cerebellum in normal speech production, owing to the lack of viable animal models, cerebellar activation during speech production has been demonstrated via positron emission tomography (Peterson, Fox, Posner, Mintun, & Raichle, 1988). It is reasonable to assume that cerebellar participation in speech motor function is similar to that reported in voluntary arm movement. This assumption is reinforced by the striking speech deficits, analogous to ataxic limb impairments, observed in patients with AD in association with cerebellar lesions (Brown, Darley, & Aronson, 1970).

The neural substrate for ataxic dysarthria was originally thought to be in the cerebellar vermis region (Holmes, 1917; Mills & Weisenburg, 1914); however, dysarthria with lesions restricted to the cerebellar hemispheres has also been reported (Holmes, 1917). Lechtenberg and Gilman (1978) examined surgical, autopsy, and radiographic data on 122 patients with focal, non-degenerative cerebellar disease, of which 32 had exhibited AD. Twenty-one of these patients had left cerebellar hemisphere damage, seven had right hemisphere damage, and two had vermal lesions. Three additional cerebellar patients who had normal speech following an initial lesion, developed AD subsequent to surgical resection of the left cerebellar hemisphere. The authors interpret these findings as strong evidence of a left hemispheric lateralization of speech function in the cerebellum. The area identified by Lechtenberg and Gilman (1978) in association with AD corresponds well on the left side to cerebellar areas reported for bilateral afferent representation of the tongue and larynx (Bowman, 1971; Lam & Ogura, 1952). Because the cerebellar-cortical projections are predominantly contralateral, it was speculated there may be a relationship between the emerging role of the nondominant right hemisphere in mediating prosody and the striking prosodic abnormalities that are characteristic of AD (Lechtenberg & Gilman, 1978). Athough the left cerebellar hemisphere may house an important subcortical center for speech production, Gilman et al (1981) have recognized that the left hemisphere localization probably does not account for all manifestations of AD occurring with cerebellar disease. Orofacial structures have somatotopic input and output representation in the right cerebellar hemisphere as well as the left, and are also represented in the anterior portion of the vermis (Thach, 1980); thus is it not surprising that some cases of AD have been observed following lesions in these areas. In addition, AD is frequently associated with damage to the input and output pathways of the cerebellum in such disorders as Friedrich's ataxia and olivopontocerebellar atrophy (Gilman & Kluin, 1984).

Ataxiogenic Disorders

The term "ataxia" is used with various connotations in specific circumstances. Sometimes it refers to difficulties with stance and gait, or it is generic heading for collective symptoms of cerebellar disease (eg, "ataxic dysarthria"); more properly it refers to a loss of motor synergy or the ability to integrate movement subcomponents in the appropriate time and space (Gilman, 1986). Etiogies of disorders that cause ataxia and related symptoms include degenerative, traumatic, vascular, infectious, metabolic, and neoplastic conditions, as well as congenital anomalies. All types of ataxiogenic disorders may be associated with AD; however, AD incidence varies greatly in different disease states. For example, AD occurs in approximately 25% of focal cerebellar lesions (Lechtenberg & Gilman, 1978) but is considered an essential criterion for diagnosis of Friedreich disease (Ackerman & Hertrich, 1993). Gilman, Bloedel, and Lechtenberg (1981) provide an extensive discussion of cerebellar disorders, from which much of the following overview (unless otherwise indicated) has been condensed.

Degenerative Ataxias

These frequently result from inherited conditions which, depending upon the specific disorder, may be autosomal-recessive or autosomal-dominant; may have their onset any time from birth to adulthood; may be associated with hyperreflexia or hyporeflexia; and characteristically include extracerebellar loci of pathology such as the cerebrum, brainstem nuclei, dorsal columns, or peripheral nerves. Friedreich disease is an example of autosomal-recessive disorder that usually has its onset between 6 and 16 years of age; involves the cerebellum, dorsal columns, and the corticospinal tracts; and exhibits hyporeflexia of the deep tendons. It presents initially as gait ataxia, then weakness and fatiguability, followed by a marked dysarthria. Autosomal-dominant diseases in which dysarthria is a prominent feature include olivopontocerebellar degenerations of the Menzel and Schute-Haymaker types. Gilman and Kluin (1984) have suggested that, while AD of both Friedreich disease and olivopontocerebellar degeneration share perceptual symptoms of slowness, dysrhythmia, excess and equalized stress, and prolonged phonemes and intervals, they can be differentiated on the basis of strained-strangled harshness and low monopitch. These features were attributed to a spastic component related to brainstem degeneration that occurs in olivopontocerebellar degeneration but not in Freidreich disease. The hypothesis of differentiated neural substrata for spastic and ataxic components within the same dysarthric patients appears to be supported by recent studies of oxygen hypometabolism via positron emission tomography (Gilman & Kluin, 1992).

Cerebellar Anomalies

Congenital malformations of the cerebellum and related structures include such factors as agenesis or dysgenesis of the vermis or of one hemisphere, hypoplasia of a particular fiber pathway (eg, pontocerebellar projections), growth of posterior fossa cysts, or atresia of the foramena of the fourth ventricle, which results in hydrocephalus. Several of these factors combine in the developmental anomalad known as Dandy-Walker malformation. The various Chiari malformations include both brainstem and cerebellar pathology.

Metabolic Disorders

A variety of metabolic conditions are known to affect the cerebellum; however, these typically affect other regions as well. Cerebellar Purkinje cells are among the most sensitive neurons in the nervous system to loss of oxygen associated with hypoxia, ischemia, or severe hyperthermia. Toxins that may affect the cerebellum include heavy metals (eg, lead and thallium), drugs (eg, certain barbituates and anticonvulsants), and alchohol. All of these toxins may have chronic, irreversible effects. Other metabolic etiologies include vitamin and trace metal deficiencies, amino acid deficiencies, and endocrine disorders. Dysarthria is typical of ataxia secondary to hypoxia, myxedema, and dilantin toxicity, and is variably present in alcoholic cerebellar degeneration (Victor & Ferrendelli, 1970).

Focal Pathologies

Focal cerebellar lesions frequently result from vascular pathology of the posterior inferior, anterior inferior, and the superior cerebellar arteries. This may take the form of transient ischemic attacks, infarction, or hemorrhage. Thrombosis is more common than embolism; but hemorrhage is more common than infarction and may result from hypertension, aneurysm and arteriovenous malformations, anticoagulant therapy, or bleeding tumors. Traumatic damage such as gunshot wounds are a frequent cause of focal cerebellar pathology (Holmes, 1917). Focal lesions may also result from abscess due to bacterial or viral infections. However, meningitis and encephalitis may cause diffuse cerebellar damage, and the slow virus *koru* causes extensive cerebellar degeneration. Cerebellar tumors are quite common, with astrocytomas and medulloblastomas occurring more frequently in children, but metastatic tumors occurring more often after middle age (French, Chou, Long, & Selyescog, 1970). Although the mechanisms are not well understood, neoplasms elsewhere in the body (in which the cancer has not spread to the cerebellum) may also cause cerebellar degeneration and associated AD (Victor & Ferrendelli, 1970).

Nonspeech Concomitants of AD

Generalized Movement Dysfunction

Hypotonia, Hyporeflexia, and Asthenia
Reduced postural muscle tone is believed to be associated with the cerebellum's role in the proprioceptive control of posture, via both cortical and spinal pathways, and may be seen in degenerative illness or most prominently following acute injury (Gilman et al, 1981). With chronic cerebellar disease the significant postural abnormalities, including abnormal postures of the head, may become entrenched. Diminished limb resistance to passive movement can be demon-

strated by grasping the patient's forearm and shaking the relaxed hand at the wrist. Hyporeflexia takes the form of "pendular reflexes," as in clinical elicitation of the patellar reflex wherein the leg swings back and forth at least three times (Gilman et al, 1981). Asthenia and muscle fatigue are also major symptoms of cerebellar disease (Eccles, 1977): affected limbs tire easily on repetitive tasks, and strength has been demonstrated by dynomometry to be as much as 50% below normal function (Holmes, 1939). Weakness is greater in proximal than in distal musculature, and facial weakness is not uncommon. Dworkin and Aronson (1986) studied tongue strength in five AD subjects as part of a broader study of dysarthria wherein anterior and lateral lingual pushing forces were transduced electronically over time and integrated under a force line curve. Inspection of the individual subject data revealed that tongue strength in the AD group ranged from 96 to 37% of average normal function based on gender matched controls, with three subjects generating less than 50% of expected normal values. Marked instability of force maintenance over time has also been reported for the finger, tongue, lip, and jaw in ataxic subjects (McNeil, Weismer, Adams, & Mulligan, 1990). One mechanism that has been hypothesized to account for voluntary motor weakness in cerebellar disease is that decreased activation of cortical upper motor neurons by the cerebellum results in similarly diminished cortical output via the pyramidal pathway to the lower motor neurons (Eccles, 1977).

Tremor, Titubation, and Myoclonus

Both static and kinetic limb tremors are common in cerebellar disease, and are greater in proximal musculature (Dichgans & Diener, 1984). Both types of tremor manifest at frequencies of 3–5 Hz (Jankovich & Fahn, 1980). Static or postural tremor may be demonstrated by extending the arms parallel to the floor when, after a few seconds, an oscillation will develop. The kinetic or "intention" tremor may be elicited by performing the

"finger-nose" or "heel-shin" tests, wherein the amplitude of the oscillation typically increases as the extremity approaches its target.

Titubation is a rhythmic rocking of the trunk or head, several times per second, in the forward-to-back, side-to-side, or rotational dimensions (Gilman, 1986). Palatal myoclonus characterized by rhythmic movements of 2–3 Hz is associated with dentate nucleus or dentato-olivary tract lesions, and may involve the pharynx, larynx, floor of the mouth, and lower face (Dichgans & Diener, 1984), or co-occur with muscular contractions at the base of the upper limbs (Rondot, Jedynak, & Ferry, 1978). Marked degrees of positional unsteadiness have been quantitatively demonstrated in ataxic subjects, using a visual cursor matching task, for both cranially and spinally innervated structures (McNeil et al, 1990). Gilman et al (1981) reported that in their series of 162 cerebellar lesioned patients, kinetic tremors were present in 56%, with hemispheric lesions affecting chiefly the ipsilateral limb and vermal lesions usually resulting in bilateral disturbance. Titubation was present in only about 9% of their patients and had little localizing significance.

Timing of Movements

Ataxic patients present an impression of pervasive slowness. Hallett, Shahani, and Young (1975) demonstrated that on a fast elbow flexion task, the average reaction time of ataxic patients was 270 msec in comparison to a normal average of 200 msec. This slowness has also been demonstrated after acute poisoning of the cerebellum by alcohol ingestion, when mean thumb flexion reaction time increased to 218 msec over a prealcohol mean of 146 msec (Marsden, Merton, Morton, Hallett, Adams, & Rushton, 1977). Marsden et al (1977) suggest that motor slowness results in disruption of agonist-antagonist muscle activity during ballistic movements, which interferes with the generation of accelerative and decelerative forces. Termination or breaking of movement is also impaired (Vilis & Hore, 1980).

Prolonged delay times for the attainment of peak force generation have also been observed in ataxic patients for lingual pushing activities (Dworkin & Aronson, 1986).

Most authors agree that the motor slowness should not be attributed solely to underlying hypotonia, but rather interpret it as part of a central timing and programming deficit (Eccles, 1977; Hallett et al, 1975; Marsden et al, 1977). Timing abnormalities contribute to the decomposition of movements; however, ataxic patients do not merely move through life in "slow motion." Hallet et al (1975) report that at times on their fast elbow flexion task the arm would move in the opposite direction from that intended and that movement would occur inappropriately at the shoulder joint in inappropriately active muscles that should have fixed the limb. Similar reciprocity abnormalities have also been reported during slow ramp visuomotor elbow tracking (Beppu, Suda, & Tanaka, 1983).

Dysmetria, Check, and Rebound
Dysmetria refers to inappropriate trajectory toward a target during a goal directed movement. Hypometria, or "undershoot," falls short of the intended target, while hypermetria, or "overshoot," surpasses the target (Hallett et al, 1975). A patient with cerebellar ataxia may on repeated occasions hit the target normally, overshoot and undershoot the same target. Upper limb dysmetrias can be assessed using the "finger-nose" test in which the forefinger of the outstretched arm is used to touch the nose. In hypometria the finger does not reach the nose; in hypermetria the finger points past the nose, perhaps poking the patient in the eye. A dysmetric movement may be erratic throughout, but tends to culminate with a crescendo of tremorlike corrective movements around the target. Gilman et al (1981) reported dysmetria in 74% of their cerebellar damaged patients in association with left hemisphere, right hemisphere, and vermal lesions. Check and rebound abnormalities are conceptually similar to dysmetria. Normally, when a limb is flexed strongly against

resistance and the resistance is released, the resulting movement is quickly checked. Impaired check is the inability to counteract that resulting forceful movement opposite the direction of the resistance.

One clinical test (Gilman, 1986) requires the patient to extend the arms forward in space with hands pronated while keeping the eyes closed. The examiner taps the wrists (strongly enough to displace the arms). A normal individual exhibits a small displacement but rapidly returns to the original position. Impaired check appears as a wide excursion away from the displacement, with *rebound* occurring as a significant overshoot of the original position on the return swing. Dichgans and Diener (1984) speculate that a similar mechanism may underlay dysmetria and impaired check/rebound phenomena due to "a pronounced delay in or absence of the agonist pause and antagonist burst resulting in inappropriate deceleratory forces" (p 129).

Diadochokinetic Impairments
Decomposition of movement in cerebellar ataxia includes errors in movement direction, off-course deviations during movement, discontinuous movement, dysmetria, and tremor (Dichgans & Diener, 1984). These phenomena can be strikingly demonstrated on tasks involving alternating rapid movements at a single joint or repetitive fine movement sequences. Dysdiadochokinesis appears as slowness and incompleteness of sequence on tasks such as rapid pronation-supination of the hand or apposition of each finger against its thumb in rapid succession (Gilman et al, 1981). Irregularity of the rhythm of repetitive movements is also quite characteristic of ataxic patients. Slow and irregular diadochokinesis of the speech musculature has been demonstrated quantitatively using computer-automated analysis of rapidly repeated monosyllables (Portnoy & Aronson, 1982). It should be noted that diadochokinetic abnormalities are common in various neuromotor disorders and are not, therefore, differentially diagnostic in and of themselves. They do, however, afford a use-

ful mechanism for highlighting the disintegration of complex motor processes in ataxia during clinical evaluation.

Other Associated Deficits

Abnormalities of Stance and Gait

Difficulties with walking and standing are among the most prominent signs of cerebellar disease, occurring frequently as isolated symptoms of vermal damage or in association with other disturbances following damage to the cerebellar hemispheres (Gilman, 1986). Postural instability manifests when standing as excessive swaying (ie, anterior-posterior, lateral, or multidirectional), which is exacerbated by closing the eyes (Dichgans & Diener, 1984). These patients adopt a wide-based stance, which tends to be maintained when walking, to compensate for truncal instability; nevertheless, falling is common (Gilman et al, 1981). Gilman (1978) has described the ataxic gait pattern as "a series of steps irregularly placed, some too far forward, some not sufficiently far forward, and some too far to the left or right" (p 415). Clinical maneuvers for assessing gait disturbance include walking a straight line; heel-to-toe placement, or "tandem walking"; walking on heels or toes only; or walking backwards (Dichgans & Diener, 1984; Gilman et al, 1981).

Oculomotor Dysfunction

Abnormal eye movements associated with cerebellar disease are many and varied. Among the most prominent are gaze-evoked nystagmus, rebound nystagmus, ocular dysmetria, and abnormal optokinetic nystagmus. Gaze-evoked nystagmus manifests as a series of jerking, to-and-fro eye movements when attempting conjugate gaze that deviates from the midline position: the eyes drift slowly back to midline, but there is a rapid corrective movement toward the intended direction of gaze (Gilman et al, 1981). Rebound nystagmus occurs following a prolonged attempt at holding an eccentric gaze (eg, extreme lateral deviation), during which the gaze evoked nystagmus gradually disap-

pears, then returning the gaze to midline where upon a nystagmus occurs in the opposite direction from the previous gaze evoked nystagmus (Dichgans & Diener, 1984). Similar to nystagmus is ocular dysmetria wherein small, rapid oscillating eye movements emerge as the gaze approaches a target and the patient attempts to correct for overshoot and undershoot of the fixation point (Gilman et al, 1981). Optokinetic nystagmus occurs normally when one observes the telephone poles on the roadside from a moving vehicle and clinically when attempting to count the stripes on a moving strip of cloth: The eyes follow the leading stripe then jerk back to the next. According to Gilman et al (1981) patients with chronic cerebellar disease may exhibit enhanced amplitude of optokinetic nystagmus, but patients with acute cerebellar lesions may have inconsistent or diminished optokinetic nystagmus. Smooth visual pursuit of a moving target is also frequently impaired in cerebellar ataxia patients (Dichgans & Diener, 1984).

Nondysarthric Communication Disorders

Other nonspeech factors affecting communication in patients with AD include disorders of writing, cognition and hearing. In their patient series, Gilman et al (1981) observed dysgraphia in 33 percent (not surprisingly given the extent of limb impairments); and more than ten percent had overt psychotic symptoms including visual hallucinations, paranoid ideation, and confabulation, all of which may result in language of confusion. Dementia sometimes occurs in degenerative diseases which affect the cerebellum, but is generally attributed to damage to other structures. While not a direct consequence of cerebellar damage itself, hearing loss commonly co-occurs with a variety of cerebellar diseases including tumors and vascular occlusions (Gilman et al, 1981).

Implications for Speech Production

The striking variety of motoric abnormalities that are associated with cerebellar disorders affect not only the movement capabilities of the limbs and torso, but also the functions of the cranially innervated structures involved in speaking. Thus, the neurophysiological bases of AD have been postulated to be of essentially the same character as motor abnormalities found elsewhere in the body and during nonspeech functions (Brown, Darley, & Aronson, 1970). Netsell and Kent (1976) proposed three hypotheses concerning the cerebellum's role in the execution of skilled movements, including speech, all of which may be operative to different degrees in different types of cerebellar lesions.

First, the cerebellum affects sensorimotor integration by biasing muscle spindles which provide continuous feedback concerning states of muscular contraction. Depression of spindle activity deprives the motor system of proprioceptive feedback about evolving movements, and reduces expected background level of muscular activation that would normally facilitate alpha motor neuron discharge. This could inhibit the strength, speed, and accuracy of movement leading to compensatory slowing. Second, the cerebellum is important to the interpretation of afferent proprioceptive information for ongoing motor control by translating the "language of tensions" into the "language of movements." Impairment of this interpretative function could result in de-automaticity of movement, leading to errors of direction, timing, and range. Third, cerebellar-cerebral interaction involves the regulation and facilitation of cortical motor commands ongoingly by the cerebellum. This could lead to the phenomenon of the presence of motor gestures that are preserved in some form but lacking in precision. It is clear that much of the underlying sensorimotor symptomatology of cerebellar disease observable during nonspeech functions is also distinctively manifested during speech activities.

Speech Characteristics of AD

Studies of ataxia have utilized either single subjects with well-documented lesions limited to the cerebellum/peduncle apparatus (eg, Kent and Netsell, 1975) or groups heterogeneous in etiology and severity (Kent, Netsell, & Abbs, 1979). The problem with case studies is that it is difficult to determine the idiosyncronicity of the observed deficits and whether the findings are generalizable to a broader group of subjects. Group studies that have focused primarily on subjects with diverse etiologies (eg, Darley, Aronson, & Brown, 1969) or degenerative lesions such as Friedreich's ataxia (Ackerman & Hertrich, 1993) or multiple sclerosis (Darley, Brown, & Goldstein, 1972; Farmakides & Boone, 1960) show damage outside the cerebellum and make it difficult to isolate deficits attributable to the cerebellum alone. Morever, as noted by Kent, Netsell, and Abbs (1979), it is difficult to separate speech behaviors due to the lesion from motor control compensations that are a response to the impairment. These qualifications withstanding, we will present speech characteristics of ataxics.

Early descriptions of ataxic dysarthria are rooted in the context of the clinical neurological examination. Charcot (1877) described slow, scanning speech; Holmes (1917) noted the monotonous vocal characteristics and indistinct production of consonants and vowels. Brown et al (1970), in a review of medical textbooks of neurology, used the adjectives of "slow, slurred, irregular, labored, intermittent, jerky, explosive, staccato, singsong, and scanning" (p 302) to describe the disorder. Speech deficits in ataxia are due to errors in the timing, force, range, and direction of movements which would be expected to affect respiratory, laryngeal, and articulatory structures. The first large-scale perceptual study of ataxic dysarthria with lesions specific to the cerebellum was included in a series of reports from Mayo Clinic (Darley, Aronson, & Brown, 1968, 1969a,b; Brown, Darley, & Aronson, 1970) that provided a comprehensive description of the primary characteristics of the disorder. Darley et al. (1969a,b) studied 212 patients divided into seven groups, one group being subjects with cerebellar damage from a wide range of etiologies (stroke, progressive degeneration, trauma). Ratings on 38 dimensions were completed from speech and reading samples.

Prominent dimensions for ataxic dysarthria included imprecise consonants, irregular articulatory breakdown with errors that were inconsistent, and sudden "telescoping" of a syllable or syllables. Also prominent were excess and equal stress ("scanning speech"), prolonged phonemes and intervals, and slow rate interactively encompassing prosodic abnormalities tied to the equalization and increase in stress. Based on the perceptual ratings, Darley et al (1969b) divided the 10 most deviant dimensions into three clusters: articulatory inaccuracy (irregular articulatory breakdown, imprecise consonants, distorted vowels); prosodic excess (excess and equal stress, prolonged phonemes, prolonged intervals, slow rate); and phonatory-prosodic insufficiency (monoloudness, monopitch, harsh voice), which have served as a focus of subsequent studies of electromyography, kinematics, and speech acoustics in ataxic dysarthria.

Despite myriad motoric difficulties that are observable in AD, disturbances of *motor programming* do not appear to be the primary source of the speech movement abnormalities. The cortically programmed serial speech gestures are not disturbed in ataxic dysarthria although there are abnormalities in speech movement rate, range, and direction (Netsell, 1973). As noted by Netsell and Kent:

> The preservation of the desired successional patterns in the face of conspicuous abnormalities in individual structural movements and speaking rate might be explained by assuming that the successional pattern for speech movements is programmed at the cortical level and that cerebellar dysfunction results in the delayed and inaccurate execution of the required submovements. In short, the coordination of articulatory movements is not destroyed, even though the overall movement pattern is slowed and individual movements may be misdirected (p 106).

Respiration

Respiratory activity is compromised in ataxic speakers including vital capacity (Brown, Darley, & Aronson, 1970) and total lung capacity (Murdoch, Chenery, Stokes, & Hardcastle, 1991). Speech respiration is characterized by abnormal synchrony in the respiratory apparatus (Gilman & Kluin, 1984; Hiller, 1929). Abbs, Hunker, and Barlow (1983), in a kinematic study, described paradoxical respiratory activity in an ataxic speaker in which abdominal contributions to lung volume changes were inspiratory while rib cage contributions were expiratory. They suggested that the asynchrony of rib cage and abdomen could potentially interfere with lung volume control and subglottal pressure. Murdoch et al (1991), using strain gauge pneumographs, found "bizarre" movements of the abdomen and rib cage in a study of 12 ataxics. Abdominal paradoxing was found, with one exception, during the performance of sustained vowel and syllable repetition tasks. The paradoxing was most notable on demanding syllable repetition tasks compared to sustained vowels. Rib cage paradoxing (circumference of the rib cage increasing while the lung volume and circumference of the abdomen are decreasing) also was found in addition to motion jerks which originated from the rib cage and abdomen; and abrupt changes in the chest wall contributions to lung volume displacements. The majority of the ataxics initiated reading and conversation below expected lung volume levels. However, they expired through a large portion of their vital capacity on vowels and syllable repetitions.

Studies of respiratory kinematics suggest that ataxics have difficulty regulating the output of the respiratory apparatus for speech due to discoordinated rib cage/abdomen movements. Respiratory hypofunction in the form of subnormal vital capacity and forced expiratory volumes occurred in a significant minority of AD patients (Murdoch et al, 1991). Netsell (1973), however, found that a 60-year-old ataxic patient was able to maintain intraoral pressures of $5\,cm/H_2O$ and $10\,cm/H_2O$ and concluded that this subject did not have a respiratory component to her speech deficits. There is little doubt that the coordinated activity of the respiratory unit in ataxia is compromised. The effects of the incoordination of rib cage and abdomen on generation of sustained subglottal pressure for speech, however, have not been systematically investigated, a major research shortfall given the phonatory and prosodic abnormalities described as characteristic of the disorder.

Phonation

Early instrumental studies focused on the utility of acoustic analysis for differential diagnosis. Scripture (1916) utilized a phonoautograph—an instrument constructed of a mouthpiece that led to a metal tube covered with a flexible membrane. Movements of the membrane were recorded on a blackened cylinder. He reported that 20 patients with disseminated sclerosis, whether speech was affected or not, demonstrated waveforms consistent with jerky irregularities of tension of the vocal folds occurring at the beginning and end of a vowel. He interpreted these findings as a difficulty in the ability to make adjustments in laryngeal tension. Similarly, Janvrin (1933) and Janvrin and Worster-Drought (1932) utilized "sound tracks" to demonstrate upward jerks in the laryngeal waveform of a patient with disseminated sclerosis which were interpreted as incoordination in laryngeal muscle function due to ataxia. Scripture (1933) believed waveform analysis was a reliable means of differential diagnosis, but Haggard (1969) demonstrated that there was significant overlap between multiple sclerosis and normal subjects in waveform variation and noted that the claim of differential diagnosis should be viewed as a historical curiosity.

"Harshness" is most frequently used to describe phonatory function in ataxic dysarthria (Darley et al, 1969b; Gilman & Kluin, 1984; Joanette & Dudley, 1980). Kent and Netsell (1975) noted the frequent appearance of aperiodic vocal pulse striations in their ataxic speaker, which is typically believed to be due to hypotonia. Some patients may engage in excessive starining or squeezing in an attempt to compensate for weak-ened laryngeal function. Highly variable phonation with sudden bursts of loudness and irregular pitch and loudness increases might also be expected as a result of discoordination (Zwirner, Murry, & Woodson, 1991). Gentil (1990) reported abnormally unsteady phonation of sustained vowels in terms of both fundamental frequency and intensity contours in all of his 14 Friedreich ataxia subjects. He concluded that this was due to respiratory-phonatory asynergy. Zwirner et al (1991) acoustically evaluated sustained vowel productions in terms of fundamental frequency, the standard deviation of fundamental frequency, jitter, shimmer, and signal-to-noise ratio in groups of Parkinsonian, ataxic, and Huntington's subjects. They found a significant correlation between perceptual judgments of severity of dysphonia and all measures of phonatory variability for the cerebellar subjects. The cerebellar subjects differed significantly from normals on standard deviation of fundamental frequency and jitter, which may be respectively interpreted as indications of long-term and short-term variability in vocal fold vibration. However, the distributional overlap with the normal subjects on the acoustic measures was large. They concluded that as vocal instability increases, perceived severity of dysphonia increases for individuals with cerebellar lesions.

Articulation

Electromyography

Hypotonia is a primary neuromuscular characteristic of ataxia in speech musculature although it may not account for all observed movement deficits (Netsell & Kent, 1976). Based on data from Abbs, Barlow, and Cole (1979) and Netsell and Abbs (1977), Netsell (1982) identified two types of electromyographic patterns in subjects with cerebellar lesions. One pattern is characterized by a gradual buildup of amplitude that approximates normal levels, but which then is prolonged with a corresponding increase in the duration of movement. A second pattern shows repetitive bursts of excitation and quieting, producing fluctuations in the degree of force between articulatory structures. Netsell summarized muscle function in ataxia as follows:

> In short, the cerebellar subject is slow, or slow plus irregular, in building up the requisite muscle force in the prime mover and, once the force is achieved, cannot rapidly suppress the activity... [and] ... cerebellar failure slows, or makes discontinuous, the normally phasic and precise muscle forces. As a consequence, all muscle contractions tend to have a uniformly long duration, yielding slow velocities to all movements and uniform duration to the syllables (pp 43–44).

The finding of irregularity in muscle activation and suppression was demonstrated by Hirose et al (1978), who found that EMG patterns in two ataxic patients were irregular in shape and timing with a plateau of activity during a period of suppression with disturbed repetitive syllable production. Gentil (1990), in a investigation of muscle function in antagonistic facial muscles plus the anterior belly of the digastric, observed increased reaction times between an auditory stimulus and the onset of muscular activity. There also was a loss of reciprocity between antagonistic muscles in eight of the 13 subjects studied, expanded mean durations of anticipatory muscle activity, and prolonged muscle activity on syllable segments which he attributed to hypotonia. Interestingly, Forrest, Adams, McNeil, and Southwood (1991) did not find differences in electromyography between various neurogenic groups (including cerebellar lesion subjects) on the basis of co-contraction and reciprocal activity in antagonistic facial muscles.

The neuromuscular features of ataxic dysarthria, then, appear to be hypotonia associated with deficits in graded muscle force development and corresponding disruptions in the synchrony of muscle activation/suppression. Kent and Netsell (1975) suggested that hypotonia may be the primary source of speech abnormalities in ataxic dysarthria

that produces delays in muscle force generation producing prolongation, reduced rates of muscular contraction causing slowed movement, and reduced range of movements producing telescoping. These observations are consistent with kinematic studies of ataxia.

Kinematics

Speech movement data in ataxia are limited primarily to case studies of paroxysmal ataxic dysarthria (Netsell & Kent, 1976) or generalized degeneration of the cerebellum (Kent & Netsell, 1975; Kent, Netsell, & Bauer, 1975). In these studies cinefluorography was used to measure displacements of the lip, jaw, and tongue during the production of sustained vowels and phrases. Primary findings included reduced articulatory velocities, prolongation of consonant constrictions and vowel steady states, inappropriate or missed articulatory targets, and poor tongue positioning for vowels. Microbeam-based measurement of lip and jaw movement (Hirose et al, 1978) also has revealed inconsistent velocities of lower lip movements and times when lip movement was dependent entirely on jaw movement. However, lip velocities in contrast to Kent and Netsell, were not markedly slowed for the ataxic subject. They concluded that ataxic dysarthria was characterized by "a difficulty in the initiation of purposeful movements and an inconsistency of articulatory movements, particularly in the repetitive production of a monosyllable" (p 96). McNeil and Adams (1991) employed movement transducers affixed to the lips and jaw, in conjunction with the co-occuring acoustic signal, to examine speech movement capabilities of four AD patients in comparison to normal controls, aphasic and apraxic subjects. The AD subjects were significantly slower than normal on durations of opening and closing phases of a /b/ segment and time to peak velocity for the opening gesture. These studies suggest that the primary movement characteristics of ataxia are reduced articulatory velocities and inaccuracy of movement.

Acoustics

Acoustical analysis has been the primary vehicle for inferences about movement-related deficits in ataxia and for examining the prosodic abnormalities characteristic of the disorder. Individuals with ataxic dysarthria demonstrate longer syllable durations, longer formant transitions, and, at times, longer voice onset times (Kent, Netsell, & Abbs, 1979). Kent et al (1979) noted, however, that the slowed rate of the ataxic speaker may allow additional time to reach vowel targets. They also found that word durations for ataxic speakers were longer with a relative lengthening of both consonant clusters and word nuclei, and a loss of durational distinctions between tense and lax vowels was documented that nearly neutralized their differences. Differences in variability of segment durations were not large considering they were four to seven times longer than normal speakers', but there appeared to be highly variable lax vowels in the more severely involved patients. In the production of base words they demonstrated instances of lengthening, inconsistent reductions, and small reductions compared to normal speakers. Kent et al (1979) concluded that a fundamental feature of ataxia was the lengthening of segments with some segments lengthened more than others, resulting in a disruption in the normal speech rhythm and timing. Duration appeared to reflect the severity of ataxia with longer segments reflecting more severe involvement. Gentil (1990) examined the production of one-, two-, and three-syllable nonsense utterances to investigate variability. He found larger coefficients of variability in patients with Friedreich's ataxia, and concluded that inconsistency of segment duration was a feature of the speech disorder. Other findings included increased durations of single word and phrase productions, and reduced diadochokinetic rates. Keller (1990) also reported higher variability of vowels, occlusions, syllable durations, and voice onset times in monosyllable repetition for three ataxic subjects. Ouellon, Ryalls, Lebeuf, and Joanette (1991) reported, in patients with Friedreich's ataxia, an increase in voice onset time variability resulting in a reduction of the voicing lead-lag differences for cognate pairs of French initial plosives (eg, /p - b/), which in turn led to the percept of inconsistent substitution errors.

These findings were consistent, in part, with a study of seven subjects with Friedreich's ataxia (Ackermann & Hertrich, 1993). Twelve German sentences were produced from which target words were available for analysis. Syllable durations, with two exceptions, were outside the normal range. However, variation coefficients, with the exception of one syllable, were within the normal 95% confidence intervals for normal subjects. Duration ratios of stressed syllable to sentence duration were greater for the ataxic subjects. In spite of reduced stressed syllable duration, stress was marked by duration, suggesting that encoding of linguistic prosody was not impaired. No significant differences in intrasyllabic timing, as reflected in voice onset time, were observed for voiceless consonants, although variation coefficients were greater for the ataxic group. However, occlusion durations were increased. Primary findings, then, were increased syllable, vowel and occlusion segment durations, normal or near-normal voice onset times, and preservation of the timing of speech segments as reflected in variation coefficients.

Resonance

Variables related to resonance, an interactive acoustic byproduct of phonation and articulation, have not been well studied in AD. Oral resonances, or formants, appear to be normal if allowances are made for slowness in acheiving target values and inconsistent overshoot and undershoot (Kent & Netsell, 1975). Perceptual reports of hypernasal resonance relating to palatal function suggest that it is usually only minimally impaired (Darley et al, 1975; Enderby, 1983). Grunewell and Huskins (1979) reported inconsistent articulation errors (eg, substitution of /b/ for /m/ or /m/ for /b/)

associated with the phonetic feature of nasality in AD, which she interpreted to be due to coordination and timing difficulties. Yorkston and Beukelman (1981) reported that, prior to treatment, one of their AD subjects was perceived to be significantly hypernasal, and this was supported by airflow and pressure measurements. However, the hypernasality proved to be attributable to discoordination of palatal movement with that of other articulators, since it was eliminated in response to slowing of the speaking rate (Yorkston & Beukelman, 1981a).

Prosody

Increased duration of syllables and segments and loss of durational distinctions between stressed and unstressed syllables, coupled to reduced control of fundamental frequency and intensity parameters, mark the prosodic abnormalities of ataxic speakers. Kent et al (1979) described two fundamental frequency patterns characteristic of ataxics. One pattern was typified by fundamental frequency which falls within each syllable as if each syllable contained its own declarative form. A second pattern included a flat fundamental frequency contour like a monotone. Large sweeps in fundamental frequency (Gentil, 1990; Kent & Netsell, 1975) also have been reported as characteristic of the disorder. Kent and Rosenbek (1982) described sweeping patterns with pronounced shifts in fundamental frequency accompanied by abnormalities in syllable durations, dissociated patterns with homogeneous intrasyllabic features characterized by segregated syllables of nearly uniform duration, and segregated syllabic patterns in which some prosodic cohesion is maintained as characteristic of AD.

Odell, McNeil, Rosenbek, and Hunter (1991) reported that cerebellar subjects demonstrate more substitution than distortion errors, more errors in polysyllabic than monosyllabic words, and more errors in noninitial positions of words. However, abnormal prosodic features at the single word level including syllabic stress errors, and initiating and completing word productions were not characteristic of ataxic subjects based on perceptual judgements. Murry (1983) suggested that ataxic dysarthrics use compensatory activity in the production of stress as a function of word position. Yorkston, Beukelman, Minifie, and Sapir (1984) examined sentence level stress patterns in three AD patients using a combination of perceptual scaling and acoustical analyses of fundamental frequency, intensity, and duration. One patient exhibited inconsistent perceptible stress errors, one used exaggerated fundamental frequency differences to mark stress, and one used compensatory lengthening of stressed syllables. Linebaugh and Wolfe (1984) compared articulation rate, intelligibility, and naturalness in ataxic and spastic speakers. Both groups differed from normal controls on all three measures, but they did not differ from each other. However, correlations between naturalness, intelligibility, and rate were significant for the spastic, but not the ataxic speakers.

In summary, all speech subsystems may be significantly deficient in AD. Speech is marked by hypotonia and discoordination with reduced velocities and inaccuracy of articulatory movements in the presence of grossly normal programming of speech sequences. Segments and syllables are variable and increased in duration with a loss of durational distinctions between stressed and unstressed syllables. Slow rate and flat fundamental frequency contours, at times marked by wide sweeps or syllable specific declinations, characterize the prosody of these speakers.

Assessment Considerations

The overall organization of the motor speech evaluation for AD does not differ conceptually from that of other types of dysarthria and need not be reiterated here (see chapters 2 through 7 of this volume). Some special considerations for assessing patients with AD are worth highlighting, however, because they feed directly into the planning, implementation, and monitoring of AD-specific treatment.

First, there are sufficient discrepancies in findings, across studies and between patients within studies, of the speech characteristics of AD to suggest the likelihood of differential subsystem impairments contributing to the variability of dysarthrias exhibited by different AD patients. This should not be surprising when dealing with a neural organ of the size, complexity, and connectivity of the cerebellum. (Consider for comparison the facetious proposition that all cerebral lesions should yield highly similar speech disturbances!) Functional localization and multiple somatotopic representation within the cerebellum have been established (Dichgans & Diener, 1984; Gilman, 1977; Thatch, 1980). Behaviorally, outside of the speech mechanism, it is known that not all elements of possible cerebellar symptomotology (eg, dysmetria, hypotonia, or tremor) will occur in a given patient; furthermore, distal vs proximal musculature, upper vs lower extremities, and left vs right sides may all be differentially affected (Gilman et al, 1981). By analogy, therefore, it is critical that each speech subsystem be evaluated for basic dysfunctions in the areas of muscular strength and tonus, coordination, speed, accuracy, and steadiness. Similarly, extremity functions should be examined, not only to support the diagnosis of ataxia, but to determine the extent to which they may be capitalized upon for treatment approaches that involve intersystemic reorganization (eg, manual pacing) or other augmentation (eg, alphabet board).

Second, the stereotype that AD speakers are intelligible, while often true, in not universally the case. Darley et al (1975) found AD to be the most intelligible of seven dysarthric subtypes, despite the fact that imprecise consonants and irregular articulatory breakdowns were among their most prominent deficiencies. Enderby (1983) observed her AD group to be the second most intelligible of five dysarthric subtypes. Mean intelligibility ratings on the 9-point interval scale used in the Frenchay Dysarthria Assessment

were approximately two scale values below "normal function," but were described as "abnormal but intelligible" (Enderby, 1983). As Enderby points out, however, it is also important to examine the standard deviations of such group ratings: AD patients falling near the -2 standard deviation benchmark would be characterized as 50% intelligible. Yorkston, Beukelman, Hammen, and Traynor (1990) report that the average percentage of sentence intelligibility (viz words that were actually understood) for a group of four AD patients at habitual speaking rate was approximately 41%. In order to acheive greater intelligibility, enormous trade-offs in the form of compensatory slowing are usually necessary, which will affect the efficiency of information exchange (ie, intelligible words per minute) and make AD speech sound peculiarly unnatural. Therefore, careful intelligibility assessments at different speaking rates using an instrument such as the Assessment of Intelligibility of Dysarthric Speech (Yorkston & Beukelman, 1981a,b) is routinely recommended.

Third, the evaluation of prosodic naturalness is particularly important in AD. Naturalness is the degree to which speech sounds acceptable and avoids bizarre behaviors. This is not to say that AD is the least natural sounding of the dysarthrias: it was in fact ranked second least bizarre by Darley et al (1975). The dilemma is that naturalness may be dramatically impaired in AD to an extent that would not be expected based on judgments of intelligibility or overall severity of deficit. Linebaugh and Wolfe (1984) demonstrated that, whereas naturalness, intelligibility, and rate were all interrelated in spastic dysarthria, these variables seem to operate independently in patients with AD. Perhaps this is because slowness as a motor symptom in cerebellar disease may be disassociated from other components such as dysmetria and directional inaccuracy, or because it occurs as a primary deficit in some patients and a compensatory strategy in others. Thus it cannot be assumed that a slow AD speaker is less natural-sounding than a fast one, nor that more intelligible AD speakers use slower or faster rates than those who are less intelligible. Finally, abnormal prosodic factors including stress patterning, intonation, and pausal phenomena are particularly relevant in AD because they can lead both to decreased intelligibility and to decreased naturalness in the presence of relatively spared intelligibility (Yorkston, Beukelman, Minifie, & Sapir, 1984). Moreover, for AD patients who are stimulatable, the manipulation of prosodic variables can facilitate striking speech improvements (Yorkston & Beukelman, 1981). Proper assessment of these variables requires careful integration of perceptual and instrumental methodology, particularly acoustic measures of fundamental frequency, intensity, and duration (Yorkston et al, 1983). Such measurements are increasingly available in everyday clinical settings with the growing utilization of commercial analysis systems, such as the Kay Elemetrics Visipitch or IBM Speech Viewer, and viable clinical protocols for prosodic assessment are beginning to emerge (Robin, Klouda, & Hug, 1991).

Treatment of AD

As with other forms of dysarthria, treatment approaches for AD can be subdivided into those which maximize the physiological substrate for support of speech production versus those designed to effect compensated intelligibility (Rosenbek & Lapointe, 1985). Within the treatment sequence, improvement of underlying physiological support logically precedes speech specific therapy activities. Exceptions to this principle can be made when trying to provide a patient with some functional communication strategies during the early stages of treatment. Maximization of physiological support includes such factors as surgical, pharmacological, and prosthetic interventions that improve the structure or function of the speech apparatus, as well as specific behavioral therapies to increase the strength, speed, stability, and accuracy of movement of component structures and muscles of the vocal tract. When the patient's underlying physiology has been

improved to an appropriate extent, the patient is best able to learn compensatory speaking strategies. Compensated intelligibity, the primary goal of most dysarthria treatment, can be acheived through componential or symptomatic approaches which address specific aspects of respiration, phonation, resonation, articulation, and prosody; however, it can also be acheived through generic approaches wherein some strategic manipulation, often of a simplistic nature (eg, slowing the speaking rate), may have beneficial consequences that reverberate throughout the speaking system. It is further recognized that enhancement of physiology may in itself improve intelligibility, and that speech or speechlike exercises might similarly ameliorate nonspeech muscle dysfunction. The remainder of this section will address the distinction between physiological enhancement vs compensated intelligibility, as well as the related issues of prosodic naturalness and augmentative communication as they apply to the treatment of AD.

Physiological Enhancement

Enhancement Through Medical Intervention
Unlike some other forms of dysarthria (eg, flaccid velopharyngeal paralysis), there are no AD-specific surgical procedures that may be recommended to enhance vocal tract structure underlying speech. Similarly, specific pharmacologic treatments for cerebellar ataxia have been unimpressive (Young & Penney, 1986). However, limited positive findings have been reported for the effects of isoniazid on limb intention tremor (Sabra, Hallett, Sudarsky, & Mullally, 1982) and physostigmine on ataxia (Kark, Budelli, & Wachsner, 1981). The beta blockers clonazepam (Klonopin) and propranolol (Inderal) may also be helpful in controlling vocal intention tremor (Dworkin, 1991).

Appropriate medical interventions for the cerebellar disease states that have caused the dysarthria, which vary on the basis of etiology, may in many cases have a beneficial influence on speech. In *Disorders of the*

Cerebellum (1981), Gilman, Boedel, and Lechtenberg discuss medical management of various pathologic states providing illustrative case examples in which dysarthria and other communicative behavior improved following treatment. Surgical excision is an appropriate treatment for some forms of abscess, hemorrhages, and tumors; endarterectomy may be indicated in cases of complete arteriole occlusion, which results in emboli formation leading to recurrent transient ischemic attacks. Gilman et al (1981) report two cases in which significant dysarthria secondary to vascular lesions cleared completely following surgical decompression with hematoma evacuation of the left cerebellar hemisphere. They also report the case of a 14-year-old girl in whom a medulloblastoma, filling the the fourth ventricle and infiltrating part of the vermis, was removed and followed with radiotherapy. Six months postsurgery her significant presurgical impairments in speech and mentation had improved to a normal level of functioning. Limb ataxia, which had affected handwriting, had also improved significantly.

According to Gilman et al (1981), several toxic and metabolic conditions that cause AD may respond favorably to nonsurgical interventions. Thallium poisoning may be corrected with removal of the toxin from the body; however, in severe caes this may require hemodialysis with cathartic agents and gastric lavage. Effects of alchohol-induced cirrhosis and hepatic disease may be reversed by reducing blood toxin levels while maintaining respiratory, cardiovascular, and renal support. AD and other related symptoms which developed in progressive systemic sclerosis patients, who were fed histadine resulting in zinc deficiency, experienced complete reversal when treated with zinc supplements. Nicotinamide deficiency is corrected by administration of that vitamin. AD associated with endocrine disorders results from diseases of the hormone-producing organs, and is correctable with correction of the endocrine disturbance. In some toxic conditions, early withdrawal of

the offending substance may result in partial or complete reversal of ataxic symptoms. In a study of sway patterns in patients with chronic alcoholism and malnutrition, stance improved dramatically in patients who were abstinent, but continued to decline in those who were not (Dichgans & Diener, 1984). This is not always the case; however, as in some instances of long term use of anticonvulsant medication (eg, dilantin) wherein AD and other symptoms may persist after withdrawal and may continue to increase insidiously.

Enhancement Through Behavioral Therapy
This approach emphasizes direct physical exercise of specific muscles or muscle groups to improve the strength, accuracy, and timing of movements of the speech apparatus, while not targeting speaking per se as the treatment variable (Netsell & Daniel, 1979). Thus someone with weak respiratory musculature, for example, may exhibit short phrases and decreased loudness: It is assumed that by improving respiratory muscle function, phrase length, and loudness should also improve, or have greater potential for improvement (Rosenbek & LaPointe, 1985). It should be noted that exercises to enhance underlying physiological support for speech are not restricted to nonspeech motor activities. Many clinicians utilize speechlike stimuli (eg, sustained vowels or repetitive monosyllables) during this phase of therapy; however, their intent is to improve function for a particular motoric process (eg, steadiness) within a subsystem (eg, respiration) rather than to perfect the production of individual speech sounds or teach specific compensatory speaking strategies. Throughout the implementation of a physical exercise approach, the careful use of baselining and charting procedures, as well as routine probing for generalization to connected speech, are strongly recommended. At present there are no available data on the efficacy for AD of exercise regimens intended to enhance physiological substrates for support of speech. The following section is therefore extrapolated from a combination of logical

inferences based on known information about motor system dysfunction in AD, treatment data available on other neuromotor disorders, and treatment suggestions offered by experienced clinicians in existing literature.

Strengthening exercises to improve *hypofunction* may be important to the treatment of some patients with AD. Despite the fact that greater clinical attention has been focused on dysprosodic aspects of AD (Edwards, 1984), hypotonia is a significant component of some ataxiogenic disorders, bearing in mind that weakness and fatiguability are greatest in proximal musculature (Holmes, 1939). In addition, especially for the degenerative ataxias, less prominent spastic or flaccid weakness elements may be inextricably intermingled with the primary AD (see Gilman & Kluin, 1984). Hypotonia may negatively impact posture and respiratory, phonatory and articulatory muscle function in AD. Hypotonic postural abnormalities of the trunk and head may interfere with effective speech production and should be managed accordingly (Murry, 1983). Existing case study data for treatment of muscular hypofunction in other neuromotor disorders may provide a basis for experimental treatment in AD cases wherein hypofunction is found to be a significant variable. For example, Netsell and Daniel (1979) report the successful use of a U-tube manometer equiped with a "leak tube" as a visual feedback device for remediating flaccid respiratory hypofunction. The patient was trained to generate subglottal pressure levels over time that would be similar to those required for the production of phonated speech. The use of visual feedback from devices such as the Respitrace, which transduces rib cage and abdominal circumference (see Watson & Alphonso, 1991) or a manometric system interfaced with a storage oscilloscope (see Rubow, 1984) may provide a means to instruct hypofunctional AD patients to initiate speech at higher lung volumes. For AD patients with significant hypotonia or weakness of the articulatory musculature, specific strengthening exercises may be useful (Dworkin, 1991). For example, the use of tongue-strengthening exercises involving lingual pushing against "resistance blocks" has been described by Dworkin (1991) as part of a general exercise physiology sequence for hypofunctional articulation. In addition, EMG-derived electronic feedback signals, in the visual and auditory modalities, have been sucessfully employed to remediate facial weakness associated with flaccid dysarthria (Rubow, 1984).

Of even greater signifcance than hypofunction for the treatment of AD is the phenomenon of *decomposition of movement*, which includes problems with timing, stability, force development and termination, directional accuracy, and integration of motoric gestures. Kinematic analysis of AD patients' expiration during speech reveals frequent aberrations such as paradoxical breathing and intention tremor (Murdoch et al, 1991). Murry (1983) suggests that steadiness of exhalation is a primary goal of respiratory training for AD, although this may be complicated by shallow expiration. He proposes three phases of treatment at the respiratory level. In the first stage, 3–4 seconds of steady exhalation is alternated with 3–4 seconds of rest. Expiration may be augmented by the use of manual self-monitoring by placing the palm of the hand on the abdomen and by using slight glottal frication to decrease the rate of expiratory airflow. In stage 2, steady vowel phonation is added to the expiration which may be augmented by a visual feedback device. Part of the goal at this stage is to overcome inappropriate bursts of loudness, voicing interruptions and initiation struggle. Once steady vowel phonation is habitual, the consistently steady and unexplosive production of individual one-syllable words is targeted. The third stage of treatment involves producing sequences of syllables on a single exhalation, moving gradually from repetitive monosyllables to multisyllabic words.

Ataxic dysphonia during speaking has been described perceptually as being monopitch, monoloud, and harsh (Brown, Darley, & Aronson, 1970); however, acoustical analyses have demonstrated increased variability of both fundamental frequency and intensity during sustained vowel, syllable, and sentence productions (Gentil, 1990a,b; Kent & Netsell, 1975; Zwirner et al, 1991). The precepts of excessive pitch changes and abnormal pitch fluctuations (Gilman & Kluin, 1984; Murry, 1983) and excessive loudness variation (Brown et al, 1970) have also been described. Heterogeneity among AD patients and among observational methods may account for some apparent discrepancies. Nevertheless, decomposition of laryngeal movements often occurs, yielding marked aberrations in phonatory control. Phonatory dysmetria may well take the forms of pitch and loudness overshoot or undershoot in the same individuals saying the same thing at different times. Thus the goal of physiological therapy for the phonatory subsystem is to bring these aberrant mechanisms under greater volitional control. Basic phonatory steadiness is a natural outgrowth of the type of expiratory steadiness exercises described above (Murry, 1983). In addition, timing and coordination of laryngeal movements may be developed through specific repetitive production drills. Murry (1983) therefore emphasizes pitch change exercises in which the patient learns to decrease and increase pitch differences voluntarily in real words and phrases in accordance with appropriate demands of meaning, and to smooth the pitch contour of any extreme or abrupt fluctuations. Visual biofeedback devices that depict fundamental frequency and intensity contours, such as the Kay Elemetrics Visipitch or the IBM Speech Viewer, can be quite useful in this context.

The need for remediation of voice onset time abnormalities in AD has been suggested by Ouellon et al (1991), who argue that inconsistently perceived voicing substitution errors, resulting from the overlapping of VOT categories in AD, are in reality phonetic distortions related to laryngeal timing and coordination difficulties. They suggest that phonological process remediation would therefore be inappropriate, but favor exploit-

ing the AD patient's intact knowledge of the voice-voiceless distinction to progressively move production toward more normal phonemic boundaries. Dworkin (1991) describes in detail a sequence of six exercises designed to improve laryngeal timing and coordination in AD that relies heavily upon the use of an adaptation of the inexpensive Pro-Ed See Scape apparatus to visually monitor oral airflow during production drills. In steps 1 and 2, this program initially employs prolongation of the vowel for 3 seconds in repetetive CV syllables, then alternating the prolonged CV syllables with 1-second glottal breath-holding pauses. Steps 3 and 4 involve the production of a vowel sequence [u: a: i: E: o: I:], which takes the form of a sustained vowel of changing resonance, wherein each vowel target position is maintained for about 2 seconds. Subsequently, the durations of the component vowel targets are varied systematically. Step 5 involves prolonging the vowel duration of meaningful CV and CVCV words, while varying the duration of glottal breath-holding pauses between the words. Finally, in step 6, specific practice is incorporated as needed on producing sequences of words and sentences with progressively more normal voice quality.

Slowness and dysmetria of the articulatory subsystem have been reported by various investigators (Dworkin & Aronson, 1986; Gentil, 1990; Kent & Netsell, 1975; McNeil & Adams, 1990). Murry (1983) describes the phenomenon of *target velocity* as "the speed utilized in reaching the point of articulation, and then continuing on, through and away from the target once it has been reached" (p 86). He suggests that target velocity, which is impaired in AD, is particularly important to articulatory precision. He further suggests the use of articulatory drills conducted at a speaking rate that is moderately faster than the patient's usual productions. These employ repetitive CV sequences, incorporating various consonants and vowels, initially with repetition of single monosyllables (eg, /pi pi pi pi pi/) and subsequently with alternation of more complex syllable sequences exemplifying vowel or consonant contrasts (eg, /pi pa pi pa pi pa/ or /pi ti pi ti pi ti/). Similar word and phrase level drills follow, systematically increasing in complexity. Augmentation by manual tapping or the use of a metronome is recommended to establish a rhythmical pattern for these exercises, and to develop in the patient a "metronomic sense" that should enhance conversational intelligibility (p. 88). Finally, for significantly hypotonic patients, Murry (1983) further recommends the use of vowel drills augmented with visual feedback using a mirror as a preliminary to the CV sequencing activities described above. These progress from sustained vowel productions, emphasizing visible features, to sequences of alternating vowel productions that maximize articulatory movements (eg, /i a i a/) at increasing rates.

Dworkin (1991) presents a distinctive program of lingual, labial, and mandibular force physiology training as well as phonetic stimulation which may be useful as treatments for the widespread incoordination deficits of the articulatory subsystem in AD. In his force physiology regimen, visual feedback is provided via mirror and auditory stimulation via metronome is employed. In addition, special assistive devices—such as bite blocks (to decouple jaw movement from that of lip and tongue) and a "cross bar apparatus" constructed from tongue depressors—are used to present slight levels of resistance to the various articulators. Oral exercises, including such activities as raising/lowering the tongue tip, protruding/spreading the lips, and raising/lowering the mandible, are performed in time with metronome beats progressing from slow to fast and then variable rates. Specific efficacy data for force physiology treatment are provided for a flaccid dysarthria case, who reportedly improved articulatory precision from a pretreatment score of 3.5 to a posttreatment score of 2.0 on a 7-point interval scale. Phonetic stimulation activities, described at length in Dworkin (1991), are an elaboration and extension of traditional phonetic placement techniques. Phonetic stimulation treatment is augmented with the use of simple positioning devices such as tongue depressors and cotton applicators for articulator positioning, as well as the Pro-ED SEE Scape apparatus, mirror feedback, and audiotape recording.

Ultimately, the utility of exercise programs such as those described by Murry (1983), Dworkin (1991), and others for treatment of AD must await confirmation through single-subject and group efficacy research designs. In the meantime, such programs appear to enjoy both face and content validity, and lend themselves well to accepted accountability procedures such as baselining, charting, and probing for generalization to connected speech. Thus, if an AD patient demonstrates deficit areas such as hypotonia and dysmetria of the speech apparatus and has the ability to perform the requisite procedures, physiological enhancement exercises seem warranted to the extent that he or she continues to demonstrate measurable improvement within the task *and on objective measures of connected speech* (eg, percent intelligibility). It should also be appreciated that the appropriate use of improvement of residual support for speech has an upper limit, and that there is a range beyond which it can be exaggerated to the detriment of the therapeutic process (Rosenbek & Lapointe, 1985).

Compensated Intelligibility and Prosodic Naturalness

Intelligibility

Although adjunctive treatment outcomes such as decreasing bizarre behaviors or improving prosodic naturalness are clearly legitimate objectives, most clinicians agree that the primary goal of dysarthric speech therapy is to acheive a level of speech intelligibility that may be used for functional communicative purposes (which may vary depending upon the specific needs and impairment severity of the individual patient). Assuming that physiological support has been enhanced through medical and/or behavioral interventions to an appropriate degree, it is crucial to assist the patient to make more optimal use of this available residual support when talking. This involves direct work on naturalistic connected speech production (ie, words, phrases, sentences, and discourses) wherein respiratory, phonatory, resonatory, articulatory, and prosodic processes are integrated with each other and with linguistic, pragmatic, and emotional demands of communicative situations. Such work follows as a logical outgrowth of physical exercise programs that have incorporated speechlike stimuli of increasing complexity within their later stages (eg, see Murry, 1983).

In contrast to the physical exercise approaches, there now exists a published database of small sample studies of compensatory strategies for directly addressing the intelligibility of AD speech. All of these studies have emphasized the manipulation of prosodic variables, especially speaking rate, as the preferred compensatory strategy for improving intelligibility (Berry & Goshorn, 1983; Calliguri & Murry, 1983; Garcia & Dongili, 1985; Simmons, 1983; Yorkston & Beukelman, 1981a; Yorkston, Hammen, Beukelman, & Traynor, 1990). Slowing of the speaking rate may, at first glance, seem counterintuitive as a treatment for AD: these patients are already using habitual rates that are markedly slower than average values reported for normal adult speakers (see Johnson, 1961). However, attempts to increase speaking rate in AD subjects have resulted in markedly increased errors which negatively impact intelligibility (Gentil, 1990; Yorkston & Beukelman, 1981; Yorkston et al, 1984). In contrast, slowing of the speaking rate is known to enhance the intelligibillity of normal speech under degraded listening conditions. For example, Picheney, Durlach, & Braida (1985, 1986) have demonstrated that speaking rates as slow as 91 words per minute, produced with clear articulation by normal speakers, significantly improved receptive intelligibility test results of hearing-impaired listeners in comparison with casually articulated speech at conversational rates. A variety of clinical techniques have been employed to control rate in the treatment of AD. For example, Rosenbek and LaPointe (1985) suggest that

delayed auditory feedback may enhance articulation time, articulation adequacy, and prosody for some patients with AD. They indicate that delay intervals of 50 msec have been the most beneficial.

Berry and Goshorn (1983) employed immediate visual feedback to enhance sentence production in a 60-year-old male patient with AD secondary to multiple cerebrovascular accidents. The patient was judged to be "overdriving" the speech mechanism by speaking too loudly and too rapidly. A four-channel storage oscilloscope provided a clinician model, an intensity target line, and a visual representation of the patient's own productions. Treatment was initiated wherein the patient was instructed to maintain intensity below the target line and fill up more than half the screen during the production of sentences. Sentence productions recorded before and after treatment, and at follow-up, were presented to 12 normal listeners in the presence of noise to evaluate intelligibility. Overall sentence intelligibility improved from pre- to posttreatment, from approximately 67 to 85% but declined to about 77% at follow-up. All three time intervals differed significantly from each other. Temporal acoustic measurements were obtained from oscillographic tracings for overall sentence duration, key word duration, and total pause time. For all three measures, there was a significant increase in duration from pre- to posttreatment, and a slight decrease in duration from posttreatment to follow-up. The durations at the follow-up recording session remained significantly longer than at pretreatment.

Garcia and Dongili (1985) presented intelligibility data for short-term results of treatment of two AD patients using traditional, noninstrumented therapy techniques. The first patient was a 73-year-old female with cerebellar dysfunction secondary to meningitis. Her treatment employed the use of slow rate via "syllable timed speech" with continuous phonation, and establishing appropriate stress patterns for polysyllabic words. Intelligibility was evaluated prior to and at 2 weeks following the onset of treatment by administering the Assessment of Intelligibility of Dysarthric Speech to two listeners. Although sentence intelligibility for this patient remained stable at about the 50% level before and after treatment, single-word intelligibility had increased from 31 to 70%. The second patient was an 84-year-old male with cerebellar dysfunction secondary to viral encephalitis. After 3 weeks of sentence level drills contrasting overall loudness levels, pitch and stress patterns, his single-word intelligibility increased from 68 to 89% while sentence intelligibility increased from 70 to 95%.

Yorkston and Beukelman (1981) provide long-term treatment data on four AD subjects who experienced ataxia secondary to acute nondegenerative etiologies. Each patient received a comprehensive treatment program consisting of rate control, development of self monitoring skills, specific "point-place" assessment and treatment, and maximization of normal prosody. Rate control strategies included (1) the rigid imposition of rate using a manual pacing board or by pointing to the first letter of each word on an alphabet board; (2) rhythmic cueing by the clinician, who pointed to printed words for time intervals approximating normal speech rhythms; and (3) oscilloscopic feedback in the form of intensity tracings over time. All four patients were using habitual rates too rapid for their residual capabilities, and the optimum rate for enhancing intelligibility was initially established at about 60–65 words per minute. Self-monitoring skills were emphasized to enable the patient to generalize the slower speaking rate to nonclinical situations and to habituate the slower speaking rate. Point-place assessment and treatment was used as needed to address idiosyncratic difficulties such as context-specific vowel distortions in individual patients. Maximizing normal prosody involved the use of sentence level contrastive stress drills to increase intelligibility and reduce bizarreness. This was accomplished by increasing the duration of stressed syllables while reducing extreme loudness peaks and fundamental frequency shifts. All four sub-

jects improved dramatically from pre- to posttreatment measures of intelligibility, with a pretreatment mean of 18.5 percent and a posttreatment mean of 90.75. However, only one subject was able to eventually achieve a speaking rate approximating the pretreatment value of 132 words per minute. The others continued to use extremely slow rates, of 60–74 words per minute.

Yorkston et al (1990) described the influence of computer-implemented rate control strategies on the intelligibility and naturalness of ataxic and hypokinetic dysarthric speech. Four dysarthric patients of each type were examined under four experimental rate conditions: (1) additive metered, in which one word at a time was added using equal durations for each word; (2) additive rhythmic, in which one word at a time was added with word durations approximating the patterns of normal speech; (3) cued metered, in which the entire passage was presented and each word successively underlined for equal durations; and (4) cued rhythmic, in which the entire passage was presented and each word underlined for durations approximating normal speech. These conditions were presented to each subject at 100%, 80%, and 60% of the speaker's habitual rate. For both dysarthric subgroups, intelligibility increased as speaking rate decreased. The AD patients' sentence intelligibility improved from a mean 40.9% at their habitual rates to a mean of 73.7% at 60% of the habitual rate. The additive conditions were more beneficial than the cued, and the metered conditions were more beneficial than the rhythmic (ie, cued rhythmic was the least effective strategy). Although the results were impressive, it should be recognized that this was a single-shot experiment rather than an ongoing treatment efficacy study. A commercial software program replicating in part the pacing conditions used in this experiment is available for clincal application (Beukelman, Yorkston, & Tice, 1988).

Naturalness
Yorkston et al (1990) also reported that both of their dysarthric subgroups sounded quite

unnatural. The average naturalness rating for habitual rate of the AD group was 3 of 7 scale values below normal. Differences in naturalness ratings between speaking rates and pacing conditions were negligible. These findings are consistent with the lack of relationship between naturalness speaking rate reported by Linebaugh and Wolfe (1984). Yorkston et al (1990) concluded:

> Presumably dysarthric speech is already so unnatural that changing rate did not have a further detrimental effect. In the clinical setting a slight reduction in speech naturalness may be an acceptable price to pay for a substantial improvement in intelligibility (p 558).

Some clinical research data have addressed prosodic naturalness in AD. Based on a perceptual-acoustic assessment protocol, Yorkston et al (1984) recommended a decision algorithm for implementing prosodic treatment: (1) Does the patient know where the stress should be located? (If not, train stress locus recognition); (2) Does the patient adequately mark primary stress on target syllables? (If not, identify and train strategies that can be reliably employed); (3) Do the strategies contribute to the naturalness of speech? (If not, train to modify bizarre-sounding strategies); (4) Establish strategies that enhance naturalness in all speaking situations.

Simmons (1983) reported results of a year-long prosodic treatment program for a 26-year-old male closed head injury patient who exhibited severe ataxia, with primary speech characteristic of excess and equal stress, slowed rate, monoloudness, and monopitch. Prior therapy had enabled him to slow his rate and avoid slurring words; however, he complained of sounding "computerlike." A four-phase treatment program was initiated that consisted of the following sequence: (1) training loudness and pitch variation; (2) altering word and sentence stress patterns by (a) inserting pauses prior to stressed units, (b) shortening unstressed syllables, and (c) decreasing loudness on unstressed syllables; (3) shortening syllable durations overall,

while maintaining stress patterns; (4) improving naturalness by (a) decreasing exaggerated pitch and loudness variations, (b) reducing the clipped and choppy quality caused by shortening words, and (c) smoothing out transitions between words. Ninety percent accuracy as judged by the clinician was the criterion for completion of each phase.

Spectrographic analysis of the first sentence of a standard reading passage was employed to monitor the ongoing effects of treatment. At the initial baseline, spectrographic measurements confirmed that there was a flat fundamental frequency with relatively equal syllable durations and little variation in pause time, in addition to an overall slow rate of production (ie, 136% of normal). Recalling that the patient was achieving target treatment goals by the completion of each phase, the resultant durational changes proved quite interesting. Following phase 1, the patients speech became markedly slower than at baseline (ie, 203% of normal), presumably because more time was needed to make necessary changes in pitch and loudness. At completion of phase 2, speech was even more prolonged (ie, 231% of normal). After stage 3, however, which targeted shortening duration, speech became less prolonged (ie, 187% of normal). By the completion of the phase 4 it became even shorter, approaching pretreatment values (ie, 144% of normal). The spectrograms also demonstrated that the patient had achieved a more normal distribution of syllable and pause durations. This study demonstrated that the patient's prosody became worse in treatment before it became better. While this study does provide limited support for the potential efficacy of prosodic treatment in AD, the actual extent of improvement is difficult to evaluate in the absence of quantified perceptual judgments.

A perceptual study of prosodic treatment in AD has been provided by Calliguri and Murry (1983), who presented immediate visual feedback to enhance prosodic control in two patients with AD. One patient was a 59-year-old male who exhibited AD secondary to cerebellar infarct, the other a 61-year-old male with a mixed dysarthria in which AD predominated secondary to multiple sclerosis. A storage oscilloscope was employed to provide a clinician model and visual feedback about word duration, vocal intensity, and intraoral air pressure associated with target stress. Speech production tasks progressed systematically from CV nonsense syllables through increasing levels of length and complexity to sentences varying with pragmatic intent. Contrastive stress techniques were employed at various stages. The 15-week treatment sequence involved an intensive visual feedback phase, a treatment withdrawal phase, and a no-visual-feedback treatment phase. Pre- to posttreatment changes in overall prosodic functioning in connected speech were evaluated by two reliable normal listeners using the perceptual method of paired comparison. The cerebellar infarct patient demonstrated 100% improvement in prosody following the visual feedback phase, but declined to 50% following the no-visual-feedback phases. The multiple sclerosis patient demonstrated 100% improvement following both the visual feedback and no-visual-feedback phases. Ratings of accuracy of word stress were found to improve following both treatment phases in the cerebellar infarct patient, and were associated with increased duration. The multiple sclerosis patient improved on word stress ratings, associated with pitch and intensity changes, only following the no-visual-feedback condition.

Augmentative Considerations

In most forms of ataxia there is the capability of movement with at least a crude degree of accuracy, providing an opportunity for the use of devices using manual activation or pointing. The unique coordination problems of the ataxic patient, including dysmetria, directional errors, and the terminal crescendos of intention tremor, pose special challenges for the patient and clinician working in the augmentative domain. Pharmaceutical intervention with physiosigmine or ionazide may help improve limb ataxia or intention tremor in some patients with degenerative illnesses (Kark et al, 1981; Sabra et al, 1982). Weighting of the limbs with heavy wristbands may also significantly reduce limb intention tremor in some patients for tasks involving pointing, and even drawing and writing (Hewer, Cooper, & Morgan, 1972). Increasing surface areas of manually activated switches and target surface areas on pointing boards may help to compensate for past pointing and corrective oscillating movement problems. Fortunately, not all patients with AD have co-occurring limb disorders, and many of those who do have them only in one extremity. Examination of incidence data reported by Gilman et al (1981) suggests that for patients with focal cerebellar lesions there is a better than 85% chance that at least one extremity will be spared and, due to the left-hemispheric lateralization of AD- producing lesions, that one will usually be dominant. In addition, in some cases of degenerative illness the upper extremities deteriorate more slowly and to a lesser extent than the lower extremities (Gilman et al, 1981). Preservation of upper- extremity function may provide an important communicative modality for AD patients with moderate to severe degrees of unintelligibility, for whom nonspeech augmentation may be employed as a strategy to facilitate better speech production and better listener comprehension. Intersystemic reorganization of speech either through manual pacing or gestures can be a viable treatment option for some dysarthric patients (Rosenbek, 1984). The use of "top-down," or knowledge-driven, strategies to provide listeners with supportive information may also enhance comprehension of dysarthric speech (Vogel & Miller, 1991). Such techniques include providing for the listener the initial letters of intended word productions by pointing to an alphabet board (Beukelman & Yorkston, 1977). Some strategies may accomplish both goals simultaneously. Crow and Enderby (1989) demonstrated that the use of an alphabet board that wasn't visible to listeners significantly improved the intelligibility of an AD pa-

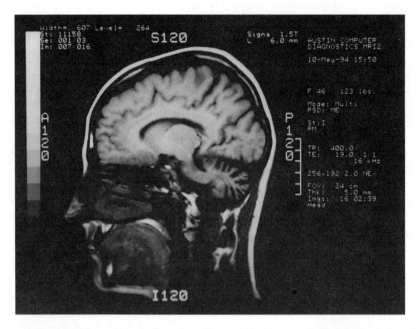

Figure 10–1. MRI scan of sagittal section demonstrating atrophy of the right cerebellar hemisphere in an individual with ataxic dysarthria.

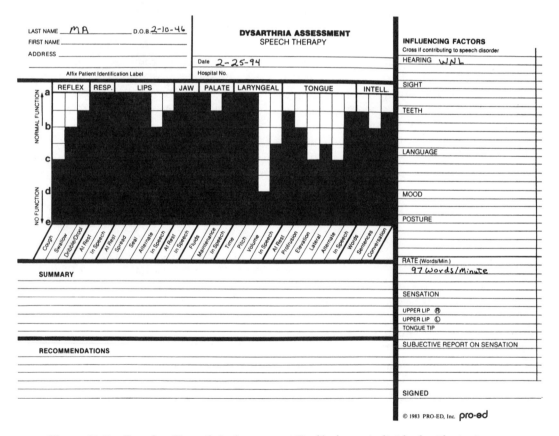

Figure 10–2. Frenchay Dysarthria Assessment Profile for an individual with ataxic dysarthria.

tient's speech, apart from any "top-down" facilitation it may have provided.

Case Study

An illustrative case study may be helpful in elucidating characteristics of ataxic dysarthria. The subject is a 49 year old woman with a 9 year history of cerebellar degeneration with progressive weakness and incoordination. CT scan at diagnosis in 1985 revealed diffuse cerebellar atrophy with a small hyperdense lesion in the right cerebellar hemisphere. A repeat CT scan in 1988 showed an increase in the lesion size. When referred in 1994, the neurological examination reported slowed movement, muscle weakness, slurred speech, an equivocal Babinski reflex, weak eye muscles, and problems with coordination and balance. Ambulation was characterized by a shuffling gate. An MRI scan was completed that included saggital T1 weighted images followed by

transaxial proton density and T2 weighted fast spin echo images. A coronal MPGR sequence was then performed followed by a post Gadolinium T1 weighted sequence. The scan sequence revealed a severe atrophy of the cerebellum (Fig. 10–1) that affected both hemispheres as well as the vermis. The pons and medullary olives were normal in size and signal intensity. The basal ganglia, tegmentum and long tracts demonstrated normal signal intensity, the cerebrum was unremarkable in appearance, the ventricles were normal, and no midline shift or mass effect could be observed. Skull base, orbits, and sinuses also were unremarkable. The scan summary suggested a severe cerebellar atrophy with otherwise normal findings.

During the case history interview, speech was slow and scanning. Vocal quality was moderately breathy with reduced loudness and pitch variation. Breathiness and pitch breaks were particularly apparent at the end of longer phrases. The speech and language

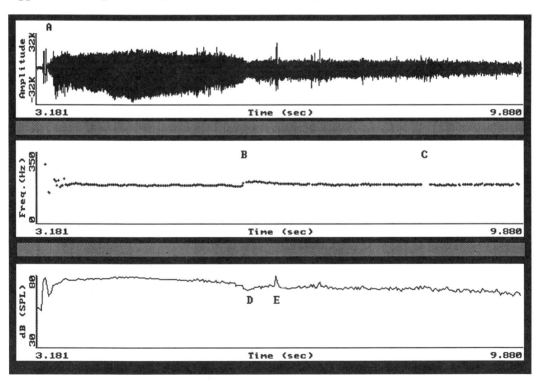

Figure 10–3. Acoustic analysis of sustained vowel /a/ produced by an individual with ataxic dysarthria. Upper view, acoustic waveform; middle view, pitch track; lower view, intensity track. See text for explanation of labels A-E.

241

evaluation included administration of the Frenchay dysarthria assessment (Enderby, 1983), an oral-peripheral examination of the speech mechanism, and audio-tape recording of the Rainbow Passage. The dysarthria profile from the Frenchay Assessment is shown in Figure 10–2. Primary areas of reduced performance were in oral pharyngeal reflexes, tongue movement, and intensity variation. Speech intelligibility was approximately 100% in single words and 95% in sentences. Reading rate was reduced to 97 words per minute.

The subject reported mild dysphagia, which was subsequently evaluated. The evaluation found decreased speed of oral structural movement for speech, eating, and drinking. Swallowing appeared within functional limits, but was significant for increased oral preparation time, decreased coordination, and multiple swallows per bolus. Auditory acuity was within normal limits bilaterally.

Diadochokinesis for monosyllables and syllable sequences was slow and irregular. With encouragement by the examining clinician, the patient was able to increase diadochokinetic rate; however, this resulted in marked deterioration of articulatory accuracy. Maximally sustained vowels exhibited reduced duration of approximately 7 to 8 seconds. Figure 10–3 provides an example of one of the patient's sustained vowels. In addition to reduced duration, other abnormal characteristics are evident. These include: (A) hard attack pattern of phonatory initiation observable in the waveform (upper view) which is associated with random occurrence of fundamental periods at voice onset in the pitch track (middle view), and an abrupt burst of intensity at onset in the intensity track (lower view). These phenomena

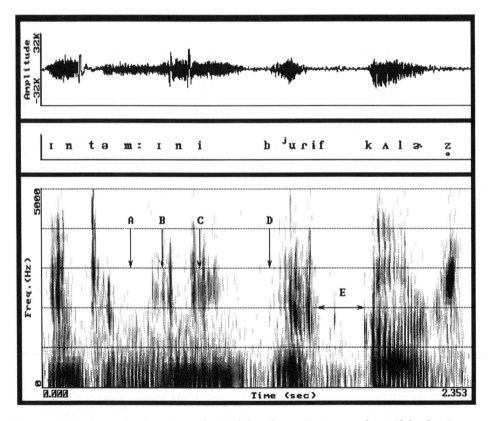

Figure 10–4. Acoustic phonetic analysis of the phrase "into many beautiful colors" produced by an individual with ataxic dysarthria. Upper view, acoustic waveform; middle view, IPA transcription; lower view, spectrogram. See text for explanation of labels A-E.

242

may reflect glottal dysmetria or overshoot of vocal fold adduction. Other acoustic symptoms include (B) an upward pitch break from 186 to 211 hertz occurring from 2.763 to 2.887 seconds into the vowel, as well as (C) an episode of aperiodic phonation which appears as a gap in the pitch track, but is not associated with loss of signal energy in the intensity track. Finally, there is evidence of excess loudness variation (D and E) in which there is a downward deflection (D) from 75.45 dB to 71.01 dB approximately timed to the pitch break (B), followed by an excessive burst of loudness (E) at 3.203 seconds into the vowel that reaches 80.9 dB. Pitch breaks and excess loudness variation may reflect respiratory and phonatory instability and incoordination. Collectively, these phenomena lend an impression of harshness to the patient's sustained phonation.

A sample of speech from the Rainbow Passage is shown in Figure 10–4. This reading of the phrase "into many beautiful colors" exhibited several acoustic features of AD which have been identified in the spectrogram (lower view). These include a slow rate of 3.40 syllables per second, reflected by (A) prolonged segment duration of /m:/ of 203 milliseconds and a prolonged between word interval (E) of 250 milliseconds. Equalization of syllable stress is exhibited in the word "many" in which there was a reversal of expected duration relationships for the stressed and unstressed vowels. The normally stressed vowel /ɪ/ was 134 milliseconds duration in comparison to the normally unstressed vowel /i/ which was prolonged to 295 milliseconds in duration. Irregular articulatory breakdowns occurred on the word "beautiful" in the form of (D) a weak pressure consonant /b/ and reduction of the unstressed syllable /fʊl/ to /f/ just prior to the prolonged interval (E). Increased breathiness is also in evidence throughout the phrase.

Conclusion

This chapter has described the neuromotor mechanisms and etiologies underlying AD,

and reviewed available literature pertaining to its characteristics and their remediation. While substantial progress has occurred, there remain important questions facing speech clinicians working with these patients: Are there different AD subtypes stemming from differential subsystem impairments? Can hypotonia be ameliorated through exercise programs to enhance the physiological support for speech? Does such enhancement influence intelligibility or naturalness of AD speech? What long-term strategies for rate control are most effective, and what factors govern the ability to eventually increase speaking rate toward a more naturalistic level? How much practical benefit may be ultimately derived from treatments focused on prosodic naturalness and augmentative facilitation? It is hoped that the synthesis presented here will stimulate further research in these areas to improve the outlook for patients with AD.

References

Abbs J, Hunker C, Barlow S. (1983). Differential speech motor subsystem impairments with suprabulbar lesions: Neurophysiological framework and supporting data. In: Berry W, ed. *Clinical Dysarthria*. San Diego: College-Hill Press, pp 21–56.

Abbs J, Barlow S, Cole K. (1979). Impairments of rapid muscle contraction as a physiologic feature of ataxic dysarthria. Presented to the American Speech-Language-Hearing Association, San Francisco.

Ackermann H, Hertrich I. (1993). Dysarthria in Friedreich's ataxia: Timing of speech segments. *Clin Linguist Phonet* 7:75–91.

Alexander GE, Delong MR. (1986). In: Ansbury AK, McKhann GM, McDonald WI, eds. *Diseases of the Nervous System: Clinical Neurobiology*. Philadelphia: W.B. Saunders, pp 352–369.

Beppu H, Suda M, Tanaka R. (1983). Slow visuomotor tracking in normal man and in patients with cerebellar ataxia. In: Desmedt JE, ed. *Motor Control Mechanisms in Health and Disease*. New York: Raven Press, pp 889–895.

Berry WR, Goshorn EL. (1983). Immediate visual feedback in the treatment of ataxic dysarthria:

A case study. In: Berry WR, ed. *Clinical Dysarthria.* San Diego: College-Hill Press, pp 253–265.

Beukelman D, Yorkston K. (1977). A communication system for the severely dysarthric speaker with an intact language system. *J Speech Hear Disord* 42:265–270.

Beukelman D, Yorkston K, Tice R. (1988). *Pacer/Tally.* Tuscon: Communication Skill Builders.

Bowman JP. (1971). *The Muscle Spindle and Neural Control of the Tongue: Implications for Speech.* Springfield, IL: Charles Thomas.

Brooks VB, Thach WT. (1981). Cerebellar control of posture and movement. In: Brooks VB, ed. *Handbook of Physiology, Section 1: Neurophysiology,* Vol. 2: Motor Control, Part 2. Bethesda: American Physiological Society.

Brown J, Darley F, Aronson A. (1970). Ataxic dysarthria. *Int J Neurol* 7:302–318.

Caliguri M, Murry T. (1983). The use of visual feedback to enhance prosodic control in dysarthria. In Berry W, ed. *Clinical Dysarthria.* San Diego: College-Hill Press, pp 267–282.

Charcot JM. (1877). *Lectures on the Diseases of the Nervous System* (Vol. 1). London: New Sydenham Society.

Crow E, Enderby P. (1989). The effects of an alphabet chart on the speaking rate and intelligibility of speakers with dysarthria. In: Yorkston KM, Beukelman DR, eds. *Recent Advances in Clinical Dysarthria.* Boston: College-Hill, pp 99–107.

Darley F, Aronson A, Brown J. (1969a). Differential diagnostic patterns of dysarthria. *J Speech Hear Res* 12:246–269.

Darley F, Aronson A, Brown J. (1969b). Clusters of deviant speech dimensions in the dysarthrias. *J Speech Hear Res* 12:462–496.

Darley F, Brown J, Goldstein N. (1972). Dysarthria in multiple sclerosis. *J Speech Hear Res* 15:229–245.

Darley F, Aronson A, Brown J. (1975). *Motor Speech Disorders.* Philadelphia: Saunders.

Dichgans J, Diener HC. (1984). Clinical evidence for functional compartmentalization of the cerebellum. In: Bloedel JR, Dichgans J, Precht W, eds. *Cerebellar Functions.* Berlin: Springer-Verlag, pp 126–147.

Dworkin JP. (1991). *Motor Speech Disorders: A Treatment Guide.* St. Louis: Mosby Year Book.

Dworkin JP, Aronson AE. (1986). Tongue strength and alternate motion rates in normal and dysarthric subjects. *J Commun Disord* 19:115–132.

Eccles J. (1977). Cerebellar function in the control of movement (with special reference to the pioneer work of Sir Gordon Holmes). In: Rose FC, ed. *Physiological Aspects of Clinical Neurology.* Oxford: Blackwell, pp 157–178.

Edwards M. (1984). *Disorders of Articulation.* Vienna: Springer-Verlag.

Enderby PM. (1983). *Frenchay Dysarthria Assessment.* Austin: PRO-ED.

Farmikides M, Boone D. (1960). Speech problems in patients with multiple sclerosis. *J Speech Hear Disord* 25:385–390.

Forest K, Adams S, McNeil M, Southwood H. (1991). Kinematic, electromyographic, and perceptual evaluation of speech apraxia, conduction aphasia, ataxic dysarthria, and normal speech production. In: Moore, C, Yorkston K, eds. *Dysarthria and Apraxia of Speech: Perspectives on Management.* Baltimore: Paul. H. Brookes.

French LA, Chou SN, Long DM, Seljeskog EL. (1970). Clinical management of cerebellar neoplasms. In: Fields WS, Willis WD, eds. *The Cerebellum in Health and Disease.* St. Louis: Warren H. Green, pp 502–518.

Garcia J, Dongilli P. (1985). Ataxic dysarthria: Case study reviews of treatment strategies. Presented to the American Speech-Language-Hearing Association: Washington, DC.

Gentil M. (1990a). EMG analysis of speech production of patients with Friedreich disease. *Clin Linguist Phonet* 4:107–120.

Gentil M. (1990b). Dysarthria in Friedreich disease. *Brain Language* 38:438–448.

Gilman S. (1986). Cerebellum and motor dysfunction. In: Asbury AK, McKhann, McDonald WI, eds. *Diseases of the Nervous System: Clinical Neurobiology.* Philadelphia: W.B. Saunders, pp 402–422.

Gilman S, Bloedel JR, Lechtenberg R. (1981). *Disorders of the Cerebellum.* Philadelphia: F.A. Davis Company.

Gilman S, Kluin K. (1984). Perceptual analysis of speech disorders in Friedreich disease and olivopontocerebellar atrophy. In: Bloedel JR, Dichigans J, Precht W, eds. *Cerebellar Functions.* Berlin: Springer Verlag, pp 148–163.

Gilman S, Kluin K. (1992). Speech disorders in cerebellar degeneration studied with positron emission tomography. In: Blitzer A, Brin MF, Sasaki CT, Fahn S, Harris KS, eds. *Neurologic Disorders of the Larynx.* New York: Thieme Medical Publishers, pp 279–285.

Granit R. (1977). Reconsidering the 'alpha-gamma switch' in cerebellar action. In: Rose FC, ed. *Physiological Aspects of Clinical Neurology*. Oxford: Blackwell, pp 201–213.

Grunwell P, Huskins S. (1979). Intelligibility in aquired dysarthria—A neuro-phonetic approach: Three case studies. *J Commun Disord* 12:9–22.

Haggard M. (1969). Speech waveform measurements in multiple sclerosis. *Folia Phoniatr* 21:307–312.

Hallett M, Shahani B, Young RR. (1975). EMG analysis of patients with cerebellar deficits. *J Neurol Neurosurg Psychiatry* 38:1163–1169.

Hewer RL, Cooper R, Morgan MH. (1972). An investigation into the value of treating intention tremor by weighting the affected limb. *Brain* 95:579–590.

Hiller F. (1929). A study of speech disorders in Friedreich's ataxia. *Arch Neurol Psychiatry* 2:75–90.

Hirose H, Kiritani S, Tatsujiro U, Sawashima M. (1978). Analysis of abnormal articulatory dynamics in two dysarthric patients. *J Speech Hear Res* 43:96–105.

Holmes G. (1917). The symptoms of acute cerebellar injuries due to gunshot injuries. *Brain* 40:461–535.

Holmes G. (1939). The cerebellum of man. *Brain* 62:1–30.

Ito M. (1984). *The Cerebellum and Neural Control*. New York: Raven Press.

Jankovic J, Fahn S. (1980). Physiologic and pathologic tremors. *Ann Intern Med* 93:460–465.

Janvrin F, Worster-Drought C. (1932). Diagnosis of disseminated sclerosis by graphic registration and film tracks. *Lancet* 2:1384.

Janvrin R. (1933). Diagnosis of a nervous disease by sound tracks. *Nature* 132:642.

Joanette Y, Dudley J. (1980). Dysarthric symtomatology of Friedreich's ataxia. *Brain Language* 10:39–50.

Johnson W. (1961). Measurements of oral reading and speaking rate and disfluency of adult male and female stutterers and nonstutterers. *J Speech Hear Disord* 7:(Monograph suppl):1–20.

Kark R, Budelli M, Wachsner R. (1981). Double-blind, triple-crossover trial of low doses of oral physostigmine in inherited ataxias. *Neurology* 31:288–292.

Keller E. (1990). Speech motor timing. In: Hardcastle WJ, Marchal A, eds. *Speech Pro-*

duction and Speech Modeling. Dordrecht: Kluwer.

Kent R, Netsell R. (1975). A case study of an ataxic dysarthric: Cineradiographic and spectrographic observations. *J Speech Hear Disord* 40:115–134.

Kent R, Netsell R, Abbs J. (1979). Acoustic characteristics of dysarthria associated with cerebellar disease. *J Speech Hear Res* 22:627–648.

Kent R, Netsell R, Bauer L. (1975). Cineradiographic assessment of articulatory mobility in dysarthrias. *J Speech Hear Disord* 40:467–480.

Kent R, Rosenbek J. (1979). Prosodic disturbance and neurologic lesion. *Brain Language* 15:259–291.

Kornhuber H. (1975). Cerebral cortex, cerebellum, and basal ganglia: An introduction to their functions. In Evarts E, ed. *Central Processing*. Cambridge: M.I.T. Press, pp 267–280.

Lam RL, Ogura (1952). An afferent representation of the larynx in the cerebellum. *Laryngoscope* 62:486–495.

Lechtenberg R, Gilman S. (1978). Speech disorders in cerebellar disease. *Ann Neurol* 3:285–290.

Leiner HC, Leiner AL, Dow RS. (1991). The human cerebro-cerebellar system: Its computing, cognitive, and language skills. *Behav Brain Res* 44:113–128.

Linebaugh C, Wolfe V. (1984). Relationships between articulation rate, intelligibility, and naturalness in spastic and ataxic speakers. In: McNeil M, Rosenbek J, Aronson A, eds. *The Dysarthrias*. San Diego: College-Hill Press.

Marsden CD, Merton PA, Morton HB, Hallett M, Adam J, Rushton DN. (1977). Disorders of movement in cerebellar disease in man. In: Rose FC, ed. *Physiological aspects of clinical neurology*. Oxford: Blackwell, pp 179–199.

McNeil MR, Adams S. (1990). A comparison of speech kinematics among apraxic, conduction aphasic, ataxic dysarthric, and normal geriatric speakers. In: Prescott T, ed. *Clinical Aphasiology* (Vol. 19). Austin: PRO-ED, pp. 279–293.

McNeil M, Weismer G, Adams S, Mulligan M. (1990). Oral structure nonspeech motor control in normal, dysarthric, aphasic, and apraxic speakers: Isometric force and static position control. *J Speech Hear Res* 33:255–268.

Mills CK, Weisenburg TH. (1914). Cerebellar symptoms and cerebellar localization. *JAMA* 63:1813–1818.

Mortimer JA. (1975). Cerebellar responses to teleceptive stimuli in alert monkeys. *Brain Res* 83:369–390.

Murdoch B, Chenery H, Stokes P, Hardcastle W. (1991). Respiratory kinematics in speakers with cerebellar disease. *J Speech Hear Res* 34:768–780.

Murry T. (1983). The production of stress in three types of dysarthric speech. In: Berry W, ed. *Clinical Dysarthria*. San Diego: College-Hill Press, pp 69–83.

Murry T. (1983). Treatment of ataxic dysarthria. In: Perkins W, ed. *Current Therapy of Communication Disorders—Dysarthria and Apraxia*. New York: Thieme-Stratton, pp 79–89.

Netsell R. (1973). Kinesiology studies of the dysarthrias. Unpublished paper, Speech Research Laboratory, University of Wisconsin, Madison.

Netsell R. (1986). *A Neurobiologic View of Speech Production and the Dysarthrias*. San Diego: College-Hill Press.

Netsell R. (1982). Speech motor control and selected neurologic disorders. In: Grillner S, Lindblom B, Lubker J, Persson A, eds. *Speech Motor Control*. New York: Pergamon Press, pp. 247–261.

Netsell R, Abbs J. (1977). Some possible uses of neuromotor speech disturbances in understanding normal mechanism. In: Sawashima M, Cooper FS, eds. *Dynamic Aspects of Speech Production: Current Results, Emerging Problems, and New Instrumentation: Proceedings*. Tokyo: University of Tokyo Press, pp 369–398.

Netsell R, Daniel B. (1979). Dysarthria in adults: Physiologic approach to rehabilitation. *Arch Physical Med Rehabil* 60:502–508.

Netsel R, Kent R. (1976). Paroxymal ataxic dysarthria. *J Speech Hear Disord* 41:93–109.

Odell K, McNeil M, Rosenbek J, Hunter L. (1991). Perceptual characteristics of vowel and prosody production in apraxic, aphasic, and dysarthric speakers. *J Speech Hear Res* 34:67–80.

Ouellon M, Ryalls J, Lebeuf J, Joanette Y. (1991). Le "Voice Onset Time" chez des dysarthriques de Friedreich. *Folia Phonatr* 43:295–303.

Peterson SE, Fox PT, Posner MI, Mintun M, Raichle ME. (1989). Positron emission tomographic studies of the processing of single words. *J Cogn Neurosci* 1:153–170.

Picheny MA, Durlach NI, Braida .D. (1985). Speaking clearly for the hard of hearing I: Intelligibility differences between clear and conversational speech. *J Speech Hear Res* 28:96–103.

Picheny MA, Durlach NI, Braida LD. (1986). Speaking clearly for the hard of hearing II: Acoustic characteristics of clear and conversational speech. *J Speech Hear Res* 29:434–446.

Portnoy R, Aronson A. (1982). Diadochokinetic syllable rate and regularity in normal and in spastic and ataxic dysarthric subjects. *J Speech Hear Disord* 47:324–328.

Robin DA, Klouda GV, Hug LN. (1991). Neurogenic disorders of prosody. In: Vogel D, Cannito MP, eds. *Treating Disordered Speech Motor Control for Clinicians by Clinicians*. Austin: PRO-ED, pp 241–271.

Rondot R, Jedynak CP, Ferrey G. (1978). Pathological tremors: Nosological correlates. *Prog Clin Neurophysiol* 5:95–113.

Rosenbek J. (1984). Selected alternatives to articulation training for the dysarthric adult. In: Winitz H, ed. *Treating Articulation Disorders for Clinicians by Clinicians*. Austin: PRO-ED, pp 249–262.

Rosenbek JC, LaPointe LL. (1985). The dysarthrias: Description, diagnosis and treatment. In: Johns DF, ed. *Clinical Management of Neurogenic Communication Disorders*. Boston: Little, Brown, pp. 97–152.

Rubow R. (1984). A clinical guide to the technology of treatment in dysarthria. *Semin Speech Language* 5:315–335.

Rubow R. (1984). Role of feedback, reinforcement, and compliance on training and transfer in biofeedback-based rehabilitation of motor speech disorders. In: McNeil MR, Rosenbek JC, Aronson AE, eds. *The Dysarthrias: Physiology, Acoustics, Perception, Management*. San Diego: College-Hill Press, pp 207–229.

Sabra AF, Hallett M, Sudarsky L, Mullally W. (1982). Treatment of action tremor in multiple sclerosis with isoniazid. *Neurology* 32:912–913.

Sasaki K. (1984). Cerebro-cerebellar interactions and organization of a fast and stable hand movement: Cerebellar participation in voluntary movement and motor learning. In: Bloedel JR, Dichigans J, Precht W, eds. *Cerebellar Functions*. Berlin: Springer-Verlag, pp 70–85.

Schell GR, Strick PL. (1984). The origin of thalamic inputs to the arcuate premotor and supplementary motor areas. *J Neurosci* 4:539.

Scripture WE. (1916). Records of speech in disseminated sclerosis. *Brain* 39:455–477.

Scripture WE. (1933). Diagnosis by sound tract. *Nature* 132:821–822.

Simmons N. (1983). Acoustic analysis of ataxic dysarthria: An approach to monitoring treatment. In: Berry W, ed. *Clinical Dysarthria.* San Diego: College-Hill Press, pp 283–294.

Thach WT. (1975). Timing of activity in cerebellar dentate nucleus and cerebral motor cortex during prompt volitional movement. *Brain Res* 88:233–241.

Thach WT. (1978). Correlation of neural discharge with pattern and force of muscular activity, joint position, and direction of the intended next movement in motor cortex and cerebellum. *J Neurophysiol* 4:654–676.

Thach WT. (1980). The cerebellum. In: Mountcastle VB, ed. *Medical Physiology,* Vol. I. St. Louis: C.V. Mosby, pp 722–746.

Victor M, Ferrendelli JA. (1970). The nutritional and metabolic diseases of the cerebellum. Clinical and pathological aspects. In: Fields SW, Willis WD, eds. *The Cerebellum in Health and Disease.* St. Louis: Warren H. Green, pp 412–449.

Vilis T, Hore J. (1981). Characteristics of saccadic dysmetria in monkeys during reversible lesions of medial cerebellar nuclei. *J Neurophysiol* 46:82–838.

Vogel D, Miller L. (1991). A top-down approach to treatment of dysarthric speech. In: Vogel D, Cannito MP, eds. *Treating Disordered Speech Motor Control for Clinicians by Clinicians.* Austin: PRO-ED, pp 87–109.

Watson BC, Alfonso PJ. (1991). Noninvasive instrumentation in the treatment of stuttering. In: Vogel D, Cannito MP, eds. *Treating Disordered Speech Motor Control for Clinicians by Clinicians.* Austin: PRO-ED, pp 319–340.

Yorkston K, Beukelman D. (1981a). *Assessment of Intelligibility of Dysarthric Speech.* Austin: PRO-ED.

Yorkston K, Beukelman D. (1981b). Ataxic dysarthria: Treatment sequences based on intelligibility and prosodic considerations. *J Speech Hear Res* 46:398–404.

Yorkston K, Beukelman D, Minifie F, Sapir S. (1984). Assessment of stress patterning. In: McNeil MR, Rosenbek JC, Aronson AE, eds. *The Dysarthrias: Physiology, Acoustics, Perception, Management.* San Diego: College-Hill Press.

Yorkston K, Hammen V, Beukelman D, Traynor C. (1990). The effect of rate control on the intelligibility and naturalness of dysarthric speech. *J Speech Hear Disord* 55:550–560.

Young AB, Penney JB. (1986). Pharmacologic aspects of motor dysfunction. In: Asbury AK, McKhann GM, McDonald WI, eds. *Diseases of the Nervous System: Clinical Neurobiology,* Vol. 1. Philadelphia: W.B. Saunders.

Zwirner P, Murry T, Woodson G. (1991). Phonatory function of neurologically impaired patients. *J Commun Disord* 24:287–300.

Chapter *11*

Hyperkinetic Dysarthria

Richard I. Zraick and Leonard L. LaPointe

Neither from nor towards;
at the still point there the dance is,
But neither arrest nor movement.
Words strain,
Crack and sometimes break, under the burden,
Under the tension, slip, slide, perish,
Decay with imprecision, will not stay in place,
Will not stay still.
—T.S. Eliot, *Collected Poems*, 1936

Eliot may not have intended it, but he captures aspects of disrupted movement and the subsequent effect of this motion disorder on speech. When the mysterious domain of the extrapyramidal or indirect nervous system exerts its influence on such a complex act as speech, the result can be finely orchestrated and a marvel of coordination; or can be neither from nor towards; with cracks, strains, slips, slides, and imprecision. This chapter delves into this synchrony of movement and speech production, and especially what happens when the fine coordination and regulation exerted by the extrapyramidal system goes awry. The results can take away from movement efficiency, or more dramatically, can add involuntary and bizarre elements that are represented by jerks, tics, tremor, writhing, slow contractions, or stoppages.

The Extrapyramidal System

"Extrapyramidal" began as a wastebasket term and remains ambiguous. Back in the days prior to World War I, in the year that Arizona became a state, the first successful parachute jump was made, and the Titanic sank in the North Atlantic, S.A.K. Wilson, the noted British neurologist, introduced the term "extrapyramidal" motor system and introduced it without specific definition (Wilson, 1912). He included the term in his classic description of hepatolenticular degeneration, a familial disorder of copper metabolism that resulted in its unfortunate victims of liver cirrhosis, "flapping tremor," muscular rigidity, and a golden-brown pigmentation of the cornea (Carpenter, 1985).

While the citizens and boundaries of the so-called extrapyramidal system have been debated and bathed in controversy for generations, there is little doubt that the primary components are those related to the subsystems called the "corpus striatum" and "basal ganglia." In order to carry out motor acts properly, the pyramidal system, which originates in the primary motor strips of the cerebral cortex, needs coordination and cooperation from at least three other sources: the vestibular system (including elements that subserve proprioception); the cerebellar system; and the corpus striatum. While all of these truly are "extra" pyramidal, it is usually the basal ganglia and corpus striatal systems that are meant when the name "extrapyramidal system" is used without further qualification (Gatz, 1966).

Traditional anatomists have included the caudate nucleus, the putamen, the globus pallidus, and sometimes the internal capsule within the striatal system. The basal ganglia include the caudate nucleus, the putamen, the globus pallidus, the amygdala, and the claustrum. Overlap and inconsistency are apparent in most descriptions of the extrapyramidal system, but in all descriptions a rich series of linkages interrelate the nuclei of the basal ganglia and corpus striatum with the thalamus, subthalamic nuclei, and the motor systems of the pyramidal tract and cerebellum.

While the boundaries and names of this important motor system seem to be as unclear and changing as the boundaries of Eastern Europe, there is little doubt that damage to the extrapyramidal system exerts distinctive clinical pictures. Two basic types of disturbances are apparent: (1) a gamut of abnormal involuntary movements, sometimes referred to generally as *dyskinesia*, and (2) disturbances of muscle tone (Carpenter, 1985). Dyskinesia types include tremor, athetosis, chorea, and ballism. Sometimes dystonia is classified as a type of dyskinesia, though dystonia can be comprised of a combination of disturbed involuntary movement as well as disrupted muscle tone. Not all types of extrapyramidal disease result in hyperkinetic dysarthria, and it is apparent to the informed reader that other types of dysarthria (hypokinetic, for example) can result from diseases and conditions that create dyskinesia (Parkinsonism, for example).

Tremor

The most common form of dyskinesia is tremor, usually a rhythmical, alternating, abnormal involuntary activity with a regular frequency and amplitude. Various subtypes of tremor (such as "action tremor" or "tremor at rest") have been described and associated with different disease processes or conditions.

Athetosis

Slow, writhing, serpentine involuntary movements, particularly involving the arms and legs, are referred to as athetosis. Generally, these movements blend with each other in a continual mobile spasm of muscular contraction.

Chorea

Chorea is a brisk, sometimes graceful series of successive involuntary movements. They may be complex and resemble fragments of purposeful voluntary movements. Mostly the distal portions of the extremities are involved (hands and feet), but the muscles of facial expression, the tongue, or the swallowing muscles can be involved. When the tongue is involved, the ticlike choreiform movements can mimic the fly-catching tongue activities of frogs and other reptiles. The disconcerting nature of this type of disorder is immediately apparent when one considers the psychosocial, let alone the speech, ramifications of it.

Ballism

Ballism is a sudden, violent, forceful flinging movement usually involving the upper extremity. It may involve only one side (hemiballism) or it may be bilateral. One author (L.L.L.) is reminded of the evaluation of his first case of motor speech impairment with accompanying hemiballism in a young Vietnam-era veteran who suffered extrapyramidal system disturbance from a shrapnel head wound. In addition to hyperkinetic dysarthria, the veteran presented an occasional hemiballistic flinging of his left arm, one of which caught the examiner alongside the face. Certain adjustments needed to be made in the close quarters of a small clinical examining room during the assessment in order to prevent the unpredictable striking of a file cabinet or further battery of the examiner.

Hyperkinetic Dysarthria

Hyperkinetic dysarthria, like the other types of neuromotor speech disorders, results from disorders of movement; in fact, the derivation of the term is from "hyper" (too much or excessive) and "kinetic" (movement). Most of the movement disorders that create hyperkinetic dysarthria arise from excessive, involuntary, and restrict movement or posture. Hyperkinetic dysarthria is characterized by variable articulatory imprecision, vocal harshness, and prosodic abnormalities. It is associated with damage to the extrapyramidal system, more specifically, lesions in the basal ganglia and their major pathways, which are important in the planning and programming of learned movements.

Movement disorders leading to hyperkinetic dysarthria can be classified into two general groups: (1) quick forms, and (2) slow forms, which describes the speed of the involuntary abnormal movements. Salient features of the "quick" forms are unsustained involuntary movements, slowness of movement, and variable muscle hypertonus; features of the "slow" forms are sustained involuntary movements, slowness of movement, and variable muscle hypertonus. Chorea, myoclonus, and tic disorders are the most common of the quick forms, and athetosis, dyskinesia, and the dystonias commonly constitute the slow forms. Speech profiles of the different patient populations with hyperkinetic dysarthria can be drawn and are presented below.

Quick Forms

Chorea

In the Mayo Clinic Study of 30 adult subjects with chorea (Darley, Aronson, & Brown, 1969), it was reported that all basic motor-speech processes were disturbed. From listener judgments, the five most prominent dysarthric features included imprecise consonants, prolonged intervals, variable speaking rate, monopitch, and harsh voice quality. Of the four general clusters of features that were identified (resonatory incompetence; articulatory incompetence; prosodic insufficiency; and prosodic excess), the prosodic deviations proved to be the most distinctive features. Two common forms of chorea are Sydenham's chorea and Huntington's chorea (Huntington's chorea is now generally labeled Huntington's disease). Sydenham's chorea, which is associated with rheumatic fever, results in choreiform movements such as grimacing, fidgeting, and dropping things (Espir & Rose, 1983). A retrospective study of 240 individuals with Sydenham's chorea (Nausieda, Grossman, Koller, Weiner, & Klawans, 1980) revealed that 39% had dysarthria. Swedo et al (1993) examined 11 children with Sydenham's chorea and found the presence of dysarthria as well as adventitious movements of the face, neck, trunk, and extremities.

Huntington's disease, which has a strong genetic/familial link, is fatal within 10–20 years, and also results in choreiform movements and dementia (Espir & Rose, 1983). Perhaps one of the most notable Americans who had Huntington's disease was the late Woody Guthrie, the songwriter and balladeer.

Zwirner, Murry, and Woodsen (1991) compared the vocal tract steadiness of individuals with Huntington's chorea to that of normal control subjects and found that affected subjects displayed greater fundamental frequency variability and formant frequency variability. Ramig (1986) also studied the acoustic-speech characteristics of subjects with Huntington's chorea and found that during sustained vowel production, abrupt drops in fundamental frequency, adductor and abductor phonatory arrests, and reduced vowel duration were noted. Ramig attributed her findings to the choreiform movements of the laryngeal musculature. Caligiuri and Murry (1984), however, in their acoustic-perceptual study of five individuals with Huntington's chorea found no correlation between limb chorea and the presence or severity of dysarthria, with these findings attributed to generalized pathophysiologic changes associated with basal ganglia disease rather than a manifestation of underlying chorea.

Myoclonus

The soft palate, larynx, and diaphragm may all be affected by the sudden, jolting, unsustained muscle contractions characteristic of myoclonus. Palatal myoclonus, which can occur rhythmically at a rate of 1–4 Hz, may result in temporary hypernasality and articulatory imprecision. Laryngeal myoclonus frequently occurs in combination with palatal myoclonus, and can have the additional effect of temporarily interrupting phonation. Diaphragmatic myoclonus can be detected during sustained phonation, and can result in slight interruptions of airflow. A relationship may exist between palato-pharyngeaolaryngeal myoclonus and essential tremor. The two conditions share a number of perceptual and physical characteristics, including intermittent voice arrests during contextual speech, rhythmical voice arrests during vowel prolongation, movements of the pharynx and larynx beneath the skin, and abnormal adduction/abduction of the vocal folds (Aronson, 1980).

Tic Disorders

Movements or vocalizations that are brief, rapid, stereotyped, and nonpurposeful are defined as tics. They are constant in morphology and location (eyelid blinks, head twitches, shoulder shrugs, grunting) and occur at irregular frequencies and intervals. They are enhanced by anxiety and are reduced if the individual is distracted (McDowell & Cederbaum, 1988; Weisberg, 1987).

The tic disorder most likely to affect motor-speech processes is Tourette's syndrome. The signs and symptoms of this most unusual disorder, first described by the Frenchman Gilles de la Tourette in 1885, may include sudden inarticulate vocalizations (grunting or barking), coprolalia (lewd speech, eg, "Fuck you," "Up yours"), and echolalia (echoic speech; eg, Examiner: "Touch your nose." Patient: "Touch your nose."). The signs and symptoms of the syndrome tend to evolve and become more elaborate with age. Tourette described three stages to the syndrome: In the first stage only multiple tics occur; in the second stage inarticulate vocalizations are added; in the third stage coprolalia and echolalia are observed. These behaviors have been shown to occur in pauses, before and after clauses, and on typically deemphasized words (Frank, 1978).

Fortunately, the incidence of Tourette's syndrome is less than 1 in 100,000 (Friedhoff & Chase, 1982), and drug therapy utilizing antidopaminergic agents such as haloperidol has been shown to be effective in many cases. The exact pathophysiology of the speech and language associated with Tourette's remains to be explored fully.

Slow Forms

Athetosis

Athetoid movements may be observed in a number of conditions, including congenital cerebral palsy and tardive dyskinesia (Goetz & Klawans, 1984; Molnar, 1973; Neilson & O'Dwyer, 1984). These "writhing" movements also may result from anoxia, trauma, and vascular disease (Darley et al, 1975).

The articulatory abnormalities noted in athetoid individuals include wide-ranging jaw movements, inappropriate tongue placement, intermittent velopharyngeal closure, retrusion of the lower lip, and prolonged transition time for articulatory movements (Kent & Netsell, 1978). Intelligibility of connected speech has been reported to be markedly decreased though phonemic competence is intact, suggesting that athetoid individuals lack the neuromuscular control for articulatory precision (Platt, Andrews, & Howie, 1980; Platt, Andrews, Young, & Quinn, 1980). This lack of neuromuscular control may not result in purely involuntary movements. Neilson and O'Dwyer (1984) have reported that involuntary movements typically occur between, rather than during, production of syllables, suggesting that abnormal voluntary movements may be the significant contributor to the hyperkinetic dysarthria observed.

Dyskinesia

While the term "dyskinesia" has been used to refer to a variety of movement disturbances, it has been used frequently in the literature to refer to a subtype of "slow" movement disorder. Tardive ("late-occurring" or "tardy") dyskinesia can manifest itself in the oral musculature as well as the laryngeal-pharyngeal and respiratory musculature (Faheem, Brightwell, Burton, & Struss, 1982; Flaherty & Lahmeyer, 1978; Jankovic & Nour, 1986; Weiner, Goetz, Nausieda, & Klawans, 1978). Orofacial dyskinesia has been reported to occur spontaneously without cause (Klawans & Barr, 1982), following dental extractions (Koller, 1983), and in the chronically mentally ill (Portnoy, 1979). It may decrease with drowsiness or disappear during sleep, and may be aggravated by emotional tension. Various drugs can affect motor processing by altering neurotransmission at the level of the neuromuscular junction (Gawel, 1981; Waskow, 1966). The pharmacologic effects of such drugs on general nervous system functioning is becoming more well known, as are the effects of specific drugs on motor-speech processes. (Portnoy, 1979; Rosenfield, 1991).

In the Mayo Clinic study (Darley et al, 1969) articulatory deviations were reported to be the most prominent features noted in individuals with tardive dyskinesia. Other studies have reported that temporal, prosodic, and phonatory deviations, as well as articulatory deviations, may occur (Gerratt, Goetz, & Fischer, 1984). In fact, hyperkinetic dysarthria may be an early indicator of impending tardive dyskinesia, particularly in individuals who have chronically ingested neuroleptic agents (Portnoy, 1979).

Dystonia

Dystonia ("abnormal muscle tone") is a collective term for a variety of neurogenic disorders of posture and movement characterized by abnormal muscle contractions which may be accompanied by irregular repetitive movements (Zraick, LaPointe, Case, & Duane, 1993). Dystonia may affect most of the body or related body parts, and a common classification of the disorder is by body distribution. Classification by body distribution includes *generalized dystonia*, affecting at least one or both legs plus another area of the body; *segmental dystonia*, affecting two or more contiguous areas of the body; and *focal dystonia*, affecting only one area or part of the body (Fahn, 1988).

Focal dystonias which may affect speech and voice include orolingual-mandibular dystonia (OLMD), and spasmodic torticollis (ST). These focal dystonias (see Table 11–1) result in unique speech and voice profiles, which bear closer examination.

Individuals with orolingual-mandibular dystonia have abnormal movements of the vocal tract, including sustained tongue movements, clenched jaw, and/or forced jaw opening (Schulz & Ludlow, 1991). These signs often occur with blepharospasms (uncontrolled eye blinks), and this complex has been referred to as focal cranial dystonia or Meige syndrome (Jankovic, 1988a,b). Phonation, prosody, and articulation all are disturbed (Darley et al, 1975), and slow speech rate, inappropriate silences and pauses, abnormal stress, and imprecise consonants have been documented (Golper, Nutt, Rau, & Coleman, 1983; Tolosa, 1981).

Individuals with spasmodic torticollis (ST), sometimes called cervical dystonia, have tonic or intermittent hypercontractions of their neck muscles that typically cause involuntary deviation of the head from its normal position. Until recently very little was known about speech and voice characteristics associated with ST. A recent impetus in attempting to understand ST has come about by an ongoing collaborative study between the Arizona Dystonia Institute and Arizona State University. More than 300 subjects with a variety of dystonic impairment have been evaluated by this team over the past 5 years. Detailed reports of acoustic and speech characteristics of individuals with

Table 11–1. Classification of focal dystonia according to distribution on parts of body affected (from Fahn, 1988).

Type of focal dystonia	Body part affected
Blepharospasm	Eyelid
Oromandibular	Mouth
Adductor dysphonia	Larynx
Writer's cramp	Arm
Spasmodic torticollis	Neck

spasmodic torticollis have been presented in several sources (Case, LaPointe, & Duane, 1990; LaPointe, Case, & Duane, 1993; Zraick, LaPointe, Case, & Duane, 1993). Compared to normal control subjects, individuals with cervical dystonia have been found to have lower habitual pitch, restricted pitch range, shorter maximum phonation time, slower phonatory reaction time, larger s/z ratios, increased jitter and shimmer values, and smaller harmonic-to-noise ratios. Table 11–2 summarizes these findings.

Evaluation of Hyperkinetic Dysarthria

Evaluation of dysarthric speech is often undertaken with the eventual goal of differential description and diagnosis of dysarthria subtypes. Historically, classification systems such as the Mayo Clinic system (Darley et al, 1969) have been taught in college courses, have been widely used clinically, and have been used to describe subjects in research studies (Kent, 1994). However, issues regarding the reliability of the Mayo Clinic system have been raised (Kent, 1994; Zyski &

Table 11–2. Acoustic voice-speech parameters significantly different from normal individuals in persons with cervical dystonia (from Case, LaPointe, & Duane, 1991; LaPointe, Case, & Duane, 1993; Zraick, LaPointe, Case & Duane, 1993).

Parameter	Gender
Lower habitual fundamental frequency	Females
Lower ceiling fundamental frequency	Females
Restricted frequency range	Females
Shorter /s/ duration	Both
Shorter /z/ duration	Both
Shorter maximum phonation duration	Both
Slower sequential movement rates	Both
Slower alternate movement rates	Both
Longer phonatory reaction time	Both
Slower reading rate (WPM)	Both
Lower overall intelligibility rating	Both
Increased jitter values	Both
Increased shimmer values	Both
Decreased harmonic-to-noise ratio	Females

Weisiger, 1987), with many of these issues revolving around the use of perceptual techniques to describe and classify disordered speech production.

As reviewed by Kent (1994), perceptual techniques such as rating scales have many shortcomings, including poor reliability for some rated dimensions, possible interactions among rated dimensions, uncertain definition of rated dimensions, psychometric unsuitability, and limited analytic potential. What may be required for the future development of sensitive and effective clinical evaluation is an integration of human perceptual judgment with instrumental evaluation (Collins, 1984; Kent, 1994).

Systematic evaluation of the speech production of individuals with movement disorders can provide both an indirect means of studying the neuromotor mechanisms underlying their dysarthria and provide clinically useful information for improved differential diagnosis and treatment. A useful overall scheme for evaluation of the speech production system is the "functional component," or "point-place" system. This means of viewing speech production components has been advocated and outlined in many sources (Netsell, 1986; LaPointe & Katz, 1994; Rosenbek & LaPointe, 1985). As noted by Hartman and Abbs (1988), motor speech disturbances may be the first and occasionally the only symptoms and signs of a movement disorder.

Perceptual judgments can be supplemented with data from acoustic, aerodynamic, electromyographic, and kinematic analyses. An historic, if rudimentary, attempt to analyze the speech signal was presented more than 100 years ago . . .

> Abbot Rouselot, professor at the Carmelite School, has succeeded in creating the series of apparatus necessary for registering, one by one, the motions whose ensemble constitutes a word or phrase. Evidently, every time that, for any cause whatever, the air contained in the rubber tube enters into vibrations, the vibrations will be communicated to the air of the drum, and after this the rubber and then the polate and lever will enter into motion. If

the cylinder is revolving at the same time, the line that will be inscribed thereon by the point of the lever, instead of being straight, will become a tracing of the vibrations. It will be possible hereafter to note the pronunciation of any language, dialect or idiom, without relying upon the testimony of the ear, which distinguishes but slight differences between the modes of speaking of several individuals.

Scientific American, 1892
[Cited in *Scientific American,* September, 1992, p. 16]

Abbot Rouselot's speech machine has undergone considerable refinement over the years. The benefit of acoustic, aerodynamic, electromyographic, and kinematic analyses have been well documented in the literature (Barlow & Abbs, 1983, 1984; Bellaire, Yorkston, & Beukelman, 1986; Dworkin, Aronson, & Mulder, 1980; Eskanazi, 1988; Gracco & Muller, 1981; Hixon, 1982, 1984; Kent & Rosenbek, 1982; Kent, Netsell, & Abbs, 1979; Ludlow & Bassich, 1984; McClean, Beukelman, & Yorkston, 1987; Murdoch, Cheney, Bowler, & Ingram, 1989; Netsell, 1969, 1973, 1983; Prosek, Montgomery, & Hawkins, 1987; Putnam & Hixon 1984; Rosenbek & LaPointe, 1985; Warren, 1982; 1992; Weismer, 1984a; Yorkston, Beukelman, & Bell, 1988; Yorkston, Beukelman, Minifie, & Sapir, 1984; Yumoto, Sasaki, & Okamura, 1984; Zraick et al, 1993).

These methods are appropriate to hyperkinetic dysarthria as well, and general principles and methods are presented elsewhere in this text.

General Treatment Principles

Precise clinical and physiological determination of the nature and extent of motor-speech subsystem disturbances is the basis of an effective treatment plan for hyperkinetic dysarthria. Once a differential diagnosis has been made, objective therapy goals can be set, procedures for achieving those goals can be chosen, and measures for testing the efficacy of the treatment plan can be employed. In many cases, medical management, either surgical or pharmacological, is a vital first order of treatment.

As has been well documented in this book, speech production results from the coordination and integration of five subsystems: (1) respiration, (2) phonation, (3) articulation, (4) resonation, and (5) prosody. Persons with hyperkinetic dysarthria may present with deficits in each of these subsystems, thus requiring a comprehensive and well-integrated therapy plan.

Dworkin (1991) has identified the following respiration subsystem disturbances in hyperkinetic dysarthria: poor posture, neck and trunk rigidity, shallow inhalations, reduced exhalation control, rapid breaths, antagonistic muscular contractions, involuntary muscular contractions, irregular patterns, and sudden-forced inhalations/exhalations. A hierarchy of respiration subsystem treatment exercises might include:

1. Muscle relaxation and postural adjustment
2. Air pressure generation
3. Prolonged inhalations/exhalations
4. Quick breathing
5. Inhalatory/exhalatory synchronization
6. Isolated sound productions
7. Connected speech breathing

For more detailed information on the objectives of the above exercises and specific techniques for achieving those objectives, the reader is encouraged to refer to Dworkin (1991).

Disturbances of the phonatory subsystem are exhibited by most dysarthric patients and may coexist with other subsystem disturbances. The voice characteristics of hyperkinetic dysarthria can be generally described as variable, fluctuating, and unpredictable. Dworkin (1991) has identified the following voice characteristics of the hyperkinetic dysarthria resulting from the various groups of movement disorders:

Group of Disorders	Characteristics
Quick forms:	Harsh-strained quality, intermittent breathiness, ar-

255

Slow forms: rests of phonation, and pitch and loudness variations.

Slow forms: Strained-strangled/hoarse-breathy quality, aperiodic arrests of phonation, loudness variations, and monopitch.

As with many neurogenic disorders of voice, a combination of behavioral, surgical, and pharmacological treatments may be employed. The random, variable, and fluctuating voice characteristics of hyperkinetic dysarthria result from abnormal patterns of vocal fold vibration, including hypoadduction, hyperadduction, and fluctuating adduction. Specific techniques for treating hyperadduction may include relaxation of laryngeal musculature, yawn-sigh phonation, and vowel prolongations; techniques for treating hypoadduction may include holding the breath, nonspeech vocal fold valving, phonatory vocal fold valving, and hard attack phonation; techniques for treating fluctuating adduction may include voice motor planning and laryngeal timing and coordination (Boone & McFarland, 1993; Case, 1991; Dworkin, 1991).

Disturbances of the articulatory subsystem rarely occur in isolation, and articulation proficiency may be adversely affected by deficits in other speech subsystems. This is particularly true in hyperkinetic dysarthria, where the involuntary respiratory and phonatory disturbances as described in the preceding paragraphs may influence articulatory proficiency and overall intelligibility of speech. Labial, lingual, and mandibular movements may correspond to the overall class of movement disorder—ie, quick, slow, or tremulous. Therapy techniques may include muscle tone reduction, muscle strengthening, force physiology training, and phonetic stimulation in various contexts (Dworkin, 1991).

Disturbances of the resonatory subsystem are usually seen in individuals with flaccid dysarthria, spastic dysarthria, or mixed dysarthrias including one of those types, but are not typically seen in patients with hyperkinetic dysarthria. However, disruptions in resonance certainly can occur in forms of myoclonus, athetosis, or oromandibular dystonia.

In general, prosodic/suprasegmental disturbances may include variations in pitch, loudness, silence and segment duration, and rhythm, stress, and intonation. Individuals with hyperkinetic dysarthria may exhibit disturbances such as variable rate, prolonged intervals, prolonged pauses, excess loudness, reduced loudness and pitch variation, and flattened affect. The interested reader is again referred to Dworkin (1991) for specific therapy techniques.

As with nearly all communication disorders, the effects and progress of intervention should be documented and plotted. Many systems exist for plotting and measuring the course of behavioral or instrumental treatment. Baseline and periodic audio and video recordings can be used throughout a treatment course, and these days computer-based files can be maintained as part of instrumental periodic analysis of the components of speech or voice. The *Base-10 Response Form* approach to recording and evaluating treatment change can be useful for all of the neuromotor speech disorders, including hyperkinetic dysarthria (LaPointe, 1991). This system is used to clearly specify, score, and plot countable communication behaviors of clients enrolled in treatment programs. The rise in third-party reimbursement and the increasing recognition of the importance of quality assurance and accountability of services underscored the development of this approach to documenting aspects of treatment efficacy and the approach remains appropriate for the dysarthrias.

Additionally, other components of sensitive and humanistic clinical management are an integral part of intervention for hyperkinetic dysarthria. This includes adequate client and family counseling. Throughout the course of treatment, families and individuals need to be provided with information [few know or are familiar with the professional jargon and restricted and eso-teric vernacular of medical conditions—eg, "Your father has an idiopathic spasmodic torticollis which affects his jitter and shim-mer."] Translations need to be made; expla-nations need to be given; participation needs to be enlisted; assurance and encouragement need to be an intimate part of the rehabilita-tion challenge. Individualism and human-ism need to guide all intervention efforts and the medical caregiver blunder of viewing the human being as a disorder needs to be avoided at all costs. Careful and sensitive clinical management interweaves all of these humanistic elements and principles into the tapestry of the special skills and knowledge required to understand and treat these unfa-miliar and alien conditions.

Conclusion

Hyperkinetic dysarthria is a challenging neuromotor speech disorder. It arises from and is associated with disorders of move-ment, including chorea, myoclonus, tic disor-ders, athetosis, dyskinesia, dystonia, and tremor. These conditions are believed to re-sult from neuropathology in the extrapyra-midal system, more specifically the basal ganglia and their major pathways—impor-tant centers and roadways for the planning and programming of learned movements. Hyperkinetic dysarthria can be intrusive, disruptive, and disabling and can affect all of the major components of speech production. We are in the embryonic stages of under-standing these disorders, but the efforts of science and enlightened clinical hypothesis testing as well as the emergence and refine-ment of technology bode well for the future.

References

Aronson A. (1980). *Clinical Voice Disorders: An Interdisciplinary Approach.* New York: Thieme-Stratton, Inc.

Barlow S, Abbs J. (1983). Force transducers for the evaluation of labial, lingual and mandibular motor impairments. *J Speech Hear Res* 26:616–621.

Bellaire K, Yorkston K, Beukelman D. (1986). Modification of breath patterning to increase naturalness of dysarthric speakers. *J Commun Disord* 19:271–280.

Boone D, McFarland S. (1993). *The Voice and Voice Therapy* (5th Ed.). Englewood Cliffs: NJ: Prentice–Hall.

Caligiuri M, Murry T. (1984). Identification of a performance deficit in dysarthria associated with Huntington's disease. Presented at the Clinical Dysarthria Conference, Tucson, AZ.

Carpenter M. (1985). *Core Text of Neuroanatomy* (3rd Ed.). Baltimore: Williams and Wilkins.

Case J. (1991). *Clinical Management of Voice Disorders* (2nd Ed.). Austin: Pro-Ed.

Case J, LaPointe L, Duane D. (1990). Speech and voice characteristics in spasmodic torticollis. Presented at the International Congress of Movement Disorders, Washing-ton, DC. (Abstract in *Movement Disorders*, 1990;5:84).

Collins M. (1984). Integrating perceptual and in-strumental procedures in dysarthria assess-ment. *J Commun Disord* 5:159–170.

Darley F, Aronson A, Brown J. (1969). Differential diagnostic patterns of dysarthria. *J Speech Hear Res* 12:246–269.

Darley F, Aronson A, Brown J. (1975). *Motor Speech Disorders.* Philadelphia: W.B. Saunders.

Dworkin P. (1991). *Motor Speech Disorders: A Treatment Guide.* St. Louis: Mosby—Year Book.

Dworkin P, Aronson A, Mulder D. (1980). Tongue force in normals and dysarthric patients with amyotrophic lateral sclerosis. *J Speech Hear Res* 23:828–837.

Eskanazi L. (1988). Acoustic correlates of voice quality and distortion measure for speech processing. Unpublished doctoral disserta-tion, University of Florida, Gainesville.

Espir M, Rose F. (1983). *The Basic Neurology of Speech and Language* (3rd Ed.). Oxford: Blackwell Scientific.

Faheem A, Brightwell D, Burton G, Struss A. (1982). Respiratory dyskinesia and dy-sarthria from prolonged neuroleptic use: Tardive dyskinesia? *Am J Psychiatry* 139:517–518.

Fahn S. (1988). Concept and classification of dystonia. In Fahn S, Marsden C, Calne B, eds. *Advances in Neurology* (Vol. 50) (Dystonia 2). New York: Raven Press, p 4.

Flaherty J, Lahmeyer W. (1978). Laryngeal pharyngeal dystonia as a possible cause of asphyxia with haloperidol. *Am J Psychiatry* 135:1414–1415.

Frank S. (1978). Psycholinguistic findings in Gilles de la Tourette syndrome. *J Commun Disord* 11:349–363.

Friedhoff A. (1982). Gilles de la Tourette syndrome. *Adv Neurol* 35:335–339.

Gatz A. (1966). *Manter's Essentials of Clinical Neuroanatomy and Neurophysiology.* Philadelphia: S.A. Davis.

Gawel M. (1981). The effects of various drugs on speech. *Br J Disord Commun* 16:51–57.

Gerratt B, Goetz C, Fischer H. (1984). Speech abnormalities in tardive dyskinesia. *Arch Neurol* 41:273–276.

Goetz C, Klawan H. (1984). Tardive dyskinesia. In: Jankovic J, ed. *Neurologic Clinics: Movement Disorders.* Philadelphia: W.B. Saunders, pp 605–614.

Golper L, Nutt J, Rau M, Coleman R. (1983). Focal cranial dystonia. *J Speech Hear Disord* 48:128–134.

Gracco V, Muller E. (1981). Analysis of supraglottic air pressure variations in spastic dysarthria. Paper presented at the Convention of the American Speech-Language-Hearing Association, Los Angeles.

Hartman D, Abbs J. (1988). Dysarthrias of movement disorders. In: Jankovic J, Tolosa E, eds. *Advances in Neurology, Facial Dyskinesias* (Vol. 49). New York: Raven Press, pp 289–306.

Hixon T. (1982). Speech breathing kinematics and mechanism interferences therefrom. In Grillner S, Persson A, Lindbolm B, Lubker J, eds. *Speech Motor Control.* New York: Pergamon Press.

Hixon T. (1984). Parameter-based evaluation of speech breathing functions in dysarthria. Presented at the Annual Convention of the American Speech-Language-Hearing Association, San Francisco.

Jankovic J. (1988a). Cranial-cervical dyskinesias: An overview. In: Jankovic J, Tolosa E, eds. *Advances in Neurology, Facial Dyskinesias* (Vol. 49). New York: Raven Press, pp 289–306.

Jankovic J. (1988b). Etiology and differential diagnosis of blepharospasm and oromandibular dystonia. In: Jankovic J, Tolosa E, eds. *Advances in Neurology, Facial Dyskinesias* (Vol. 49). New York: Raven Press, pp. 289–306.

Jankovic J, Nour F. (1986). Respiratory dyskinesia in Parkinson's disease. *Neurology* 36:303–304.

Kent R. (1994). The clinical science of motor speech disorders: A personal assessment. In: Till J, Yorkston, K, Beukelman D, eds. *Motor Speech Disorders: Assessment and Treatment.* Baltimore: Paul H. Brooks, pp 3–18.

Kent R, Netsell R. (1978). Articulatory abnormalities in athetoid cerebral palsy. *J Speech Hear Disord* 43:353–373.

Kent R, Netsell R, Abbs J. (1979). Acoustic characteristics of dysarthria associated with cerebellar disease. *J Speech Hear Res* 22:627–648.

Kent R, Rosenbek J. (1982). Prosodic disturbance and neurologic lesion. *Brain Language* 15:259–291.

Klawans H, Barr A. (1982). Prevalence of spontaneous lingual-facial-buccal dyskinesias in the elderly. *Neurology* 32:558–559.

Koller W. (1983). Edentulous dyskinesia. *Ann Neurol* 13:97–99.

LaPointe L. (1991). *Base-10 Response Form* (revised manual). San Diego: Singular.

LaPointe L, Case J, Duane D. (1993). Perceptual-acoustic speech and voice characteristics of subjects with spasmodic torticollis. In: Till J, Yorkston K, Beukelman D, eds. *Motor Speech Disorders: Advances in Assessment and Treatment.* Baltimore: Paul H. Brooks, pp 40–45.

LaPointe L, Katz R. (1994). Neurogenic disorders of speech. In: Shames G, Wiig E, Secord W, eds. *Human Communication Disorders: An Introduction* (4th Ed.). New York: Macmillan, pp 480–518.

Ludlow C, Bassich C. (1984). Relationships between perceptual ratings and acoustic measures of hypokinetic speech. In: McNeil M, Rosenbek J, Aronson A, eds. *The Dysarthrias: Physiology, Acoustics, Perception, Management.* San Diego: College-Hill Press.

McClean M, Beukelman D, Yorkston K. (1987). Speech muscle visuomotor tracking in dysarthric and non-impaired speakers. *J Speech Hear Res* 30:276–282.

McDowell F, Cedarbaum J. (1988). The extrapyramidal system and disorders of movement. In: Joynt R, ed. *Clinical Neurology* (Vol. 3). Philadelphia: J.B. Lippincott.

Molnar G. (1973). Clinical aspects of cerebral palsy. *Pediatr Ann* 2:10–27.

Murdoch B, Cheney H, Bowler S, Ingram J. (1989). Respiratory function in Parkinson's subjects exhibiting a speech deficit: A kinematic and spirometric analysis. *J Speech Hear Disord* 54:610–626.

Nausieda P, Grosman B, Koller W, Weiner W, Klawan H. (1980). Sydenham chorea: An update. *Neurology* 30:331–334.

Neilson P, O'Dwyer N. (1984). Reproducibility and variability of speech muscle activity in athetoid dysarthria of cerebral palsy. *J Speech Hear Res* 27:502–517.

Netsell R. (1969). Evaluation of velopharyngeal function in dysarthria. *J Speech Hear Disord* 34:113–122.

Netsell R. (1973). Speech physiology. In: Minifie F, Hixon T, Williams F, eds. *Normal Aspects of Speech, Language and Hearing*. Englewood Cliffs, NJ: Prentice-Hall.

Netsell R. (1983). Speech motor control: Theoretical issues with clinical impact. In: Berry W, ed. *Clinical Dysarthria*. San Diego: College–Hill Press.

Netsell R. (1986). *A Neurobiological View of Speech Production and the Dysarthrias*. San Diego, CA: College-Hill Press.

Platt L, Andrews G, Howie P. (1980). Dysarthria of adult cerebral palsy: II. Phonemic analyses of articulation errors. *J Speech Hear Res* 23:41–45.

Platt L, Andrews G, Young M, Quinn P. (1980). Dysarthria of adult cerebral palsy: I. Intelligibility and articulatory impairment. *J Speech Hear Res* 23:28–40.

Portnoy R. (1979). Hyperkinetic dysarthria as an early indicator of impending tardive dyskinesia. *J Speech Hear Disord* 44:214–219.

Prosek A, Montgomery and Hawkins D. (1987). An evaluation of residue features as correlates of voice disorders. *J Commun Disord* 20:105–117.

Putnam A, Hixon T. (1984). Respiratory kinematics in speakers with motor neuron disease. In: McNeil M, Rosenbek J, Aronson A, eds. *The Dysarthrias: Physiology, Acoustics, Perception, Management*. San Diego: College-Hill Press.

Ramig L. (1986). Acoustic analyses of phonation in patients with Huntington's disease. *Ann Otol Rhinol Laryngol* 95:288–293.

Rosenbek J, LaPointe L. (1985). The dysarthrias: Description, diagnosis and treatment. In: Johns D, eds. *Clinical Management of Neurogenic Communication Disorders*. Boston: Little, Brown, pp 97–152.

Rosenfield D. (1991). Pharmacologic approaches to speech motor disorders. In: Vogel D, Cannito M, eds. *Treating Disordered Speech Motor Control*. Austin: Pro-Ed, pp 111–152.

Schulz G, Ludlow C. (1991). Botulinum treatment for orolingual-mandibular dystonia: Speech effects. In: Moore C, Yorkston K, Beukelman D, eds. *Dysarthria and Apraxia of Speech: Perspectives on Management*. Baltimore: Paul H. Brookes, pp 227–241.

Swedo S, Leonard H, Schapiro M, Casey B, Mannheim G, Lenane M, Rettew D. (1993). Sydenham's chorea: Physical and psychological symptoms of St. Vitus dance. *Pediatrics* 91:706–713.

Tolosa E. (1981). Clinical features of Meige's disease (idiopathic orofacial dystonia): A report of 17 cases. *Arch Neurol* 38:147–151.

Warren D. (1982). Aerodynamics of speech. In: Lass N, McReynolds L, Northern J, Yoder D, eds. *Handbook of Speech Pathology and Audiology*. Philadelphia: W.B. Saunders, pp 191–213.

Warren D. (1992). Aerodynamic measurements of speech. In: Cooper J, ed. *Assessment of Speech and Voice Production: Research and Clinical Applications, NIDCD Monograph*. Bethesda, MD: National Institute on Deafness and Other Communication Disorders, pp 103–111.

Waskow I. (1966). The effects of drugs on speech: A review. *Psychopharmacol Bull* 3:1–20.

Weiner W, Goetz C, Nausieda P, Klawans H. (1978). Respiratory dyskinesias: Extrapyramidal dysfunction and dyspnea. *Ann Intern Med* 88:327–331.

Weisberg L. (1987). Abnormal involuntary movement. In: Weisberg L, Strub R, Garcia C, eds. *Decision Making in Adult Neurology*. Toronto: B.C. Decker, pp 38–39.

Weismer G. (1984a). Acoustic descriptions of dysarthric speech: Perceptual correlates and physiological inferences. *Semin Speech Language* 5:293–314.

Wilson S. (1912). Progressive lenticular degeneration: A familial nervous disease associated with cirrhosis of the liver. *Brain* 34:295–509.

Yorkston K, Beukelman D, Minifie F, Sapir R. (1984). Assessment of stress patterning. In: McNeil M, Rosenbek J, Aronson A, eds. *The Dysarthrias: Physiology, Acoustics, Perception, Management*. San Diego: College-Hill Press, pp 131–162.

Yorkston K, Beukelman D, Bell K. (1988). *Clinical Management of Dysarthric Speakers*. San Diego: College-Hill Press.

Yumoto E, Sasaki Y, Okamura H. (1984). Harmonics-to-noise ratio and psychophysical measurement of the degree of hoarseness. *J Speech Hear Res* 27:2–6.

Zraick R, LaPointe L, Case J, Duane D. (1993). Acoustic correlates of vocal quality in spas-

modic torticollis. *J Med Speech-Language Pathol* 1:261–269.

Zwirner P, Murry T, Woodson G. (1991). Phonatory function of neurologically impaired patients. *J Commun Disord* 24:287–300.

Chapter 12

Hypokinetic Dysarthria in Parkinson's Disease

Scott G. Adams

Introduction

The term *hypokinetic dysarthria*, first introduced by Darley, Aronson, & Brown (1969a), refers to the speech characteristics observed in patients with parkinsonism (1969a,b). Darley et al (1969a,b, 1975) called this motor speech disorder *hypokinetic*, based on their view that the physiologic basis of the dysarthria involved a reduction in the mobility of movements for speech. While hypokinetic dysarthria is most commonly observed in idiopathic Parkinson's disease (PD), it also occurs in a wide range of parkinson-like, akinetic rigid syndromes including progressive supranuclear palsy, Wilson's disease, postencephalitic parkinsonism, MPTP-induced parkinsonism, and atherosclerotic parkinsonism. Whereas few studies have examined the speech manifestations of these akinetic rigid syndromes (Darley et al, 1975; Grewel, 1957; Metter & Hanson, 1991), there is an extensive literature on speech in idiopathic PD. As such, the present chapter will focus exclusively on the nature and treatment of the hypokinetic dysarthria associated with idiopathic PD. In particular, this chapter will attempt to (1) provide a general discussion of the pathophysiology and nonspeech symptoms associated with PD; (2) summarize the perceptual, acoustic, and physiologic data related to speech production in PD; and (3) describe a number of approaches that have been used in the treatment of hypokinetic dysarthria in PD.

Parkinson's Disease: History, Pathophysiology, Symptoms

In 1817, James Parkinson first described the major clinical features of a progressive neurological disorder that is now referred to as Parkinson's disease (Parkinson, 1817). He noted the presence of resting tremor, gait disturbances, and a general slowness of movement. Later, Charcot (1880) named the disease after Parkinson, and added the feature of rigidity to the clinical description of PD.

The prevalence of PD in the general population has been estimated to be between one and two cases per 1000 (Weiner & Lang, 1989). However, in the segment of the population that is 70 years or older the prevalence of PD rises to approximately 15 in 1000 (Scott, Caird, & Williams, 1985). The cause of PD is not known, and genetic studies have been fairly inconclusive. The current consensus appears to be that PD involves a genetic susceptibility in combination with certain undetermined environmental factor(s) (Golbe & Langston, 1993; Weiner & Lang, 1989). Lesions in the part of the basal ganglia referred to as the substantia nigra, and the associated loss of the dopaminergic nigrostriatal pathways, have come to be accepted as the primary explanations for most of the motor symptoms observed in PD (Weiner & Lang, 1989).

Recognition of the role of the nigrostriatal dopaminergic pathways in PD led to the discovery, in the 1960s, that levodopa medication could reduce many of the major symptoms of PD (Barbeau, Sourkes, & Murphy, 1962; Birkmayer & Kiewicz, 1962; Cotzias, Papauasiliou, & Gellene, 1969; Cotzias, Van Woert, & Schiffer, 1967). Following this discovery, there was a dramatic increase in research related to the pharmacological and neurochemical aspects of PD. This work has led to numerous refinements in current levodopa therapy (ie, carbidopa/levodopa, controlled-release levodopa), and the development of a number of dopamine-enhancing medications (dopamine-receptor agonists, monoamine oxidase inhibitors) (see Jankovic & Marsden, 1993; Poewe, 1993; Weiner & Lang, 1989, for details).

Prior to levodopa therapy, approximately 50% of PD patients became severely disabled or died within the first 10 years after diagnosis (Weiner & Lang, 1989). Since the introduction of levodopa, the mortality rate among PD patients has decreased to approximately that of the normal population. Furthermore, levodopa therapy has been shown to significantly delay the development of major disabilities in PD (Weiner & Lang, 1989).

The neurologist's diagnosis of PD is based on the presence of four major signs: tremor, rigidity, akinesia, and postural instability. Tremor typically occurs at rest and at a frequency of approximately 4 to 7 Hz. Rigidity is characterized by an involuntary resistance to passive movement that may be released momentarily during testing (cogwheel rigidity). Akinesia refers to a reduction in the range, complexity, and speed of movement. Reduced movement speed, referred to as bradykinesia, is an important component of akinesia. Postural instability is reflected in the PD patient's unsteady gait and reduced ability to compensate for being pushed off balance. Other secondary signs of PD include stooped posture, reduced arm swing, micrographia, reduced facial expression, and difficulties initiating movement.

Because there are no confirmatory laboratory procedures for PD, neurologists must rely on their observations of these four major motor signs of PD. The presence of resting tremor and rigidity, in the absence of akinesia and postural instability, appears to be sufficient to make a diagnosis of PD (this is assuming an absence of specific etiological factors such as exposure to MPTP, encephalitis, etc). However, the presence of rigidity and akinesia (bradykinesia) in the absence of tremor usually causes the neurologist to delay the diagnosis of PD while continuing to search for the signs and symptoms of other akinetic rigid syndromes (PSP, Wilson's disease, Shy-Drager, olivopontocerebellar or striatonigral degeneration) (Weiner & Lang, 1989).

The typical profile of a PD patient in the early stages of the disease (1 to 5 years) includes a unilateral resting tremor, usually involving the hand, complaints of a loss of dexterity for fine movements (ie, manipulating of small objects), and hand writing that has become difficult and small (micrographia). In addition, the patient may have mild complaints of stiffness, slowness, or a lack of power in one limb. There may also be a reduction in facial expression, a reduction in arm swing during walking, and a slightly stooped and asymmetrical posture; and speech may be characterized by reduced intensity and expressiveness.

In the later stages of the disease (+15 years), the early symptoms become progressively more severe. The resting tremor usually becomes bilateral and extends to all limbs, as well as the trunk, neck, and jaw. The stiffness, slowness, and loss of coordination and power extend to include a wider range of movements. The patient often cannot perform most fairly simple skilled movements. Periods of immobility, in which the patient appears to be frozen, become more frequent and prolonged. Immobile periods are often separated by periods of hyperactivity involving uncontrolled, rapid movements of the limbs, trunk, and head. These so-called dyskinesias resemble the hyperkinetic movements of patients with Huntington's disease, and are associated with the higher doses of levodopa medication required to overcome the severe immobility that can occur in the later stages of PD. It has been estimated that 80 to 90% of PD patients will develop dyskinesias within the first 5 to 10 years after diagnosis (Weiner & Lang, 1989). Patients also begin to have increasing impairments of gait and balance, such that they may eventually require a wheelchair. Swallowing problems may lead to alterations in diet or methods of feeding. Dementia, memory loss, and depression may also become apparent in the later stages of PD.

Presenting Perceptual, Acoustic, and Physiologic Speech Signs and Symptoms in Parkinson's Disease

Perceptual Findings

It is estimated that between 60 and 80% of PD patients will develop speech symptoms as the disease progresses (Atarashi & Uchida, 1959; Mutch, Strudwick, & Roy, 1986; Selby, 1968; Streifler & Hofman, 1984; Uziel, Bohe, & Cadilhac, 1975). In the early stages of PD, many patients complain of a reduction in speech intensity, or "hypophonia." These patients can become extremely frustrated by the increasingly frequent requests that they receive to speak louder and repeat themselves. In addition to reduced speech intensity, several clinical reports have noted that PD patients demonstrate reduced stress and intonation patterns, abnormal voice qualities, distorted consonantal sounds, and abnormally rapid or slow speaking rates (see Canter, 1963, 1965a,b, for reviews of the early literature based largely individual clinical impressions of speech in PD).

Over the past 20 years, several researchers have conducted systematic perceptual studies of speech in PD. These perceptual studies have verified many of the earlier clinical impressions and have added a number of new dimensions to the clinical profile of hypokinetic dysarthria in PD.

Loudness Level

Although reduced loudness is generally recognized as one of the major speech symptoms in PD, it has rarely been examined in systematic perceptual studies. In Darley et

al's (1975) extensive perceptual study of seven dysarthria groups, they found that in the 15 PD patients they examined the average speech loudness levels were lower than those of the other dysarthric groups. This finding suggests that reduced speech loudness is a distinctive characteristic of speech in PD and, as such, may have a useful role in the differential diagnosis of hypokinetic dysarthria.

Nevertheless reduced speech loudness does not appear to be present in all dysarthric PD patients. Ludlow and Bassich (1984) reported that only 42% (5/12) of their dysarthric PD patients were perceived as having reduced speech loudness. However, this value may underestimate the actual proportion of dysarthric PD patients who are hypophonic, given that many PD patients appear to be able to compensate for their hypophonia during formal speech testing.

Pitch and Loudness Variation

Reduced pitch and loudness variation were among the most prominent speech deficits observed in Darley, Aronson and Brown's (1969a,b, 1975) perceptual studies of speech in PD. Based on their average perceptual rating scale scores, the following hierarchy of deviant dimensions was observed in 32 PD patients:

1. Monopitch
2. Reduced stress
3. Monoloudness
4. Imprecise consonants

All of the above dimensions, except imprecise consonants, were judged to be more deviant in PD patients than in any of the other six neurologic groups examined. The authors summarized their results thus:

> Characteristics most distinctive of hypokinetic dysarthria comprise significantly reduced variability in pitch and loudness, reduced loudness level overall, and decreased use of all vocal parameters for achieving stress and emphasis. (p 195)

Ludlow and Bassich (1984) reported that, within their sample of 12 PD patients, most were judged to have significant prosodic abnormalities including monopitch, mono-loudness, pitch breaks, inappropriate si-lences, and reduced stress. Specifically, 67% of the PD patients were perceived as being abnormally monopitch, while 58% were per-ceived as monoloud.

Voice Quality
It appears that many PD patients experience changes in voice quality. Logemann, Boshes, & Fisher (1973, 1978) found that voice disor-ders such as breathiness, hoarseness, rough-ness, and tremor were among the most frequent speech symptoms, occurring in 89% of their sample of 200 PD patients. More-over, in approximately 45% of these patients, a voice disorder was the only symptom of dysarthria.

Darley et al (1975) reported that many PD patients were perceived as either harsh or breathy, and that these characteristics oc-curred with about an equal degree of sever-ity. In contrast, Ludlow and Bassich (1984) found that 83% of their PD patients had ab-normally harsh voices, while only 17% were judged to have abnormally breathy voices. Similarly, Logemann et al (1978) found that only 15% of their PD patients had abnor-mally breathy voices. Ludlow and Bassich (1984) speculated that differences between their results and those of Darley et al's re-garding breathiness may be related to the fact that patients in the Ludlow and Bassich study were receiving levodopa medication while patients in the Darley study were not. Specifically, they suggested that levodopa-related dyskinesias and hyperkinesia, when present in the laryngeal system, may pro-duce an abnormally harsh voice quality in some PD patients. This interesting hypoth-esis needs to be examined in PD patients who are experiencing drug-cycle-related voice changes and dyskinesias (see Winckel & Adams, 1992).

Consonant Articulation
In an early description of imprecise conso-nant articulations in PD, Cramer (1940) noted that plosives appeared to lack precision and were produced almost like fricatives.

Logeman et al (1973, 1978) reported that in the 200 PD patients they examined, 45% demonstrated articulatory disorders. In a later study, Logemann and Fisher (1981) pro-vided a detailed description of the speech articulation errors in PD, based on phonetic transcriptions of 90 patients' speech. Their analysis revealed that stops, affricates, and fricatives were often distorted and that these distortions appeared to be the result of an inadequate narrowing of the vocal tract. That is, stops and affricates became more fricative-like, and fricatives showed a gen-eral reduction in frication energy.

Logeman et al (1973, 1978) hypothesized that in PD there is a relationship between the severity of an articulatory disorder and the predominant place of the articulation errors. For example, PD patients with the mildest articulatory disorders had difficulties prima-rily with consonants involving placement of the tongue dorsum (/k/ and /g/), whereas the articulatory errors of the more severe PD patients involved more anterior vocal tract placements such as the tongue blade, lips, and tongue tip. These authors further sug-gest that there may be a progression of dys-function in PD, beginning with the laryngeal system and subsequently involving the pos-terior tongue, more anterior portion of the tongue, and finally the labial articulators. They suggested that this progression, from more posterior vocal tract (voice) deficits, to deficits involving more anterior portions of the vocal tract, may be related to a predict-able pattern of neural degeneration in the somatotopic representations of the speech articulators in PD.

While this progressive vocal tract degen-eration hypothesis is intriguing, other inter-pretations are possible. It is conceivable that the capacity of two different vocal tract struc-tures to produce the movements necessary for speech could be differentially reduced by an equivalent motor impairment. For ex-ample, a 50% increase in both laryngeal and lip rigidity may severely disrupt the normal patterns of vocal fold vibration but have rela-tively minor effects on lip movements re-quired for speech. Similarly, equivalent motor impairments may have differential effects on articulatory precision and the perceived clarity of speech. For example, a 50% reduction in the range of tongue tip movements may have a more dramatic impact on perceived speech clarity than an equivalent 50% reduction in the range of jaw movements.

Rate of Speech

A number of previous studies have indicated that PD patients can demonstrate abnormal speaking rates. In his review of the early studies of PD speech, Canter (1963) observed that, while some authors reported abnormally rapid speech in PD, a more common observation was that PD patients had "slow rates of speaking." Logemann et al (1978) found that the proportion of PD patients who demonstrate either an abnormally rapid or slow speech rate was only about 20%. Darley et al (1975) noted that while slow speech is a common feature of most dysarthric groups, rapid speech only occurred in the patients with PD. This suggests that rapid speech can

Table 12–1. Proportion of PD patients demonstrating rapid speech.

Darley et al (1975) (4/32 pts)	13%
Ludlow & Bassich (1984) (1/12 pts)	8%
Canter (1963) (1/17 pts)	6%
Logemann et al (1978) (21/200 pts)	11%

be a useful diagnostic sign in PD; however, it appears that the proportion of PD patients who demonstrate rapid speech is relatively small. An examination of the results from several previous studies (Table 12–1) suggests that between 6 and 13% (mean 10.5%) of PD patients may demonstrate an abnormally rapid rate of speech.

In contrast to the finding that only a small proportion of PD patients demonstrate a rapid "habitual" speaking rate, it appears that a large percentage of PD patients have difficulty making adjustments in their rate of speech. For example, Ludlow and Bassich (1984) found that 83% of their PD patients had difficulty increasing their rate of speech when asked to speak rapidly. This difficulty in modifying speaking rate was found to be one of the most frequent and severe speech characteristic in the PD patients that Ludlow and Bassich (1984) examined (see Table 12–2).

Acoustic Findings

Intensity Level and Variability

As discussed in the previous section, perceptual studies have suggested that PD patients are perceived as speaking with decreased loudness and a reduced range of loudness. Interestingly, the acoustic correlates of these perceptual features have been difficult to find. For example, various authors have reported no differences between PD patients and normals on measures of average peak

Table 12–2. Summary of Ludlow and Bassich's (1984) perceptual analysis of PD speech.

	Average scale score	% of PDs scores ≥3
1. Problems modifying speaking rate	3.77	83%
2. Monopitch	3.71	67%
3. Pitch breaks	3.70	67%
4. Monoloudness	3.66	58%
5. Harsh voice	3.48	83%
6. Imprecise consonants	3.28	33%
7. Inappropriate silences	3.12	50%
8. Hypernasality	2.90	42%
9. Reduced stress	2.78	33%

speech intensity (Canter, 1963; Ludlow & Bassich, 1984) and average peak intensity range (Canter, 1963), or relative speech intensity (Metter & Hanson, 1986) obtained during connected speech. The apparent lack of agreement between these acoustic and perceptual findings suggests that additional parameters of the acoustic speech signal may be contributing to the perception of reduced loudness in PD. For example, acoustic parameters that relate to the resonance of the vocal tract, such as relative upper formant intensity, formant bandwidth, and nasal formants, as well as acoustic measures of voice quality, for example, vocal perturbations, and signal/noise ratio, may be important variables in the perception of reduced loudness in PD.

As mentioned previously, PD patients may not use their habitual speech loudness levels in the speech clinic. Therefore, methods for obtaining acoustic measures of speech intensity outside of the clinical setting need to be developed in order to establish valid estimates of hypophonia in PD.

Fundamental Frequency (F0) Level and Variability

Canter (1963) reported that F0 was significantly higher in PD patients than normal speakers. In contrast, more recent studies have reported no differences in the F0 levels of PD and normal subjects (Metter & Hanson, 1986; Zwirner, Murry, & Woodson, 1991). It is noteworthy that Canter's study was conducted several years before levodopa therapy was available for the treatment for PD, whereas the more recent studies included PD patients who were on levodopa medication. Although it is possible that levodopa had a direct effect on F0 levels, it has also been suggested that F0 may increase with the clinical severity of PD (Metter & Hanson, 1986). Thus, the non-levodopa-medicated PD patients in Canter's study may have had higher F0 values because they were demonstrating increased levels of clinical severity.

Acoustic studies of F0 variation have been consistent with the numerous perceptual

studies demonstrating that monopitch is a feature of the dysarthria in PD speech. That is, PD patients have been found to have a reduced range of F0 in connected speech (Canter, 1965; Ludlow & Bassich, 1984) and on tests of maximum F0 range (Canter, 1965a; Ludlow & Bassich, 1984), when compared to normal speakers. In addition, it appears that there may be a gradual reduction in the range of F0 in connected speech as the severity of PD increases (Metter & Hanson, 1986).

Voice Quality/Phonatory Function

Maximum phonation time (MPT). The results of studies of MPT in PD have been inconsistent. While some studies have indicated that PD patients have reduced MPTs (Boshes, 1966; Canter, 1965b), others have suggested that PD patients have MPT values similar to those of age-equivalent normal subjects (Buck & Cooper, 1956; Kruel, 1972; Ramig, Horii, & Rosenbek, 1987). While these differences may reflect differences in the characteristics of the patient populations that were studied (ie, severity level, symptom profiles, etc), it is also likely that the methods of testing MPT influenced these results. Previous reports suggest that MPT values are highly variable and significantly influenced by the testing procedures and the amount of practice that subjects receive (Kent, Kent, & Rosenbek, 1987).

Standard deviation of F0 (SDF0). SDF0 is one of a number of acoustic measures of voice quality that has been examined in PD. Unlike measures of F0 variation over phrase-length or sentence-length utterances, SDF0 is a measure of F0 variation over a short period (1 to 3 seconds) of steady phonation (ie, prolonged vowel). SDF0 values have been found to be higher and more variable in PD patients than in normal speakers (Ramig, Scherer, & Titze, 1988; Zwirner et al, 1991). In addition, SDF0 is significantly correlated with perceptual judgments of dysphonia in PD (Zwirner et al, 1991).

Jitter and shimmer. These acoustic measures reflect cycle-to-cycle variations in the duration (jitter) and amplitude (shimmer) of the voice signal. PD patients have been found to have significantly higher and more variable (across patient) jitter values than normals (Ramig et al, 1988; Zwirner et al, 1991). Shimmer values have been reported to be either higher (Ramig et al, 1988) or equal to those of normals (Zwirner et al, 1991). In addition, when repeated measures were obtained over a period of several hours, PD patients were found to demonstrate more variable jitter and shimmer values than age-equivalent normals (Winckel & Adams, 1992).

Signal/Noise Ratio (S/N). The acoustic voice signal contains a certain amount of noise energy. Normal voices have low levels of noise whereas many abnormal voices show greater noise levels (Colton & Casper, 1990). S/N is a measure of the relative amount of noise energy that is present in the voice signal. S/N was originally developed as an acoustic measure of vocal hoarseness (Yumoto, 1983). S/N values have been found to be either higher (Ramig et al, 1988) or not significantly different from those of normal subjects (Zwirner et al, 1991).

Vocal tremor. Tremor, in the range of 3 to 7 Hz, has been observed in the acoustic voice signals of PD patients (Ludlow, Bassich, Connor, & Coulter, 1986; Philippbar, Robin, & Luschei, 1989; Ramig et al, 1988). When present, the tremor is more likely to affect the frequency domain than the amplitude domain of the acoustic voice signal (Ludlow et al, 1986; Philippbar et al, 1989). The presence of vocal tremor in the acoustic signal can create problems in the interpretation of other acoustic measures, such as jitter and shimmer; however, a number of procedures have been developed to deal with this problem (Ludlow et al, 1986; Winholtz & Ramig, 1992).

Imprecise Consonant Articulation
Several acoustic studies have provided information regarding the potential acoustic correlates of imprecise consonant articulation in PD speech. Three such acoustic correlates are spirantization, spectral tilt, and the tim-

ing of vocal onsets and offsets. Spirantization is the presence of fricative-like, aperiodic noise during stop closures. PD patients have been found to produce an abnormal amount of spirantization particularly during bilabial stops (Weismer, 1984). Spectral tilt refers to the relative distribution of energy (ie, high versus low frequencies) in the spectra of stop and fricative consonants. PD patients appear to produce fricatives such as /s/ and /sh/ with an abnormal distribution of spectral energy. In particular, the fricative spectra obtained from PD patients can show an overall tilt toward the lower frequencies (Uziel et al, 1975; Weismer, 1984). It is possible that both spirantization and low frequency spectral tilt are the acoustic correlates of the stop and fricative distortions that have been described in previous perceptual studies (Cramer, 1940; Logemann et al, 1978). Future studies are required to further elucidate the relationship between these perceptual and acoustic variables.

Weismer (1984) reported that PD patients produce a significant amount of voicing during the normally voiceless closure interval of voiceless stops. Consistent with this, Ackermann and Ziegler (1991) showed that sound intensity levels during stop closures are significantly higher in PD patients than in normals (presumably due to voicing into closure). Furthermore, these higher intensity levels during stop closures were significantly correlated ($r = .64$) with perceptual ratings of the PD patients' severity of articulatory imprecision (Ackermann & Ziegler, 1991).

Forrest et al (1989) reported longer voice onset times (VOT) in PD patients, relative to normal subjects, and suggested that this may reflect a movement initiation problem (a classic movement deficit in PD) at the level of the larynx. Similarly, Ludlow and Bassich (1984) and Kruel (1972) found that PD patients were significantly impaired on vowel repetition tasks that required the rapid repetition of on-off phonations.

Diadochokinetics (DDKs). Studies of diadochokinesis provide additional information about consonant articulations in PD. Several studies have examined the DDK rate of stop consonant syllables in PD (Canter, 1965a; Kruel, 1972; Ludlow, Conner, & Bassich, 1987). Two of these studies found no differences between PD patients and normals for DDKs involving the voiceless plosives /p/, /t/, and /k/ (Kruel, 1972; Ludlow et al, 1987). In contrast, a third study found that PD patients had significantly reduced repetition rates for DDKs involving the voiced plosives /b/, /d/, and /g/, relative to normal speakers (Canter, 1965a). A number of factors could have given rise to these discrepant results, including the use of voiced versus voiceless DDKs, and other factors related to DDK testing procedures (for further discussion see Kent et al, 1987).

Rate of Speech
Consistent with the results of perceptual studies, acoustic studies have indicated that a small proportion of PD patients produce speech segments that are shorter in duration and therefore more rapid than those of normals. For example, Canter (1963) found that although PD patients as a group had median phrase and syllable durations that were no different from those of normals, 1 of 17 PD patients examined had abnormally short segment durations. Both short segment and transition durations have been reported in the speech of a small proportion of PD patients (Forrest et al, 1989; Uziel et al, 1975; Weismer, 1984; Weismer et al, 1985).

As mentioned previously, PD patients have difficulty modifying their speech rate when they are requested to speak more rapidly. However, when PD patients do achieve faster rates of speech, the relative timing of words within phrases is preserved and remains equivalent to that of normal (Ludlow et al, 1987; Volkmann, Hefter, & Lange, 1992).

Physiological Findings

Respiratory/Aerodynamic

PD patients have been reported to show reduced values on many measures of aerodynamic function including (1) a reduction in the total amount of air expended during maximum phonation tasks (Mueller, 1971); (2) reduced intraoral air pressure during CV productions (Marquardt, 1973; Mueller, 1971; Solomon & Hixon, 1993); and (3) reduced vital capacity (Cramer, 1940; De la Torre, Mier, & Boshes, 1960; Laszewski, 1956). It has been suggested that PD patients may fail to generate sufficient aerodynamic energy necessary for normal speech (Mueller, 1971).

In addition to overall reductions in aerodynamic function, there is also evidence of increased aerodynamic variability and abnormal airflow patterns in PD (Schiffman, 1985; Vincken, Gauthier, & Dollfuss, 1984). For example, Vincken et al (1984) identified two types of airflow abnormalities in PD patients during maximal inspiratory and expiratory tasks: Type A involved regular, tremor-like oscillations (4 to 8 Hz) in airflow, while Type B was characterized by an irregular, rapidly changing pattern of airflow and brief periods of zero airflow. Vincken et al (1984) suggested that these airflow abnormalities may reflect variations in airflow resistance caused by abnormal movements of glottic and supraglottic structures. However, respiratory kinematic and EMG studies suggest that these airflow abnormalities may also be the result of irregularities in chest wall movement and respiratory muscle activation patterns (Estenne, Hubert, & Troyer, 1984; Murdoch, Chenery, & Bowler, 1989). For example, Murdoch et al (1989) noted that PD patients demonstrated highly unusual chest wall kinematics including marked irregularities in the rate and amplitude of individual respiratory excursions, and "paradoxical" inspiratory events during sustained vowels and syllable repetitions. More recently, Solomon and Hixon (1993) noted that, at the initiation of speech breath groups, PD patients had relatively smaller rib cage volumes and larger abdominal volumes than normal subjects. It was suggested that this may reflect a relative reduction in the compliance of the rib cage in PD. Increases in abdominal excursions were suggested to reflect the PD patient's attempt to compensate for this reduction in rib cage compliance.

Interestingly, Solomon and Hixon (1993) found little variation in the PD patients' respiratory patterns across different points in the levodopa drug cycle. They suggested that drug-cycle-related fluctuations in motor performance may not have a substantial effect on speech breathing in PD.

Laryngeal

Few physiologic data are available on laryngeal function in PD. A small number of electroglottographic and laryngoscopic studies have reported (1) alterations in vocal fold kinematics, (2) vocal fold asymmetry and bowing, and (3) vocal fold paralysis in PD.

Electroglottography (EGG)
Gerratt, Hanson, and Berke (1987) provided a description of the EGG signals obtained from one PD patient. The patient had an abnormally large speed quotient value (opening/closing ratio = 2.9), and a poorly defined closing period, suggesting that the vocal folds were opening slowly, relative to the rate of closure, and that there may have been inadequate or incomplete closure of the vocal folds. In Uziel et al's (1975) study of 18 PD patients, EGG waveforms were reported to be reduced in amplitude relative to those of normals. It was hypothesized that these reduced EGG signals reflected reduced laryngeal movements caused by a hypertonia of the laryngeal musculature.

Laryngoscopy
Hanson, Gerratt, and Ward (1984) observed abnormal laryngeal signs in PD patients who underwent laryngoscopic examinations. The most prominent sign was bowed vocal folds which occurred to varying degrees in 30 of the 32 PD patients examined. During phonation, the bowed vocal folds were noted to vibrate with a greater width and a greater amount of glottic aperture than is normally observed. In 26/30 of the PD patients a laryngeal asymmetry was noted. This asymmetry was frequently associated with one side showing (1) a more posterior position of the vocal process, (2) a more posterior and

lateral position of the apex of the arytenoid, and (3) a more contracted ventricular fold than is seen in normal speakers. The side demonstrating these laryngeal signs consistently corresponded to the side of the body that was most affected by the disease. With disease progression, it is known that PD patients experience an increasing degree of bilateral limb impairment, and this tendency toward bilateral involvement appears to be paralleled in the laryngeal system. A number of studies have reported bilateral vocal fold paralysis, particularly in the late stages of PD (Holinger, Holinger, & Holinger, 1976; Huppler, Schmidt, & Devine, 1955; Plasse & Liberman, 1981; Schley, Fenton, & Niimi, 1982).

Velopharyngeal

Aerodynamic and kinematic studies have indicated that the amplitudes of velopharyngeal movements are reduced in PD (Hirose, Kiritani, & Ushijima, 1981; Hoodin & Gilbert, 1989a,b). Furthermore, the degree of velopharyngeal impairment appears to be positively correlated with disease severity (Hoodin & Gilbert, 1989a,b).

Orofacial

Jaw Kinematics
Several studies have described abnormalities in the lip and jaw movements of PD patients during speech and nonspeech tasks (Caligiuri, 1987, 1989; Conner & Abbs, 1991; Conner et al, 1989; Forrest et al, 1989; Hirose, 1986; Hirose et al, 1981; Hunker, Abbs, & Barlow, 1982). Studies of jaw movement have consistently reported that, relative to normals, PD patients show a significant reduction in the size and peak velocity of jaw movements during speech (Conner et al, 1989; Forrest et al, 1989). Forrest et al (1989) indicated that jaw movements of PD patients were, on average, approximately half the size of the jaw movements observed in normal subjects. Interestingly, the durations of jaw movements during speech produced by PD patients and normals were not significantly

different. Thus, the PD group exhibited normal speed of speech-related jaw movements. This finding is of interest in comparison to data reported by Connor and Abbs (1991). When PD patients were asked to produce visually-guided, nonspeech jaw movements, their jaw movements were significantly slower than those of normal subjects. Taken together, the studies by Forrest et al (1989) and Connor and Abbs (1991) suggest the possiblity that certain kinematic impairments in PD, in this case bradykinesia, may be task-dependent. This notion of task specificity may help to explain the clinical observation that PD patients with significant limb and oral nonspeech bradykinesia frequently demonstrate speech rates that are within normal limits.

Lip Kinematics
Studies of lip movements in PD have been somewhat inconsistent. While reduced amplitude and peak velocity of lower lip movements during speech have been reported in PD (Caligiuri, 1987, 1989a,b; Forrest et al, 1989; Hirose et al, 1981; Hunker et al, 1982), normal lower lip kinematic patterns for speech also have been observed (Conner et al, 1989). This inconsistency may reflect the fact that different experimental approaches have been employed across studies, including bite-block versus non-bite-block speech, connected speech versus syllable repetitions, and jaw-referenced versus non-jaw-referenced lower lip movements.

Other movement abnormalities of the lower lip that have been noted in PD include (1) an increase in the ratio of movement amplitude to peak velocity (Forrest et al, 1989); (2) reductions in the deceleration phase of movements (Forrest et al, 1989); and (3) reversals in the normal sequencing of lower lip and jaw movements (Conner et al, 1989).

Two studies have examined the relationship between reduced size of lower lip movements and rigidity in PD, by measuring passive lip stiffness (Caligiuri, 1987, 1989b; Hunker et al, 1982). Whereas Hunker et al (1982) reported a significant positive relationship between passive lip stiffness and la-

bial hypometria (ie, decreased movement amplitude), Caligiuri (1987, 1989b) failed to observe a relationship. Taken together, these findings support the view that, while rigidity and hypometria may co-occur in PD, the two variables do not appear to be causally related.

To date, only one investigation has examined the effects of antiparkinsonian levodopa medication on oral speech kinematics (Caligiuri, 1989b). Caligiuri (1989b) reported that PD patients who exhibited reduced lip displacements and peak velocities prior to medication showed significant increases in both parameters shortly after levodopa medication. Additional research is needed to determine a comprehensive profile of the effects of various levels of levodopa on the movement patterns involved in speech production in PD.

Force Stability and the Effects of Tremor
Studies of orofacial force control have indicated that PD patients produce decreased maximum voluntary lip closing forces (Wood, Hughes, & Hayes, 1992) and increased instability on isometric force tasks (Abbs, Hartman, & Vishwanat, 1987; Barlow & Abbs, 1983). Increases in force instability appear to become more pronounced when PD patients were required to produce increasingly higher levels of isometric force. Furthermore, the degree of force instability differs across various orofacial structures. For example, Abbs et al (1987) reported that, for a given target isometric force, the tongue showed greater force instability than the lip, which, in turn, showed greater instability than the jaw (Abbs et al, 1987; Barlow & Abbs, 1983). While these isometric force studies have been interpreted as showing differential force impairments across orofacial structures in PD, it also has been suggested that force instability measures may be differentially affected by the degree of tremor present in each structure (Abbs, 1990; Weismer, 1990). This possibility is supported by the results of a study by Philippbar et al (1989). They found that, in PD patients with tremor in two or more

structures, there was a different dominant tremor frequency in each structure. Based on this finding, they suggest that a peripheral mechanism, as opposed to a central mechanism, may play an important role in the generation of PD postural tremor (see Rack & Ross, 1986, for a further discussion of peripheral mechanisms in PD tremor). In contrast, Hunker and Abbs (1984) examined orofacial resting tremor, and reported that PD patients showed similar resting tremor frequencies across different orofacial structures. They interpreted the finding as an indication that PD resting tremor may be caused by a central mechanism possibly involving an aberrant neural oscillator (Hunker & Abbs, 1984).

Electromyographic (EMG)
Orofacial EMG studies of speech in PD have reported two major abnormalities: (1) increased levels of tonic resting and background EMG activity in both lip and jaw muscles (Hunker & Abbs, 1984; Leanderson, Meyerson, & Persson, 1971, 1972; Moore & Scudder, 1989; Netsell, Daniel, & Celesia, 1975); and (2) loss of reciprocity with increased EMG coactivation patterns in functionally antagonistic lip and jaw muscle groups (Hirose, 1986; Hirose et al, 1981; Hunker & Abbs, 1984; Leanderson et al, 1971, 1972). Some authors have suggested that these abnormal EMG patterns are associated with the Parkinsonian symptom of rigidity. In addition, there is evidence that these abnormal EMG patterns become more apparent as the disease progresses (Leanderson et al, 1971). Levodopa medication is reported to produce a reduction in these abnormal EMG patterns in some PD patients (Leanderson et al, 1971).

Another finding to emerge from EMG studies is that there may be deficits in orofacial reflex function in PD. Caligiuri and Abbs (1987) measured lower lip EMG activity (orbicularis oris inferior) and found that the magnitude of the short-latency component of the perioral reflex was greater in PD patients than in normals. They suggested that this apparent increase in the sensitivity of the perioral reflex may be related to a more generalized impairment in oral sensorimotor function in PD (Caligiuri & Abbs, 1987; Caligiuri, Heindel, & Lohr, 1992).

Sensorimotor Testing
Whereas PD traditionally has been viewed as primarily a disease of motor output, recent evidence suggests the presence of sensory and sensorimotor deficits in PD (Koller, 1984; Schneider & Lidsky, 1987; Schneider, Diamond, & Markham, 1986; Snider, Fahn, & Isgreen, 1976; Tatton, Eastman, & Bedinghm, 1984). Tatton et al (1984) have proposed a causal link between sensorimotor impairment and the major motor symptoms of PD. More specifically, they hypothesized that bradykinesia, rigidity, and decreased movement repertoire in PD are related to an abnormal processing of the mechanoreceptor sensory inputs used in the generation and execution of movements. Subsequent studies in the orofacial system have provided support for this sensorimotor hypothesis (Schneider & Lidsky, 1987; Schneider et al, 1986). Relative to normals, PD patients have been found to produce a greater number of errors on tests of orofacial sensorimotor integration such as jaw proprioception, lingual localization, and motor tracking of orofacial stimuli (Schneider et al, 1986). Additional studies are required to determine what impact these sensorimotor deficits have on orofacial motor performance in PD.

Of potential importance to our understanding of PD speech disorders is the investigation of auditory-motor integration deficits in PD. Recent studies of auditory function in PD indicate that PD patients exhibit a hyperactive stapedial reflex (Murofushi, Yamane, & Osanai, 1992) and deficits in the temporal discrimination of auditory stimuli (Artieda, Pastor, & Lacruz, 1992). The relationship between these abnormalities in auditory function and the speech production deficits associated with PD remains poorly understood. While a number of reports have addressed the relationship between PD patients' speech prosody deficits and their perception of speech prosody (Blonder, Gur, & Ruben, 1989; Caekebeke,

1991; Darkins, Fromkin, & Benson, 1988; Hartman & Abbs, 1985; Scott & Caird, 1985; Scott, Caird, & Williams, 1984), no clear relationship has emerged.

Given the evidence suggesting sensory and sensorimotor deficits in PD, it would seem important for future treatment studies to examine the influence of sensory manipulations on speech performance in PD.

Treatment of Hypokinetic Dysarthria in Parkinson's Disease

Pharmacological and Surgical Treatments

Prior to the discovery in the late 1960s that levodopa medication could be used to treat most of the major symptoms of PD (Cotzias et al, 1967, 1969), a surgical procedure referred to as thalamotomy was commonly used in the treatment of PD. Thalamotomy typically involves the placement of a lesion in the region of the ventrolateral thalamus using high frequency electrical current passed through a stimulating electrode (Van Buren & Ratcheson, 1982). Several studies have reported significant speech impairments in PD patients following both unilateral and bilateral thalamotomy (Bell, 1968; Gillingham, Kalyanaraman, & Donaldson, 1964; Jenkins, 1968; Laitinen, 1972; Selby, 1967; Van Buren, Li, & Shapiro, 1972). For example, Bell (1968) noted that dysarthria developed in more than 50% (34/72) of his thalamotomy cases. In a comparison of the effects of thalamotomy and levodopa, Quaglieri and Celesia (1977) found that PD patients who had undergone thalamotomy had more severe speech impairments than PD patients who had received only levodopa therapy.

During the early 1970s, when many PD patients were beginning to receive levodopa medication, a number of studies examining the effects of levodopa on speech were reported (Critchley, 1981; Mawdsley, 1973; Mawdsley & Gamsu, 1971; Nakano, Zubick, & Tyley, 1973; Rigrodsky & Morrison, 1970; Wolfe, Garvin, & Bacon, 1975; Yaryura-Tobias, Diamond, & Merlis, 1971). Most of these studies measured speech based on perceptual evaluations. Levodopa medication was associated with the following perceived changes in the PD patients' speech: (1) increased intelligibility (Mawdsley & Gamsu, 1971; Nakano et al, 1973); (2) increased overall adequacy of speech (Mawdsley, 1973); (3) improved speech rate and fluency (Rigrodsky & Morrison, 1970); and (4) improved voice quality, articulation, and pitch variation (Wolfe et al, 1975).

Improvements in several acoustic measures of speech also were associated with levodopa medication, including (1) more regular periods of phonation and more distinct pauses between periods of phonation (Mawdsley & Gamsu, 1971); (2) increased verbal response time (Yaryura-Tobias et al, 1971); and (3) increased maximum phonation time and vocal intensity (Mawdsley & Gamsu, 1971).

The results from most of these early studies provide fairly consistent evidence of the beneficial effects of levodopa medication on speech in PD. However, several investigators have also noted that levodopa medication can be associated with speech deficits such as palilalia, oral dyskinesias, and dysphonia in isolated cases (Ackermann, Ziegler, & Oertel, 1989; Critchley, 1976). Furthermore, levodopa-related improvements in PD speech symptoms are often much less apparent than the improvements observed in most of the other physical symptoms of PD (Rigrodsky & Morrison, 1970; Wolfe et al, 1975). Interestingly, recent studies have suggested that, for patients who have had PD for more than 10 years, speech symptoms can begin to show a selective resistance to levodopa medication (Bonnet, Loria, & Saint-Hilaire, 1987; Klawans, 1986). This finding underscores the potential importance of speech management during the later stages (+10 years) of PD.

Behavioral, Biofeedback, and Prosthetic Treatments

A variety of methods have been employed in attempts to improve the speech of PD patients including traditional, perceptually based behavioral speech therapy, instrumentally based biofeedback therapy, and prosthetic or assistive speech devices. Regardless of the method of choice, treatment typically has aimed at one or several of the following: (1) increasing speech intensity, (2) improving speech prosody (ie, monotonous/monoloud speech), (3) reducing rapid speech, and (4) increasing articulatory mobility and precision.

Behavioral Treatments

Prior to 1980, very few studies addressed the use of behavioral speech therapy in PD (Allen, 1970; Sarno, 1968). Those that did typically did not provide detailed descriptions of the treatment methods and the measures of treatment outcome employed. For example, Sarno (1968) reported on the treatment of over 300 PD patients who had received 6 months of biweekly behavioral speech therapy focused on intensity control, facial mobility, and speech articulator mobility. However, the specific treatment protocol was not described, and treatment outcome was limited to general clinical impressions. Sarno (1968) suggested that the PD patients showed some improvements in speech production during the treatment sessions but failed to transfer these changes to situations outside the clinical setting. While Sarno (1968) did not provide evidence in support of this conclusion, the problem of "transfer of treatment" has been addressed by several other investigators and appears to be one of the most important issues in the treatment of PD speech. This issue will be discussed in more detail in a separate section.

Since 1980, several treatment studies have provided more detailed descriptions of the speech therapy procedures and measures of treatment outcome employed with PD patients (Perry & Das, 1981; Ramig et al, 1991; Robertson & Thomson, 1984; Scott & Caird, 1981, 1983). Robertson and Thomson (1984) reported on 12 PD patients who received 2 weeks (30 to 40 hours) of intensive group speech therapy focused on improving (1) respiratory control and capacity; (2) control of pitch variation and vocal loudness; (3) range, strength, and speed of speech and nonspeech oral movements; and (4) control of speech rate. A perceptual rating (0–4 scale) of eight dysarthric speech parameters was used to measure treatment outcome. Each patient's speech was rated, in the clinic, prior to therapy, immediately following therapy, and at 3 months posttherapy. The results of the study suggested that these PD patients showed significant improvements on all eight speech parameters immediately following therapy and at 3 months posttreatment.

Ramig et al (1991) studied 40 PD patients who received 4 weeks of intensive speech therapy (1 hour/day, 4 days/week) focused on: (1) increasing vocal loudness and vocal fold adduction through pushing and lifting techniques; (2) increasing maximum phonation time; (3) increasing fundamental frequency range; and (4) improving vocal steadiness during vowel prolongations. Audio recordings of the patients' speech were made in the clinic before and after the therapy program. Two speech pathologists' perceptual ratings (visual analogue scale) of the patients' recorded speech revealed significant improvements in loudness (31.5%), monotony of speech (30%), and intelligibility (20.5%). Acoustic analyses revealed significant increases in (1) maximum phonation time (26%); (2) maximum fundamental frequency range (14%); (3) F0 variation (12%, males only); and (4) average F0 (5%, males only). In addition to these measures, which were determined from the patients' speech in the clinic, patients' self-ratings and spouses' ratings were also obtained. These latter measures could be expected to reflect the PD patients' speech performance outside the clinical setting. The results from these rating scales were equivocal. Only 27/40 of the treated patients provided self-ratings. For these 27 patients, the only measure to show a significant increase was loudness (12%). Interestingly, the untreated control group of 12 PD patients also had a 6% increase on the self-rating of loudness. The spousal ratings, which were obtained from only 17/40 spouses, indicated a significant increase (13%) in the patients' intelligibility. The untreated PD patients also showed a significant improvement of 11% on their spousal ratings of intelligibility.

In summary, the literature on behavioral speech treatment in PD indicates that significant improvements in speech can be obtained on a wide variety of measures within the speech clinic setting. What remains unclear, however, is the extent to which PD patients are able to transfer these improvements to situations outside of the clinic.

Instrumental Biofeedback Treatments

Several reports have examined the effectiveness of biofeedback for the treatment of PD speech disorders (Hand, Burns, & Ireland, 1979; Johnson & Pring, 1990; Netsell & Cleeland, 1973; Rubow & Swift, 1985; Scott & Caird, 1981, 1983; Yorkston, Beukelman, & Bell, 1988). Many of the speech dimensions that are most impaired in PD, such as pitch variation, speech loudness, and speech rate, can be easily transduced and displayed using a variety of simple laboratory instruments. These include pitch meters, sound pressure meters, and oscilloscopes. In addition, a variety of relatively inexpensive computer-based programs which provide real-time displays of pitch and loudness, such as Kay Elemetrics' Visipitch (see Fig. 12–1), are becoming standard instruments in the clinical setting.

Scott and Caird (1983) compared the effectiveness of speech therapy with and without visual biofeedback. The therapy involved an intensive period of prosodic exercises (10 1-hour sessions in 2 weeks) aimed at improving pitch and loudness variation. A voice-operated light source (Vocalite) provided visual biofeedback about these prosodic dimensions. Ratings of the patients' prosodic abnormality (0–7 scale), obtained before and after treatment, indicated that patients who received prosodic exercises alone showed a 33% improvement, while patients who received prosodic exercises plus visual biofeedback demonstrated a 45% improvement on ratings of speech prosody.

Johnson and Pring (1990) used intensive visual biofeedback therapy in attempts to

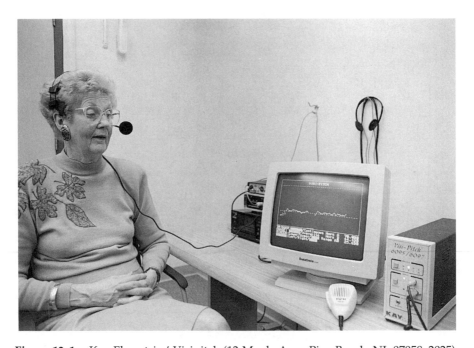

Figure 12–1. Kay Elemetrics' Visipitch (12 Maple Ave., Pine Brook, NJ, 07058–2025).

modify abnormal speech prosody and re-duced speech intensity in six PD patients. Patients received 10 1-hour therapy sessions over a 4-week period. Biofeedback was provided through a computer program (Visispeech), and audio recordings of the patients' speech, before and after therapy, were used to obtain perceptual ratings (Frenchay Dysarthria Scale) and acoustic measures. Following therapy, the PD patients showed significant improvements on the perceptual ratings and on a number of acoustic measures including maximum intensity level and range, intensity during conversation and reading, and maximum pitch range.

These studies suggest that: (1) improvements in the speech of PD patients can be achieved through biofeedback therapy; (2) these improvements can be measured in the clinical setting through the use of both perceptual and acoustic procedures; and (3) improvements achieved through behavioral therapy plus biofeedback are greater than improvements achieved with behavioral therapy alone. As in the case of the behavioral treatment studies discussed previously, reports on the use of biofeedback generally have not demonstrated that improvements in speech are transferred beyond the clinical setting. One exception is a study by Rubow and Swift (1985) in which objective, instrumental measures of PD speech outside of the clinic following treatment were provided. Rubow and Swift (1985) used intensive visual biofeedback therapy to treat one PD patient whose speech was characterized by low speech intensity. The patient received 18 sessions of visual biofeedback regarding his speech intensity and progressed through a hierarchy of structured tasks until he demonstrated improved speech intensity within the clinical setting. In order to obtain measures of speech outside of the clinic, the patient was fit with a small portable computer that recorded his speech intensity throughout the day. Out-of-clinic measures of speech intensity were obtained before and after the period of intensive biofeedback therapy. Rubow and Swift (1985) reported that intensive biofeedback therapy produced little

improvement in the patient's speech intensity outside of the clinical setting. While this study was limited to the examination of only one PD patient, it is extremely important because it provides the first objective, instrumental evidence that PD patients may be experiencing significant difficulty transferring the beneficial effects of speech therapy into speaking situations outside of the clinical setting.

Determining that there has been a transfer of treatment to conversational situations outside of the clinic is a common concern in the treatment of most communication disorders. However, some of the cognitive and sensorimotor deficits associated with PD suggest that the generalization of new speech strategies into habitual speech may be particularly difficult for these patients (McNamara, Obler, & Durso, 1992; Saint-Cyr, Taylor, & Lang, 1988; Schneider et al, 1986). For example, Saint-Cyr et al (1988) found that PD is characterized by a specific cognitive deficit wherein the patient has difficulty learning new procedures or "habits." It is possible that this "procedural learning deficit" is the reason that many PD patients have difficulty generalizing new speech behaviors into situations outside the clinic. If this is the case, then the use of traditional, behaviorally oriented speech therapy techniques that rely on the patient's ability to establish new habitual patterns of speech, may need to be reconsidered.

Assistive Device Treatments
One means of circumventing the transfer of treatment problem in PD is through the use of assistive speech devices. Like other prosthetic devices (eg, eye glasses, hearing aids), assistive speech devices can provide an immediate benefit to the patient's communication, and they will remain effective for as long as the patient continues to wear them. In addition, most assistive devices require a minimum amount of patient instruction and training. This means that the patient is not required to establish new habitual patterns of behavior. Because of this, assistive devices may prove to be particularly effective forms

of treatment for parkinsonian speech disorders.

One of the most commonly prescribed assistive devices used in the treatment of speech deficits associated with PD is the portable voice amplifier (see Fig. 12–2). In spite of their widespread use, very little data is available on the prevalence of voice amplifier use among PD patients or on the relative effectiveness of the various voice amplifiers that are currently being recommended to PD patients. Yorkston et al (1988, p 264) described one PD patient with low voice intensity who was provided with a voice amplifier after he failed to transfer the gains made in therapy to situations outside of the speech

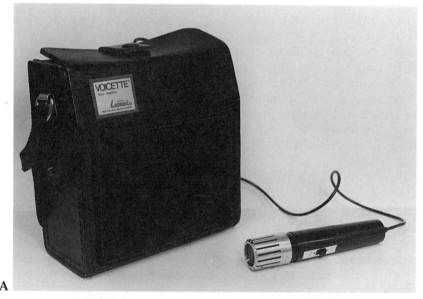

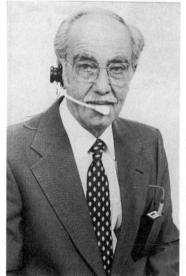

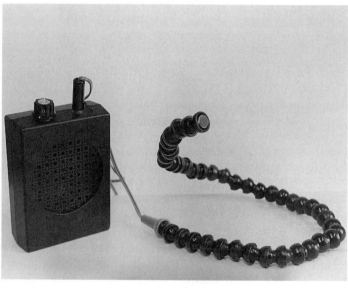

Figure 12–2. Voice amplifiers: (a) Voicette Amplifier (A.S. Telecom, 9915 St. Vital, Montreal, Quebec, Canada H1H 4S5); (b) Park Surgical JM010 Amplifier (5001 New Utrecht Ave., Brooklyn, NY 11219). (c) Flex-mike amplifier (Audiology Associates, 5991 Spring Garden Rd., Suite 230, Halifax, Nova Scotia, Canada B3H 1Y6).

clinic. While this case report suggests that the voice amplifier may have provided a solution to this patient's transfer of treatment difficulties, no data regarding the patient's effective use of this device were presented. In PD patients who have been fit with voice amplifiers, it would be useful to examine (1) the amount of time that the amplifier is worn each day, (2) the average level of speech intensity that is produced, and (3) the level of communicative success (ie, the number of requests to repeat or clarify) that is attained while wearing the amplification device.

Rubow and Swift (1985) used a portable assistive (biofeedback) device with one PD patient in order to facilitate the transfer of increased speech intensity into situations outside of the clinic setting. The assistive device monitored the patient's conversational speech and provided a warning tone, through a miniature earphone, whenever his intensity level fell below a predetermined (60 dB) intensity level. The authors monitored the patient's out-of-clinic conversations, through the use of a portable microcomputer, and determined the amount of time that his speech intensity fell below the target level (60 dB). Out-of-clinic measures, made before and after fitting the assistive biofeedback device, demonstrated a significant improvement in the patient's out-of-clinic speech intensity when he was wearing the assistive device. While this study was limited to a single patient, the recent development of a commercially available portable intensity biofeedback device, by Wintronix (see Fig. 12–3), will make it relatively easy for clinicians to evaluate the efficacy of this type of assistive device on larger numbers of PD patients.

Another assistive speech device that has been used in treating the rapid speech that is associated with PD is the portable delayed auditory feedback (DAF) device (see Fig. 12–4) (Adams, 1993; Downie, Low, & Lindsay, 1981a,b; Hanson & Metter, 1983; Yorkston et al, 1988). Auditory feedback delays in the range of 50 to 150 msec have been shown to produce a dramatic slowing of speech rate. For example, Hanson and Metter (1983) ex-

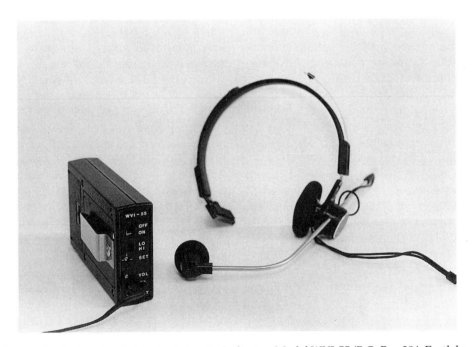

Figure 12–3. Wintronix's Voice Intensity Indicator, Model WVI-55 (P.O. Box 384, Eastlake, CO 80614).

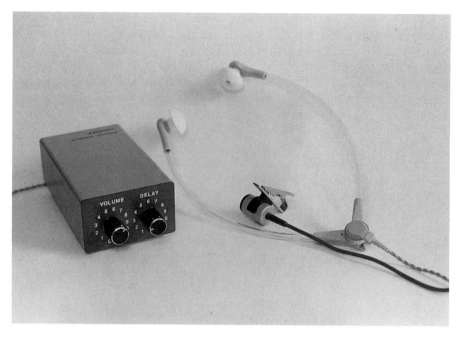

Figure 12–4. Phonic Ear's Delayed Auditory Feedback device, Model PM505 (250 Camino Alto, Mill Valley, CA 94941).

amined the effects of DAF (150 ms delay) in two PD patients with rapid speech. Measures of speech rate, speech intensity, and intelligibility (rated on a 1–7 scale) were obtained four times over a 3-month interval. Across the 3 months of testing, DAF produced consistent and significant reductions (25 to 30%) in the patients' speech rates and also improved the patients' speech intensity and intelligibility. As with behavioral and biofeedback approaches to speech therapy, out-of-clinic measures of the effect of the DAF device are needed. However, reports that have included PD patients' personal accounts suggest that the benefits of DAF can be maintained outside of the clinic for periods of at least 2 years (Adams, 1993; Downie et al, 1981a).

DAF appears to require little patient instruction beyond the procedures for fitting and operating the device. Yorkston et al (1988) have suggested that, in order to maximize the effectiveness of DAF, patients should be instructed to (1) produce the first word of a sentence with relatively strong in-

tensity; (2) speak in full sentences rather than single words; and (3) avoid trying to "overdrive" the effects of DAF. This third point refers to the observation that some patients may attempt to compensate for the DAF by speaking more rapidly. While this initial resistance to DAF is usually brief, some patients may need to be instructed to "allow" the DAF to slow their speech.

Several other assistive devices have been offered as alternatives to DAF for the treatment of rapid speech in PD (Beukelman & Yorkston, 1977; Hammen, Yorkston, & Beukelman, 1989; Helm, 1979; Lang & Fishbein, 1983; Yorkston et al, 1988, 1990). Helm (1979) reported improvements in one PD patient's rapid speech and palilalia when he employed a pacing board. The pacing board consisted of a narrow board with seven dividers equally spaced along its one foot length. The patient tapped from left to right between the dividers as he spoke each syllable. This syllable-by-syllable tapping caused a significant reduction in the patient's speaking rate. The pacing board has the ad-

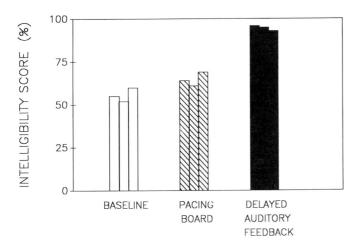

Figure 12–5. Intelligibility scores obtained for one patient with hypokinetic dysarthria during baseline, pacing board, and DAF conditions (the three bars correspond to the scores from three listeners).

vantage of being less expensive than DAF devices (DAF is approximately $700) (Lang & Fishbein, 1983).

Recent studies in the author's laboratory have focused on comparing the relative effectiveness of these rate reduction techniques. The intelligibility scores for one patient's speech (patient is described in a previous study [Adams, 1993]) while using either a DAF device or a pacing board are shown in Figure 12–5. DAF was associated with significantly higher intelligibility scores. This appeared to be related to the patient's production of rapid and festinating finger tapping movements which interfered with his consistent use of the pacing board.

Another pacing technique involving finger tapping while speaking is the paced alphabet board technique (Beukelman & Yorkston, 1977; Yorkston et al, 1988). In this technique, the patient must touch the first letter of each word on a small portable alphabet board before it is spoken. The time taken to find and move to each new letter will produce a significant reduction in speaking rate. This pacing procedure may be useful for PD patients who demonstrate both rapid speech and festinating limb movements.

A final rate reduction technique that has been used in attempts to reduce speaking rate in PD involves the use of computer-generated pacing procedures (Yorkston et al, 1988, 1990). In this technique, PD patients read aloud sentences as they are presented on a computer screen. Yorkston et al (1990) examined several methods of sentence presentation and found that, in the four hypokinetic dysarthric patients they examined, the most effective method was an additive metered presentation. In the additive metered procedure, a sentence was presented word by word across the computer screen, with each word receiving an equal presentation duration. This pacing procedure resulted in significant reductions in speaking rate and increased speech intelligibility scores. Because this assistive device relies on a computer-generated pacer, it is unlikely that it can be incorporated into a portable assistive device. Therefore, its application will largely be restricted to the clinical setting, or possibly to a home computer for the purpose of extended practice. The extent to which PD patients can generalize the gains achieved through this rate reduction procedure to out-of-clinic settings remains to be determined.

Suggested Reading

General Parkinson's Disease

Weiner WJ, Lang AE. (1989). *Movement Disorders; A Comprehensive Survey.* Mount Kisko, NY: Futura.

Jankovic J, Tolosa E. (1993). *Parkinson's Disease and Movement Disorders.* Baltimore: William & Wilkins.

Schneider JS, Lidsky TI. (1987). *Basal Ganglia and Behavior: Sensory Aspects of Motor Functioning.* Toronto, Hans Huber Pub.

Levodopa Medication in Parkinson's Disease

Poewe W. (1993). L-dopa in Parkinson's disease: mechanisms of action and pathophysiology of late failure. In: Jankovic J, Tolosa E, eds. *Parkinson's Disease and Movement Disorders.* Baltimore: William & Wilkins, pp 103–111.

Neurosurgery in Parkinson's Disease

Goetz CG, DeLong MR, Penn RD, et al. (1993). Neurosurgical horizons in Parkinson's disease. *Neurology* 43:1–7.

Hypokinetic Dysarthria

Darley FL, Aronson AE, Brown JR. (1975). *Motor Speech Disorders.* Philadelphia, W.B. Saunders, pp 192–197.

Scott S, Caird FI, Williams BO. (1985). *Communication in Parkinson's Disease.* Rockville: An Aspen Publication, pp 1–113.

Mlcoch AG. (1987). Diagnosis and Treatment of Parkinsonian Dysarthria. In: Koller WC. *Handbook of Parkinson's Disease.* New York: Marcel Dekker Inc., pp 181–207.

Putnam AHB. (1988). Review of Research in Dysarthria. In: Winitz H. ed. *Human Communication and its Disorders, a Review.* Norwood: Ablex Pub., pp 107–223.

Ramig LO. (1992). The role of phonation in speech intelligibility: a review and preliminary data from patients with Parkinson's disease. In: Kent RD. ed. *Intelligibility in Speech Disorders.* Amsterdam, pp 119–155.

References

Abbs JH, Hartman DE, Vishwanat B. (1987). Orofacial motor control impairment in Parkinson's disease. *Neurology* 37:394–398.

Abbs JH. (1990). Orofacial impairment in Parkinson's disease: Reply from the author. *Neurology* 40:192–193.

Ackermann H, Ziegler W, Oertel WH. (1989). Palilalia as a symptom of levodopa induced hyperkinesia in Parkinson's disease. *J Neurol Neurosurg Psychiatry* 52:805–807.

Ackermann H, Ziegler W. (1991). Articulatory deficits in parkinsonian dysarthria: An acoustic analysis. *J Neurol Neurosurg Psychiatry* 54:1093–1098.

Adams SG. (1993). Accelerating speech in a case of hypokinetics dysarthria: Descriptions and treatment. In: Till JA, Beukelman DR, Yorkston KM, eds. *Motor Speech Disorders: Advances in Assessment and Treatment.* Baltimore: Brookes.

Allen CM. (1970). Treatment of non fluent speech resulting from neurological disease—treatment of dysarthria. *Br J Disord Commun* 5(1):3–5.

Artieda J, Pastor MA, Lacruz F. (1992). Temporal discrimination is abnormal in Parkinson's disease. *Brain* 115:199–210.

Atarashi J, Uchida E. (1959). A clinical study of parkinsonism. *Recent Adv Res Nerv Syst* 3:871–882.

Barbeau A, Sourkes TL, Murphy CF. (1962). Les Catecholamines de la Maladie de Parkinson. In: Ajuriaguerra J, ed. *Monoamines et Systeme Nerveux Central.* Geneve: George, pp 247–262.

Barlow SM, Abbs JH. (1983). Force transducers for the evaluation of labial, lingual, and mandibular motor impairments. *J Speech Hear Res* 26(4):616–621.

Bell DS. (1968). Speech functions of the thalamus inferred from effects of thalamotomy. *Brain* 91:619–638.

Beukelman DR, Yorkston KM. (1977). A communication system for the severely dysarthric speaker with an intact language system. *J Speech Hear Disord* 42:265–270.

Birkmayer W, Kiewicz GH: Oder l-dioxyphenylalanin (l-dopa) effekt deim parkinson-syndrom des menschen. *Arch Psychiatr Nervenkr* 203:560–574.

Blonder LX, Gur RE, Ruben CG. (1989). The effects of right and left hemiparkinsonism on prosody. *Brain Language* 36:193–207.

Bonnet AM, Loria Y, Saint-Hilaire MH, et al. (1987). Does long-term aggravation of Parkinson's disease result from nondopaminergic lesions? *Neurology* 37;1539–1542.

Boshes B. (1966). Voice changes in parkinsonism. *J Neurosurg* Suppl 24(1):286–288.

Buck JF, Cooper IS. (1956). Speech problems in Parkinsonian patients undergoing anterior choroidal artery occlusion or chemopallidectomy. *J Am Geriatr Soc* 4:1285–1290.

Caekebeke JFV, Jennekens-Schinkel A, van der

Linden ME, et al. (1991). The interpretation of dysprosody in patients with Parkinson's disease. *J Neurol Neurosurg Psychiatry* 54:145–148.

Caligiuri MP (1989b). Short-term fluctuations in orofacial motor control in Parkinson's disease. In: Yorkston KM, Beukelman DR, eds. *Recent Advances in Clinical Dysarthria.* Boston: College-Hill Press, pp 199–212.

Caligiuri MP, Abbs JH. (1987). Response properties of the perioral reflex in Parkinson's disease. *Exp Neurol* 98:563–572.

Caligiuri MP, Heindel WC, Lohr JB. (1992). Sensorimotor disinhibition in Parkinson's disease: effects of levodopa. *Ann Neurol* 31:53.

Caligiuri MP. (1987). Labial kinematics during speech in patients with parkinsonian rigidity. *Brain* 110:1033–1044.

Caligiuri MP. (1989a). The influence of speaking rate on articulatory hypokinesia in parkinsonian dysarthria. *Brain Language* 36:493–502.

Canter GJ. (1963). Speech characteristics of patients with Parkinson's disease: I. Intensity, pitch, and duration. *J Speech Hear Disord* 28(3):221–229.

Canter GJ. (1965a). Speech characteristics of patients with Parkinson's disease: III. Articulation, diadochokinesis, and over-all speech adequacy. *J Speech Hear Disord* 30(3):217–224.

Canter GJ. (1965b). Speech characteristics of patients with Parkinson's disease: II. Physiological support for speech. *J Speech Hear Disord* 30(1):44–49.

Charcot JM. (1880). *De la paralysie agitante. Lecons sur les maladies du systeme nerveux.* Paris: Recueillies et Publiees par Bourneville.

Colton RH, Casper JK. (1990). *Understanding Voice Problems: A Physiological Perspective for Diagnosis and Treatment.* Baltimore: Williams & Wilkins.

Conner NP, Abbs JH, Cole KJ, et al. (1989). Parkinsonian deficits in serial multiarticulate movements for speech. *Brain* 112:997–1009.

Conner NP, Abbs JH. (1991). Task-dependent variations in parkinsonian motor impairments. *Brain* 114:321–332.

Cotzias GC, Papauasiliou PS, Gellene R. (1969). Modification of parkinsonism—chronic treatment with L-dopa. *N Engl J Med* 280:337–345.

Cotzias GC, Van Woert MH, Schiffer LM. (1967). Aromatic amino acids and modification of parkinsonism. *N Engl J Med* 276:374–378.

Cramer W. (1940). De spaak bij patienten met Parkinsonisme. *Logop Phoniatr* 22:17–23.

Critchley EMR. (1976). Peak-dose dysphonia in parkinsonism. *Lancet* 544.

Critchley EMR. (1981). Speech disorders of parkinsonism: a review. *J Neurol Neurosurg Psychiatry* 44:751–758.

Darkins AW, Fromkin VA, Benson DF. (1988). A characterization of the prosodic loss in Parkinson's disease. *Brain Language* 34:315–327.

Darley FL, Aronson AE, Brown JR. (1969a). Clusters of deviant speech dimensions in the dysarthrias. *J Speech Hear Res* 12(3):462–496.

Darley FL, Aronson AE, Brown JR. (1969b). Differential diagnostic patterns of dysarthria. *J Speech Hear Res* 12(2):246–269.

Darley FL, Aronson AE, Brown JR. (1975). *Motor Speech Disorders.* Philadelphia: W.B. Saunders, pp 192–297.

De la Torre R, Mier M, Boshes B. (1960). Evaluation of respiratory function—preliminary observation. *Q Bull Northwestern Univ Med School* 34:232–236.

Downie AW, Low JM, Lindsay DD. (1981a). Speech disorder in parkinsonism: Usefulness of delayed auditory feedback in selected cases. *Br J Disord Commun* 16.2:135–139.

Downie AW, Low JM, Lindsay DD. (1981b). Speech disorder in parkinsonism: Use of delayed auditory feedback in selected cases. *J Neurol Neurosurg Psychiatry* 44:852–853.

Estenne M, Hubert M, Troyer AD. (1984). Respiratory-muscle involvement in Parkinson's disease. *N Engl J MedI* 311(23):1516.

Forrest K, Weismer G, Turner GS. (1989). Kinematic, acoustic, and perceptual analyses of connected speech produced by parkinsonian and normal geriatric adults. *J Acoust Soc Am* 85(6):2608–2622.

Gerratt BR, Hanson DG, Berke GS. (1987). Glottographic measures of laryngeal function in individuals with abnormal motor control. In: Baer T, Sasaki C, Harris K, eds. *Laryngeal Function in Phonation and Respiration.* Boston: College-Hill Press, pp 521–532.

Gillingham J, Kalyanaraman S, Donaldson A. (1964). Bilateral stereotaxic lesions in the management of parkinsonism and the dyskinesias. *BMJ* 2:656–659.

Golbe LI, Langston JW. (1993). The etiology of Parkinson's disease: New directions for research. In: Jankovic J, Tolosa E, eds.

Parkinson's Disease & Movement Disorders. Baltimore: Williams & Wilkins, pp 93–101.

Grewel F. (1957). Dysarthria in post-encephalitic parkinsonism. *Acta Psychol Neurol Scand* 32(4)440–449.

Hammen VL, Yorkston KM, Beukelman DR. (1989). Pausal and speech duration characteristics as a function of speaking rate in normal and Parkinsonian dysarthric individuals. In: Yorkston KM, Beukelman DR, eds. *Recent Advances in Clinical Dysarthria.* Boston: College-Hill Press, pp 213–224.

Hand CR, Burns MO, Ireland E. (1979). Treatment of hypertonicity in muscles of lip retraction. *Biofeedback Self-Regul* 4(2):171–181.

Hanson DG, Gerratt BR, Ward PH. (1984). Cinegraphic observations of laryngeal function in Parkinson's disease. *Laryngoscope* 94:348–353.

Hanson WR, Metter EJ. (1983). DAF Speech Rate Modification in Parkinson's disease: A report of two cases. In: Berry WR, ed. *Clinical Dysarthria.* San Diego: College-Hill Press, pp 231–251.

Hartman DE, Abbs JH. (1985). Letter to the editor. The response of the apparent receptive speech disorder of Parkinson's disease to speech therapy. *J Neurol Neurosurg Psychiatry* 48:606.

Helm NA. (1979). Management of palilalia with a pacing board. *J Speech Hear Disord* 44:350–353.

Hirose H, Kiritani S, Ushijima T, et al. (1981). Patterns of dysarthric movements in patients with parkinsonism. *Folia Phoniatr* 33:204–215.

Hirose H: Pathophysiology of motor speech disorders (dysarthria). *Folia Phoniatr* 38:61–88.

Holinger LD, Holinger PC, Holinger PH. (1976). Etiology of bilateral vocal cord paralysis: Review of 389 cases. *Ann Otol Rhinol Laryngol* 85:425–436.

Hoodin RB, Gilbert HR. (1989a). Nasal airflows in parkinsonian speakers. *J Commun Disord* 22:169–180.

Hoodin RB, Gilbert HR. (1989b). Parkinsonian dysarthria: An aerodynamic and perceptual description of velopharyngeal closure for speech. *Folia Phoniatr* 41:249–258.

Hunker CJ, Abbs JH, Barlow SM. (1982). The relationship between parkinsonian rigidity and hypokinesia in the orofacial system: A quantitative analysis. *Neurology* 32:749–754.

Hunker CJ, Abbs JH. (1984). Physiological analyses of Parkinsonian tremors in the orofacial system. In: McNeil MR, Rosenbek JC, Aronson AE, eds. *The Dysarthrias: Physiology, Acoustics, Perception, Management.* San Diego: College-Hill, pp 69–100.

Huppler EG, Schmidt HW, Devine K. (1955). Causes of vocal cord paralysis. *Mayo Clin Proc* 30:518–521.

Jankovic J, Marsden D. (1993). Therapeutic strategies in Parkinson's disease. In: Jankovic J, Tolosa E, eds. *Parkinson's Disease & Movement Disorders.* Baltimore: Williams & Wilkins, pp 115–144.

Jenkins A. (1968). Speech following stereotaxic operations for the relief of tremor and rigidity in parkinsonism. *Med J Aust* 7:585–588.

Johnson JA, Pring TR. (1990). Speech therapy and Parkinson's disease: A review and further data. *Br J Disord Commun* 25:183–194.

Kent RD, Kent JF, Rosenbek JC. (1987). Maximum performance tests of speech production. *J Speech Hear Disord* 52:367–387.

Klawans HL. (1986). Individual manifestations of Parkinson's disease after ten or more years of levodopa. *Movement Disord* 1(3):187–192.

Koller WC. (1984). Sensory symptoms in PD. *Neurology* 34:957–959.

Kruel EJ. (1972). Neuromuscular control examination (NMC) for parkinsonism: Vowel prolongations and diadochokinetic and reading rates. *J Speech Hear Res* 15:72–83.

Laitinen L. (1972). Surgical treatment, past and present in Parkinson's disease. *Acta Neurol Scand Suppl* 51:43–58.

Lang AE, Fishbein B. (1983). The "pacing board" in selected speech disorders of Parkinson's disease. *J Neurol Neurosurg Psychiatry* 46:789.

Laszewski Z. (1956). Role of the department of rehabilitation in preoperative evaluation of parkinsonian patients. *J Am Geriatr Soc* 4:1280–1284.

Leanderson R, Meyerson BA, Persson A. (1971). Effect of L-dopa on speech in Parkinsonism an EMG study of labial articulatory function. *J Neurol Neurosurg Psychiatry* 43:679–681.

Leanderson R, Meyerson BA, Persson A. (1972). Lip muscle function in parkinsonian dysarthria. *Acta Otolaryngol* 74:350–357.

Logemann J, Boshes B, Fisher H. (1973). The steps in the degeneration of speech and voice control in Parkinson's disease. In: Siegfried J, ed. *Parkinson's Diseases: Rigidity, Akinesia, Behavior.* Vienna: Hans Huber, pp 101–112.

Logemann JA, Fisher HB, Boshes B, et al. (1978). Frequency and cooccurrence of vocal tract dysfunctions in the speech of a large sample of Parkinson patients. *J Speech Hear Disord* 43:47–57.

Logemann JA, Fisher HB. (1981). Vocal tract control in Parkinson's disease: Phonetic feature analysis of misarticulations. *J Speech Hear Disord* 46:348–352.

Ludlow CL, Bassich CJ, Connor NP, Coulter DC. (1986). Phonatory characteristics of vocal fold tremor. *J Phonet* 14:509–515.

Ludlow CL, Bassich CJ. (1984). Relationships between perceptual ratings and acoustic measures of hypokinetic speech. In: McNeil MR, Rosenbek JC, Aronson AE, eds. *The Dysarthrias: Physiology, Acoustics, Perception, Management.* San Diego, College-Hill, pp 163–192.

Ludlow CL, Conner NP, Bassich CJ. (1987). Speech timing in Parkinson's and Huntington's disease. *Brain Language* 32:195–214.

Marquardt TP. (1973). Characteristics of speech in Parkinson's disease: Electromyographic, structural movement, and aerodynamic measurements. Unpublished doctoral dissertation, University of Washington, Seattle.

Mawdsley C, Gamsu CV. (1971). Periodicity of speech in parkinsonism. *Nature* 231:315–316.

Mawdsley C. (1973). Speech and levodopa. *Adv Neurol* 3:33–47.

McNamara P, Obler LK, Durso R, et al. (1992). Speech monitoring skills in Alzheimer's disease, Parkinson's disease, and normal aging. *Brain Language* 42:38–51.

Metter EJ, Hanson WR. (1986). Clinical and acoustic variability in hypokinetic dysarthria. *J Commun Disord* 19:347–366.

Metter EJ, Hanson WR. (1991). Dysarthria in progressive supranuclear palsy. In: Moore CA, Yorkston KM, Beukleman DR, eds. *Dysarthria and Apraxia of Speech; Perspectives on Management.* Baltimore: Paul H. Brookes, pp 127–136.

Moore CA, Scudder RR. (1989). Coordination of jaw muscle activity in Parkinsonian movement: Description and response to traditional treatment. In: Yorkston KM, Beukelman DR, eds. *Recent Advances in Clinical Dysarthria.* Boston: College-Hill Press, pp 147–163.

Mueller PB. (1971). Parkinson's disease: Motorspeech behavior in a selected group of patients. *Folia Phoniatr* 23:333–346.

Murdoch BE, Chenery HJ, Bowler S, et al. (1989). Respiratory function in Parkinson's subjects exhibiting a perceptible speech deficit: A kinematic and spirometric analysis. *J Speech Hear Disord* 54:610–626.

Murofushi T, Yamane M, Osanai R. (1992). Stapedial reflex in Parkinson's disease. *J Oto-Rhino-Laryngol Rel SpecialtiesI* 54(5):255–8.

Mutch Wj, Strudwick A, Roy SK, et al. (1986). Parkinson's disease: disability review and management. *BMJ* 293:675–677.

Nakano KK, Zubick H, Tyley HR. (1973). Speech defects of parkinsonian patients. *Neurology* 23:865–870.

Netsell R, Cleeland CS. Modification of lip hypertonia in dysarthria using EMG feedback. *J Speech Hear Disord* 38:131–140.

Netsell R, Daniel B, Celesia GG. (1975). Acceleration and weakness in parkinsonian dysarthria. *J Speech Hear Disord* 40(2):170–178.

Parkinson J. (1817). *An Essay on the Shaking Palsy.* London: Sherwood, Neely and Jones.

Perry AR, Das PK. (1981). Speech assessment of patients with Parkinson's disease. In: Rose FC, Capildeo R, eds. *Research Progress in Parkinson's Disease.* Kent: Pitman, pp 373–383.

Philippbar SA, Robin DA, Luschei ES. (1989). Limb, jaw, and vocal tremor in Parkinson's patients. In: Yorkston KM, Beukelman DR, eds. *Recent Advances in Clinical Dysarthria.* Boston: College-Hill Press, pp 165–197.

Plasse HM, Liberman AN. (1981). Bilateral vocal cord paralysis in Parkinson's disease. *Arch Otolaryngol* 107:252–253.

Poewe W. (1993). L-dopa in Parkinson's disease: Mechanisms of action and pathophysiology of late failure. In: Jankovic J, Tolosa E, eds. *Parkinson's Disease & Movement Disorders.* Baltimore: William & Wilkins, pp 103–111.

Quaglieri CE, Celesia GG. (1977). Effect of thalamotomy and levodopa therapy on the speech of Parkinson patients. *Eur Neurol* 15:34–39.

Rack PMH, Ross HF. (1986). The role of reflexes in the resting tremor of Parkinson's disease. *Brain* 109:115–141.

Ramig LO, Horii Y, Bonitati CM. (1991). The efficacy of voice therapy for patients with Parkinson's disease. *NCVS Status Prog Rep* 1:61–86.

Ramig LO, Scherer RC, Titze IR, et al. (1988). Acoustic analysis of voices of patients with neurologic disease: Rationale and preliminary data. *Ann Otol Rhinol Laryngol* 97:164–172.

Rigrodsky S, Morrison EB. (1970). Speech changes in parkinsonism during L-dopa therapy: Preliminary findings. *J Am Geriatr Soc* 18(2):142–151.

Robertson SJ, Thomson F. (1984). Speech therapy in Parkinson's disease: A study of the efficacy and long term effects of intensive treatment. *Br J Disord Commun* 19:213–224.

Rubow R, Swift E. (1985). A microcomputer-based wearable biofeedback device to improve transfer of treatment in parkinsonian dysarthria. *J Speech Hear Disord* 50:178–185.

Saint-Cyr JA, Taylor AE, Lang AE. (1988). Procedural learning and neostriatal dysfunction in man. *Brain* 111.

Sarno MT. (1968). Speech impairment in Parkinson's disease. *Arch Physical Med Rehabil* 269–275.

Schiffman PL. (1985). A "saw-tooth" pattern in Parkinson's disease. *Chest* 87(1):124–126.

Schley WS, Fenton E, Niimi S. (1982). Vocal symptoms in Parkinson disease treated with levodopa. A case report. *Ann OtolI* 91:119–121.

Schneider JS, Diamond SG, Markham CH. (1986). Deficits in orofacial sensorimotor function in Parkinson's disease. *Ann Neurol* 19:276–282.

Schneider JS, Lidsky TI. (1987). *Basal Ganglia and Behavior: Sensory Aspects of Motor Functioning.* Toronto: Hans Huber.

Scott S, Caird FI, Williams B. (1984). Evidence for an apparent sensory speech disorder in Parkinson's disease. *J Neurol Neurosurg Psychiatry* 47:840–843.

Scott S, Caird FI, Williams BO. (1985). *Communication in Parkinson's Disease.* Rockville, MD: An Aspen Publication, pp 1–113.

Scott S, Caird FI. (1981). Speech therapy for patients with Parkinson's disease. *BMJ* 283:1088.

Scott S, Caird FI. (1983). Speech therapy for Parkinson's disease. *J Neurol Neurosurg Psychiatry* 46:140–144.

Scott S, Caird FI. (1984). The response of the apparent receptive speech disorder of Parkinson's disease to speech therapy. *J Neurol Neurosurg Psychiatry* 47:302–304.

Scott S, Caird FI. (1985). Reply to letter to the editor. The response of the apparent receptive speech disorder of Parkinson's disease to speech therapy. *J Neurol Neurosurg Psychiatry* 48:606.

Selby G. (1967). Stereotactic surgery for the relief of Parkinson's disease. II. An analysis of the results in a series of 303 patients. *J Neurol Sci* 5:343–375.

Selby G. (1968). Parkinson's disease. In: Vinken PJ, Bruyn GW, eds. *Handbook of Clinical Neurology.* Amsterdam: North Holland.

Snider SR, Fahn S, Isgreen WP, et al. (1976). Primary sensory symptoms in Parkinsonism. *Neurology* 26:423–429.

Solomon NP, Hixon TJ. (1993). Speech breathing in Parkinson's disease. *J Speech Hear Res* 36:294–310.

Streifler M, Hofman S. Disorders of verbal expression in Parkinsonism. In: Hassler RG, Christ JF, eds. *Advances in Neurology.* New York: Raven Press, pp 385–393.

Tatton WG, Eastman MJ, Bedingham W, et al. (1984). Defective utilization of sensory input as the basis for bradykinesia, rigidity and decreased movement repertoire in Parkinson's disease: A hypothesis. *Can J Neurol Sci* 11:136–143.

Uziel A, Bohe M, Cadilhac J, et al. (1975). Les troubles de la voix et de la parole dans les syndromes parkinsoniens. *Folia Phoniatr* 27:166–176.

Van Buren JM, Li C, Shapiro DY, et al. (1973). A qualitative and quantitative evaluation of parkinsonians 3 to 6 years following thalamotomy. *Confinia Neurol* 35:202–235.

Van Buren JM, Ratcheson RA. (1982). Principles of stereotaxic surgery. In: Youmans JR, ed. *Neurological Surgery*, Vol 6: *A Comprehensive Guide to the Diagnosis and Management of Neurological Problems.* Philadelphia: W.B. Saunders, pp 3785–3820.

Vincken WG, Gauthier SG, Dollfuss RE, et al. (1984). Involvement of upper-airway muscles in extrapyramidal disorders, a cause of airflow limitation. *N Engl J Med* 311(7):438–442.

Volkmann J, Hefter H, Lange HW, et al. (1992). Impairment of temporal organization of speech in basal ganglia diseases. *Brain Language* 43:386–399.

Weiner WJ, Lang AE. (1989). *Movement Disorders; A Comprehensive Survey.* Mount Kisko, NY: Futura.

Weismer G, Kimelman MDZ, Gorman S. (1985).

More on the speech production deficit associated with Parkinson's disease. *J Acoust Soc Am* 78(Suppl 1):S55.

Weismer G. Acoustic descriptions of dysarthric speech: Perceptual correlates and physiological inferences. *Semin Speech Language* 5:293–314.

Weismer G. (1984). Articulatory characteristics of Parkinsonian dysarthria: Segmental and phrase-level timing, spirantization, and glottal-supraglottal coordination. In: McNeil MR, Rosenbek JC, Aronson AE, eds. *The Dysarthrias: Physiology, Acoustics, Perception, Management.* San Diego: College-Hill Press, pp 101–130.

Weismer G. (1990). Orofacial impairment in Parkinson's disease: Letter to the editor. *Neurology* 40:191–192.

Winckel J, Adams SG. (1992). Drug-cycle related voice changes in parkinsonian patients. *Am Speech Hear Assoc* 34:158.

Winholtz WS, Ramig LO. (1992). Vocal tremor analysis with the vocal demodulator. *NCVS Status Prog Rep* 2:119–137.

Wolfe VI, Garvin JS, Bacon M, et al. (1975). Speech changes in Parkinson's disease during treatment with L-dopa. *J Commun Disord* 8:271–279.

Wood LM, Hughes J, Hayes KC, et al. (1992). Reliability of labial closure force measurements in normal subjects and patients with CNS disorders. *J Speech Hear Res* 35:252–258.

Yaryura-Tobias JA, Diamond B, Merlis S. (1971). Verbal communication with L-dopa treatment. *Nature* 234:224–225.

Yorkston KM, Beukelman DR, Bell KR. (1988). *Clinical Management of Dysarthric Speakers.* Boston: College-Hill Press.

Yorkston KM, Hammen VL, Beukelman DR, et al. (1990). The effect of rate control on the intelligibility and naturalness of dysarthric speech. *J Speech Hear Disord* 55:550–560.

Yumoto E. (1983). The quantitative evaluation of hoarseness: A new harmonics to noise ratio method. *Arch Otolaryngol* 109:48–52.

Zwirner P, Murry T, Woodson GE. (1991). Phonatory function of neurologically impaired patients. *J Commun Disord* 24:287–300.

Chapter 13

Spastic Dysarthria

Bruce E. Murdoch, Elizabeth C. Thompson, and Deborah G. Theodoros

Introduction and History

Darley, Aronson, and Brown (1969a,b) used the term "spastic dysarthria" to describe the speech disturbance seen in association with damage to the upper motor neurons that convey nerve impulses from the motor areas of the cerebral cortex to the lower motor neurons originating from the bulbar cranial nerve nuclei. The lesions associated with spastic dysarthria can involve either the cortical motor areas from which the descending motor pathways originate (primarily the precentral gyrus and premotor cortex) or the descending tracts themselves as they pass through the internal capsule, cerebral peduncles, or the brainstem. The resulting speech disturbance reflects the clinical signs of upper motor neuron damage which include spastic paralysis or paresis of the involved muscles, hyperreflexia (eg, hyperactive jaw-jerk), little or no muscle atrophy (except for the possibility of some atrophy associated with disuse), and the presence of pathological reflexes (eg, sucking reflex). The reference to spastic in the term "spastic dysarthria" reflects the hypertonic state of the bulbar musculature.

Pathophysiology

Neurological Disorders Associated with Upper Motor Neuron Lesions

Two major syndromes can be attributed to upper motor neuron damage: pseudobulbar palsy (supranuclear bulbar palsy) and spastic hemiplegia. Both are characterized by spasticity and impairment or loss of voluntary movements. Pseudobulbar palsy takes its name from its clinical resemblance to bulbar palsy (pseudo = "false") and is associated with a variety of neurological disorders which bilaterally disrupt the upper motor neuron connections to the bulbar cranial nerves. In this condition, the bulbar muscles, including the muscles of articulation, the velopharynx, and larynx are hypertonic and exhibit hyperreflexia. In addition, there is a reduction in the range and force of movement of the bulbar muscles as well as slowness of individual and repetitive movements. The rhythm of repetitive movements, however, is regular and the direction of movement normal. Symptoms of pseudobulbar palsy, depending of course on the precise location and size of the lesions, often include bilateral facial paralysis, dysarthria (including dysphonia), bilateral hemiparesis, incontinence, and bradykinesia. Drooling from the corners of the mouth is common, and many of these patients exhibit excessive emotional responses (eg, uncontrolled outbursts of laughing or crying) to otherwise normal emotional or environmental stimuli. A hyperactive jaw reflex and positive sucking reflex are also evident. Swallowing problems are also a common feature, and there is a definite danger of aspiration and choking in the more severe cases.

The etiology of pseudobulbar palsy varies but may include multiple strokes, brain damage sustained as the result of open or closed head injuries acquired in accidents, especially those injuries with elevated intracranial pressure and a midbrain or upper brainstem shearing injury; extensive brain tumors; multiple sclerosis; cerebral palsy of infancy; or a variety of progressive degenerative diseases. In childhood, the most common cause of pseudobulbar palsy is hypoxic ischemic encephalopathy. In most cases this is associated with intrapartum asphyxia, although severe anoxic brain damage at any stage can cause the same disorder. Brainstem ischemia with infarction resulting from embolization in association with congenital heart disease can also cause pseudobulbar palsy in children. Although a common cause of pseudobulbar palsy in adolescents and young adults, multiple sclerosis is not a common cause of spastic dysarthria in prepubertal children. Degenerative disorders such as metachromatic leukodystrophy can also cause childhood pseudobulbar palsy. In this chapter, discussion will be restricted to pseudobulbar palsy associated with acquired brain lesions rather than congenital conditions such as cerebral palsy.

Although lesions that cause spastic dysarthria can be located in a number of different regions of the brain, including the cerebral cortex, the internal capsule, cerebral peduncles, or brainstem, for such lesions to produce a persistent spastic dysarthria, they need to disrupt the upper motor neuron connections bilaterally. To understand the need for bilateral lesions, an understanding of the neuroanatomy of the upper motor neuron pathways is required. The neuroanatomy of the upper motor neuron system is described in the following section.

Unilateral upper motor neuron lesions produce spastic hemiplegia, a condition in which the muscles of the lower face and extremities on the contralateral side of the body are primarily affected. The bulbar muscles are not greatly affected (for reasons explained further below) with weakness being confined to the contralateral lips, the lower half of the face, and the tongue. The forehead, palate, pharynx, and larynx are largely unaffected. Consequently, unlike pseudobulbar palsy, spastic hemiplegia is not associated with problems in mastication,

swallowing, velopharyngeal function, or laryngeal activity. The tongue appears normal in the mouth but deviates to the weaker side on protrusion. Only a transitory dysarthria comprised of a mild articulatory imprecision rather than a persistent spastic dysarthria is present.

Neuroanatomy of the Upper Motor Neuron System

Two major components comprise the upper motor neuron system, including a direct and an indirect component. The direct component, also known as the pyramidal system, is comprised of neurons that project their axons from their cell bodies located in the cortical motor areas directly to the level of the lower motor neurons without synapsing along the way. In contrast, the indirect component or extrapyramidal system involves multisynaptic pathways that originate from the motor cortex but then pass to the level of the lower motor neurons via multisynaptic connections that involve structures such as the basal ganglia, various brainstem nuclei, the reticular formation, cerebellum, and thalamus. For instance, many of the extrapyramidal fibers descend from the motor cortex in the internal capsule and cerebral peduncles to the pons and are then relayed to the cerebellum, from which projections then pass to either the brainstem or back to the cerebral cortex via the thalamus. Many other extrapyramidal fibers descend from the motor cortex via the internal capsule to the basal ganglia, where they are relayed by a variety of pathways to the excitatory and inhibitory centers of the brainstem. Overall, the extrapyramidal system is said to comprise all of those tracts, besides the pyramidal system, that transmit motor signals from the cortical motor areas to the lower motor neurons. The final pathways for transmission of extrapyramidal signals to the lower motor neurons include the vestibulospinal tracts, the tectospinal tracts, the rubospinal tracts, and the reticulospinal tracts. The extrapyramidal system is thought to be primarily responsible for postural arrangements and the orientation of movement in space, whereas the pyramidal system is chiefly responsible for controlling the far more discrete and skilled voluntary aspects of a movement.

Anatomically, the pyramidal and extrapyramidal systems lie in close proxmity to one another. Consequently acquired brain lesions that affect one system also usually involve the other, and disorders restricted to only one component of the upper motor neuron system are rarely seen in clinical neurology.

Based on their projections to either the midbrain, bulbar region of the brainstem, or spinal cord, three major fiber groups are recognized as comprising the pyramidal system: the corticomesencephalic tracts, the corticobulbar tracts, and the corticospinal tracts (pyramidal tracts proper). In that they terminate by synapsing with lower motor neurons in the nuclei of cranial nerves v, vii, ix, x, xi, and xii, the corticobulbar tracts are those of concern with regard to the occurrence of spastic dysarthria. The clinical outcome of lesions that disrupt the corticobulbar tracts, however, depends very much upon whether the lesion is unilateral or bilateral. This is particularly the case with respect to the effect on speech production, with permanent spastic dysarthria only resulting from bilateral corticobulbar lesions. The reason for this lies in the nature of the upper motor neuron innervation of the bulbar cranial nerve nuclei. Although there is a predominance of corticobulbar fibers that cross to innervate cranial nerve motor nuclei on the contralateral side, there is also considerable ipsilateral (uncrossed) innervation. To state this another way, most of the motor nuclei of the cranial nerves in the brainstem receive bilateral upper motor neuron connections.

Based on the clinical signs observed in cases of unilateral upper motor neuron lesions, it would appear that the ipsilateral upper motor neuron connection is adequate to maintain near-normal function in most muscles controlled by the bulbar cranial nerves with the exception of the tongue and muscles in the lower half of the face. Consequently, unilateral corticobulbar lesions are not associated with spasticity or weakness in the forehead, muscles of mastication, soft palate (ie, no hypernasality), pharynx (ie, no swallowing problems), or larynx (ie, no dysphonia). There is, however, demonstrable weakness in the lower face, lips, and tongue on the opposite side as well as weakness in the extremities of the opposite side. Although unilateral upper motor neuron lesions may therefore be associated with a mild transient dysarthria due to weakness of the contralateral orbicularis oris and tongue, the weakness is usually thought to be too mild to impair speech permanently.

Clinical Features of Spastic Dysarthria

All aspects of speech production including respiration, phonation, resonation, and articulation are affected in pseudobulbar palsy but to varying degrees. Overall spastic dysarthria is characterized by slow, labored speech that is produced with some effort.

Perceptual and Acoustic Features of Spastic Dysarthria

On the basis of a perceptual analysis, the deviant speech characteristics of spastic dysarthria have been reported to cluster primarily in the areas of articulatory-resonatory incompetence and prosodic insufficiency (Darley et al, 1969a,b). In particular, Darley and co-workers identified the following features to be the most prominent perceptible deviant speech dimensions exhibited by persons with pseudobulbar palsy: imprecise consonants, monopitch, reduced stress, harsh voice quality, monoloudness, low pitch, slow rate, hypernasality, strained-strangled voice quality, short phrases, distorted vowels, pitch breaks, continuous breathy voice, and excess and equal stress. Similar findings were reported by Chenery, Murdoch, and Ingram (1992). Using the Frenchay Dysarthria Assessment (Enderby, 1983), Enderby (1986) identified the major aspects of spastic dysarthria (in decreasing order of frequency of occurrence) as including: poor movement of the tongue in speech;

slow rate of speech; poor phonation and intonation; poor intelligibility in conversation; reduced alternating movements of the tongue; poor lip movements in speech; reduced maintenance of palatal elevation; poor intelligibility of description; hypernasality; and lack of volume control.

In support of the findings of Darley et al (1969a,b), other groups of researchers have also identified a slow rate of speech in spastic dysarthric speakers based on their performance when reading a standard passage (Linebaugh & Wolfe, 1984; Ziegler & Von Cramon, 1986). As a measure of articulation rate, Linebaugh and Wolfe (1984) used the mean syllable duration which was obtained by dividing the audible speech emission time by the number of syllables produced during a standard reading passage. Using this method they found that spastic dysarthric speakers had significantly longer mean syllable durations than normal speakers and that the mean syllable duration significantly correlated with both intelligibility and naturalness for the spastic dysarthric speakers. In an attempt to make Darley and co-workers' concepts of slow rate, imprecise consonants, and distorted vowels more precise and quantifiable, Ziegler and Von Cramon (1986), using a computerized signal processing technique, reported spastic dysarthric speakers to have increased word and syllable durations (indicative of a slow rate), a reduction of sound pressure level contrast in consonant articulation (indicative of imprecise consonants), and centralization of vowel formants (indicative of distorted vowels). In addition to a slower rate of speech, spastic dysarthric speakers have also been reported to have significantly slower syllable repetition rates than normal subjects (Dworkin & Aronson, 1986; Portnoy & Aronson, 1982).

Physiological Features of Spastic Dysarthria

Darley, Aronson, and Brown (1975) identified four major symptoms of muscular dysfunction subsequent to disruption of the upper motor neuron supply to the speech musculature as reflecting in the speech output, spasticity, weakness, limited range of movement, and slowness of movement. Information concerning the functioning of various components of the speech production apparatus in spastic dysarthria has been gained from both oromotor and instrumental assessments.

An oromotor assessment usually reveals the presence of weakness in the muscles of the lip and tongue in people with pseudobulbar palsy. Movement of the tongue in and out of the mouth is usually performed slowly, and the extend of tongue movement is usually limited. Often the patient is unable to protrude the tongue beyond the lower teeth. Lateral movements of the tongue are also restricted, although the tongue is of normal size. Voluntary lip movements are also usually slow and restricted in range. These findings are consistent with the consonant imprecision and slow articulation rate noted in perceptual studies of spastic dysarthric speech (Chenery et al, 1992; Darley et al, 1975). Instrumental studies have also confirmed a reduced range of articulatory movement and a slowed rate of speech in patients with pseudobulbar palsy. Hirose (1986) used a range of different instrumental techniques, including cineradiography and X-ray microbeam systems, fiberoptic and photoglottographic recording, ultrasonic techniques, position-sensitive detector, and electromyographic assessment to investigate a variety of dysarthric patients. A reduced range of articulatory movements and a slow rate of speech were observed in subjects with pseudobulbar palsy. However, the consistency of the dynamic pattern of articulatory movements as observed in syllable repetition tasks tended to be preserved. This latter finding is consistent with the perceptual findings of Darley et al (1969a,b) that spastic dysarthric patients have regular rhythm of syllable repetition. Dworkin and Aronson (1986) used a semiconductor strain-gauge force transducer to assess tongue strength in a group of 18 dysarthric subjects, including three with spastic dysarthria. They found that the dysarthric group demonstrated reduced and unsustained levels of maximum tongue force compared to normal controls.

Velopharyngeal function is also usually compromised in spastic dysarthria. Although symmetrical, elevation of the soft palate during phonation appears to be slow and may be incomplete. Consequently, hypernasality is a usual finding in pseudobulbar palsy. As pointed out by Darley et al (1975), however, the degree of hypernasality associated with upper motor neuron lesions tends to be less than in conditions (such as bulbar palsy) that involved damage to the lower motor neurons. In the latter conditions nasal emission frequently accompanies the compromise in velopharyngeal function. Nasal emission, however, is an infrequent finding in pseudobulbar palsy. Based on observations made during cineradiography, Aten (1983) reported that, following initial elevation, there is progressive failure of velar closure in spastic dysarthric patients when counting or during production of serial speech. Unfortunately, to date, however, no comprehensive group studies of velopharyngeal function in pseudobulbar palsy based on quantifiable, physiological measures appear to have been reported in the literature. Consequently the pathophysiology of the perceived hypernasality in this group of subjects remains speculative. It is assumed that the noted reduction in speed and range of movements of the palate, such as those reported by Aten (1983), are the product of spasticity in the muscles responsible for palatal elevation.

Since the descriptions of the perceptual features of spastic dysarthria provided by Darley et al (1969a,b), it has been presumed that bilateral upper motor neuron lesions are manifest at the laryngeal level primarily by increased tone of the laryngeal muscles leading to narrowing of the laryngeal aperture. This narrowing is supposedly the result of hyperadduction of the vocal cords. Hypertonic changes in the vocal cords, however, cannot be easily visualized, so laryngoscopy of pseudobulbar cases often does not reveal any obvious abnormality in their structure or function. The presence of hypertonicity in the laryngeal adductor muscles is suggested, however, by the observed harsh voice quality and strained-strangled sound of the voice in pseudobulbar palsy.

These features are thought to be caused by the exhaled breath stream during speech being squeezed through the stenosed laryngeal valve. Aerodynamically, stenosis of the laryngeal aperture would be expected to manifest as increased glottal resistance, increased subglottal pressure, decreased laryngeal airflow during phonation, and a decrease in abadduction rate of the vocal folds (Hillman, Holmberg, Perkell, Walsh, & Vaughan, 1989; Smitheran & Hixon, 1981). Unfortunately there is a lack of reports in the literature of quantitative, instrumental studies of laryngeal function in pseudobulbar palsy. In a study recently completed by us at the Motor Speech Research Unit at the University of Queensland (Murdoch, Thompson, & Stokes, 1994), we investigated laryngeal activity in patients with upper motor neuron lesions following cerebrovascular accidents using electroglottography in combination with a computerized airflow/air pressure analysis system (Aerophone II). Unexpectedly, we found that only half of our cases with upper motor neuron damage exhibited a predominance of laryngeal features classically associated with hyperfunctional laryngeal activity including increased glottal resistance, elevated subglottal pressures, and decreased laryngeal airflow. The other 50% of the subjects with upper motor neuron lesions demonstrated hypofunctional laryngeal activity, with lower than normal glottal resistance and higher than normal laryngeal airflow during phonation. Despite being an unexpected finding, the presence of hypofunctional laryngeal activity seemed to be best explained as a compensatory device to reduce the muscular effort needed to produce speech against hypertonic vocal folds.

Impaired respiratory support for speech has been identified as one of the predominant perceptual features of speech disorders associated with upper motor neuron damage

291

(Darley et al, 1975; Enderby, 1983). As in the case of laryngeal function, few quantitative instrumental studies have been reported on speech respiration in pseudobulbar palsy. Murdoch, Noble, Chenery, and Ingram (1989) used a strain-gauge belt pneumograph system to investigate speech breathing in patients with pseudobulbar palsy following cerebrovascular accidents. They reported that four of their five pseudobulbar palsy cases had below normal vital capacities. In addition, their pseudobulbar palsy subjects had irregularities in chest wall movements during speech, which they speculated could possibly be attributed to spasticity and weakness of the muscles of the chest wall. In a more recent study using larger subject numbers, we (Thompson & Murdoch, 1993) confirmed the presence of reduced lung volumes and capacities (including reduced vital capacity and forced expiratory volume one second) in subjects with upper motor neuron lesions following cerebrovascular accidents. In addition we observed distinctive kinematic patterns of chest wall movements during speech including reduced lung volume excursions, reduced abdominal volume initiation levels and excursions, and significantly lower abdominal contributions to expiration during speech production. Overall, the kinematic patterns indicated that the upper motor neuron dysarthric subjects presented with reduced abdominal contributions to speech breathing, especially in speech tasks (eg, vowel prolongations) requiring maximal respiratory efforts.

In general, the acoustic and physiological studies that have been carried out tend to support the perceptual analysis of spastic dysarthria reported by Darley et al (1969a,b). These studies have shown that spastic dysarthric speakers have a slow rate of speech most probably caused by longer durations of syllables and perhaps longer pauses within and between words. There is evidence that the articulators move through a reduced range and that tongue strength in spastic dysarthria is reduced compared to normal. Although observations made during cineradiography of spastic dysarthric

speakers suggest that velopharyngeal function is impaired, objective instrumental validation is needed. Those instrumental studies reported to date have indicated that impairments in speech breathing may contribute to the overall speech problem in spastic dysarthria. Although it is thought that the disturbed functioning of the various components of the speech mechanism is the product of the spasticity associated with bilateral upper motor neuron lesions, this interpretation remains speculative, and further objective validation of this hypothesis is required.

Treatment of Spastic Dysarthria

Currently patients with spastic dysarthria receive treatment procedures based on the assumption that the perceived speech deficits are a result of spasticity in the various components of the speech mechanism. As is evident from the previous section, however, few studies based on objective physiological assessment of the speech mechanism in spastic dysarthric speakers have been reported in the literature. To enable the design of specific treatments for various forms of dysarthria, information regarding their physiological basis is required. As stated by Abbs and DePaul (1989), "The quality of clinical treatment for dysarthria generally is related to the degree of knowledge of the pathophysiology and extent to which reliable assessment procedures can be devised to exploit that knowledge" (p 207). It follows, then, that the efficiency and effectiveness (such as the generalization of skills to untrained tasks, etc) of dysarthria treatment can only be improved when the therapy techniques are selected to remedy specific physiological deficits. As Orlikoff (1992) stated, "a custom made assessment leads to a custom fit therapy program" (p 37). One outcome, therefore, of the dearth of physiological data relating to the speech mechanism in spastic dysarthria is that few authors have developed programs designed specifically for remediation of the speech disorder in this population.

The following section on therapy techniques for spastic dysarthria is therefore based on a collection of therapy techniques and therapeutic issues which have either been effectively used in intervention with subjects with spastic dysarthria or which have been used with other dysarthric groups but could have high applicability for the intervention of spastic dysarthria. It is unfortunate that the majority of articles that have assessed dysarthria treatment and management using a variety of treatment procedures have often had limited subject numbers and have included subjects with a variety of types of dysarthria resulting from different etiologies. A true evaluation of the use of certain therapy techniques for subjects with spastic dysarthria is therefore difficult at this time.

A number of the treatment strategies for the functional components of the motor speech system have already been well discussed in the literature (Halpern, 1986; Netsell & Rosenbek, 1986; Rosenbek & LaPointe, 1978); however, it is hoped that the present chapter can highlight some of the new instrumental techniques available for the therapist and how these techniques may be useful in the treatment of patients with spastic dysarthria.

Prognostic Issues

Predicting the prognosis of a patient is often difficult owing the wide range of variables that can influence progress. Authors have listed factors such as neurological status and history, time postonset, age, motivation, personality, intelligence, associated language, cognitive and sensory problems, severity of the dysarthric involvement, skill of the clinician, type of treatment, and home environment as just some of the points to be considered (Kearns & Simmons, 1990; Rosenbek & LaPointe, 1978).

One of the most influential of the prognostic factors is the clinician's ability to implement the most appropriate and efficient therapy approach to ensure a better outcome for the patient. Netsell and Rosenbek (1986)

discussed six main factors which can influence the treatment decisions the clinician must make, with reference to treating the dysarthrias in general: (1) the severity of neurological insult; (2) underlying pathophysiology; (3) the medical status; (4) available methods and tools; (5) time available; and (6) the patient's need to communicate. A number of these factors have a great influence over the treatment decisions which need to be made for subjects with spastic dysarthria. In particular, the severity of the insult and the underlying pathophysiology of the dysarthria can greatly influence treatment decisions. Langworthy and Hesser (1940) noted that subjects with pseudobulbar palsy show varying abnormalities in their speech depending on the amount of strength of voluntary control lost and the condition of either increased or decreased tone in the muscles. Treatment must therefore be based on a thorough pathophysiological assessment to determine the status of the muscular impairment, whether it be increased or decreased tone, in each of the speech subsystems. Therapy techniques must then be selected to correspond to this physiological state. As therapy techniques that can effect change in several spastic muscle groups, such as the larynx, are limited, the severity of impairment in each subsystem also dictates the availability of techniques that can be the most effective for the patient.

At the more detailed level of planning and scheduling of therapy sessions, there are still more factors the clinician must consider for therapy to be efficient and effective for the patient. In their chapter on the dysarthrias, Rosenbek and LaPointe (1978) provide a excellent summary of therapy level planning considerations. Factors such as scheduling of sessions, use of drill work, the decision for individual vs group therapy, the hierarchical organization of symptoms, the setting of the specific treatment goals, and how to help the person to be a productive patient are well discussed. Such factors, however, are relevant to the treatment of all dysarthric patients and therefore do not require further specific evaluation here.

Treatment of Specific Speech Processes

Rosenbek and LaPointe (1978) state that the goal of dysarthria therapy is not to achieve normal speech, but rather, through therapy, it is hoped that the patient can achieve *compensated intelligibility*. A number of different approaches to the treatment of motor speech disorders can be utilized by clinicians, including behavioral techniques, instrumental therapy techniques, or surgical or prosthetic types of intervention; more recently, a pragmatic approach to the treatment of dysarthria (Kearns & Simmons, 1988) has also been discussed. These approaches allow the therapists' treating motor speech disorders to modify structure, increase function, and teach the patients new compensatory behaviors (Caligiuri & Murry, 1983).

The behavioral approach to dysarthria management includes the attempt to teach patients new skills, compensations, or adjustments that utilize traditional treatment techniques involving stimulus presentation, patient responding, and response contingencies (Kearns & Simmons, 1990). Some of the difficulties with using the behavioral therapy techniques, however, include the lack of sensitivity, calibration, and quantitative nature of the data obtained. For this reason, much of the recent research interest into therapy for dysarthria has been focused on studies investigating the use of instrumental approaches involving biofeedback techniques.

The growth of commercially available instrumentation designed to provide feedback on a number of different physiological parameters is increasing. Netsell and Daniel (1979) note that most adult dysarthric patients can actually improve the function of their individual speech components when given biofeedback. Biofeedback instrumentation transforms covert physiologic processes of speech production into precisely expressed signals via auditory, visual, or tactile pathways (Nemec & Cohen, 1984) and thereby allows the patient to focus on the key elements of a specific problem through instantaneous and simplified comparison between their muscle actions and normal muscle control (Netsell & Daniel, 1979). Research has shown that therapy using biofeedback can assist with the return of function even after subject performance has plateaued using traditional therapy techniques (Nemec & Cohen, 1984). Consequently, the use of biofeedback techniques provides a promising approach for the remediation of a variety of aspects of speech disorders.

Rubow (1980) discussed the need for research focusing on the development of reliable, valid instrumental technology and the need for greater understanding of biofeedback methodology (ie, in what order should the components be treated, does nonspeech training generalized to speech tasks, and which tasks can be learned through training and for which types of dysarthrias). While research to date has done much to validate the importance of biofeedback, there still exists a need for efficacy studies to be undertaken, based on greater subject numbers and focusing on specific dysarthric groups to establish reliable and effective biofeedback techniques which can help effect change in the clinical setting. Specific details of the behavioral, instrumental, and prosthetic therapy techniques available for the intervention of disorders of respiration, articulation, phonation, resonance, and prosody in subjects with spastic dysarthria are detailed below.

Classifying therapy techniques as *pragmatic approaches* is relatively new. The treatment procedures in this category include therapy techniques that involve helping the patient to maximize communication within situations and contexts of daily life (Kearns & Simmons, 1990). Kearns and Simmons (1990) note that taking a pragmatic approach requires the clinician to work closely with the patients and their families to evaluate environmental obstacles to communication and to find solutions. The focus, therefore, of this type of approach is to develop strategies to help the client, and which will generalize into their communicative environment (Kearns & Simmons, 1990).

In the pragmatic approach, treatment does not focus on the dysarthric impairment but rather on the patient as a communicator in various contexts (Kearns & Simmons, 1988). Kearns and Simmons (1988) outlined some examples of pragmatic treatments, including:

1. Environmental manipulation. This involves the alteration of the communicative environment in order to enhance communication. Examples of this are strategies such as avoiding communication in dark or noisy places, reducing the distance between dysarthric speaker and listener or compensate for volume deficits, learning to maximize situational, nonverbal, and gestural cues to aid the listener.
2. Utterance length. Modifying the length of utterances.
3. Repair strategies. Teaching effective repair strategies, such that a request for clarification by the listener, is not met by the dysarthric speaker simply repeating the utterance without modifications.
4. Self-monitoring. This is linked with the repair strategies and involves teaching the patient to listen to their output and learn to monitor the need to make adjustments.
5. Topic and attention getting. Teaching the dysarthric speaker to ensure that the listener is orientated to the topic at hand can help improve the conversational situation.

Effective treatment of patients with spastic dysarthria is therefore dependent on the skills of the clinician to thoroughly assess the physiological bases of the presenting speech deficit and then to select and combine treatment approaches best suited to effect change in the patient. The following section involves the discussion of techniques available for the therapist, for disorders of respiration, phonation, articulation, resonance, and prosody.

Respiration

Physiological investigations of the speech breathing abilities of subjects with spastic dysarthria have found deficits in the speech breathing process which could conceivably contribute to the perceived respiratory deficits of these patients (Murdoch et al, 1989; Thompson & Murdoch, 1993). In a recent study conducted in the Motor Speech Research Unit, at the University of Queensland, kinematic and spirometric assessments of 18 subjects with dysarthria due to upper motor neuron damage following cerebrovascular accident (CVA) revealed that the dysarthric group had reduced lung volumes and capacities compared to the controls as well as reduced lung volume excursions during speech tasks (Thompson & Murdoch, 1993). In addition, on comparison to the control group, the CVA group demonstrated reduced contributions of the abdominal muscles during speech production.

Traditionally, regardless of the type of approach taken (behavioral, instrumental, etc), therapy for respiratory deficits has been directed toward increasing the subjects vital capacity and generally improving strength and coordination of the lungs (Robertson & Thompson, 1986). The results of our study (Thompson & Murdoch, 1993), indicate that while the dysarthric subject group may benefit from a component that concentrates on strengthening and coordinating the rib cage and abdominal muscles, a particular emphasis should be placed on improving the contributing role of the abdominal muscles in the respiratory process for speech. Indeed, this study emphasizes the important role instrumental evaluations play in determining the nature of the physiological impairment, and directing therapy specifically to the underlying bases for the perceived respiratory deficits in each subject.

Traditional therapy. Speech production requires the controlled, sustained, and smooth flow of a sufficient air supply (Kearns & Simmons, 1990). Consequently, the main aim of respiratory therapy is to help the patient achieve controlled exhalation for speech (Boone, 1977; Eisenson, 1985; Kearns & Simmons, 1990; Robertson & Thompson, 1986; Rosenbek & LaPointe, 1978). Some of the specific treatment goals that can help the patient achieve improved breath support for speech include increasing breath control, increasing the depth of inspiration, and improving breath control and air wastage during speech production (Moncur & Brackett, 1974).

A number of researchers have suggested a variety of techniques that may help improve the breath support and control for speech. Shimizu, Watanabe, and Hirose (1992) discussed the use of the "accent method" with seven subjects with motor speech disorders. Five of these subjects had pseudobulbar type speech disorders, and two had ataxic dysarthria. Training took place during 30-minute sessions over 14 to 20 months, during which time the emphasis of therapy was to make the patient relax his neck, shoulders, and upper chest and to transfer the respiratory effort to the abdominal level during breathing. After 4 months an improvement in speech was noted, and by the end of therapy, it was found that phonation time had extended, oral diadochokinetic rate for /pa/ had increased, duration of syllables was shorter and more stable, and speech intelligibility had improved (Shimizu et al, 1992). While it is diffcult to evaluate Shimizu et al's (1992) procedure based on the information provided in the conference proceedings alone, it would appear that focusing respiratory therapy on improving the role of the abdominal muscles during speech can be beneficial for subjects with spastic dysarthria. This finding supports the suggestions by Thompson and Murdoch (1993) that the respiratory process of subjects with spastic dysarthria could benefit from therapy specifically designed to improve the abdominal contribution to the speech breathing process.

Netsell and Hixon (1992) described the use of another technique designed to help breath control called "inspiratory checking" with six head-injured, dysarthric subjects. The technique consists of a two-part instruction to "take a deep breath" and "now let the air out slowly," which effectively trains the patient to regulate the flow of air and volume loss during speech. By following the instruction, the subject inhales more air and there-fore can make use of the passive recoil pressures available for speech. The task of letting the air out slowly also forces the subjects to use the inspiratory muscle forces to maintain a relatively constant subglottal air pressure (Netsell & Hixon, 1992). Of the six subjects taking part in the trials, three showed improvement using this technique; consequently, Netsell and Hixon (1992) concluded that the technique of inspiratory checking was a viable method for some individuals with speech breathing dysfunction.

Aten (1983) specifically outlined the use of "breathy sighs" with subjects with spastic dysarthria to help establish an easy air flow. The intent of this technique is that, once established, the breathy sigh can be shaped into breath support for voice. Aten (1983) describes the technique as using "the least amount of breath possible to allow the subjects to produce a briefly sustained relaxed phonation that is audible but essentially voiceless" (p 73).

Other behavioral techniques that may benefit subjects with spastic dysarthria are the adjustment of posture and the self-monitoring of their respiratory supply. Netsell and Rosenbek (1986) note that some patients experience increases in loudness either when lying or sitting, or in supine or prone positions. Consequently, adjusting the posture of the patient into a position that makes respiratory control easiest can be very beneficial, especially for patients who are not ambulatory (Netsell & Rosenbek, 1986). Relaxation of the head, neck, and shoulders can also help decrease tension and improve respiration.

Providing abdominal support by pushing on the abdominal muscles during exhalation is a simple but useful technique to improve respiratory support for speech (Rosenbek & LaPointe, 1978). By pushing on the abdominal muscles, the pressure provides a means of passive breath release and therefore can further help a subject with spastic dysarthria increase respiratory support while at the same time reduce tension in the respiratory musculature.

Instrumental therapy. Some of the better known of the instrumental techniques for increasing respiratory support for speech include the use of an air pressure transducer coupled to an oscilloscope, and the U-tube water manometer (Rosenbek & LaPointe, 1978). These devices and their construction are described in detail elsewhere (Rosenbek & LaPointe, 1978). Both techniques are based on the principle of encouraging the patient to produce consistent low pressure exhalation over a period of time. Daniel-Whitney (1989) reported the successful use of the U-tube manometer to provide biofeedback of intraoral air pressure for a child with dysarthria following traumatic brain injury. Using this technique, the child was able to progress from being able to sustain $1\,cm\,H_2O$ for no more than 1 sec, to achieving $5\,cm\,H_2O$ for 2.5 sec with the help of visual feedback. The biofeedback technique therefore helped the child achieve almost normal performance on this task, as a person is considered to have adequate respiratory support for speech when they can generate $5\,cm\,H_2O$ and maintain this at a steady level of 3 to 5 sec (Netsell & Daniel, 1979).

While the use of instrumental devices such as the U-tube manometer may be beneficial for some patients, there may also be the tendency for these tasks to actually increase tension in subjects with spastic dysarthria, due to the nature of the task. It has been noted that taking in too much air in inspiration can actually exaggerate tension of the thorax and the throat (Froschels & Jellinek, 1941). Consequently, tasks such as these, which encourage taking deep breaths, may actually trigger an increase in tension, and their use may therefore need to be monitored closely with the spastic dysarthric patient. It is important that the therapist adequately assess the point at which taking in a deep breath may trigger an increase in tension, and then encourage the patient to breathe as deeply as possible without exerting past this point. Additionally, the presence of other factors such as oral weakness, incoordination, hyperactive abnormal reflexes, or involuntary movements (not necessarily associated with spastic

dysarthria) may also contraindicate the use of these techniques with some patients with spastic dysarthria.

Hixon, Goldman, and Mead (1973), in their study of the chest wall kinematics of normal subjects, noted that "subjects given feedback in the form of a storage oscilloscope display of a relative motion diagram could voluntarily trace out a wide variety of prescribed motion pathways while speaking, including those where they used either all rib cage or all abdomen when instructed to do so" (p 108). There is the potential, therefore, for respiratory kinematics to be modified into a feedback treatment. In the Motor Speech Research Unit at the University of Queensland, we are currently investigating the efficacy of using respiratory kinematic methods as a biofeedback therapy tool. Using an ABAB design, the efficacy of traditional therapy and kinematic biofeedback therapy was examined on two subjects with mixed dysarthrias (spastic-flaccid, spastic-ataxic) following closed head injury. The preliminary results of the study have revealed that while both the traditional and the instrumental methods were effective in remediating abnormal respiratory patterns in the two subjects, the biofeedback method effected a greater and more consistent change in the respiratory parameters under treatment in both subjects.

Surgical/prosthetic therapy. Prosthetic techniques for improving respiratory support for speech in subjects with spastic dysarthria concentrate on improving and enhancing the abdominal contribution to the exhaled breath stream. Aten (1983) reported that some patients with spastic dysarthria benefit greatly from providing a more natural posture for speech by supporting or "girdling" (Rosenbek & LaPointe, 1978) the abdominal musculature with an elastic bandage. Through the use of this technique, subjects with spastic dysarthria have been noted to produce better airflow with less effort as well as having reduced strained-strangled phonation (Aten, 1983). Aten (1983), however, reported that caution must be taken not to restrict thoracic movement with the girdle, as this may disturb the natural pattern of breathing. Consequently, the use of a thick leather belt 2 to 3 inches in diameter positioned and stabilized around the waist beneath the ribs is suggested as a preferable method (Aten, 1983).

Rosenbek & LaPointe (1978) also suggested the use of a board, which could be attached to the patient's wheelchair at the level of the abdominal muscles, which the patient could lean into to help the airflow. The use of this technique, however, has been reported to be less than successful with subjects with spastic dysarthria (Aten, 1983). One other prosthetic approach that may prove beneficial with subjects with spastic dysarthria involves elevating the arms with the use of slings, thus allowing the patient to initiate and sustain breath with less overall effort (Rosenbek & LaPointe, 1978; Aten, 1983).

Phonation

Arguably, the strained-strangled voice quality of patients with spastic dysarthria is often the least responsive of the motor speech subsystems to therapeutic intervention. There is, therefore, a need for a better understanding of the motor physiology at the laryngeal level for subjects with spastic dysarthria, in addition to a greater number of efficacy studies reporting trialed treatments for this population. Unfortunately, though, reviews of the voice research literature by Moore (1977), Perkins (1985), and Hillman, DeLassus Gress, Hargrave, Walsh, and Bunting (1990) have concluded that over the years there has been very little change in the practices of voice therapy. Additionally, there have been few published reports of research evaluating the efficacy of intervention for voice disorders (Hillman et al, 1990). The following section on treatment of the phonatory deficits for patients with spastic dysarthria reflects the need for research to provide the therapist with more knowledge about the physiological functioning of the larynx and a greater number of therapy options on which they can base their therapy.

Traditional therapy. Behavioral techniques that can contribute to reducing laryngeal hyperadduction in subjects with spastic dysarthria include: general body and specific head and neck relaxation exercises; specific vocal exercises to decrease laryngeal tension in the vocal cords; and techniques designed to decrease tension in the laryngeal musculature by altering the focus of voice production. Moncur and Brackett (1974) recommended a number of relaxation techniques, both general and specific, which can be applied to reduce whole body, head, and neck tension in voice-disordered patients. Theoretically, it is believed that incorporating relaxation techniques into the therapy program for subjects with spastic dysarthria may help to decrease some of the increased muscular tension in these patients. Training the patient to be able to achieve by themselves a state of relaxation can be beneficial to help them counteract periods of spasticity when they occur.

One of the most widely used techniques to reduce hyperadduction at the level of the vocal folds is the use of breathy onset phonation. Aten (1983) reported that initiating phonation after a breathy sigh is a useful technique for decreasing the perceived strain-strangled quality in the voice of subjects with spastic dysarthria. With this technique, therapy begins with producing a relaxed, breathy sigh of short duration, which can be gradually shaped into a relaxed /a/ vowel, which then can progress to the production of single-syllable, CVC words. Aten (1983) suggests that the CVC words begin with the letter *h* and are followed by open-mouth vowels and nasal consonants or continuants (eg, harm, half) while avoiding the use of plosives and affricates due to the excess pressure and musculature movement required. It is also important to encourage the patient to produce all movements in a relaxed and slow manner, without force or excess effort, to avoid triggering hyperactive reflexes.

Chewing and yawning techniques have been discussed in the literature as beneficial in reducing laryngeal tension in subjects with hyperfunctional laryngeal activity (see Moncur & Brackett [1974] and Boone [1977] for more detail). Their application with subjects with spastic dysarthria, however, may be restricted by the musculature effort involved in the chewing and yawning, which may trigger an increase in tension in the musculature rather than relaxation.

Possibly one other important behavioral technique the patient must learn is the ability to use their auditory skills to monitor their own voice production. Having the ability to effectively listen and evaluate the quality of the vocal productions can enable the patient to recognize examples of the desired voice quality when it is produced. Being able to make judgments about voice production and knowing techniques that can be used to modify the production provides the patient with the ability to generalize this quality to other speech tasks and settings outside the clinic.

Instrumental therapy. One instrumental therapy technique that may be applicable for disorders of phonation in subjects with spastic dysarthria is the use of EMG biofeedback techniques to reduce laryngeal tension. Stemple, Weiler, Whitehead, and Komray (1980) discussed the use of EMG biofeedback with seven subjects who had vocal nodules due to increased laryngeal tension and found that these subjects could reduce tension levels with EMG biofeedback training. Prosek, Montgomery, Walden, and Schwartz (1978) also investigated using the EMG technique on decreasing laryngeal tension for subjects with functional voice disorders, and reported some success with the technique with half their subject group. While the subjects in these EMG studies did not have the same underlying physiological deficits as subjects with spastic dysarthria, EMG biofeedback to reduce hypertonia in other aspects of the speech mechanism (Nemec & Cohen, 1984) has been successful for subjects with spastic dysarthria. Consequently, there is enough evidence to advocate the use of the EMG technique to help decrease laryngeal tension for spastic dysarthric patients.

Other instrumental assessment techniques that could have beneficial application as therapy tools include the VisiPitch (Kay Elemetrics) and the Laryngograph. As a feedback system, the VisiPitch computer system provides instantaneous visual feedback for a number of target behaviors including fundamental frequency and intensity, average fundamental frequency and intensity, perturbation, and voice onset time. Using this system, the patient can receive visual feedback of performance as well as compared performance to the clinician's model. The Laryngograph is an electroglottographic technique that utilizes electrical impedance to estimate vocal cord contact during phonation. Again, the patient can receive visual feedback through observing the glottal wave recorded by the equipment and displayed on the computer screen. Hard glottal attacks are represented in the waveforms as a short steep closing phase as opposed to more breathy onsets of phonation which are represented by a more gradual gentle slope. The combination of this technique of feedback with behavioral therapy for breathy onsets could be a beneficial therapy technique. There are no reports in the literature of treatment using the VisiPitch or the Laryngograph as biofeedback tools; however, there are certainly opportunities for them to be incorporated as a therapeutic method for subjects with spastic dysarthria.

Surgical/prosthetic therapy. Surgical management is not an intervention approach that is regularly taken for hyperfunctional voice disorders. The possibility of reducing severe spastic dysphonic conditions through reducing laryngeal innervation unilaterally, however, may warrant investigation. The induction of unilateral vocal cord paralysis through the reduction of innervation is a technique that has been used for subjects with spastic (spasmodic) dysphonia (Dedo & Shipp, 1980). More recently, injections of botulinum toxin into the laryngeal muscles have been used to temporarily paralyze one of the vocal cords in the attempt to relieve the symptoms of strangled phonation in subjects with spasmodic dysphonia (Blitzer & Brin, 1992; Zwirner, Murry, Swenson, & Woodson, 1991; Zwirner, Murry, Swenson, & Woodson, 1992). There are no reports in the literature, however, to support the effectiveness of either of these surgical procedures in reducing the strained-strangled phonation of subjects with spastic dysarthria.

Articulation

Rosenbek and LaPointe (1978) stated that the aim of articulation treatment is "to improve the patients volitional-purposive control of speech sound production to the limits imposed by his physiologic support for speech" (p 295). In the case of subjects with spastic dysarthria, Aten (1983) redefined this goal as "achieving modest improvements in articulatory precision without overflow of tension into the oral or laryngeal/respiratory musculature" (p 75).

The patient with spastic dysarthria is described as having labored jaw closure, restricted tongue movements (particularly isolated velar contacts), and lip closures that "at best are crude with very limited flexibility" (Aten, 1983, p 75). The articulatory abilities of patients with spastic dysarthria are therefore often quite impaired, due in part to both the compromised function of the articulators and the coexisting deficits of impaired respiration, phonation, and resonance. Consequently, articulation therapy for subjects with spastic dysarthria must be preceded by therapy for disorders of voice onset and voice control, and improving oral flow, through the reduction of nasal resonance and emission prior to successful intervention work with the articulators (Aten, 1983).

Traditional therapy. While a number of authors have discussed orofacial treatment procedures in great detail (Rosenbek & LaPointe, 1978; Netsell & Rosenbek, 1986), much of the information discussed by the authors has been concentrated on training procedures to increase tone and the speed, range, and accuracy of the articulatory muscles. Due, however, to the already exist-

ing increased tone in the articulators of subjects with spastic dysarthria, work on speed, rate, and force is not appropriate for these subjects, as abrupt transitions and quick articulatory movements tend only to increase tension and trigger difficulties (Aten, 1983). Aten (1983) outlined treatment strategies designed to improve intelligibility for subjects with spastic dysarthria which involved stressing the concepts of gentle approximation of consonants and emphasizing clear vowel productions with minimum constriction and tension. The hierarchy of tasks involves beginning with open-mouth vowels and then progressing to high tongue-jaw vowels (eg, /i/). Following this, the patient is encouraged to produce CVC words beginning with *h* and, initially, only containing continuant or liquid sounds. Later when these have been produced successfully, more demanding sounds including voiced, then unvoiced plosives, and finally affricates can be included. In each case, Aten (1983) states that approximation of sound production is the realistic objective for these patients.

Instrumental therapy. The most popular instrumental technique for modifying the function of the articulators is EMG feedback of muscle function and tone. The use of EMG biofeedback techniques has been discussed in the literature as providing beneficial intervention for modifying tone in orofacial muscles. Daniel-Whitney (1989) reported the successful use of EMG biofeedback to increase tone in the obicularis oris muscle of a child with severe spastic-ataxic dysarthria. The child presented with weak lips and poor lip closure, and the results of EMG recordings of the lip muscles demonstrated no evidence of spasticity. Therapy using the EMG biofeedback was focused on increasing lip muscle tone and was successful in helping the child attain lip closure.

EMG biofeedback techniques have also been successful in reducing tension in subjects with spastic dysarthria. Nemec and Cohen (1984) used EMG biofeedback techniques with a male subject with spastic dysarthria to increase awareness of generalized tension in the facial muscles involved in elevation and depression of the mandible. Training focused on generalized reduction of tension in the facial muscles and gaining conscious control over the desired response. Speech intelligibility for the subject was noted to improve, due to appropriate lingual postures accompanying mandibular closure, and follow-up assessments revealed good generalization of the newly acquired skills (Nemec & Cohen, 1984).

The movement of the articulators in subjects with spastic dysarthria is often restricted by increased tone. Another approach to reduce this tone, other than EMG, is the use of vibration therapy to improve the state of relaxation of the muscles. Daniel-Whitney (1989) discussed the use of vibration therapy for a child with severe spastic-ataxic dysarthria. The child presented with reduced jaw opening, and trials with prosthetic management only achieved some increased jaw opening. Relaxation of the masseter using bilateral vibration for periods of 20 min was found to be successful in further increasing jaw opening from 12 mm to 25 mm (Daniel-Whitney, 1989).

Another instrumental technique that may have therapeutic application for subjects with spastic dysarthria is the electropalatograph. The technique of electropalatography (EPG) involves the use of artificial palate that contains a number of electrodes exposed to the lingual surface. When the artificial palate is in place, it can provide details of the timing and location of the tongue with the hard palate during continuous speech. By using the artificial palate as a training tool, it can help provide the patient with visual feedback of the location of the tongue during articulation and how this positioning needs to be adjusted to achieve a closer approximation of the sound. One possible detrimental factor to this technique, however, is the cost and time involved in constructing the palate. An article by Hardcastle, Gibbon, and Jones (1991) provides a good description of the electropalate and its functions.

Surgical/prosthetic therapy. Types of prosthetic management for articulation disorders discussed in the literature for use with all types of dysarthria include the use of items such as jaw slings, which can help maintain jaw closure (Kearns & Simmons, 1988), and bite blocks, which stabilize the jaw and effectively force the patient to make lip and tongue movements without assistance from the jaw (Rosenbek & LaPointe, 1978; Netsell & Rosenbek, 1986). In the Daniel-Whitney (1989) case study, improving jaw opening was an important treatment goal. Using increasing numbers of tongue depressors inserted between the teeth, he reported success with increasing jaw opening from 2 mm to 12 mm. Following this technique a bite block was also trialed in the attempt to obtain additional opening; however, this was unsuccessful as the child demonstrated extensor spasm on insertion of the block. While prosthetic management was useful to some extent, this case study report demonstrates that the increased tone in subjects with spastic dysarthria may often prevent or at least restrict the use of some types of treatment.

Resonance
Disorders of resonance in the dysarthrias can result from abnormal tongue positioning, an increase or lack of tension in the articulatory muscles, or an impairment in coordination of the velopharyngeal mechanism (Rosenbek & LaPointe, 1978). Subjects with spastic dysarthria, therefore, may have disorders of resonance as a result of spasticity or weakness in any one or all of these muscle groups. Disruptions of resonance stemming from deficits in articulatory posturing or tension can be remediated using techniques discussed in the above section on articulatory deficits. The following section, therefore, will address the intervention strategies useful in remediating disruptions of velopharyngeal function.

The most prominent disorder of resonance associated with spastic dysarthria is hypernasality. Hypernasality in spastic dysarthria results from spasticity and weakness of the velopharyngeal muscles which, in turn, may result in the subject having either an inconsistent or an incomplete closure of the velopharyngeal port during speech. In his chapter on treatment in spastic dysarthria, Aten (1983) reported that, in his experience of observing the velum of spastic dysarthric subjects using cineradiography, the initial elevation of the velum in these patients is soon followed by a progressive failure of the velum to elevate during serial speech activities. In subjects with more severe resonance disorders, Aten (1983) describes an "inertia in initiating speech activities" (p 70). Aten accounts for these velar movements as not actually weaknesses, but rather "a rapid onset of increased resistance to stretch" (p 70), which results in blocking the movement pattern.

Determining the need for therapeutic intervention for velopharyngeal dysfunction is often difficult due to coexisting deficits in other aspects of the speech production mechanism. A thorough assessment of the velopharyngeal muscles' structure and function, as well as determining the degree to which the hypernasality is disrupting speech production in subjects with spastic dysarthria is therefore critical to accurate therapeutic intervention. While the therapy decisions for the milder and more severe cases can be made with relative confidence, Netsell and Rosenbek (1986) suggest that some guidelines are needed to help make the decisions for those patients who fall into what they describe as the "gray area." The decision to treat these cases can be aided by considering the following factors: (1) the relative severity of involvement in the other functional components; (2) whether the treatment of the velopharynx would enhance function in other areas (eg, tax the respiratory system less); and (3) whether the velopharyngeal function would benefit from treating other components first or simply having the patient speak more slowly and with greater effort (Netsell & Rosenbek, 1986).

Traditional therapy. Many of the traditional approaches to the treatment of hypernasality have been based on the principles of increasing velopharyngeal muscle strength, learning to direct airflow, and increasing patient awareness of velopharyngeal function. Pushing techniques, which involve the patient attempting velopharyngeal closure while simultaneously pushing with the hands against an object or simply tensing other muscles, and tasks that encourage the patient to control and modify the airstream using balls, whistles, candles, fluff, powder, paper, bubbles, straws, etc have been discussed at length elsewhere (Halpern, 1986). There have, however, been reports that such therapy techniques, on the whole, are not effective (Powers & Starr, 1974), possibly because they do not provide the patient with information on the timing of articulatory gestures during speech (Kunzel, 1982). The relevance of these techniques with subjects with spastic dysarthria has not been specifically assessed; however, if, as Aten (1983) suggests, the problems with velopharyngeal control is a progressive failure of the velum to elevate as the resistance to stretch increases, single-sound tasks and nonspeech tasks will possibly be of little benefit for these patients. Pushing techniques, which effectively increase tension, may also adversely affect the patient with spastic dysarthria for whom the aim is to decrease the amount of tension in the speech system.

Another behavioral approach for modifying disorders of resonance is "oral resonance" therapy. Having a raised mandible and retracted tongue during speech can actually enhance nasal resonance. Consequently, speech exercises that emphasize increased jaw widening and tongue movements can help to open the oral cavity as a resonator and provide additional reduction in the perceived levels of hypernasality. Examples and specific tasks for oral resonance therapy can be found elsewhere in vocal therapy texts such as Moncur and Brackett (1974).

Instrumental therapy. A major contributing factor to the problem of treating hypernasality stems from the inability of the subject to perceive velopharyngeal movements and receive adequate feedback. Due to the difficulties of receiving feedback about the muscle functioning using traditional therapy approaches, the use of biofeedback techniques for hypernasality therapy has proven to be very beneficial for patients. Over the past years, a number of different instrumental systems have been designed and trialed with a variety of patients to provide the dysarthric speaker with feedback on veolpharyngeal functioning during speech and nonspeech tasks. In the literature to date, however, there are very few reports of the efficacy of biofeedback techniques with dysarthric subjects. As a result, we can again only speculate the effectiveness of such therapy techniques for spastic dysarthric subjects.

In the late 1970s and early 1980s a number of researchers introduced some of the first instrumental biofeedback techniques for velopharyngeal dysfunction. Shelton, Paesani, McClelland, and Bradfield (1975) and Shelton, Beaumont, Trier, and Furr (1978) discussed the use of an endoscope with visual feedback of the movements of the lateral pharyngeal walls provided on a closed circuit monitor. Siegel-Sadewitz and Shprintzen (1982) and Witzel, Tobe, and Salyer (1988) used flexible fiberoptic nasopharyngoscopes to obtain close observations of the velopharyngeal sphincter during connected speech. Velographs (Künzel, 1982), palatal training appliances (Tudor & Selly, 1974), and the use of displacement transducers (Moller, Path, Worth, & Christiansen, 1973) have also been demonstrated to be effective in increasing palatal movements during phonation.

While these instrumental methods have been found to effect change in the velopharyngeal function of a number of different speech-disordered patients, mainly cleft palate subjects, generalization and long-term maintenance of the skills acquired using these techniques have not been documented. In addition, the ability to use this equipment in a clinical setting is restricted by factors such as cost, complexity of equipment, and,

in some cases, such as nasoendoscopy and endoscopy, the need for a physician to be present.

There are some instrumental techniques, however, that are less invasive and more easily incorporated into clinical use. One such system is the Nasometer (Kay Elemetrics), which provides an indirect measure of velopharyngeal function through measuring acoustic energy output. The Nasometer is a microcomputer-based instrument designed for the assessment and treatment of patients with disorders of nasality; unlike many of the instrumental techniques previously discussed, this program is simple to use, is comparatively inexpensive, and has applications for both children and adults. The equipment consists of two directional microphones set onto a horizontal sound separator plate which rests against the patient's top lip, creating a shelf between the nose and the mouth. During speech production, information regarding the relative amount of nasal acoustic energy in a patient's speech is then displayed on the computer screen expressed as a "nasalance" score. In addition to evaluating the degree of nasality, the nasometer program also provides visual displays such as bar displays and real-time screen displays of the degree of nasalance the person produces during speech. This provides the patient with feedback about the degree of nasal acoustic output during tasks and consequently allows the patient to attempt to monitor and control velopharyngeal functioning. Studies of the effectiveness of the system as a therapy tool, however, are still required.

The accelerometer is another assessment tool based on indirectly measuring velopharyngeal function which also have applications as a system to provide feedback. Horii and Monroe (1983) outline the use of accelerometers coupled with visual feedback via an oscilloscope display and auditory feedback through a microphone/headset as a simple and cost-effective feedback tool for velopharyngeal therapy.

One other possible biofeedback aid which has only recently been mentioned in the literature is the Exeter Bio-Feedback Nasal An-emometer (EBNA) (Bioinstrumentation Ltd Exter) (Hutters & Bronsted, 1992). This system consists of a flow sensing device which contains an electrically heated bead which works on the same principles as a hot wire anemometer which is then placed in a mask which is positioned over the nose. The EBNA system is being defined as much less expensive and more convenient than other airflow systems (Hutters & Bronsted, 1992). Its efficacy as a clinical tool, however, remains undetermined.

Surgical/prosthetic therapy. The decision to use invasive, prosthetic intervention to remedy hypernasality must be based on a number of general factors, including (1) the severity of the hypernasality, (2) the degree to which hypernasality is affecting other aspects of the speech mechanism, (3) attempts at therapeutic intervention using behavioral and instrumental methods having been unsuccessful, and (4) the absence of contra-indicating factors for the surgery and/or postsurgical therapy. Indeed, while there have been no specific criteria lists compiled which predict the success of prosthetic management, investigations into palatal lift prosthetic intervention have indicated that it is a successful method for subjects with severe velopharyngeal dysfunction (Lotz & Netsell, 1984, cited in Netsell & Rosenbek, 1986). How long the lift is effective, though, is a matter that requires investigation, as Aten (1983) reported that the positive effects of palatal lifts with severely spastic dysarthric patients do tend to dissipate over time due to increased tension in the hypopharyngeal and laryngeal musculature. Subjects with less severe deficits, however, have been found to benefit over a longer period of time, and may not require the lift after a few months (Aten, 1983).

A palatal lift prosthesis is designed to help compensate for reduced or incoordinated movement of the velophayrngeal muscles. Consequently, subjects with severe spastic dysarthria, which is affecting the functioning of the velopharyngeal musculature, may in-volve the use of a palatal lift prosthesis. The lift is usually designed to attach to the teeth and consists of a hard plastic shelf attached to the posterior section of the plate which projects posteriorly under the soft palate and maintains elevation. The aim of using a palatal lift is to allow the lateral pharyngeal walls to move toward the midline and contact with the velum, which is being artificially raised by the prosthesis. Individual differences in VP anatomy, muscle action, and patterns of VP closure mean that prosthetic management of velopharyngeal incompetence must be based on a thorough instrumental observation of muscle function. Construction of a palatal lift can be found elsewhere (Schweiger, Netsell, & Sommerfeld, 1970; Spratley, Chenery, & Murdoch, 1988); however, in general, the construction of the lift is designed so that when the prosthesis is in place, the velum is continually raised, yet the subject can breath comfortably through the nose when the lateral edges of the life have been extended maximally (Netsell & Daniel, 1979).

Gonzalez and Aronson (1970) investigated the use of the palatal lift prosthesis for the treatment of both anatomic and neurologic velopharyngeal insufficiency. Of the 19 patients in a neurologic subgroup investigated, 10 had spastic paresis of the velopharyngeal musculature resulting from upper motor neuron damage, five had flaccid paresis, and four subjects had mixed spastic-flaccid paresis. All subjects at the immediate, 3-month, and 1-year assessments showed moderate to marked improvements in the reduction of hypernasality and nasal emission, as well as an increase in speech intelligibility due to the improved ability to build intraoral air pressure. In addition to this finding, reassessment, at 2 years post the initial fitting of the prosthesis of four (three neurological, one anatomical) of the original subjects showed improved palatopharyngeal efficiency with the prosthesis removed. This finding demonstrated that, in addition to being used to correct and improve palatopharyngeal closure, the prosthesis may in fact stimulate palatopharyngeal musculature and function as a supportive type of prosthesis until the muscles gain strength and activity to effect palatopharyngeal closure (Gonzalez & Aronson, 1970). Unfortunately, as Lotz and Netsell (1984, cited in Netsell & Rosenbek, 1986) reported, the long-term effects of palatal lifts have not been documented, and therefore further research into the long-term effects of palatal lift prosthetic management is required to evaluate the role it has in stimulating palatopharyngeal movement.

Gonzalez and Aronson (1970) noted a number of selection criteria to be considered to optimize successful prosthetic intervention. In their study, subjects were selected for the lift prosthesis after oral and cineradiographic examinations determined the residual muscular activity in the palatopharyngeal region and the presence of adequate retention for the prosthesis. Physiologic, psychologic, and economic status were also considered. Based on their experience, Lotz and Netsell (1984, cited in Netsell & Rosenbek, 1986) suggested some more physiologically based selection criteria for successful prosthetic intervention. These included:

1. If nasal air flow on oral sounds is consistently above 200 cc/sec, successful treatment of the velopharynx should increase speech intelligibility.
2. If nasal flows are in the range of 100 cc/sec they do not have a major impact on intelligibility if intraoral air pressures for oral sounds are 5 to 10 cm H_2O and orofacial articulation is reasonable.
3. If intraoral air pressures are below 4 cm H_2O for oral sounds, nasal flows of 100 cc/sec can be clinically significant, and treatment of the velopharynx may be necessary.

There are also a number of other factors to be taken into consideration, which contraindicate the fitting of a palatal lift, especially for subjects with spastic dysarthria.

Daniel (1982) found that hypersensitivity of the gag reflex is another factor to be considered, after noting that some of their patients, even following successful desensitization of the gag reflex, could not tolerate the prosthesis. As a possible solution to this problem, Aten (1983) discussed the use of palatal lift with spastic dysarthric patients which has flexible twin wire extensions from the denture acrylic which can easily be adjusted in the anterior-posterior and vertical planes to allow graduated support to the velum. The flexibility of the structure of this lift thus allowed patients to gradually become accustomed to the lift and help extinguish the gag reflex.

Gonzalez and Aronson (1970) also noted that a palatal lift should not be used when a person has a very spastic or stiff soft palate that does not tolerate elevation. Strong velar, palatoglossus, or pharyngeal contractions can also inhibit the subject from retaining the device (Netsell & Rosenbek, 1986).

Prosody
Disruptions of the suprasegmental and prosodic features of speech may result in affected intelligibility. Consequently, prosodic features should receive equal attention in dysarthria treatment and management. It is often the case, however, that prosodic intervention is initiated in the final stages of therapy or not at all. The three prosodic features of rhythm, stress, and intonation are the result of the interaction of suprasegmental factors such as pitch, loudness, articulation time, and pause time (Rosenbek & LaPointe, 1978). Rhythm is defined as "the perception of the time program applied to the phonetic events" (p 224), while stress is considered to be "the perception of syllable emphasis, relative to the emphasis perceived on other syllables in the same sentences or phrase" (p 224) (Netsell, 1973). Rosenbek and LaPointe (1978) suggest that the treatment of rhythm and stress can be achieved using a common method, as stress is a result of changes in pitch, loudness, articulation time, and pause time, while

305

rhythm is considered the timing of speech, which also results, in part, from changes in pause time. Intonation, which is defined as "the perception of changes in the fundamental frequency of vocal fold vibration during speech production" (p 224), in contrast, requires separate intervention strategies. The prosodic features of subjects with spastic dysarthria are often impaired due to the combination of characteristic low, monotonous pitch, monotony of loudness, shortness of phrases, and a slow rate of speech characterized by labored articulation.

Traditional therapy. The variables that affect the elements of prosody are complex and interrelated (Kearns & Simmons, 1988). Consequently, many of the behavioral therapy techniques discussed previously in the articulation, phonation, and respiration sections of this chapter will have some effect on the prosodic elements of speech (eg, increased respiratory support with relaxed phonation may have a carry over effect to increase phrase length). There are some specific intervention techniques, however, that can be applied to modify aspects such as stress and intonation.

Aten (1983) reported that therapy involving stress and contrast exercises may be useful toward the end of treatment for patients with less severe spastic dysarthria. Contrastive stress drills, involve the production of the same sentence, however, each time the focus of the stress is changed, such that the meaning of the sentence changes (eg, Bob bit *Bill*, *Bob* bit Bill). These drills can also be effectively combined with rate control and articulation work to improve intelligibility. Therapy tasks that target intonation patterns include reading aloud text that has been marked with the natural intonation patterns and pause times appropriate for the passage. Moncur and Brackett (1974) have written an excellent chapter on therapy for prosodic disruption which outlines a number of treatment techniques and stimuli.

Aten (1983) reported little success eliminating monotony or increasing rate in the moderate to severely involved spastic dysarthric patients. The use of a pacing technique

to regulate the rhythm of speech has been suggested as a possible technique to improve rate and intelligibility in spastic dysarthria (Nailling & Horner, 1979). Other, more simplified techniques include instructing the patient to speak at a slower rate. Articulating at a slower rate and pausing between words can often prevent triggering of increased spasticity in the speech system and, therefore, improve intelligibility. Unfortunately, such techniques often result in producing equalized stress patterns which differ from normal speech production (Barnes, 1983).

Monotonous quality in speech is often perceived as a deficit in fundamental frequency variation. It has been suggested in the literature, however, that attempting to reduce a monotonous voice quality through the modification of pitch and intonation alone may be insufficient. Soloman, Ludolph, and Thompson (1984; cited in Bellaire, Yorkston, and Beukelman, 1986) acoustically analyzed the fundamental frequency of speech samples of normal subjects and subjects defined as having monotonous speech, and found that the range of fundamental frequency excursion for each group was not different. Bellaire et al (1986) reported that therapy to improve "breath patterning" in a subject with mild dysarthria following closed head injury resulted in a reduction of the patient's monotonous voice quality. Bellaire et al (1986) therefore concluded that the perception of monotony must include other factors other than fundamental frequency. From the results of the investigation, it appeared that the speech of the patient Bellaire et al (1986) had investigated was judged to be monotonous, at least in part, as a consequence of his short, regular breath groups. These results emphasize the need to assess the breath patterns of speech and the role of the breath group as a unit of prosody that requires intervention. Specific tasks and exercises for breath patterning can be found in Moncur and Brackett (1974).

Instrumental therapy. There have been reports in the literature of the use of biofeedback techniques for the intervention of prosodic disturbances. Caligiuri and Murry (1983) demonstrated the effectiveness of biofeedback training on articulatory precision, speaking rate, and prosody for three subjects with dysarthria. In their study, Caligiuri and Murry displayed intensity and duration information as well as intraoral air pressure information on a four-channel storage oscilloscope. Results of 9 weeks of visual feedback therapy revealed improvements in speaking rate and prosodic control, and a reduction in the overall severity of the speech disorder (Caligiuri & Murry, 1983).

The VisiPitch (Kay Elemetrics) is a commercially available biofeedback tool, which can provide the patient with performance feedback on a number of target behaviors including pitch, range, vocal intensity, speech rate, intonation, and stress patterns. Through the computer system the clinician can demonstrate the target behavior, and then have the patient practice the task with the aid of the visual feedback on the screen. There have been no reports cited in the literature of the effectiveness of this equipment in the treatment of prosody for subjects with spastic dysarthria, so its application for this population can only be assumed.

Summary

Spastic dysarthria results from bilateral disruption of the upper motor neuron connections to the bulbar cranial nerves. The resulting speech disturbance has been described as slow, labored speech which is produced with some effort. To date, few specific treatments for spastic dysarthria have been proposed, largely reflecting a lack of published reports concerning the physiological functioning of the various components of the speech production mechanism in spastic dysarthric speakers. It is thought that the deviant speech dimensions perceived to be present in spastic dysarthria are the products of spasticity in the speech musculature. Although some confirmatory studies have been reported in the case of many components of the speech production system, this interpretation remains speculative. Until such time as comprehensive studies of the physiological functioning of the speech production mechanism of spastic dysarthric speakers are reported, further development of effective treatment procedures for this condition will be hampered. The current chapter provides a commentary on the application of techniques used in dysarthria treatment in general to the rehabilitation of disordered speech in spastic dysarthria. In addition, the few reported treatments that have been trialed with spastic dysarthric speakers are reviewed.

References

Abbs JH, De Paul R. (1989). Assessment of dysarthria: A critical prerequisite to treatment. In: Leahy MM, ed. *Disorders of Communication: The Science of Intervention*. London: Taylor & Francis.

Aten JA. (1983). Treatment of spastic dysarthria. In: Perkins W, ed. *Dysarthria and Apraxia*. New York: Thieme-Stratton, pp 69–77.

Barnes GJ. (1983). Suprasegmental and prosodic considerations in motor speech disorders. In: Berry W, ed. *Clinical Dysarthria*. San Diego: College Hill, pp 57–68.

Bellaire K, Yorkston K, Beukelman DR. (1986). Modification of breath patterning to increase naturalness of a mildly dysarthric speaker. *J Commun Disord* 19:271–280.

Blitzer A, Brin MF. (1992). Treatment of spasmodic dysphonia (laryngeal dystonia) with local injections of botulinum toxin. *J Voice* 6(4):365–369.

Boone DR. (1977). *The Voice and Voice Therapy*. NJ: Prentice-Hall.

Caligiuri MP, Murry T. (1983). The use of visual feedback to enhance prosodic control in dysarthria. In: Berry WR, ed. *Clinical Dysarthria*. San Diego: College-Hill Press.

Chenery HJ, Murdoch BE, Ingram JCL. (1992). The perceptual speech characteristics of persons with pseudobulbar palsy. *Aust J Hum Commun Disord* 20:21–31.

Daniel B. (1982). A soft palate desensitization procedure for patients requiring a palatal lift prosthesis. *J Prosthet Dent* 48:565–566.

Daniel-Whitney B. (1989). Severe spastic-ataxic dysarthria in a child with traumatic brain injury: Questions for management. In: Yorkston KM, Beukelman DR, eds. *Recent Advances in Clinical Dysarthria*. Boston: Little, Brown.

Darley FL, Aronson AE, Brown JR. (1969a). Differential diagnostic patterns of dysarthria. *J Speech Hear Res* 12:246–269.

Darley FL, Aronson AE, Brown JR. (1969b). Clusters of deviant speech dimensions in the dysarthrias. *J Speech Hear Res* 12:462–496.

Darley FL, Aronson AE, Brown JR. (1975). *Motor Speech Disorders*. Philadelphia: W.B. Saunders.

Dedo H, Shipp T. (1980). *Spastic Dysphonia*. Houston: College-Hill Press.

Dworkin JP, Aronson AE. (1986). Tongue strength and alternate motion rates in normal and dysarthric subjects. *J Commun Disord* 19:115–132.

Eisenson J. (1985). *Voice and Diction. A Program for Improvement* (5th Ed.). New York: Macmillan.

Enderby P. (1983). *Frenchay Dysarthria Assessment*. San Diego: College Hill Press.

Enderby P. (1986). Relationships between dysarthric groups. *Br J Disord Commun* 21:189–197.

Froschels E, Jellinek A. (1941). *Practice of Voice and Speech Therapy*. Boston: Expression Company.

Gonzalez JB, Aronson AE. (1970). Palatal lift prosthesis for treatment of anatomic and neurologic palatopharyngeal insufficiency. *Cleft Palate J* 7:91–104.

Halpern H. (1986). Therapy for agnosia, apraxia and dysarthria. In: Chapey R, ed. *Language Intervention Strategies in Adult Aphasia*. Baltimore: Williams & Wilkins.

Hardcastle WJ, Gibbon FE, Jones W. (1991). Visual display of tongue-palate contact: Electropalatography in the assessment and remediation of speech disorders. *Br J Disord Commun* 26:41–74.

Hillman RE, DeLassus Gress G, Hargrave J, Walsh M, Bunting G. (1990). The efficacy of speech-language pathology intervention: Voice disorders. *Semin Speech Language* 11(4):297–309.

Hillman RE, Holmberg EB, Perkell JS, Walsh M, Vaughan C. (1989). Objective assessment of vocal hyperfunction: An experimental framework and initial results. *J Speech Hear Res* 32:373–392.

Hirose H. (1986). Pathophysiology of motor speech disorders (dysarthria). *Folia Phoniatr* 38:61–68.

Hixon TJ, Goldman M, Mead J. (1973). Kinematics of the chest wall during speech production: Volume displacements of the rib cage, abdomen, and lung. *J Speech Hear Res* 16:78–115.

Horii Y, Monroe N. (1983). Auditory and visual feedback of nasalization using a modified accelerometric method. *J Speech Hear Res* 26:472–475.

Hutters B, Brondsted K. (1992). A simple nasal anemometer for clinical purposes. *Eur J Disord Commun* 27(2):101–119.

Kearns KP, Simmons NN. (1988). Motor speech disorders: The dysarthrias and apraxia of speech. In: Lass NJ, McReynolds IV, Northern JL, Yoder DE, eds. *Handbook of Speech-Language Pathology and Audiology*. Toronto: B.C. Decker.

Kearns KP, Simmons NN. (1990). The efficacy of speech-language pathology intervention: Motor speech disorders. *Semin Speech Language* 11(4):273–295.

Künzel H. (1982). First applications of a biofeedback device for the therapy of velopharyngeal incompetence. *Folia Phoniatr* 34:92–100.

Langworthy OR, Hesser FH. (1940). Syndrome of pseudobulbar palsy: An anatomic and physiologic analysis. *Arch Intern Med* 65:106–121.

Linebaugh CW, Wolfe VE. (1984). Relationships between articulation rate, intelligibility and naturalness in spastic and ataxic speakers. In: McNeil MR, Rosenbek JC, Aronson AE, eds. *The Dysarthrias: Physiology, Acoustics, Perception, Management*. San Diego: College Hill Press.

Moller K, Path M, Werth L, Christiansen R. (1973). The modification of velar movement. *J Speech Hear Disord* 38:323–334.

Moncur JP, Brackett IP. (1974). *Modifying Vocal Behaviour*. New York: Harper & Row.

Moore GP. (1977). Have the major issues in voice disorders been answered by research in speech science? A fifty year retrospective. *J Speech Hear Disord* 42:152–160.

Murdoch B, Noble J, Chenery H, Ingram J. (1989). A spirometric and kinematic analysis of respiratory function in pseudobulbar palsy. *Aust J Hum Commun Disord* 17(2):21–35.

Murdoch BE, Thompson EC, Stokes PD. (1994). Phonatory and laryngeal dysfunction following upper motor neuron vascular lesions. *J Med Speech-Lang Pathol* 2(3):177–189.

Nailling K, Horner J. (1979). Reorganizing neurogenic articulation disorders by modifying prosody. Paper presented at the convention of the American Speech-Language-Hearing Association, Atlanta.

Nemec RE, Cohen K. (1984). EMG biofeedback in the modification of hypertonia in spastic dysarthria: Case report. *Arch Physical Med Rehabil* 65:103–104.

Netsell R. (1973). Speech physiology. In: Minifie F, Hixon T, Williams F, eds. *Normal Aspects of Speech, Hearing and Language*. New Jersey: Prentice-Hall.

Netsell R, Daniel B. (1979). Dysarthria in adults: Physiologic approach to rehabilitation. *Arch Physical Med Rehabil* 60:502–508.

Netsell R, Hixon TJ. (1992). Inspiratory checking in therapy for individuals with speech breathing dysfunction. *ASHA* 34:152.

Netsell R, Rosenbek J. (1986). Treating the dysarthrias. In: Netsell R, ed. *A Neurobiologic View of Speech Production and the Dysarthrias*. San Diego: College-Hill Press, pp 123–152.

Orlikoff RF. (1992). The use of instrumental measures in the assessment and treatment of motor speech disorders. *Semin Speech Language* 13(1):25–37.

Perkins W. (1985). Assessment and treatment of voice disorders: State of the art. In: Costello J, ed. *Speech Disorders in Adults*. San Diego: College-Hill Press.

Portnoy RA, Aronson AE. (1982). Diadochokinetic syllable rate and regularity in normal and in spastic and ataxic dysarthric subjects. *J Speech Hear Disord* 47:324–328.

Powers G, Starr C. (1974). The effects of muscle exercises on velopharyngeal gap and nasality. *Cleft Palate J* 11:28–35.

Prosek RA, Montgomery AA, Walden BE, Schwartz DM. (1978). EMG biofeedback in the treatment of hyperfunctional voice disorders. *J Speech Hear Disord* 43:282–294.

Robertson SJ, Thompson F. (1986). *Working with Dysarthrics: A Practical Guide to Therapy for Dysarthria*. Oxon: Winslow Press.

Rosenbek JC, LaPointe LL. (1978). The dysarthrias: Description, diagnosis, and treatment. In: Johns D, ed. *Clinical Management of Neurogenic Communicative Disorders*. Boston: Little, Brown, pp 251–310.

Rubow R. (1980). Biofeedback in the treatment of speech disorders. Speech Motor Control Laboratories Preprints (Autumn), Waisman Center, University of Wisconsin, Madison.

Schweiger J, Netsell R, Sommerfeld R. (1970). Prosthetic management and speech improvement in individuals. *JADA* 80:1348–1353.

Shelton RL, Paesani A, McClelland K, Bradfield S. (1975). Panendoscopic feedback in the study of voluntary velopharyngeal movements. *J Speech Hear Disord* 40:232–244.

Shelton R, Beaumont K, Trier W, Furr M. (1978). Videoendoscopic feedback in training velopharyngeal closure. *Cleft Palate J* 15:6–12.

Shimizu M, Watanabe Y, Hirose H. (1992). Use of the accent method in training for patients with motor speech disorders. Paper presented at the 22nd World Congress of the Internation Association of Logopedics and Phoniatrics, Hannover, Germany.

Siegel-Sadewitz VL, Shprintzen RJ. (1982). Nasopharyngoscopy of the normal velopharyngeal sphincter: An experiment of biofeedback. *Cleft Palate J* 19:194–200.

Smitheran JR, Hixon TJ. (1981). A clinical method for estimating laryngeal airway resistance during vowel production. *J Speech Hear Disord* 46:138–146.

Spratley MH, Chenery HJ, Murdoch BE. (1988). A different design of palatal lift appliance: Review and case reports. *Aust Dent J* 33(6):491–495.

Stemple JC, Weiler E, Whitehead W, Komray R. (1980). Electromyographic biofeedback training with patients exhibiting a hyperfunctional voice disorder. *Laryngoscope* 90:471–476.

Thompson EC, Murdoch BE. (1993). Impaired speech breathing in dysarthria following vascular lesions of supranuclear origin. Paper presented at the 11th International Australasian Winter Conference on Brain Research, Queenstown, New Zealand.

Tudor C, Selly W. (1974). A palatal training appliance and a visual aid for use in the treatment of hypernasal speech. *Br J Disord Commun* 9:117–123.

Witzel M, Tobe J, Salyer K. (1988). The use of nasopharyngoscopy biofeedback therapy in the correction of inconsistent velopharyngeal closure. *Int J Pediatr Otorhinolaryngol* 15:137–142.

Zwirner P, Murray T, Swenson M, Woodson GE. (1991). Acoustic changes in spasmodic dysphonia after botulinum toxin injection. *J Voice* 5(1):78–84.

Zwirner P, Murray T, Swenson M, Woodson GE. (1992). Effects of botulinum toxin therapy in patients with adductor spasmodic dysphonia: Acoustic, aerodynamic, and videoendoscopic findings. *Laryngoscope* 102:400–406.

Ziegler W, von Cramon D. (1986). Spastic dysarthria after acquired brain injury: An acoustic study. *Br J Disord Communic* 21:173–187.

Chapter 14

Apraxia of Speech: Definition, Differentiation, and Treatment

Malcolm R. McNeil, Donald A. Robin, and Richard A. Schmidt

Introduction

Darley (1967) is credited with the first reported observation that there was a clinical
phenomenon of neurologic origin that did
not fit into the general categories of the then
accepted neurogenic disorders of speech production (the dysarthrias and aphasia). At the
turn of the century (Liepmann, 1900), in the
recent past (Darley, 1967; Jakobson, 1968),
and in the more current and commonly accepted framework of speech pathologies
(Boone & Plante, 1993; Darley, Aronson, &
Brown, 1975a; Hegde, 1991; Palmer & Yantis,
1990), neurogenic speech production disorders have been classified as either linguistic
(ie, phonologic) or motoric. Since Darley's
observation and the subsequent accrual of
research into the phenomenon, these general
introductory and the more specialized and
dedicated texts (Duffy, 1996) subdivide motor speech disorders into the dysarthrias and
apraxia of speech (AOS).

The movement disorder termed "apraxia"
and the original description and elucidation
of the general mechanisms of the family of
apraxias are usually attributed to Liepmann
(1900, 1905, 1913). Darley's (1969) presentation at the American Speech and Hearing
Association on "apraxia of speech" appears
to have been the modern emergence of the
concept of apraxia applied to speech, although it was not the first time the term was
used to describe a phenomenon that fell outside of the accepted clinical classification

schema. Like Liepmann, Darley suggested
that the term would only be applicable when
assurance could be given that the patient had
the *intent*, the underlying *linguistic representation*, and the fundamental *motor abilities* to
produce speech, but could not do so *volition-
ally*. Darley further used the term to specify
a disorder of speech that was attributable
to a disorder of the *programming* for speech
movements. Thus were set some of the conditions for the identification and psychological specification of AOS. Since the late 1960s,
there has been a suffusal of research, to a
great measure performed by Darley and his
students, into the nature and clinical management of AOS. Histories of the term AOS
(Rosenbek, Kent, & LaPointe, 1984; Square &
Martin, 1994; Wertz, LaPointe, & Rosenbek,
1984) and its relationship to oral nonspeech
apraxia (Moore, 1975; Roy & Square, 1985;
Square-Storer, Roy, & Hogg, 1990), limb
apraxias (Duffy & Duffy, 1990; Faglioni &
Basso, 1985; Miller, 1986; Rothi & Heilman,
1985; Square-Storer & Roy, 1990), and a variety of other apraxias (eg, dressing apraxia,
writing apraxia, whole-body apraxia, ocular
apraxia, unilateral limb apraxia) have been
written elsewhere by limpid-thinking, articulate authors from both the neurology
and speech-language pathology disciplines.
These histories will not be reviewed in this
chapter. However, it is important to note
that, like all diagnostic categories, the term
AOS carries with it some very specific assumptions about its underlying neuroana-

tomic, neurophysiologic, linguistic, and motoric mechanisms. More recently, specific assumptions about its treatment have emerged (Marquardt & Cannito, 1996; Square, 1989; Wambaugh & Doyle, 1995).

In the context of proposing a revised definition of AOS, it will be necessary to examine many of these assumptions, and in doing so, to review some of the pertinent historical accounts. There are three purposes for this chapter. First we will review those clinical features that differentiate among the general classification of neurogenic speech production disorders, comprised of motor speech disorders (apraxia of speech and the dysarthrias), and phonological-level disorders (literal or phonological paraphasia). In order to do this, it is essential to contrast the phenomenology and the assumptions underlying the labels for these clinical neighbors. These pathologies include (1) the family of dysarthrias, (2) disorders of prosody, and (3) the phonemic paraphasias that cross aphasic classifications but that occur frequently in the individual with so-called conduction aphasia. Next, we will provide an evaluation of the current state of defining characteristics of AOS and will specify a tentative inventory of the necessary and sufficient behaviors and conditions used to differentiate it from its nearest clinical neighbors. Finally, we will provide a critical review of the current treatments for AOS along with an outline of the principles of treatment derived from research on motor learning.

AOS VS Dysarthria

As discussed in great detail throughout this volume, the dysarthrias are a family of disorders that are in part defined by Darley et al as "disturbances in muscular control of the speech mechanism resulting from impairment of any of the basic motor processes involved in the execution of speech." (p 2). As stated by Darley et al (1975a), the term is used generically to cover isolated or coexisting motor disorders of respiration, phonation, articulation, resonance, and prosody as well as single or multiple cranial nerve involvement. The term traditionally and explicitly excludes disorders of speech that have an anatomic structural (eg, cleft palate), psychological (eg, hysterical aphonia), learning (eg, developmental phonological disorders), stuttering, dental, or malocclusal bases. Keys to this definition are the specific set of behaviors and mechanisms implied by the words *basic motor* and *execution*. One consequence of the "basic motor processes" part of the definition implies that any movement disorder underlying speech production and dysarthria must be present in the speech apparatus when used to perform speech and similar nonspeech movements (see the chapter in this volume by Robin, Soloman, Moon, & Folkins, for a detailed discussion of this issue). The restriction of the movement deficits to those involving the "execution" level of movement, encompassed in the definition of dysarthria, are poorly specified by Darley and colleagues as well as by most others who write about sensorimotor speech disorders. However, any one or a number of the physiologic parameters of tone and reflexes along with the kinematic parameters of strength, speed, range, accuracy, and steadiness are necessarily aberrant in dysarthria. Dysarthria, therefore, can be identified in the absence or presence of any one or a combination of these kinematic/physiologic parameters. For example, dysarthria can be identified in the absence of abnormal tone (eg, hyperkinetic dysarthria) or abnormal reflexes (eg, ataxic dysarthria). It can be identified in the presence of abnormalities of movement speed (eg, bradykinesia), strength (eg, spastic or flaccid dysarthria), range (eg, hypokinetic or spastic dysarthria), accuracy (ataxic dysarthria), or steadiness (eg, quick or slow hyperkinetic dysarthria, tremor). In all cases, however, it must be identified in the *speech* of the individual. That is, dysarthria is a disorder of speech production and must be perceived by the listener or felt by the speaker. It cannot be diagnosed only by measuring an abnormal physiologic or kinematic variable in the absence of a perceptually evident disorder of speech production unless an acoustic or physiologic measure has been shown to predict with certainty that the speech would be perceived as evidencing an abnormality consistent with dysarthria. To date, these predictions have not been verified.

Tone and reflex abnormalities can be evidenced from pathology of any neural system (eg, pyramidal, extrapyramidal, cerebellar, vestibular-reticular, lower motor neuron) involved in speech production except the higher conceptual "planning" and "programming" levels (see Chapter 1 in this volume authored by Van de Merwe for a complete discussion of these issues). Traditionally, planning and programming disorders are not consistent with disorders of tone or reflexes, although disorders at the planning or programming level of motor control could evidence strength, speed, range, accuracy, and steadiness kinematic abnormalities if these discrete movement parameters were involved in the planning or programming deficit. The exact parameters of movement that are programmed and that represent the control variables for the motor programmer are not agreed upon. At the physiologic level, activation of the appropriate motoneurones at the appropriate times is a reasonable formulation of the goal (Grillner, 1982). However, this level of specification does not detail the parameters of the movement that a program is likely to control. Likely candidates at the kinematic level include the proportional assignment of movement duration and amplitude (displacement; Brooks, 1986), although such parameters as acceleration, deceleration, time to peak velocity, stiffness, or other variables may be critical parameters of a multicomponentially organized motor program. Relative timing of various speech events play the primary role in some theories of speech motor control such as Coordinative Structure Theory (Kugler, Kelso, & Turvey, 1980), Action Theory (Kelso, Tuller, & Harris, 1983), or Dynamical Theory, and replace the notion of specifically programmed parameters of movement in this conceptualization of motor control.

Although Darley et al's (1975a) definition of the dysarthrias is inadequate to differentiate AOS from dysarthria, they suggest that with the addition of the aforementioned definitional guidelines, AOS should be separable from the dysarthrias. That is, an absence of tone or reflex abnormalities during speech or nonspeech activities along with a clear differentiation between movement disorders that are manifest only in speech (AOS) and not in comparable nonspeech (unless a concomitant dysarthria or oral nonspeech apraxia were present) behaviors should aid the differential diagnosis. It should also be clear that the differentiation of AOS from dysarthria might be accomplished by perceptual analyses of the speech just as the differentiation of one form of dysarthria is differentiable from another via patterns of finite perceptible speech behaviors. Indeed it has been a major goal of a number of clinical scientists, spanning the 28 years since Darley's seminal unpublished papers in 1968 and 1969, to describe the pattern of speech behaviors that are characteristic of and isomorphic with AOS.

The first-large scale and perhaps the most comprehensive treatise on AOS was the exhaustive review and analysis of the state of the clinical science by Wertz et al (1984). Based upon the aggregate of the published research, a wealth of clinical experience, and a profusion of reason and logic, these authors proposed a definition of AOS that has been the most cited and influential on both research and clinical practice. These authors defined AOS as "a neurogenic *phonologic* disorder resulting from sensorimotor impairment of the capacity to *select*, program, and/or *execute* in coordinated and normally timed sequences, the positioning of the speech musculature for the *volitional* production of speech sounds" (p 4). Consistent with, or based upon this definition, the authors proposed that AOS was differentiable from dysarthria on anatomic grounds (AOS = unilateral and anterior; dysarthria = bilateral if cortical but usually subcortical), assumed psychophysiological level of impairment (AOS = disturbed motor programming;

dysarthria = disturbed movement execution) observed speech behavior (AOS resulting in speech initiation, selection and sequencing difficulties with a predominance of phoneme substitutions, abnormal prosody, and infrequent metathetic errors; dysarthria = predominance of sound-level distortions), speech process involvement (AOS = essentially normal in resonance, respiration, and phonation and when affected, the physiological mechanisms are different from dysarthria; dysarthria = frequent disturbance in resonance, respiration, and phonation), physiological manifestations (AOS = free from paralysis or paresis, ataxia, and involuntary movements; dysarthria = presence of paralysis or paresis, ataxia, and/or involuntary movements), the influence of nonphonologic factors (AOS = influenced by such phonetic variables as context, word length, and error inconsistency; dysarthria = less effected by context and word length and errors are more consistent), and presence of concomitant oral nonverbal apraxia (AOS = frequently present; dysarthria = absent). Table 1 summarizes these contrasts.

AOS VS Phonemic Paraphasia

It was the dissemination of the dissertation by LaPointe (1969) and the publication by Johns and Darley (1970) that set the stage for the lingering controversy into the description, the mechanisms, and even the existence of AOS. These works followed directly from Darley's (1968) observation that there was a clinical phenomenon that did not fit into the general categories of the then accepted neurogenic disorders of speech production, along with his formulation of this clinical entity as something that was consistent with the general notion of apraxia. Immediately following the Johns and Darley (1970) publication on the phonemic variability of apraxic speakers, there followed publications by Aten, Johns, and Darley (1971), Deal and Darley (1972), and Rosenbek, Wertz, and Darley (1973) that further described the auditory processing, speech characteristics, and oral sensation of the population, respectively. These publications set the stage for Martin's (1974) influential criticisms of the newly inspired AOS Zeitgeist.

Table 14–1. "Traditional" differentiating characteristics of AOS and dysarthria.

Feature	AOS	Dysarthria
Lesion location	Unilateral/anterior	Bilateral if Cortical, Usually Subcortical
Psychophysiological level/ mechanism	Motor programming	Movement Execution
Observed deviant speech behavior	Speech initiation, selection, & sequencing; phoneme substitution; abnormal prosody; infrequent metathetic errors	Sound-level Distortions
Speech processes involved	Essentially normal: 1. Resonance 2. Respiration 3. Phonation	Frequent Disturbance of: 1. Resonance 2. Respiration 3. Phonation
Physiological manifestations	Free from paralysis, paresis, ataxia, involuntary movements	Presence of Paralysis, Paresis, Ataxia, Involuntary Movements
Influence of nonphonologic (phonetic) factors	Effected by word length; error inconsistency	Less effected by word length; errors are more consistent
Oral Nonverbal Apraxia	Frequently present	Absent

Source: Wertz, LaPointe, and Rosenbek, 1984.

In his challenge to the individuals fever- ishly exploring this newly recognized clinical entity, Martin (1974) objected to the *term* AOS as it was applied to the specific subjects chosen for study by Darley and his students. It is important to note that he did not object, nor did he provide an argument that would support an objection to the existence of the clinical entity. Martin argued that the speech errors described by this series of studies could be accounted for as easily by linguistic concepts as by motor programming con- cepts. This alternative interpretation of the data was designed to inspire a reexamination of the assumptions underlying specific speech errors as evidence for linguistic ver- sus motor attribution. It accomplished this goal and inspired a torrent of studies and critical analysis of the existing data designed to support the motor or the linguistic inter- pretation. Retrospectively it appears that Martin was right to object to the term (or at least raise serious questions about its accu- racy) as applied to the populations being studied experimentally and to the clinical cases presented as prototypical exemplars of the disorder (eg, "the tornado man" case pre- sented by Darley, Aronson, and Brown, 1975b; and subsequently reported by Square (1996) to have speech symptoms similar to those of patients with parietal lobe lesions and to have had a confirmed left parietal lobe thromboembolic lesion). Numerous studies designed to investigate this alterna- tive explanation and a sudden interest in the earlier and contemporary descriptions of the speech errors of persons with aphasia followed. The question for Darley and his colleagues is the question confronted by any clinical pioneer. That is, on what bases do you select subjects for study when trying to identify and characterize a new clinical en- tity? Without established inclusional and exclusional criteria, derived from careful ex- perimentation, usually accumulated over a long period of time, and without models that specify the levels of breakdown and the po- tential mechanisms responsible for the phe- nomena (neither of which were available during Darley's early formulations of AOS),

it is difficult or impossible to have confidence that the individuals and groups actually rep- resent the subjects of interest. In other words, it is difficult or impossible to avoid experimental tautologies. Illustrative of this problem, there is some indirect evidence that Halpern, Keith, and Darley (1976) may have fallen into such a predicament. These au- thors asked the question whether aphasic patients make errors in the production of phonemes and if so, if there is a discernible pattern to the errors. Being careful research- ers, and as the article title implies ("Phone- mic behavior of aphasic subjects without dysarthria or apraxia of speech"), the authors selected subjects that would provide the best test of the hypothesis. That is, they elimi- nated potential subjects that had concomi- tant dysarthria or AOS. Twenty-eight of thirty (93%) subjects made *no* phonemic er- rors. Of those errors produced by the two subjects that did make phonemic errors, 75% were attributable to word-level errors. They concluded that "Aphasic behavior is not characterized by significant breakdown of articulatory performance" (p 371). This would indeed be an important and surpris- ing finding given the abundant literature describing and quantifying the frequent phonological errors in patients characterized as having aphasia in the absence of motor speech problems. In selecting their subjects for study the authors stated that:

> Patients were excluded from the study if (1) they made articulation errors referrable to sig- nificant weakness, slowness, incoordination, or alteration of tone of the speech musculature (dysarthria) or (2) they showed groping, off target, highly inconsistent articulatory errors— primarily substitutions, additions, prolonga- tions, and repetitions—in attempting target words in the context of islands of fluent speech, these errors being especially evident on repeti- tion tasks and increasing in incidence with increase in length of word (apraxia of speech) (p 366).

The fundamental question is whether the criteria used for eliminating potential sub- jects with AOS actually eliminated aphasic subjects that demonstrate phonological paraphasias. If one examines the typical description of "conduction aphasia," the similarities become striking. Goodglass (1992), for example, described the symptomatology of conduction aphasia:

> 1. Conversation includes runs of normally articulated words, with generally preserved use of grammatical inflections and syntactic structures. However, speech is marred by more or less frequent errors in the selection and sequencing of phonemes and syllables: these may be omitted, substituted, or transposed, creating "literal paraphasias." 2. Auditory comprehension is relatively well preserved and may even be completely normal. 3. The task of repeating words or sentences after the examiner may be particularly deficient, in comparison with the level of fluency observed in conversation (p 40).

Goodglass goes on to clarify the phonological output difficulties of the conduction aphasic. He states that:

> Because the phonological output difficulties of these patients are linked to the articulatory planning load, the objects or pictures to be named or repeated should include two-, three-, or four-syllable words. Words that involve the proper ordering of two or three consonants (e.g., baseball, elephant, pocketbook) may be insoluble tongue twisters to conduction aphasics, provoking repeated, often unsuccessful, attempts at self-correction . . . (p 41).

The *substitutions* and *omissions* errors types, *islands of fluent, normally articulated speech* and *more frequently occurring errors in repetition than in elicited or self-generated speech* are unmistakably corresponding between the descriptions of the two theoretically distinct pathological populations. The addition of the *preserved use of grammatical inflections and syntactic structures* along with *relatively well preserved auditory comprehension* in Goodglass' description of conduction aphasia goes even further toward the orthodox description of AOS that is not confounded by aphasia. The increased "planning load" of Goodglass is consistent with the increased word length effect for Darley. Further, the repeated trials and attempts at self-correction of the conduction aphasic may be consistent

with the groping, off target, reportedly highly inconsistent articulatory errors of the AOS patient. Table 2 summarizes these and other similarities between AOS and the phonologic paraphasias of the person with Conduction Aphasia.

The precise speech errors that are made by the phonological paraphasic (Kohn, 1984; Tuller, 1984) versus the AOS patient have also been proposed to differentiate the two populations. Garrett's (1880, 1884) model of language production and its modifications (Buckingham, 1990) have had a major influence on the conceptualization and characterization of the phonological-level errors, especially in Conduction and Broca aphasia. The phonetic, and particularly the motoric, levels of speech production are egregiously underspecified in Garrett's and many other such models (Bock, 1982; Dell, 1986, 1988). These levels of speech production have been entirely omitted in some discussions and models designed to explain phonological paraphasias, in spite of the fact that some errors categorized as "phonological" can be arguably assigned to the subphonemic or motoric levels. Equally notable is at least the attempt to include phonetic and motoric processes in the explanation of aphasic speech production errors by such notable speech researchers as Blumstein (1981), Blumstein and Baum (1987), Buckingham (1979, 1991), and Ryalls (1987).

The descriptions of AOS and phonological paraphasic patients are perhaps more similar than proponents of their differentiation have demonstrated. Blumstein (1981), for example, summarized the problem and the state of the two pathologies' differentiation. She wrote:

> In reality, it would not be surprising to find similar patterns of phonological disintegration whether the errors are articulatory or linguistically based, primarily because theoretical linguistic assumptions are derived from the intrinsic nature or organization. Thus, what is articulatorily simple is phonologically or linguistically simple, and what is articulatorily complex is also linguistically complex (p 135).

Table 14–2. "Traditional" characteristics of AOS and conduction aphasia.

AOS	Conduction aphasia
Physiology:	
Absence of : 1) muscle weakness, 2) movement slowness, 3) movement incoordination, 4) alterations of muscle tone	Intact movement and muscle physiology
Speech characteristics:	
Groping, off-target, highly inconsistent articulatory errors	Repeated trials, attempts at self-correction
Primarily sound errors of 1) substitution, 2) addition, 3) prolongation, 4) repetition	Sound may be 1) substitutions, 2) omissions, 3) transpositions
Islands of error-free speech	Runs of normally articulated words
Errors especially evident on repetition tasks	More frequently occurring errors on repetition
More errors with increase in word length	Difficulties are linked to the articulatory "planning load"
Preserved auditory language comprehension	Auditory comprehension is relatively well preserved and may be completely normal
Preserved syntax semantics, and morphology	Generally preserved use of grammatical inflections and syntactic structures
Speech error type:	
More consonant than vowel	More consonant than vowel
More substitutions than 1) distortions, 2) omissions, 3) additions	More substitutions than 1) distortions, 2) omissions, 3) additions
More errors in word initial than final position	More errors in word initial than final position
More error of simplification (eg, consonant cluster reduction) than complication	More error of simplification (eg, consonant cluster reduction) than complication
More single feature than multiple feature sound substitutions	More single feature than multiple feature sound substitutions

The literature attempting to describe differences between these two populations have, for the most part, selected subjects based on either lesion location (anterior vs posterior) or aphasia syndrome (eg, Broca vs Wernicke or Conduction) or both, with the assumption that Broca aphasic subjects are synonymous with the anterior, and Wernicke or Conduction aphasic subjects are synonymous with posterior. Broca Aphasia is *not* synonymous with apraxia of speech, although, depending on the exact criteria for its diagnosis, Broca patients are likely to have an accompanying motor speech problem along with their agrammatism (Marquardt & Connito, 1996; McNeil, 1984; McNeil & Kent, 1990) and typically good auditory and reading comprehension. Studies in which lesion location have been correlated with the presence of AOS have not found a relationship using Computerized Axial Tomography (Marquardt & Sussman, 1984).

Anterior vs posterior lesions inferred from neurological records and neuropsychological testing by Deutsch (1984) was reported to yield a significant difference between the two lesion groups, with the posterior group producing significantly more polysyllabic sequencing errors than the anterior group. The groups did not differ significantly on monosyllabic or polysyllabic complex errors, fluency errors, phoneme errors (eg, substitutions, omissions, additions, repetitions, and distortions), or syllable addition errors. The groups were also not different on monosyllabic sequencing errors, or total monosyllabic or polysyllabic errors. Discriminant analysis yielded three measures (percent of polysyllabic sequencing errors, percent of monosyllabic articulation errors, and total number of polysyllabic errors) that correctly classified 89% of the two groups (misclassifying one subject in each group). While the author based the premise of the investigation on the notion that there were two forms of apraxia of speech described under various names (eg, anterior or "efferent kinetic speech apraxia" and posterior or "afferent kinesthetic speech apraxia") by Liepmann (1905, 1913), Luria (1966, 1970), and Canter (1969), the error pattern of the posterior group is most consistent with our description in this chapter of what we have called and attributed mechanistically to phonemic paraphasia.

A single and focal cortical or subcortical lesion location underlying either AOS or conduction aphasia has indeed been elusive. As discussed below, patterns of speech behavior based upon *assumed* differential lesion locations underpinning AOS and conduction aphasia have been more productive in separating, both theoretically and clinically, the two neurological speech production pathologies. In spite of this failure to find differential single and focal lesions between the two populations, Square (1996) has called for a reexamination and a reclassification of AOS based on lesion location within the left hemisphere.

Phonologic Characteristics of AOS

The great majority of studies attempting to characterize AOS have used the perhaps invalid category of Broca Aphasia to select subjects. The major findings from these studies, using broad phonetic transcription of the speech, suggest that the anterior (ostensibly apraxic) patients produce: (1) more consonant than vowel errors (Darley, 1982; Keller, 1978; LaPointe & Johns, 1975; Lebrun, Buyssens, & Henneaux, 1973); (2) more substitution than distortion, omission, or addition errors (Blumstein, 1973; Dunlop & Marquardt, 1977; Johns & Darley, 1970; Klich, Ireland, & Weidner, 1979; Sasanuma, 1971; Shankweiler, Harris, & Taylor, 1968; Trost & Canter, 1974); (3) more errors in word initial than word final position (LaPointe &

Johns, 1975); (4) more errors of simplification (eg, consonant cluster reduction) than complication (Keller, 1984); (5) more single-feature than multiple-feature sound substitutions (Blumstein, 1973; LaPointe & Johns, 1975; Trost & Canter, 1974); and (6) more place than manner or voicing errors (LaPointe & Johns, 1975; Trost & Canter, 1974). Using pure AOS subjects, Odell, McNeil, Rosenbek, and Hunter (1990) found more place errors than other feature errors, more voiceless sounds substitutions for voiced sounds than the converse, and more single-feature than multiple-feature sound substitutions.

Meuse, Marquardt, and Cannito (1996) reported a phonological process analysis from the productions of 10 Broca Aphasic subjects during spontaneous word, single-word repetition, and narrative production tasks. Ninety-three percent of the total errors exhibited across the three elicitation tasks were accounted for by the 29 processes examined. However, no one process accounted for their criterion of 20% process utilization. The authors concluded that "a detailed phonological analysis failed to reveal consistent evidence that AOS subjects with Broca's Aphasia exhibit impairment in phonological ability." This is an interesting conclusion given the unsupported assumption advanced by some (Bowman, Hodson, & Simpson, 1980) and cautiously advanced by others (Kearns, 1980) that errors described by "phonological process" analysis represents phonological-level deficits. Process analysis has been shown to be a useful way of characterizing speech production errors of children with "developmental" articulation errors, however, the underlying mechanisms for the so-called phonological processes are unknown and cannot be assigned unambiguously to any level of the speech production mechanism. The cautions offered by Kearns for the utility of characterizing the speech of persons with AOS remains as valid today as it was in 1980. He stated that:

It should be noted that the results of process analyses may not represent a patient's rules for transforming abstract phonological forms into phonetic realizations. The need to establish minimal qualitative and quantitative criteria for when a process is present has only recently been recognized. There is, in fact, insufficient data available with regards to whether phonological processes are "psychologically real" (p 190).

As Blumstein (1981) pointed out, many studies of the posterior patient (both Conduction and Wernicke patients) have found the same pattern of speech errors as with the anterior patients, including more (1) consonant than vowel errors; (2) substitution errors than distortion, omission, or addition errors; (3) errors in the initial than the final position of the word; (4) errors of simplification (eg, consonant cluster reduction) than complication; and (5) single-feature than multiple-feature sound substitutions. Blumstein (1981) concluded that anterior (AOS) and posterior aphasic subjects could not be distinguished on the basis of the patterns of phonological errors.

So what speech errors can unambiguously be assigned to the phonologic level of speech production? As stated earlier, sound substitutions such as voiced for voiceless or voiceless for voiced cognates could result from the selection of the incorrect phoneme or from the mistiming of vocal fold onset with upper airway articulatory timing. Likewise, most other phoneme substitutions cannot be unambiguously attributed to either level of the mechanism. Sound omissions and additions could also be generated from either motor or linguistic mechanisms. Sound sequencing errors, on the other hand, are very difficult to assign to the motor level. That is, left-to-right, progressive assimilative or perseverative (eg, PLAYBACK → PLAYPACK OR PLAYPLACK), right-to-left, regressive assimilative or anticipatory (eg, PLAYBACK → BLAYBACK OR BAYBACK) and complete exchange or metathetic (eg, PLAYBACK → BAYPLACK OR BLAYPACK) errors that are without phonetic or motoric distortions are most consistent with the assignment of an error constructing the phonological buffer or in

filling it with misselected phonemes from the phonemic lexicon. While this may seem paradoxical, movement sequencing often described in the motor programming literature (Square, 1996; Wertz et al, 1984) does not equate to the ordering of speech sounds in the speech production process. Nonetheless, as reflected in the title of their manuscript ["Repeated trials of words by patients with neurogenic phonological selection-sequencing impairment (apraxia of speech)]," LaPointe and Horner (1976) equated phonological selection and sequencing with AOS.

Phonetic/Motoric Characteristics of AOS

While phonologic production errors have not differentiated AOS from phonemic paraphasia, perhaps phonetic patterns could. Blumstein (1981), in fact, made this prediction. Based on several studies conducted at that point in time, and later verified by additional research, she concluded that anterior aphasic (presumably AOS) patients demonstrated impairments of (1) voice onset time (VOT) (Blumstein, Cooper, Zurif, & Caramazza, 1977; Blumstein, Cooper, Goodglass, Statlender, & Gottlieb, 1980; Hoit-Dalgaard, Murry, & Kopp, 1983; Shewan, Leeper, & Booth, 1984), and (2) nasal sounds (Itoh, Sasanuma, & Ushijima, 1979; Itoh, Sasanuma, Hirose, Yoshioka, & Ushijima, 1980), because both dimensions require finite interarticulator timing. Posterior patients have been reported to show no, or only minor, deficits on these phonetic segments (Itoh, Sasanuma, Hirose, Yoshioka, & Sawashima, 1983). Following discussion of this issue, several other phonetic/motoric dimensions have been investigated.

Durations of vowels and consonants have been investigated in normal speakers, Broca, apraxic and other aphasic (typically Wernicke) patients. As summarized by McNeil and Kent (1990), between groups, differences in vowel durations have generally not been found when the stimuli were monosyllables (Bauman, 1978; Duffy & Gawle, 1984; Gandour & Dardarananda, 1984; Mercaitis, 1983; Ryalls, 1984, 1986).

Vowels in multisyllabic words or nonsense utterances have been shown to be significantly longer for apraxic than normal subjects or aphasic subjects (Collins, Rosenbek, & Wertz, 1983; Kent & Rosenbek, 1983; Mercaitis, 1983; Ryalls, 1981, 1987; Strand, 1987; Strand & McNeil, accepted for publication). McNeil and Kent (1990) have speculated that the sensitivity of vowel duration to syllabic or other aspects of utterance complexity may be an important clinical feature of AOS. Consonant durations, though less often studied than vowels, have also generally been found to be lengthened in AOS (Bauman, 1978; Kent & Rosenbek, 1983). These increased segment durations, along with increased intersegment (Mercaitis, 1983) and transition durations (Kent & Rosenbek, 1983), are consistent with the clinical impression that apraxic and Broca Aphasic speakers' speech rate is reduced (Kent & McNeil, 1987; Kent & Rosenbek, 1983; McNeil, Liss, Tseng, & Kent, 1990). Since these lengthened segments carry no meaning change, it is difficult to attribute them to a phonological or morphological level of dysregulation (McNeil & Kent, 1990). It should also be cautioned that the sheer presence or even number of vowel errors failed to differentiate AOS, Conduction Aphasic, and Ataxic Dysarthric groups by Odell, McNeil, Rosenbek, and Hunter (1991) using perceptual analyses in a single-word task. Further, the number of syllables in a word did not differentially effect the vowel error rate across groups in this study.

Force and Position Control
Movement control as well as strength of the speech articulators of persons with neurologic speech production disorders are routinely assessed clinically during speech and nonspeech activities. However, relatively few studies have been conducted to evaluate the parameters of movement, force, or position control with instruments more sensitive and potentially more reliable than the hand-and-eye typically used in the clinical evaluation. While the clinical examination of persons suspected of having AOS includes

the evaluation of muscle forces produced during nonspeech tasks, if weakness is evidenced during these tasks, the default diagnosis is usually that of dysarthria, not AOS or phonemic paraphasia. If disorders of postural control are evidenced, the diagnosis of oral-nonverbal apraxia or dysarthria (depending on its precise nature) are the likely diagnoses. In fact, it is usually part of the criteria for the diagnosis of AOS that individual articulator strength (usually measured as maximum muscle force) as well as articulatory positioning (usually measured as accurate articulatory placement and speed of movement) be judged within normal limits.

McNeil, Weismer, Adams, and Mulligan (1990) investigated the articulatory control of small nonspeech isometric forces and small static positions in normal, pure AOS, Conduction Aphasic, and Ataxic Dysarthric subjects. They found that subjects identified as having "pure" AOS without concomitant dysarthria or aphasia, tracked with visual feedback, forces and postures of the articulators that were significantly poorer (off-target and more variable) than the normal subjects but not different from the dysarthric subjects. The Conduction Aphasic subject's performance fell between the normal and other two pathological groups, but was not significantly different from either. This latter finding was interpreted as opening the possibility of a fundamental motor control deficit accompanying or perhaps accounting for the perceived speech production deficits in Conduction Aphasia.

Hageman, Robin, Moon, and Folkins (1994) compared five apraxic and 23 normal subjects on their ability to track, with visual feedback, a 0.3-, 0.6-, 0.9-Hz and a nonpredictable signal with the lower lip, jaw and voice (f_0). Although the authors did not compare the groups or the conditions statistically, the normal subjects achieved a best cross-correlation (disregarding their phase lead or lag) with the predictable targets and their highest cross-correlations were inversely related to the frequency of the predictable target. Further, the normal subjects' poorest cross-correlation occurred with the nonpredictable signals for all structures. The apraxic subjects, on the other hand, achieved their highest cross-correlations across all structures for the unpredictable targets and their correlations were variable across the three frequencies of the predictable targets. Confounding the interpretation of this finding is the fact that the actual cross-correlational values were similar for the apraxic and normal groups for the nonpredictable targets. Interpreting their results, the authors noted that movement control for the nonspeech tasks was impaired in their AOS subjects. Second, because the unpredictable target was tracked relatively better than the predictable one for the AOS subjects, the authors proposed that the AOS speakers had problems retrieving or "developing an internal model or plan of the intended movement patterns." It must be remembered that as with all of the other studies that have used "pure" apraxic subjects, the subject numbers are too small to generalize to other pure apraxic subjects or to individuals with AOS accompanied by other speech production deficits. Nonetheless, given the high confidence in accurate subject selection from these two studies, it seems clear that the nonspeech movements of individuals with AOS are not normal and that these deficits of static and dynamic force and position tracking ability are not related to the clinical detection of oral motor movement or force deficits nor to nonverbal apraxia.

Intra- and Interarticulator Kinematics
The measurement of movements within an articulator have been investigated in a variety of studies using a variety of methods and procedures. One issue addressed by many of the kinematic studies attempts to account for the slower speech of the apraxic subject found with both perceptual and acoustic analyses. For example, Itoh et al (1980) reported peak velocities for one apraxic subject that were substantively lower than a normal control subject, and were in the range of those reported for a patient with amyotrophic lateral sclerosis. Using the x-ray

microbeam system for simultaneously tracking movements of multiple articulators, Itoh et al (1980) and Itoh and Sasanuma (1984) reported inconsistent interarticulator timing abnormalities between the lip, velum, and tongue dorsum in one patient with "pure" AOS. Using fiberscopic observation of the velum, Itoh and Sasanuma (1984) reported velar timing distortions that were often perceived as sound substitutions in this same patient. Itoh and Sasanuma (1987) reported lip and jaw kinematics for 10 normal (five young and five aged), five Broca Aphasic with AOS, and three Wernicke Aphasic subjects. While the Wernicke subjects showed no abnormalities in peak velocity or displacement, the AOS subjects demonstrated inconsistent articulatory velocity and or displacement values that occasionally violated the normal reciprocal relationship between peak velocity and displacement. On these occasions, the apraxic speakers underassigned velocity to a displacement or overassigned both velocity and displacement simultaneously.

Using strain gauge transducers, McNeil, Caliguiri and Rosenbek (1989) compared labiomandibular durations, displacements, velocities, and dysmetrias in four "pure" AOS and four normal control subjects. The movement durations across the transition from the vowel /a/ in "stop" to the vowel /ae/ in "fast" in the phrase "stop fast" was significantly longer in the AOS subjects. While, the average peak velocities were not significantly different between the groups, the AOS subjects produced significantly greater lower lip + jaw displacements than the control subjects. While the finding of a normal peak velocity has been replicated by Robin, Bean, and Folkins (1989), and by McNeil and Adams (1990), the greater displacement in the AOS group has not been replicated in subsequent analyses of these same subject's productions of other utterances (McNeil & Adams, 1990). In addition to the finding of normal peak velocity, McNeil and Adams (1990) found that these subjects produced abnormally long times to reach peak velocity compared to normal, conduction aphasic, and ataxic dysarthric subjects. These authors also reported significantly longer total utterance durations for all three pathological groups compared to the normal subjects.

As mentioned above, Robin et al (1989) also found normal peak velocities in six carefully selected AOS subjects but failed to find abnormal peak velocity/displacement relationships under conditions of altered speech rate, whether the jaw was blocked or unblocked or whether the utterance was produced correctly or incorrectly. Fromm, Abbs, McNeil, and Rosenbek (1982) reported a descriptive study of three "pure" apraxic and three normal control subject's speech under simultaneous acoustic, kinematic, and electromyographic measurement. Description across structures and analysis levels revealed a variety of intra- and interarticulator temporal and spatial dyscoordinations.

Hardcastle (1987) also described a general dyscoordination of the tongue tip, blade, and body in one apraxic speaker using the electropalatograph. The dyscoordination was described as one of unsmooth transitions between successive lingual gestures with poor anticipatory coarticulation. Consistent with this interpretation of the primary deficit of AOS subjects, Forrest, Adams, McNeil, and Southwood (1991) found from a kinematic analysis of AOS, Conduction Aphasia, ataxic dysarthric, and normal control subjects, phase plane trajectories for closing gestures in the AOS speakers that were decoupled in temporal-spatial relations (ie, amplitude/velocity relations) relative to the same gestures in the normal subjects. These authors noted that these decouplings were strikingly similar to the decomposition of multiarticulate movements evidenced in complex arm trajectories in individuals with limb apraxia (Poizner, Mack, Verfaellie, Rothi, & Heilman, 1990).

Katz, Machetanz, Orth, and Schonle (1990) reported the labial and velar kinematic results from an investigation into the extent and time course of anticipatory coarticulation in the speech of two normal and two anterior German aphasic speakers.

Using Electromagnetic articulography, the anterior aphasic subject's on target productions were more variable than those of the control subjects and these differences were primarily in the spatial/displacement aspects of the movements. The temporal aspects of the anticipatory coarticulatory movements were judged to be largely intact.

Following Shankweiler et al's (1968) pioneering descriptive electromyographic (EMG) study of two patients with "phonetic disintegration", or what is most likely consistent with AOS as defined in this chapter, showing a lack of temporal differentiation (ie, reduced independent movements) among articulators, several EMG studies have followed. Fromm (1981) and Fromm et al (1982) described antagonistic muscle co-contraction, continuous undifferentiated muscle activity, and EMG shutdown from recording of orbicularis oris superior, orbicularis oris inferior, mentalis and depressor labi inferior muscles in three AOS patients. In order to replicate this descriptive study, Forrest et al (1991) compared EMG activity from the same muscles in four subjects in each of the following groups; "pure" AOS, conduction aphasia, ataxic dysarthria, and normal control. Antagonistic muscle co-contraction, continuous undifferentiated muscle activity and EMG shutdown did not differentiate any of the groups. In fact, all groups, including the normal control group, demonstrated instances of these patterns. The frequency of their occurrence was not related to the judged severity of the AOS in any group. The authors concluded, "It is difficult to conceptualize any group characteristics concerning AOS on the basis of the EMG data because each speaker displayed individual patterns of muscle activity."

Hough and Klich (1987) investigated the EMG timing of lip rounding for vowel productions in the context of the vowel shorting that normally accompanies the increase in syllable number (eg, Short/Shorten/Shortening). These authors concluded that there are measurable linguistic influences on EMG lip rounding onset activity and that these influences were preserved, although less consistently applied in the AOS subjects compared to the normal control subjects.

The conclusion reached by McNeil and Kent (1990) relative to the EMG evidence describing AOS remains valid. They suggested that the EMG studies attempting to characterize and differentiate phonemic paraphasia from AOS subjects are meager and in desperate need of replication and careful comparison with equivalent data from normal control and other pathological subjects who share speech symptoms and lesion specificity.

Speech Prosody

Relatively few studies have investigated the amplitude of AOS speech. Fewer still have investigated these attributes in patients with phonemic paraphasia, as they are rarely identified as having prosodic problems. Kent and Rosenbek (1983) investigated syllable amplitude in AOS subjects, and Lebrun et al (1973) reported on syllable amplitude in Broca Aphasic subjects. Both reported amplitude uniformity, which along with the temporal regularity, leads to neutralization of stress pattern and dysrhythmia which is part of the characteristic dysprosody often described in AOS.

F_0 variations (contour) in Broca Aphasic individuals have been reported as restricted in range for sentence-level stimuli by Ryalls (1982) and Cooper, Soares, Nicol, Michelow, and Goloskie (1984), but not for within-word level stimuli by Danly and Shapiro (1982). Additionally, Broca Aphasic subjects have been found to shorten the obligatory utterance-final lengthening (Danly, deVilliers, & Cooper, 1979).

Odell et al (1990) added to the description of the prosodic disturbance in AOS and its differentiation from the prosodic pattern found with the phonologic paraphasic and the ataxic dysarthric (Odell, McNeil, Rosenbek, & Hunter, 1991). They found that the AOS and Ataxic dysarthric subjects had substantially more errors on stressed syllables than the phonemic paraphasic subjects. Further, frequent errors involving

sound transitions, as reflected by open juncture, separated the small sample sizes of AOS from Conduction Aphasic subjects who demonstrated virtually no such errors.

Ziegler and Von Cramon (1985) investigated lingual-laryngeal, lingual-velar, and lingual-labial coarticulation. They found that in contrast to the normal speakers, the AOS subjects failed to provide the necessary coarticulatory acoustic cues for normal listeners to judge the upcoming acoustic event (eg, vowel) when it was totally or partially removed from the auditory stimulus. McNeil, Hashi, and Southwood (1994) replicated this finding for bilabial gestures for two subjects with AOS and also found a similar effect for one of two subjects with Conduction Aphasia. Using acoustic analyses, Tuller and Story (1987) and Katz (1987) investigated anticipatory coarticulation or the anticipation of an articulatory feature in advance of the production of its parent segment. While Tuller and Story found that some of their "nonfluent" aphasic subjects did *not* show evidence of anticipatory coarticulation as early as the "fluent" aphasic or normal controls, Katz failed to find evidence for a delay of coarticulatory gestures in his "anterior" aphasic speakers. Katz, Machetanz, Orth, and Shonle (1990) performed acoustic analyses on two anterior and two normal German-speaking subjects' word productions contrasting in post-consonantal vowel rounding. Anticipatory labialization was assessed by measuring frequency shift in the F2 peaks and transitions. They found anticipatory labial coarticulation in the aphasic speakers that resembled the two normal speakers. While these results are interesting, it is not possible to equate with any degree of certainty the "nonfluent," "anterior," and AOS subjects used across these studies.

Variability, Consistency, and Target Approximation Profile

The consistency of speech errors has been argued as evidence for both a basic motoric (execution level) and a linguistic representational error assignment-level. One argument, for example, suggests that because no studies have demonstrated a consistently impaired feature (eg, place) across all the phonemes in which it appears, it is evidence against a linguistic (representational) mechanism for the speech errors of aphasic or apraxic speakers. Another argument specifies that a consistent error is evidence for a motoric-level error. As stated by McNeil, Odell, Miller, and Hunter (1995), there is no shared set of criteria among clinicians or researchers regarding the direction of prediction or magnitude of effect for the three variables of consistency of error location, variability of error type, or the accuracy of attempts of the target on multiple and successive trials. Inconsistency of error location (Wertz et al, 1984), variability of error type (Wertz et al, 1984), and improvement on successive attempts to reach the phonemic/phonetic target (Aten et al, 1971; Darley, 1982; Wertz et al, 1984) are reported to be characteristic of AOS. Likewise, the phonologic paraphasic errors of the conduction aphasic have been reported to increase in accuracy with successive attempts at the target, be consistent in location of the error in the segment, as well as be nonvariable in the type of the error (Joanette, Keller, & Lecours, 1980). Though this differential consistency and variability has not been documented, it appears that these are principles used by many clinicians to guide their differential diagnosis of AOS from phonemic paraphasia. As summarized by McNeil et al (1995), dysarthric speakers are traditionally described as producing errors that are consistent in error location and nonvariable in type (Darley et al, 1975a; Wertz et al, 1984). In order to test this assumption, McNeil et al (1995) assessed the consistency of error location, variability of error type, and accuracy of successive approximations on three repeated trials of the same word, in carefully selected and "pure" subjects with AOS, Conduction Aphasia, and Ataxic Dysarthria. They reported that the consistency of location of errors was higher for the AOS and Ataxic Dysarthric subject groups than for the phonemic paraphasic

group. Conversely, the variability of error type was considerably higher for the phonemic paraphasic group than for the AOS and Ataxic Dysarthric groups, whose performances were very similar to each other. The phonemic paraphasic group produced more *attempts* (defined as "any phonemic or audible nonphonemic utterance occurring prior to the final production that was separated from it by any perceived silence") and *starters* (defined as "an audible initial sound, syllable, or word characterized by a smooth transition into the final production, with no perceivable pauses or breaks") with a greater percentage of accurately reached targets for both attempts and starters than the AOS or Ataxic Dysarthric groups. Further, the phonemic paraphasic subjects produced more attempts and starters at the word level and few at the sound level, while the AOS group produced more attempts and starters at the sound level and none at the word level. The groups produced approximately equal proportions of these "trial and error gropings" at the syllable level. While the number of subjects from which these findings are derived are extremely small, the purity of their classification can be used to form the basis from which further studies on larger numbers and perhaps less isolated impairments can be conducted. In the interim, data from carefully selected subjects with isolated impairments, using finite systems for analysis such as narrow phonetic transcription, can offer more insight into the nature and phenomenology of the disorder than the data accumulated over the previous 30 years from subjects poorly defined or with mixed disorders. In addition, data derived from individuals with isolated disorders such as "pure" AOS or phonemic paraphasia without concomitant AOS or dysarthria, provide the bases for productive hypothesis building.

In summary, the phonemic paraphasic subjects were *less* consistent in the location of their errors on repeated trials of the same utterance than the AOS subjects, *more* variable in the type of errors than the AOS subjects, and they tended to get closer to the target on successive productions of the target with more starters and attempts along the way. These findings are counter to current clinical beliefs and may offer insight into both the mechanisms of the error generators in the two populations and into their differential diagnosis. However, until appropriate numbers of carefully selected subjects with "pure" pathologies can be assessed using the same stimuli and measurement procedures along with the appropriate statistical procedures (eg, discriminant function analysis) for determining their contributions to an overall profile that differentiates the populations, these differential features will remain hypotheses for testing.

If there has been no a priori means of selecting subjects for study in order to describe the phenomenology of the disorder and to determine the underlying nature of pathology, it must follow that all of the data are suspect relative to their usefulness for setting identification criteria and their validity for assigning underlying mechanisms to the pathological behaviors. If one also examines the performance characteristics of carefully selected AOS and conduction aphasic subjects (described below), the probability is increased that the criteria employed by Halpern et al (1976) and most other researchers that have contributed to the current database, actually did eliminate the aphasic subjects that demonstrated phonological or literal paraphasias. This contamination of the AOS database has been recognized by others. For example, Itoh and Sasanuma (1984) stated:

> ... those articulatory characteristics of apraxia of speech set forward by Johns and Darley [1970] which have been confirmed by many investigators since then, in fact, might be reflecting an underlying impairment which is not confined to the level of motor programming ..., but extend into the level of linguistic (phonological) processing ... as well (p 159).

Effort

The notion of excessive effort expended in the production of speech is a frequently ap-

pearing characteristic in the sundry descriptions and definitions of AOS. As discussed by Pierce (1991), the notion of effort may be tied, to some degree, to the concepts of consistency, variability, and successive approximations discussed earlier in this chapter. Attempts to self-correct speech errors may give the impression that speech is more effortful to produce, and in fact it may be. However, the notions of consistency, variability, and successive approximations (trial-and-error behavior) toward a correct target cannot unambiguously be assigned to the AOS patient (Joanette et al, 1980; Hough, 1978; Kohn, 1984).

Solomon, Robin, and Luschei (1994), Somodi, Robin, and Luschei (1995), and Solomon, Robin, Mitchinson, VanDaele, and Luschei (in press) have recently begun a program of research investigating the relationships among motor abilities and "sense of effort" in normal and brain damaged individuals. Somodi et al (1995) had 20 normal subjects exert from 10 to 100% of their own perceived maximum tongue and hand contractions while measuring the actual pressures produced on a fluid-filled bulb. Comparisons made between their effort attempted and pressures achieved were reliable and accurately described by a third polynomial. Clark and Robin (1996) replicated the basic finding of a predictable relationship between task performance and sense of effort in normal subjects; however, they found that brain-damaged individual's sense of effort was not always reflected in the predictable relationships among task complexity, reaction time, and effort during a dual-task situation. The authors concluded that brain-damaged individuals may not be sensitive to task demands and may require external feedback to effectively allocate resources to motor or other tasks.

These studies on "sense of effort" hold as much interest as they do potential clinical importance. However, there is no literature attempting to relate the listener's judgment of the speaker's effort to the actual effort expended by the speaker. Until this enormously complex set of issues is systematically disentangled, it is very difficult to know what perceptual or linguistic features listeners are attributing to the description that apraxic speech is effortful and perhaps more effortful than individuals with phonological paraphasia, dysarthria, stuttering, or another speech or language impaired population. Until this is systematically clarified with research, it is difficult to use the term "effortful" as a necessary or differential feature of AOS.

Redefining Apraxia of Speech

Rosenbek and McNeil (1991) proposed that one worthy goal of contemporary clinical scientists interested in speech production and its pathologies is to find strong neuromotor syndromes in dysarthria and apraxia of speech. According to these authors:

> A strong syndrome is one in which neuromuscular abnormalities are identified in predictable distribution across functional components and are related to a pattern of perceptual speech abnormalities with sufficient frequency to suggest a causal relationship. If the pattern is unique, the syndrome is stronger yet (p 293).

Rosenbek and McNeil (1991) suggested that the goal of contrasting assumed mechanisms, signs, symptoms, and the presence or absence of concomitant disorders between AOS and dysarthria is to eventually work out the significant characteristics of the groups and find constant differences between them. Having begun, of clinical and experimental necessity, to use the labels of dysarthria and apraxia with their inadequately tested assumptions borrowed from neurology, the search for the defining characteristics and constant differences for AOS has been biased from the onset. The realization of this goal awaits a great deal of clinical experimentation. Similarly, and more critical to the goals of this chapter, the goal of contrasting assumed mechanisms, signs and symptoms between AOS and phonemic paraphasia is also to eventually work out the significant characteristics of the groups and find constant differences between them. The review of the phonologic, phonetic, prosodic,

and motoric characteristics above provide a beginning for such an enterprise. Table 3 summarizes a tentative list of characteristics that both define AOS and differentiate it from phonemic paraphasia. The list is tentative because it will require systematic verification on relatively large numbers of subjects who demonstrate characteristics of only one pathological group or alternatively, on very large groups of carefully described subjects with less pure pathological conditions. Further, when perceptual analyses form the dependent measure, it is essential that narrow phonetic analysis be used in order to capture the nonphonologic, as well as the phonologic characteristics of the speech errors.

Dabul (1979) proposed a list of 15 speech and nonspeech behaviors that characterize AOS, any five or more of which were sufficient for its diagnose. The list consisted of the exhibition of: (1) anticipatory phonemic errors, (2) perseverative phonemic errors, (3) phonemic transposition errors, (4) phonemic voicing substitutions, (5) phonemic vowel substitutions, (6) visible and audible searching behavior, (7) numerous and varied off-target attempts at the word, (8) highly inconsistent errors, (9) increase in errors with increase in phonemic sequence, (10) fewer errors in automatic speech than volitional speech, (11) marked difficulty initiating speech, (12) intrusion of a schwa between syllables or in consonant clusters, (13) abnormal prosodic features, (14) awareness of errors and inability to correct them, and (15) receptive-expressive gap. Pierce (1991) suggested that only three of these 15 behaviors were unique characteristics of AOS and could be used to differentiate it from phonemic paraphasic speech errors. The three unique behaviors were difficulty initiating speech, intrusion of a schwa, and abnormal prosody. Visible and audible searching, he suggested, might be useful for the differentiation of the two pathologies depending on how "searching" is defined; however, the other 11 behaviors are characteristics of both phonemic paraphasia and AOS.

Cautiously, we would both disagree with Pierce's selections identifying unique behav-

Table 14–3. Tentative list of characteristics that differentiate AOS from phonemic paraphasia.

Apraxia of speech	Phonemic paraphasia
Disturbed prosody:	
Overall rate:	
Slow rate in phonemically "on target" or "off-target" phrases and sentences.	*Near normal rate* in phonemically "on-target" phrases and sentences.
Inability to increase rate while maintaining phonemic integrity.	Variable *ability to increase rate,* but *within normal ranges,* while maintaining phonemic integrity.
Microsegmental rate:	
Variable, but *overall prolonged movement transitions.*	Variable, but *normal movement transition durations.*
Variable, but *prolonged interword intervals* in phonemically "on-target" utterances.	Variable, but *normal average interword intervals* in phonemically "on-target" utterances.
Variable, but *abnormally long vowels* in multisyllabic words or words in sentences.	Variable, but *normal vowel duration* in multisyllabic words or words in sentences.
Variable, but *increased movement durations* for individual speech gestures in the production of contextual speech.	Variable, but *average movement durations* within the ranges for normal subjects.
Successive self-initiated trials to repair an error leads *no closer to the target.*	Successive self-initiated trials to repair an error leads *closer to the target.*
Stress assignment:	
Presence of errors on stressed syllables.	*No clear relationship between syllabic stress and error frequency.*
Phonological characteristics:	
With distorted perseverative, anticipatory and exchange phoneme or phoneme cluster errors.	*With* undistorted perseverative, anticipatory and phoneme exchange or phoneme cluster errors.
With phoneme distortions.	*Without phoneme distortions.*
Presence of distorted sound substitutions—primarily of prolonged phonemes and secondarily devoiced phonemes.	*Absence of distorted sound substitutions.*
Other kinematic characteristics:	
Inability to track predictable movement patterns with speech articulators.	*Ability to track predictable movement patterns* with speech articulators.
Ability to track unpredictable movement patterns with speech articulators.	*Inability to track unpredictable movement patterns* with speech articulators.
Other Characteristics:	
The *location of errors* in the utterance *is consistent* from trial to trial.	The *location of errors* in the utterance *is not consistent* from trial to trial.
The *types of errors* in the utterance *are not variable* from trial to trial.	The *types of errors* in the utterance *are variable* from trial to trial.
Treatment characteristics:	
Positive response to "minimal pairs" treatment.	*Negative* response to "minimal pairs" treatment.
Positive response to treatment based on principles of "motor learning."	*Ineffective* response to treatment based on principles of "motor learning."

iors listed by Dabul that separate the two pathologies. That is, anticipatory, perseverative, and transposition errors belong exclusively to the phonemic paraphasic. Errors that are highly inconsistent are also most likely generated by the phonemic paraphasic. From Dabul's list, only the intrusive schwa and abnormal prosody (depending on how it is defined) belong exclusively to the individual with AOS. Errors that increase with increases of phonemic sequences, are more frequent with volitional than automatic speech (depending on how the terms "volitional" and "automatic" are operationalized), are uncorrectable with awareness (depending to a great measure on the severity of the disorder) and occur in the context of a receptive-expressive performance gap (depending on the severity of both the speech production deficit and the other aphasic symptoms), belong to both groups. Voicing and vowel substitutions, visible and audible searching, varied off-target attempts and marked difficulty initiating speech are more likely to be seen in the phonemic paraphasic; however, they can be seen in both groups.

Following their 40 pages of detailed review of the characteristics, Wertz et al (1984) condensed their discussion into the four most salient clinical characteristics of AOS:

> 1. Effortful, trial and error, groping articulatory movements and attempts at self-correction. 2. Dysprosody unrelieved by extended periods of normal rhythm, stress and intonation. 3. Articulatory inconsistency on repeated productions of the same utterance. 4. Obvious difficulty initiating utterances (p 81).

They suggested that those patients revealing these four behaviors in spontaneous and imitative speech are apraxic. While all of these behaviors are likely to be seen in AOS, only the dysprosody, in the context of these three (and other) behaviors is likely to separate it from phonemic paraphasia. It will be recalled that the phonemic paraphasic may present with inconsistent trial and error behaviors and attempts at self correction, with a great deal of effort, often at the initiation of an utterance.

It is unlikely that a "checklist" method of features can be developed that will allow the differential diagnosis of AOS. All of the behaviors that comprise the core features of the syndrome can be seen in other neurogenic speech production disorders. It is the behaviors that occur in particular clusters, likely influenced by severity, that allow the differ-

ential identification of AOS. It is unfortunate that a large enough pool of "pure" AOS subjects, or an even larger pool of not-so-pure AOS subjects have not been collected on the same appropriate tasks, using the same methods of measurement so that cluster analyses, or similar procedures could be employed to establish the patterns of behavior that differentiate AOS from its clinical pathological neighbors. Until this is done, the sifting and winnowing of information from diverse populations, using diverse tasks and measurement procedures, along with the continued sharpening of theory will constitute the grounds for our formal definition of AOS and the criteria by which it is to be identified and eventually managed. It is critical to the clinical theoretician and to the practicing clinician to remember that AOS rarely presents in isolation. Such behaviors as sound substitutions, can occur in a person with AOS because they are distortions of the intended sound or because they are phoneme substitutions that occur because of a phonological misselection. In the former case the mechanism might be consistent with the mechanism for AOS. In the later case it might be attributable to a phonological-level error. If it could be established that the mechanism was one attributable to the phonological-level of speech processing, it does not mean, and cannot be concluded that AOS is a phonological disorder. The arguments about whether AOS is a phonological disorder or a motor programming disorder are fatuous. While the exact manifestations in the speech apparatus are to a large measure yet to be specified, AOS is by definition, a motor planning/programming disorder. The issue is not one of defining "apraxia"; that has been done. The issue is one of specifying to whom the term AOS applies.

Consistent with the proposed mechanisms discussed throughout the chapter, and consistent with the characteristics discussed above and summarized in Table 3 that should eventually differentiate AOS from phonemic paraphasia, the following definition of AOS is proposed:

Apraxia of speech is a phonetic-motoric disorder of speech production caused by inefficiencies in the translation of a well-formed and filled phonologic frame to previously learned kinematic parameters assembled for carrying out the intended movement, resulting in intra- and interarticulator temporal and spatial segmental and prosodic distortions. It is characterized by distortions of segment and intersegment transitionalization resulting in extended durations of consonants, vowels, and time between sounds, syllables, and words. These distortions are often perceived as sound substitutions and as the mis-assignment of stress and other phrasal and sentence-level prosodic abnormalities. Errors are relatively consistent in location within the utterance and invariable in type. It is not attributable to deficits of muscle tone or reflexes, nor to deficits in the processing of auditory, tactile, kinesthetic, proprioceptive, or language information. In its extremely infrequently occurring "pure" form, it is not accompanied by the above listed deficits of motor physiology, perception, or language.

Requirements for Additional Research

"Pure" AOS Subjects and Narrow Phonetic Transcription

There are at least two important experimental methods, in addition to continued theoretical developments, that have clarified the assignment of specific speech errors to specific levels of the linguistic and motoric speech production process. The use of narrow phonetic transcription and the selection of subjects for study that demonstrate "pure" AOS (ie, without coexisting aphasia or dysarthria) both have allowed the continued specification of linguistic and motoric mechanisms of the speech production process. It must be recognized, however, that pure AOS (AOS in isolation from dysarthria and aphasia) and pure phonemic (literal) paraphasia (phonemic paraphasia in isolation from any convincing signs of dysarthria, AOS or other signs of aphasia such as evidence of impairments in reading, writing, auditory comprehension, lexical retrieval, etc) are extremely rare speech/language pathologies.

It must also be recognized, however, that pure subjects whose speech is transcribed narrowly may be the only convincing forms of perceptual evidence from which defining characteristics can be formulated. That is, if pathologies frequently or typically coexist, there is little assurance that the data on which the phenomenology of AOS or phonemic paraphasias can be used to set the defining characteristics of either pathological group unless certain error types or certain measurements can unambiguously be assigned to different levels of the speech production system/model. As so clearly called for by Itoh and Sasanuma (1984):

> More rigorous criteria for subject selection in research will be mandatory if we are to extract only those articulatory characteristics which are the direct acoustic results of apraxic movements per se and nothing else (p 159).

They go on to say:

> Our findings ... are clearly in support of the view that faulty programming of speech musculature constitutes the base of the symptom complex called "apraxia of speech" and that the most natural and reasonable end products of this underlying deficit are (phonetic) distortions (p 160).

It is only with narrow phonetic transcription that these distortions can be extracted from the phonemic errors that are the natural consequence of categorical speech perception (Lieberman & Studdert-Kennedy, 1978).

Treatment

Given the assumption that AOS is defined as a motor control problem, it is important to apply principles of motor control and leaning to the therapeutic process. Structuring sessions based on motor learning principles may require speech-language pathologists to reorganize treatment for the AOS patient; however, the principles are in no way inconsistent with customary or best practices in the treatment of motor speech or other neurogenic disorders. This section first briefly reviews the major treatment techniques for AOS that have developed since Darley and colleagues brought the notion and the clinical phenomenon to light. This is followed by a review of principles of motor learning that are requisite for specifying the structure of treatment sessions so as to promote the learning of skilled motor routines. Finally, a brief section is devoted to the application of more specific principles of the motor approaches to speech remediation in AOS.

Review of Traditional Remediation Approaches to AOS

Over the past 25 years a number of different approaches to the treatment of AOS in adults and children have been developed. Traditional approaches to therapy for AOS have been reviewed critically elsewhere (Pierce, 1991; Rosenbek, 1985; Square-Storer, 1989). Hall, Jordan, and Robin (1993) have also provided a critical review of "motor" approaches to articulation therapy. This section presents a summary of these treatments which the reader is encouraged to review critically and in enough detail from the original descriptions and the various published studies reporting procedural modifications as well as any available efficacy data, in order to implement them into their clinical armamentaria.

Square-Storer (1989) lists a number of traditional approaches to the treatment of AOS that she indicates have their basis in the enhancement of "spatial targeting and phasing at the segmental and syllable levels." One general approach is that of *phonetic derivation.* Phonetic derivation refers to the shaping of speech sounds based on their nonspeech postures and/or actions. Activities in this type of treatment involve such tasks as putting the lips together and then blowing to prepare for the production of bilabial plosives. Square-Storer suggests that the presence of oral apraxia would make this approach difficult. However, it may be that the nonspeech movements allow the clinician to control the complexity of the task (see Robin et al, this volume) and may work even in the face of oral apraxia.

Another traditional approach to the treatment of AOS has to do with progressive approximation. *Progressive approximation* is the process whereby the clinician gradually shapes speech segments from other speech segments (Square-Storer, 1989). This approach seems to follow as a next step from phonetic derivation and relies on the production of speech sounds as a starting place for treatment. Using progressive approximation requires the clinician to use a speech sound that the patient is able to produce, and to modify it slightly to produce a new phoneme or phonetic target. For instance, if the patients can produce the nasal /m/, the clinician might use the bilabial posture to move to a bilabial plosive such as /b/.

Phonetic placement techniques have also been used to target the segmental level of production. Here the clinician focuses on the position of the articulator during speech production and the coordination between speech production subsystems. The clinician uses graphs, models, drawings, verbal descriptions, and physical manipulation to demonstrate or explain how a given speech sound is produced.

The *key word* technique requires that the patient with AOS be able to produce, consistently, some words. The clinician has the patient produce these "key words" under conditions whereby the patient exhibits greater degrees of control and lesser degrees of automaticity in the responses. Once the patient shows fairly good control of the key words, practice is expanded to include new words that contain the same phonemes as the key words. For example, if the patient is able to produce the word "Bob," then this word would be targeted until it is produced under the control of the patient in meaningful ways. The clinician encourages the patient to think about how it feels to produce a /b/ sound and then moves to new words with minimal phonetic change such as "bib."

Another segmental technique requires the imitation of *phonetic contrasts* or *minimal pairs.* The use of this treatment technique requires the establishment of speech stimuli that vary minimally relative to features such as manner, place, and voicing. The clinician has the patient imitate minimally contrasted words. Changes in task demand might involve changing the predictability of the target phonemes in the position within the word or phrase, or imposing a delay so that the imitation is not immediate.

Another group of treatments for AOS have been categorized as targeting the *temporal schemata of speech and the sequencing of segments into longer utterances* (Square-Storer, 1989). The basic premise underlying these approaches to the treatment of AOS is that there is a temporal or rhythmic basis to the control of motor behavior, including speech. In fact, Kent and Adams (1989) have argued that speech coordination is best defined in terms of temporal constraints. They further suggested that AOS may best be viewed as a breakdown in the normal temporal coherence of speech production.

One technique that falls under the temporal schema and sequencing of speech category is *melodic intonation therapy (MIT)*, first described by Sparks, Helm, and Albert (1974) for use with patients with aphasia. MIT uses a hierarchy of four levels to help the patient develop volitional control of speech production. The basic technique requires the patient with AOS to tap out the rhythm of speech and produce speech using an exaggerated melodic line that is akin to singing earlier on in the treatment. Thus, as Sparks and Deck (1994) indicate, MIT has the patient produce an exaggerated tempo which is lengthened and lyrical. The patient also varies the pitch of the utterance in a manner that is "reduced and stylized into a melodic pattern" (p 371). Finally, emphasis is a focus of the treatment by exaggeration of the natural rhythm and stress of speech.

Another speech level technique has to do with *vibrotactile stimulation* (Rubow, Rosenbek, & Collins (1982). Rubow et al. (1982) applied a 50-Hz vibration to the patients right finger during speech production. The clinician controls the intensity, timing, and duration of the stimulation. The clinician is required to increase the intensity and duration of the stimulation during stressed

syllables. Because the information about stress comes from the finger, this method is considered a good example of intersystemic reorganization.

Prompts for restructuring oral muscular phonetic targets (PROMPT). PROMPT is one of the few treatments for AOS that is described adequately for its evaluation, and one of the few with any efficacy data supporting its use. It is a treatment that was initially aimed at AOS in children (Chumpelik, 1984). Square, Chumpelik, and Adams (1985) modified this technique for use with adults with AOS. A detailed description of this approach can be found in Square-Storer and Hayden (1989). This technique is tactile in nature and requires a highly structured set of finger placements on the face and neck of the patient with AOS that represent various oral positions of the articulators during speech (Pierce, 1991). The purpose of the finger placements is to provide feedback to the patient about the articulatory position to move toward during speech production and is used to cue the patient about such aspects of production as muscular tension, duration of production, and continuance.

A technique that has been frequently used with patients who have AOS is the *eight-step task continuum* (Rosenbek, Lemme, Ahern, Harris, & Wertz, 1973). This method incorporates the methods of several other methods and is designed to systematically move the patient from imitation to spontaneous production of phonemes. It begins with Step 1 (integral stimulation) in which the clinician says "Watch me" and "Listen to me" and the clinician and patient simultaneously produce the target. The patient is encouraged to carefully attend to how the speech feels and sounds when it is produced. The final step (8) requires a role-playing situation with the clinician and patient. Friends and family members are encouraged to participate in this aspect of therapy. The intermittent stages move the patient systematically from simultaneous imitation to role-play by delayed imitation, removal of visual cues, the addition of successive productions and so on. Deal and Florence (1978) have provided a modification of this general hierarchy, along with some efficacy data to support it.

There are a number of other "articulation" treatment techniques that fall under the category of motor approaches to Remediation, particularly with children (Hall et al, 1993). The *Moto-Kinesthetic Speech Training Method* (Stinchfield & Young, 1938) emphasizes tactile stimulation to identify the locations of muscles involved in the production of speech. The patient is also instructed to attend to the feeling of speech movements, thereby emphasizing the kinesthetic aspects of motor control.

The *Association Method* (McGinnis, Kleffner, & Goldstein, 1956) focuses on the association between speech sound learning and other "essential aspects of learning" such as attention and memory. The *Sensory-Motor Approach* (McDonald, 1964) focuses on sequential aspects of movements during speech. The patient imitates speech sound production. The sounds are modeled and described to the patient in terms of sensations during movement. The program moves from simple to complex by increasing the number of syllables and changing the phonemes that are produced.

The *Touch-Cue Method* (Bashir, Graham-jones, & Bostwick, 1984) is based on the assumption that individuals with apraxia have difficulty integrating volitional oral movements to produce speech. The treatment utilizes touch cues by the clinician to the lower face and neck for /b/, /d/, /g/, /s/, /f/, /n/, /θ/, and /l/. The cues are provided auditorily and visually. Additional cues for other phonemes are developed by the clinician.

Principles of Motor Learning

Much of what we know about the principles of motor learning have been elegantly summarized by Schmidt (1988). Below, we present an overview of the principles of motor learning and discuss how these apply to structuring speech therapy for persons with AOS. Motor learning refers to the "process

of acquiring the capability for producing skilled actions" (Schmidt, 1988). Thus, motor learning represents a relatively permanent change in the capability to produce skilled actions based on the processes associated with practice and experience. Motor learning is achieved through **practice and experience**. Skills that are learned have become permanent and are thus habitual.

The motor learning literature distinguishes between performance during practice (acquisition) and learning (retention). It is very important for the clinician to distinguish these two separate phases as well since factors that promote improved performance during practice often fail to produce learning that carries over to long-term capabilities to perform the task subsequent to practice. Thus during treatment, the facilatory effects found during a session may not be indicative of learning or permanent changes. Moreover, factors that may promote facilitation of performance during treatment sessions may not have an effect on learning and in some instances may have a negative affect on learning. Clinicians take note. During the session you may be getting great improvement and this will motivate you to continue doing similar techniques. But beware, this may not have the desired effect in terms of retention and may in fact impede learning. The review of motor learning below is designed to assist the clinician in promoting learning and does not focus on the more temporary practice effects.

There are a number of important precursors to motor learning which clinicians working with neurologically involved patients must be keenly aware. Two extremely important precursors are attention and memory. The ability to attend affects all aspects of information processing. Disrupted attentional mechanisms will have a deleterious affect on motor learning. There is a limited capacity to perform/learn various tasks (Kahneman, 1973). Attention requires effort and as such, the ability to learn must occur within the bounds of the patient's attentional ability. The amount of effort required to learn will limit the amount of learning as well as the amount of time given to a treatment session. During treatment sessions, the patient's basic attentional ability and overall capacity must be considered in terms of their potential to learn (their ultimate candidacy for treatment). Though the attentional capabilities of patients must be considered there is a growing literature suggesting that learning can occur without awareness. Thus, just because a person may have an attentional impairment, one might still be successful in improving motor skills.

Motor learning ultimately requires the storage of information in long-term memory (LTM) systems. The ultimate ability to learn requires the utilization of LTM systems and impairments of LTM can also have deleterious effects on motor learning.

Prior to beginning treatment with a person with AOS, or prior to embarking on new goals with a given patient, the clinician should consider certain principles that fall under the category of "prepractice" in the motor learning literature. The first step in prepractice is to establish the motivation for learning. The ways in which clinicians motivate their patients will vary depending on a number of factors. However, it is essential that the clinician make the task seem important. One way is to make sure the patient knows why a task is important to learn. Showing how a given task will ultimately lead to better speech is one way to improve motivation. A second way to enhance the motivation to learn is through goal setting. Goal setting should be a process that includes both the clinician and the patient. The more a patient can be part of the goal setting process, the greater the motivation for learning that will be established. In the general motor learning literature it has been found that performance is poorer and that less learning occurs when subjects are told to "do the best you can" compared to setting a standard to achieve. Thus, clinicians should set a specific level of expected performance, and not let the patient decide what is meant by "doing the best that they can."

Another important aspect of prepractice is to make sure the patient gets a general idea of the task. Motor learning is enhanced if the patient understands the task in a clear way. After providing the patient with motivation, the clinician should work to ensure that the particular skill to be learned and the ways in which learning will take place are known. In order to promote the patient's understanding of the task, careful instructions are needed. The clinician should keep instructions simple and focus only on one or two important aspects of movement. Verbal instructions are often overdone and are often unable to capture the many subtle aspects of skilled movements. Moreover, long verbal instructions place a large load on the attentional, memory, and motivational capacities of the patients. Schmidt (1991) suggests that simple instructions that "start people off on the right track" are best to promote motor learning. If longer instructions are needed, the clinician should consider giving a few added details after practice has begun. The most important message here is *do not overinstruct*.

Perhaps one of the more important principles of prepractice is to provide observational learning for the patients through modeling and demonstration. Viewing the movements to be learned allows for observation of the more subtle aspects of skilled performance that verbal instructions are unable to capture. Moreover, modeling and demonstration help ensure understanding of the task, particularly when the patient has a language impairment concomitant with the AOS. The use of pictures, videotapes, and live demonstrations may be important to include in the prepractice portions of therapy sessions. Watching others perform a task is a very good way to promote eventual skill learning.

One aspect of prepractice, called "verbal pretraining," is used to give the patient exposure to the stimuli that will be used in the task. Though called "verbal," more often than not this portion of the prepractice session is not verbal. Here the clinician systematically progresses through all of the stimuli before the patient begins practice. Thus, if working on lip closure as a precursor to the production of bilabials, the clinician would show the patient the movement a number of times. If working on a CV syllable, the clinician would produce the syllable a number of times before practice began. As noted below, practice sessions should include more than one stimulus. Therefore, verbal pretraining should cover all of the stimuli that will be targeted in the treatment session.

Prepractice sessions should also provide knowledge of how a movement is produced. Clinicians might show graphic representations of how a given sound is produced using simplified anatomical drawings or models. If targeting nonspeech tasks, drawings of the movements involved in the task could be used. Again, clinicians should be wary of using verbal instructions, and in general are encouraged to rely on visual representations.

A final aspect of prepractice is to establish a prepractice reference of correctness. The patient must be able to know when s/he is correct. In speech training this is often achieved through auditory feedback, but one can also use other sensory systems as well. Clear knowledge of what is correct for each stimulus is important, particularly if the patient is not ready to produce the sound or movement with complete accuracy initially. For example, if working on the CV syllable /pa/, the clinicians might adopt a level of correctness that the target goal has been reached when lip closure has been achieved, and not the perceptually accurate production of /pa/. As skill level improves, the reference of correctness will change and be more demanding such that eventually a perceptually accurate sound is produced. One goal of establishing a reference of correctness (error-detection capability) is to allow the patient to practice at home, away from the therapy room.

After prepractice, the practice portion of a treatment session can begin. The most important aspect of motor skill learning is practice (Schmidt, 1988, 1991). The need for practice during treatment of AOS has also been stressed (Wertz et al, 1984). In addition to large amounts of practice, the quality of the practice is important to consider. In-

creasing the efficiency of practice requires careful structuring of the sessions. A second critical aspect of practice to consider relative to motor learning is the type and structure of the feedback provided to the patient. Two types of feedback are *knowledge of results* (KR) and *knowledge of performance* (KP). Below we discuss the structure of the practice session to enhance learning efficiency, followed by a detailed discussion of how to use KR to maximize motor learning.

To become a skilled motor performer, the motor-impaired patient must be able to deal with the variability that is inherent in performance, and this is nowhere more true than during speech motor control. If one practices under unvarying conditions and variability is not systematically controlled during practice, then motor learning is likely to be diminished. Thus, it is argued that variable practice enhances motor learning. In particular, variability in practice promotes generalization and carry-over, the ultimate goal of speech treatments. Evidence suggests that variable practice enhances the ability to control the parameters of movements that are input to motor programs such as the overall speed or amplitude of the movement, but that variable training does not have much of an affect on motor program development.

Another aspect of motor learning that is extremely important to consider in treating individuals with AOS is whether practice is random or blocked. During treatment, there is rarely only one targeted goal. Rather, treatment sessions have multiple goals and multiple stimuli. For example, the clinician may target lip closure, tongue elevation and lip retraction in one session. Blocked practice would occur when each of those goals was targeted separately in the session. Thus, the patient might practice lip closure drills prior to beginning practice on tongue elevation. Random practice occurs when the clinician mixes the tasks or stimuli throughout the treatment session. Random practice would result in practice blocks with both lip closure and tongue elevation drills interspersed in a random manner throughout the practice session. Or the clinician might target three different speech sounds during practice, randomly selecting which sound the patient will produce on a given trial. Random practice facilitates the development of motor programs and thus facilitates learning and is more efficient than blocked practice.

Mental practice facilitates the learning of skilled motor routines. Thinking about an activity will enhance learning. However, the clinician cannot simply tell the patient to "think about or to practice in your head" a motor activity. That is, clinicians should not instruct their patients with AOS to go home and practice mentally how a /p/ sound is made. Rather, the clinician should provide systematic instructions that the patient follows during mental practice sessions. Schmidt (1991) suggests that the motor learner (in our case the patient) should "move to a quite, relaxing place, and focus clearly on the movement task." This will require work with the clinician in terms of relaxation exercises. The patient should then be instructed to "let the movement unfold in real time" (Schmidt, 1991). As well, the patient must be able to imagine success and avoid images of failure for mental practice to be effective.

Perhaps the most important aspect of motor learning has to do with the feedback provided during treatment sessions. Feedback can be in the form of *knowledge of results* and *knowledge of performance*. KR refers to feedback about the **outcome** of a movement pattern with reference to the environmental goal. KR is **not** feedback about the parameters of the movement pattern itself, which is termed KP. KR refers to information provided by the clinician, to the patient, about the success of the movement (e.g., "Yes, you got it." Or "No, that's not quite right.").

Clinicians need to carefully consider the temporal aspects of KR in order to best facilitate motor learning in patients with AOS. First the patient produces a response, this is followed by a *KR-delay interval*, which is the period between the response and when KR is provided. Large delays in this first interval may inhibit learning. Filling the KR-delay interval may produce detrimental effects on

performance and learning. Filling the KR-delay interval can occur in a number of different ways including the clinician or patient talking or the production of movements not related to the specific task at hand by the patient. That is, extraneous activity during this interval should be avoided.

After the KR-delay interval, the clinician provides feedback about the accuracy of the patient's response. This is followed by the *post-KR-delay interval*, which represents the period of time between KR and the subsequent response. During this interval the patient is actively processing information. There must be time for the patient to "think" about the movement response and the KR that has followed. All of this information must be assimilated and remembered. Thus, if this interval is too short, learning is inhibited. Filling this period of time has the potential to **severely** degrade performance and learning. While the length of time needed for information processing may vary from patient to patient, no less than 3 seconds is recommended before the next response is elicited. While long intervals do not necessarily interfere with motor learning, they should be kept relatively short so that motivation is maintained and memory constraints do not affect learning.

An issue to be considered is if KR is immediate or summarized over a number of trials. As a profession, speech-language pathologists typically give feedback after each response. This is termed *immediate KR*. However, investigators have examined the effectiveness of immediate versus **summary** KR in which feedback is provided after a number of responses. It has been found, perhaps contrary to intuition or to popular notions, that summary KR promotes motor learning more than immediate KR. Schmidt (1991) argues that immediate KR provides the learner with too much information. It is possible that with immediate KR the patient will rely on KR too much! As well, summary KR may help promote response variability, which is generally needed to fully acquire a motor skill. The optimal number of trials to be summarized is of crucial importance and an answer to this is not known for speech movements (or for many other movement types). Relatively simple tasks can use a summary of up to 15 trials, while for difficult tasks the optimal number is considered to be about 5. These numbers are based on the normal literature and refer to nonspeech systems. When working with patients, the task difficulty may be extremely high, even for "simple" movements (eg, production of a single syllable). When working on speech motor control with patients with AOS, clinicians might begin with summary KR over three responses and move to greater response summary feedback.

There are many forms of KR. Remember that too much information is detrimental to learning. The clinician could say "right" versus "wrong" or give some specific information about the movement such as, "Good, you got both lips together in a tight seal." Clinicians might suggest that the production is "a bit distorted" or give more precise information such as "your vowel was just a little too long on that production." Data show that providing some information about the error is good, but in a fairly general way. Too much specific information may degrade motor learning.

Frequent KR is not as facilitative in motor learning as reduced feedback. Reduced feedback is thought to decrease the dependency on the KR as well as thought to avoid overcorrection on the part of the patient. During bandwidth training a range or band of correctness is defined for the patient. The patient is told to keep out of the band of incorrect. KR is provided only when performance falls outside the band of correctness. In this way, feedback is infrequent. As well, feedback tends to fade across the learning occurs. As well, there is positive reinforcement for keeping performance within the band since the patient will know that they are doing well when feedback is not provided. Schmidt (1991) also notes that bandwidth training reduces moment-to-moment corrections by the learner in response to frequent feedback which has the positive effect of stabilizing performance.

The other form of feedback introduced earlier is KP (knowledge of performance). KP in this instance refers to feedback about specific aspects of the movement. Biofeedback or verbal feedback specifically about the movement is considered KP. For instance, using the visipitch to provide feedback about pitch change during treatment of prosody might be considered KP. Or feedback about the exact position of the lips or tongue during a task is considered KP. Many of the same constraints as discussed above for KR hold for KP.

Principles of AOS Treatment Based on Motor Training

The first principle of motor training for speech sound remediation in AOS is that intensive treatment is required. Treatment should be as intensive as possible taking the needs and circumstances of each case into consideration. The definition of intensive varies from clinician to clinician. However, massed practice that is sustained over a relatively long time period is usually necessary and consistent with general motor learning.

The second principle of motor approaches to speech treatment is that a large number of repetitions of speech or nonspeech movements are needed. That is, there must be sufficient practice to learn or re-learn motor skills. The motor learning literature does not provide an estimate of the number of repetitions that are needed to produce automaticity so the clinician should be careful in making assumptions about how many repetitions are needed relative to each patient. While there is no magic number of repetitions needed in a therapy session, clinicians should consider eliciting no fewer than 20 repetitions of a behavior in a given context. The severity of the disorder will, to a large measure, determine this and other variables. However, the structure or the practice session is extremely important to consider as noted above.

Most "motor" speech therapies suggest that the patient should come to a neutral position between attempts. In particular, after each attempt, there should be a rest period in which the patient assumes a neutral position before attempting the next response. The use of nonspeech tasks to develop motor control for speech is controversial. Schmidt (1991) suggests that when an action is divided into its component parts the action learned does not transfer back to the main task. It is presumed that this is because the individual component of the action will develop its own program that will not then become part of a larger program for the speech movement. However, in patients with AOS, reducing the degrees of freedom may be necessary. It is suggested that the clinician move to speech as soon as possible.

Another principle derived from the literature is that remediation should progress systematically through hierarchies of task difficulty. This principle implies that treatment should begin with relatively simple movement tasks and move to more complex movement patterns. With severely impaired patients, treatment might begin with nonspeech movements of the articulators (eg, tongue protrusion). As explained in the chapter in this volume on nonspeech assessment (Robin et al), nonspeech tasks reduce the degrees of freedom of movements and isolate the motor system from the constraints of the linguistic system. Since AOS is a motor control problem, treatment should be aimed at the motor system. When necessary, simple nonspeech movements should be targeted first, then more complicated control tasks that require **sequencing** of movement patterns or **tracking** targets with the oral structures could be initiated. Based on the theoretical assumptions outlined in the Robin et al chapter in this volume, the motor control capabilities that are learned during nonspeech movements should facilitate the development of speech motor skills in patients with AOS.

Consistent with the general approach advocated by Rosenbek (1985), the hierarchical order principle also suggests that treatment using speech as stimuli should begin with syllables in isolation when words or larger units of connected speech cannot be managed. If needed, the clinician can break the syllables into component movements (nonspeech movements) and target each part of the movement pattern, gradually moving towards syllables or words. For example, if targeting the /p/ phoneme, the clinician might begin with lip closure and plosive releases as separate drills. When the goals for these movement patterns are successfully completed, treatment might move to combining the two patterns, eventually adding other aspects of the speech movement until speech becomes the target.

Initial remedial speech tasks might begin with motorically less complex sounds such as vowels (/o/, /a/, /I/). Frequently occurring consonants and those that are motorically simple should be targeted first. Visible consonants are often a good starting point. Later treatment should target control of the voicing contrast. Initial work should focus on the voiceless sounds followed by the voiced cognate. Task complexity can then be increased by placing sounds in CV syllables and then increasing the number of syllables. The clinician might then change the position of the VC or the context and move to a CVC, then to a CV2C, then to a CV1C2 etc. Next treatment can move to more motorically difficult and/or less visible sounds.

Another important aspect of treatment is the focus on prosody. Prosody is not treated after all other articulatory drills are completed. Rather, treatment of rhythm, stress, and intonation should be coincident with articulation treatment. Treatment of prosody results in improved intelligibility (Yorkston, Beukelman, & Bell, 1988) and possibly better articulatory control. Prosodic Remediation may begin with nonspeech stimuli focusing on pitch or duration changes. Speech stimuli frequently start with highly contrastive prosodic patterns (Robin, Klouda, & Hug, 1991). Treatment might use different stress drills, and the clinician may want to provide visual feedback in the form of a visipitch or another device.

Treatment must provide successful experiences for the patient with AOS. However, the criterion goal may change over the course of remediation. "Perfection" is never a reasonable goal. In fact, as noted above, variability in practice is an important aspect of motor skill acquisition and having patients produce speech as movements in the same way each time may diminish motor learning.

It is critical that the clinician select targets, employ specific techniques, and use more general principles for treatment that are appropriate for the individual patient, that are theoretically consistent with the presumed nature of the disorder, and that have been demonstrated to be effective with similar patients. The final constraint, to apply treatments that have been demonstrated to be effective, is at this stage of clinical history a tall order. Treatment research programs are active in a number of locations throughout the United States, Canada, South Africa, and Europe. It will be some time before the fruits of these programs have passed peer review and have been made available to the practicing clinician. It is true that practicing what is reasonable but untested is unacceptable clinical practice. However, it is also true that patients communicatively devastated by the effects of AOS cannot, and should not wait for the important efficacy data on any of the treatments discussed above. While these data are systematically collected, evaluated and disseminated, it is the general principles discussed here that may provide the clinical compass until such time as these treatments can be offered with a reasonable degree of certainty that their benefits can be reproduced.

References

Aten JL, Johns DF, Darley FL. (1971). Auditory perception of sequenced words in apraxia of speech. *J Speech Hear Res* 14:131–143.

Bashir AS, Grahamjones F, Bostwick RY. (1984). A touch-cue method of therapy for developmental verbal apraxia. In: Perkins WH, Northern JH, eds. *Seminars in Speech and Language*. New York: Thieme-Stratton, pp 127–137.

Bauman JA. (1978). Sound duration: A comparison between performances of subjects with central nervous system disorders and normal speakers. Unpublished doctoral dissertation, University of Colorado.

Blumstein S, Cooper WE, Goodglass H, Statlender S, Gottlieb J. (1980). Production of deficits in aphasia: A voice-onset time analysis. *Brain Language* 9:153–170.

Blumstein S, Cooper WE, Zurif EB, Caramazza A. (1977). The perception and production of voice-onset time in aphasia. *Neuropsychologia* 155:371–383.

Blumstein S. (1973). *A Phonological Investigation of Aphasic Speech*. The Hague: Mouton.

Blumstein S. (1981). Phonological aspects of aphasia. In: Sarno MT, ed. *Acquired Aphasia*. New York: Academic Press, pp 129–155.

Blumstein SE, Baum S. (1987). Consonant production deficits in aphasia. In: Ryalls JH, ed. *Phonetic Approaches to Speech Production in Aphasia and Related Disorders*. Boston: College-Hill Press, pp 3–22.

Bock JK. (1982). Toward a cognitive psychology of syntax: Information processing contribution to sentence formulation. *Psychol Rev* 89:1–47.

Boone DR, Plante E. (1993). *Human Communication and Its Disorders*, 2nd Ed. Englewood Cliffs, NJ: Prentice-Hall.

Bowman CA, Hodson BW, Simpson RK. (1980). Oral apraxia and aphasic misarticulations. *Clin Aphasiol* 8:89–95.

Brooks VB. (1986). *The Neural Basis of Motor Control*. New York: Oxford University Press.

Buckingham HW Jr. (1979). Explanation in apraxia with consequences for the concept of apraxia of speech. *Brain Lang* 8:202–226.

Buckingham HW. (1990). Abstruse neologisms, retrieval deficits and the random generator. *J Neurolinguist* 5:215–235.

Buckingham HW. (1992). Phonological production deficits in conduction aphasia. In: Kohn SE, ed. *Conduction Aphasia*. Hillsdale, NJ: Lawrence Erlbaum Associates, pp 77–116.

Canter GJ. (1969). The influence of primary and secondary verbal apraxia on output disturbances in aphasic syndromes. Paper presented to the Annual Convention of the American Speech and Hearing Association, Chicago.

Chumpelik D. (1984). The prompt system of therapy: Theoretical framework and applications for developmental apraxia of speech. *Semin Speech Language* 5:139–156.

Clark HM, Robin DA. (1996). Sense of effort during a lexical decision task: Resource allocation deficits following brain damage. (Submitted for publication.)

Collins MJ, Rosenbek JC, Wertz RT. (1983). Spectrographic analysis of vowel and word duration in apraxia of speech. *J Speech Hear Res* 26:224–230.

Cooper WE, Soares C, Nicol J, Michelow D, Goloskie S. (1984). Clausal intonation after unilateral brain damage. *Language Speech* 27:17–24.

Dabul B. (1979). Apraxia Battery for Adults. Tigard, Ore: C.C. Publications, Inc.

Danly M, de Villiers JG, Cooper WE. (1979). Control of speech prosody in Broca's aphasia. In: Wolf JJ, Klatt DH, eds. *Speech Communication Papers.* Presented at the 97th Meeting of the Acoustical Society of America. New York: Acoustical Society of America.

Danly M, Shapiro B. (1982). Speech prosody in Broca's aphasia. *Brain Language* 16:171–190.

Darley FL, Aronson AE, Brown JR. (1975a). *Motor Speech Disorders.* Philadelphia: W.B. Saunders.

Darley FL, Aronson AE, Brown JR. (1975b). *Motor Speech Disorders: Audio Seminars in Speech Pathology.* Philadelphia: W.B. Saunders.

Darley FL. (1967). Lacunae and research approaches to them. IV. In: Millikan CH, Darley FL, eds. *Brain Mechanisms Underlying Speech and Language.* New York: Grune & Stratton, pp 2236–290.

Darley FL. (1968). Apraxia of speech: 107 years of terminological confusion. Paper presented to the American Speech and Hearing Association, Denver (unpublished).

Darley FL. (1969). Aphasia: Input and output disturbances in speech and language processing. Paper presented to the American Speech and Hearing Association, Chicago (unpublished).

Darley FL. (1982). *Aphasia.* Philadelphia: W.B. Saunders.

Deal JL, Darley FL. (1972). The influence of linguistic and situational variables on phonemic accuracy in apraxia of speech. *J Speech Hear Res* 15:639–653.

Deal JL, Florence CL. (1978). Modification of the eight-step continuum for treatment of apraxia of speech in adults. *J Speech Hear Disord* 43:89–95.

Dell GS. (1986). A spreading-activation theory of retrieval in sentence production. *Psychol Rev* 96(3):283–321.

Dell GS. (1988). The retrieval of phonological forms in production: Tests of prediction from a connectionist model. *J Memory Lang* 27:124–142.

Deutsch SE. (1984). Prediction of site of lesion from speech apraxic error patterns. In Rosenbek JC, McNeil MR, Aronson AE, eds. *Apraxia of Speech: Physiology, Acoustics, Linguistics, Management.* San Diego: College Hill Press, pp 113–134.

Duffy JR, Duffy RJ. (1990). The assessment of limb apraxia: The limb apraxia test. In: Roy EA, ed. *Neuropsychological Studies of Apraxia and Related Disorders.* Amsterdam: Elsevier Science Publishers, pp 503–531.

Duffy JR, Gawle CA. (1984). Apraxic speakers' vowel duration in consonant-vowel-consonant syllables. In: Rosenbek JC, McNeil MR, Aronson AE, eds. *Apraxia of Speech: Physiology Acoustics, Linguistics, Management.* San Diego: College-Hill Press, pp 167–196.

Duffy JR. (1996). *Motor Speech Disorders: Substrates, Differential Diagnosis and Management.* St. Louis: Mosby.

Dunlop J, Marquardt T. (1977). Linguistic and articulatory aspects of single word production in apraxia of speech. *Cortex* 13:17–29.

Faglioni P, Basso A. (1985). Historical perspectives on neuroanatomical correlates of limb apraxia. In: Roy EA, ed. *Neuropsychological Studies of Apraxia and Related Disorders.* Amsterdam: Elsevier Science Publishers, pp 3–44.

Forrest K, Adams S, McNeil MR, Southwood H. (1991). Kinematic, electromyographic, and perceptual evaluation of speech apraxia, conduction aphasia, ataxic dysarthria and normal speech production. In: Moore CA, Yorkston KM, Beukelman DR, eds. *Dysarthria and Apraxia of Speech: Perspectives on Management.* Baltimore: Paul H. Brookes, pp 147–171.

Fromm D, Abbs JH, McNeil MR, Rosenbek JC. (1982). Simultaneous perceptual-physiological method for studying apraxia of speech. *Clin Aphasiol* 10:155–171.

Fromm D. (1981). Investigation of movement/EMG parameters in apraxia of speech. Unpublished Masters Thesis, University of Wisconsin-Madison.

Gandour J, Dardarananda R. (1984). Prosodic disturbance in aphasia: Vowel length in Thai. *Brain Language* 23:206–224.

Garrett MF. (1880). Levels of processing in sentence production. In: Butterworth B, ed. *Lan-*

guage Production: Volume 1, *Speech and Talk.* London: Academic Press, pp 177–220.

Garrett MF. (1884). The organization of processing structure for language production: Applications to aphasic speech. In: Caplan D, Lecours AR, Smith, A, eds. *Biological Perspectives on Language.* Cambridge: MIT Press, pp 172–193.

Goodglass H. (1992). Diagnosis of conduction aphasia. In: Kohn SE, ed. *Conduction Aphasia.* Hillsdale, NJ: Lawrence Erlbaum Associates, pp 3–50.

Grillner S. (1982). Possible analogies in the control of innate motor acts and the production of sound speech. In: Grillner S, Lindblom B, Lubker J, Persson A, eds. *Speech Motor Control.* Oxford: Pergamon Press, pp 217–230.

Hageman CF, Robin DA, Moon JB, Folkins JW. (1994). Oral motor tracking in normal and apraxic speakers. *Clin Aphasiol* 22:219–229.

Hall PK, Jordan LS, Robin DA. (1993). *Development Apraxia of Speech: Theory and Clinical Practice.* Austin: PRO-ED.

Halpern H, Keith R, Darley FL. (1976). Phonemic behavior of aphasic subjects without dysarthria or apraxia of speech. *Cortex* 12:365–372.

Hardcastle WJ. (1987). Electropalatographic study of articulation disorders in verbal dyspraxia. In: Ryalls JH, ed. *Phonetic Approaches to Speech Production in Aphasia and Related Disorders.* Boston: College-Hill Press, pp 113–136.

Hegde MN. (1991). *Introduction to Communicative Disorders.* Austin: Pro-Ed.

Hoit-Dalgaard J, Murry T, Kopp HG. (1983). Voice onset time production and perception in apraxic subjects. *Brain Language* 20:329–339.

Hough MS, Klich RJ. (1987). Effects of word length on lip EMG activity in apraxia of speech. *Clin Aphasiol* 15:271–276.

Hough MS. (1978). Frequency of specific types of phonological/motor errors produced by fluent and nonfluent aphasic adults. Unpublished master's thesis, University of Florida.

Itoh M, Sasanuma S, Hirose H, Yoshioka H, Sawashima M. (1983). Velar movements during speech in two Wernicke aphasic patients. *Brain Language* 19:283–292.

Itoh M, Sasanuma S, Hirose H, Yoshioka H, Ushijima T. (1980). Abnormal articulatory dynamics in a patient with apraxia of speech:

X-ray microbeam observations. *Brain Language* 11:66–75.

Itoh M, Sasanuma S, Ushijima T. (1979). Velar movements during speech in a patient with apraxia of speech. *Brain Language* 7:227–239.

Itoh M, Sasanuma S. (1984). Articulatory movements in apraxia of speech. In: Rosenbek JC, McNeil MR, Aronson AE, eds. *Apraxia of Speech: Physiology, Acoustics, Linguistics, Management.* San Diego: College Hill Press, pp 134–165.

Itoh M, Sasanuma S. (1987). Articulatory velocities of aphasic patients. In: Ryalls JH, ed. *Phonetic Approaches to Speech Production in Aphasia and Related Disorders.* Boston: College-Hill Press, pp 137–162.

Jakobson R. (1968). *Child Language Aphasia and Phonological Universals.* The Hague: Mouton.

Joanette Y, Keller E, Lecours AR. (1980). Sequence of phonemic approximations in aphasia. *Brain Language* 11:30–44.

Johns DF, Darley FL. (1970). Phonemic variability in apraxia of speech. *J Speech Hear Res* 13:556–583.

Kahneman D. (1973). *Attention and Effort.* Englewood Cliffs, NJ: Pentice-Hall, pp 1–19.

Katz W, Machetanz J, Orth U, Schonle P. (1990). A kinematic analysis of anticipatory coarticulation in the speech of anterior aphasic subjects using electromagnetic articulography. *Brain Language* 38:555–575.

Katz W, Machetanz J, Orth U, Schonle P. (1990). Anticipatory labial coarticulation in the speech of German-speaking anterior aphasic subjects: Acoustic analyses. *J Neurolinguist* 5(2/3):295–320.

Katz WF. (1987). Anticipatory labial and lingual coarticulation in aphasia. In: Ryalls JH, ed. *Phonetic Approaches to Speech Production in Aphasia and Related Disorders.* Boston: College-Hill Press, pp 221–242.

Kearns K. (1980). The application of phonological process analysis to adult neuropathologies. *Clin Aphasiol* 8:187–195.

Keller E. (1978). Parameters for vowel substitutions in Broca's aphasia. *Brain Language* 5:265–285.

Keller E. (1984). Simplification and gesture reduction in phonological disorders of apraxia and aphasia. In: Rosenbek JC, McNeil MR, Aronson AE, eds. *Apraxia of Speech: Physiology, Acoustics, Linguistics and Management.* San Diego: College-Hill Press, pp 221–256.

Kelso JAS, Tuller B, Harris KS. (1983). A "dynamic" pattern perspective on the control and coordination of movement. In: MacNeilage PF, ed. *The Production of Speech.* New York: Springer-Verlag, pp 137–173.

Kent RD, Adams SG. (1989). The concept and measurement of coordination in speech disorders. In: Wallace SA, ed. *Perspectives on the Coordination of Movement.* Amsterdam: Elsevier Science Publishers, pp 415–449.

Kent RD, McNeil MR. (1987). Relative timing of sentence repetition in apraxia of speech and conduction aphasia. In: Ryalls JH, ed. *Phonetic Approaches to Speech Production in Aphasia and Related Disorders.* Boston: College-Hill Press, pp 181–220.

Kent RD, Rosenbek JC. (1983). Acoustic patterns of apraxia of speech. *J Speech Hear Res* 26:231–249.

Klich RJ, Ireland JV, Weidner WE. (1979). Articulatory and phonological aspects of consonant substitutions in apraxia of speech. *Cortex* 15:451–470.

Kohn S. (1984). The nature of the phonological disorder in conduction aphasia. *Brain Language* 23:97–115.

Kugler PN, Kelso JAS, Turvey MT. (1980). On the concept of coordinative structures as dissipative structures: I. Theoretical lines of convergence. In: Stelmach GE, ed. *Tutorials in Motor Behavior.* Amsterdam: North Holland, pp 1–47.

LaPointe LL, Horner J. (1976). Repeated trials of words by patients with neurogenic phonological selection-sequencing impairment (apraxia of speech). *Clin Aphasiol* 6:261–277.

LaPointe LL, Johns DF. (1975). Some phonemic characteristics in apraxia of speech. *J Commun Disor* 8:259–269.

LaPointe LL. (1969). An investigation of isolated oral movements, oral motor sequencing abilities and articulation of brain injured adults. Unpublished doctoral dissertation, University of Colorado.

Lebrun Y, Buyssens E, Henneaux J. (1973). Phonetic aspects of anarthria. *Cortex* 9:126–135.

Lieberman AM, Studdert-Kennedy M. (1978). Phonetic perception. In: Held R, Leibowitz H, Teuber HL, eds. *Handbook of Sensory Physiology,* Vol VII: *Perception.* Heidelberg: Springer-Verlag, pp 143–178.

Liepmann H. (1900). Das Krankheitsbild der apraxia (motorischen asymboli) auf Grund eines Falles von einseitiger apraxie. *Monatschrift Psychiatrie Neurol* 9:15–40.

Liepmann H. (1905). Die linke hemisphaere und das handeln. *Muchener medizinische Wochenschift* 52:2322–2326, 2375–2378.

Liepmann H. (1913). Motor aphasia, anarthria and apraxia. *Transactions of the 17th International Congress of Medicine,* Section XI, Part II, pp 97–106.

Luria AR. (1966). *Higher Cortical Functions in Man.* New York: Basic Books.

Luria AR. (1970). *Traumatic Aphasia: Its Syndromes, Psychology and Treatment.* The Hague: Mouton.

Marquardt TP, Cannito M. (1996). Treatment of verbal apraxia in Broca's aphasia. In: Wallace GL, ed. *Adult Aphasia Rehabilitation.* Boston: Butterworth-Heinemann, pp 205–228.

Marquardt TP, Sussman H. (1984). The elusive lesion—Apraxia of speech link in Broca's aphasia. In: Rosenbek JC, McNeil MR, Aronson AE, eds. *Apraxia of Speech: Physiology, Acoustics, Linguistics, Management.* San Diego: College Hill Press, pp 91–112.

Martin AD. (1974). Some objections to the term apraxia of speech. *J Speech Hear Dis* 39:53–64.

McDonald ET. (1964). *Articulation Testing and Treatment: A Sensory-Motor Approach.* Pittsburgh: Stanwiz House.

McGinnis MA, Kleffner FR, Goldstein R. (1956). Teaching aphasic children. *Volta Rev* 58:239–244.

McNeil MR, Adams S. (1990). A comparison of speech kinematics among apraxic, conduction aphasic, ataxic dysarthric and normal geriatric speakers. *Clin Aphasiol* 18:279–294.

McNeil MR, Caliguiri M, Rosenbek JC. (1989). A comparison of labiomandibular kinematic durations, displacements, velocities and dysmetrias in apraxic and normal adults. *Clin Aphasiol* 17:173–193.

McNeil MR, Hashi M, Southwood H. (1994). Acoustically derived perceptual evidence for coarticulatory errors in apraxic and conduction aphasic speech production. *Clin Aphasiol* 22:203–218.

McNeil MR, Kent RD. (1990). Motoric characteristics of adult aphasic and apraxic speakers. In: Hammond GE, ed. *Cerebral control of speech and limb movements.* Amsterdam: Elsevier Science Publishers, pp 349–386.

McNeil MR, Liss J, Tseng C-H, Kent RD. (1990). Effects of speech rate on the absolute and relative timing of apraxic and conduction aphasic sentence production. *Brain Language* 38(1):135–158.

McNeil MR, Odell KH, Miller SB, Hunter L. (1995). Consistency, variability, and target approximation for successful speech repetitions among apraxic, conduction aphasic and ataxic dysarthric speakers. *Clin Aphasiol* 23:39–55.

McNeil MR, Weismer G, Adams S, Mulligan M. (1990). Oral structure nonspeech motor control in normal, dysarthric, aphasic and apraxic speakers: Isometric force and static position control. *J Speech Hear Res* 33:355–368.

McNeil MR. (1984). Current concepts in adult aphasia. *Int Rehabil Med* 6(3):347–356.

Mercaitis PA. (1983). Some temporal characteristics of imitative speech in non-brain-injured, aphasic, and apraxic adults. Unpublished doctoral dissertation, University of Massachusetts-Amherst.

Meuse S, Marquardt TP, Cannito M. (1996). Phonological analyses of apraxia of speech in individuals with Broca's aphasia. Paper presented to the Motor Speech Conference, Amelia Island, Fla, February.

Miller N. (1986). *Dyspraxia and Its Management.* Rockville: Aspen Publishers, Inc.

Moore WM. (1975). Assessment of oral, nonverbal gestures in normal and selected brain-injured sample populations. Unpublished doctoral dissertation, University of Colorado.

Odell K, McNeil MR, Rosenbek JC, Hunter L. (1990). Perceptual characteristics of consonant productions by apraxic speakers. *J Speech Hear Disor* 55:345–359.

Odell K, McNeil MR, Rosenbek JC, Hunter L. (1991). A perceptual comparison of prosodic features in apraxia of speech and conduction aphasia. *Clin Aphasiol* 19:295–306.

Odell K, McNeil MR, Rosenbek JC, Hunter L. (1991). Perceptual characteristics of vowel and prosody production in apraxic, aphasic, and dysarthric speakers. *J Speech Hear Res* 34:67–80.

Palmer JM, Yantis PA. (1990). *Survey of Communication Disorders.* Baltimore: Williams & Wilkins.

Pierce RS. (1991). Apraxia of speech versus phonemic paraphasia: Theoretical, diagnostic, and treatment considerations. In: Vogel D, Cannito MP, eds. *Treating Disorders Speech Motor Control: For Clinicians by Clinicians.* Austin: PRO-ED, pp 185–216.

Poizner H, Mack L, Verfaellie M, Rothi LJ, Heilman KM. (1990). Three dimensional computergraphic analysis of apraxia. *Brain* 113:85–101.

Robin DA, Bean C, Folkins JW. (1989). Lip movement in apraxia of speech. *J Speech Hear Res* 32:512–523.

Robin DA, Klouda GV, Hug LN. (1991). Neurogenic disorders of prosody. In: Cannito MP, Vogel D, eds. *Treating Disordered Speech Motor Control: For Clinicians by Clinicians.* Austin: Pro-Ed, pp 241–271.

Rosenbek JC, Kent RD, LaPointe LL. (1984). Apraxia of speech: An overview and some perspectives. In: Rosenbek JC, McNeil MR, Aronson AE, eds. *Apraxia of Speech: Physiology, Acoustics, Linguistics, Management.* San Diego: College Hill Press, pp 1–72.

Rosenbek JC, Lemme M, Ahern M, Harris E, Wertz RT. (1973). A treatment for apraxia of speech in adults. *J Speech Hear Disord* 38:462–472.

Rosenbek JC, McNeil MR. (1991). A discussion of classification in motor speech disorders: Dysarthria and apraxia of speech. In: Moore CA, Yorkston KM, Beukelman DR, eds. *Dysarthria and Apraxia of Speech: Perspectives on Management.* Baltimore: Paul H. Brookes, pp 289–295.

Rosenbek JC, Wertz RT, Darley FL. (1973). Oral sensation and perception in apraxia of speech and aphasia. *J Speech Hear Res* 16:22–36.

Rosenbek JC. (1985). Treating apraxia of speech. In: Johns DF, ed. *Clinical Management of Neurogenic Communicative Disorders.* Boston: Little, Brown.

Rothi LJ, Heilman K. (1985). Ideomotor apraxia: Gestural discrimination, comprehension and memory. In: Roy EA, ed. *Neuropsychological Studies of Apraxia and Related Disorders.* Amsterdam: Elsevier Science Publishers, pp 65–74.

Roy EA, Square PA. (1985). Common considerations in the study of limb, verbal, and oral apraxia. In: Roy EA, ed. *Neuropsychological Studies of Apraxia and Related Disorders.* Amsterdam: Elsevier Science Publishers, pp 111–162.

Rubow RT, Rosenbek JC, Collins MJ. (1982). Vibrotactile stimulation for intrasystemic reorganization in apraxia of speech. *Arch Phys Med Rehabil* 63:150–153.

Ryalls JH. (1981). Motor aphasia: Acoustic correlates of phonetic disintegration in vowels. *Neuropsychologia* 19:365-374.

Ryalls JH. (1982). Intonation in Broca's aphasia. *Neuropsychologia* 20:355–360.

Ryalls JH. (1984). Some acoustic aspects of fundamental frequency of CVC utterances in aphasia. *Phonetica* 41:103–111.

Ryalls JH. (1986). An acoustic study of vowel production in aphasia. *Brain Language* 29:48–67.

Ryalls JH. (1987). Vowel production in aphasia: Towards an account of the consonant-vowel dissociation. In: Ryalls JH, ed. *Phonetic Approaches to Speech Production in Aphasia and Related Disorders.* Boston: College-Hill Press, pp 23–44.

Sasanuma S. (1971). Speech characteristics of a patient with apraxia of speech. *Annu Bull Res Inst Logoped Phoniatr* 5:85–89.

Schmidt RA. (1991). *Motor Learning and Performance: From Principles to Practice.* Champaign, Ill: Human Kinetics.

Schmidt RA. 1988. *Motor Control and Learning: A Behavioral Emphasis.* 2nd Ed. Champaign: Ill. Human Kinetics.

Shankweiler D, Harris KS, Taylor ML. (1968). Electromyographic studies of articulation in aphasia. *Arch Physical Med Rehabil* 1:1–8.

Shewan CM, Leeper HA Jr, Booth JC. (1984). An analysis of voice onset time (VOT) in aphasic and normal subjects. In: Rosenbek JC, McNeil MR, Aronson AE, eds. *Apraxia of Speech.* San Diego: College-Hill Press, pp 197–220.

Solomon NP, Robin DA, Luschei ES. (1994). Strength, endurance and sense of effort: Studies of the tongue and hand in people with Parkinson's disease and accompanying dysarthria. Paper presented to the Motor Speech Conference, Sedona, Ariz.

Solomon NP, Robin DA, Mitchinson SI, VanDaele DJ, Luschei ES. (In press). Sense of effort and the effects of fatigue in the tongue and hand. *J Speech Hear Res.*

Somodi L, Robin DA, Luschei ES. (1995). A model of "sense of effort" during maximal and submaximal contractions of the tongue. *Brain Language.*

Sparks RW, Deck JW. (1994). Melodic intonation therapy. In: Chapey R, ed. *Language Intervention Strategies in Adult Aphasia,* 3rd ed. Baltimore: Williams & Wilkins, pp 368–379.

Sparks RW, Helm N, Albert M. (1974). Aphasia rehabilitation resulting from melodic intonation therapy. *Cortex* 10:303–316.

Square PA, Chumpelik D, Adams SG. (1985). Efficacy of the PROMPT system of therapy for the treatment of acquired apraxia of speech. *Clin Aphasiol* 13:319–320.

Square PA, ed. (1989). *Acquired Apraxia of Speech in Aphasic Adults.* London: Taylor & Francis.

Square PA, Martin RE. (1994). The nature and treatment of neuromotor speech disorders in aphasia. In: Chapey R, ed. *Language Intervention Strategies in Adult Aphasia.* 3rd Ed. Baltimore: Williams & Wilkins, pp 467–499.

Square PA. (1996). Apraxia of speech reconsidered. In: Bell-Berti F, Raphael LJ, eds. *Producing Speech: Contemporary Issues for Katherine Safford Harris.* New York: AIP Press, pp 375–286.

Square-Storer PA, Hayden DC. (1989). PROMPT treatment. In: Square-Storer P, ed. *Acquired Apraxia of Speech in Adults.* London: Taylor & Francis, pp 190–219.

Square-Storer PA, Roy EA, Hogg SC. (1990). The dissociation of aphasia from apraxia of speech, ideomotor limb, and buccofacial apraxia. In: Hammond GE, ed. *Cerebral Control of Speech and Limb Movements.* Amsterdam: Elsevier Science Publishers, pp 451–476.

Square-Storer PA, Roy EA. (1990). The dissociation of aphasia from apraxia of speech, ideomotor limb, and buccofacial apraxia. In: Hammond GE, ed. *Cerebral Control of Speech and Limb Movements.* Amsterdam: Elsevier Science Publishers, pp 477–502.

Square-Storer PA. (1989). Traditional therapies for apraxia of speech-reviewed and rationalized. In: Square-Storer PA, ed. *Acquired Apraxia of Speech in Adults.* London: Taylor & Francis, pp 145–161.

Stinchfield SM, Young EH. (1938). *Children with Delayed or Defective Speech.* Palo Alto: Stanford University Press.

Strand EA, McNeil MR. (Accepted for publication). Effects of length and linguistic complexity on temporal acoustic measures in apraxia of speech. *J Speech Hear Res.*

Strand EA. (1987). Acoustic and response time measures in utterance production: A comparison of apraxic and normal speakers. Unpublished doctoral dissertation, University of Wisconsin-Madison.

Trost JE, Canter GJ. (1974). Apraxia of speech in patients with Broca's aphasia: A study of phoneme production accuracy and error patterns. *Brain Language* 1:65–79.

Tuller B, Story RS. (1987). Anticipatory coarticulation in aphasia. In: Ryalls JH, ed.

Phonetic Approaches to Speech Production in Aphasia and Related Disorders. Boston: College-Hill Press, pp 243–260.

Tuller B. (1984). On categorizing aphasic speech errors. *Neuropsychologia* 22:547–557.

Wambaugh JL, Doyle PJ. (1995). Treatment for acquired apraxia of speech: A review of efficacy reports. *Clin Aphasiol* 22:231–243.

Wertz RT, LaPointe LL, Rosenbek JC. (1984).

Apraxia of Speech in Adults: The Disorder and Its Management. Orlando: Grune and Stratton, Inc.

Yorkston KM, Beukelman DR, Bell KR. (1988). *Clinical Management of Dysarthric Speakers.* Boston: College-Hill Press.

Ziegler W, von Cramon D. (1985). Anticipatory coarticulation in a patient with apraxia of speech. *Brain Language* 26:117–130.

Chapter *15*

Speech Impairment Secondary to Hearing Loss

Sheila R. Pratt and Nancy Tye-Murray

Introduction

The study and treatment of speech problems secondary to hearing impairment have a history in the United States dating back to the early 1800s. The literature is voluminous, and this chapter represents a condensation of only portions of that literature. Much has been added to our knowledge of hearing loss and its effects on speech production. Our technological armamentarium for assessing and treating hearing loss and associated speech impairment has increased substantially over this period of time, especially in the past two decades. However, research in the treatment of speech in individuals with hearing impairment has been limited.

Although speech disorder secondary to hearing loss is traditionally not included within the category of sensorimotor speech disorders, there are numerous reasons for its inclusion. Foremost, audition is a major sensory contributor in the development of speech. It is generally believed that substantive loss of audition not only interferes with exposure to speech models but also interferes with the internal and external feedback necessary to develop speech normally. Without functional auditory skills, speakers have difficulty developing auditory and motor representations of speech. As a result, mapping of the speech sensorimotor system to the linguistic system is typically impaired. Compounding the problem is that hearing loss occurring in early childhood often results in language delay due to incomplete linguistic models. Therefore, it is often the case with prelingually impaired persons that an impaired motor-speech system interacts with an impaired linguistic system.

The role that audition plays for individuals who have developed normal speech and language is less well established. There tends to be three general beliefs. One is that in mature speakers, audition contributes to the ability of speakers to make the subtle postural and phonemic adjustments required for intra- and interarticulator coordination and that without auditory feedback speech intelligibility deteriorates over time (Cowie, Douglas-Cowie, & Kerr, 1982; Zimmermann & Rettaliata, 1981).

Others believe that the adjustments made in ongoing speech are not dependent on an intact auditory system (Goehl & Kaufman, 1984; Sapir & Canter, 1991). A more moderate view is held by Lane and his associates (Lane & Webster, 1991; Lane, Wozniak, Matthies, Svirsky, & Perkell, 1995; Perkell, Lane, Svirsky, & Webster, 1992). Lane et al (1995) suggest that auditory feedback plays a variable role. They have hypothesized that auditory feedback is used to validate the articulatory and acoustic relations within speakers' internal models of speech. Secondly, audition is used to monitor environmental conditions, such as background noise and reverberation, and ensures that accommodations are made so that acceptable speech intelligibility is maintained. Accordingly, some speech behaviors and speaking conditions require more or less access to the auditory system. The auditory system is, therefore, a contributor to the sensorimotor speech mechanism although the degree of influence is dependent on the maturity of the system, the speech behaviors being produced, and the context within which speech is occurring.

Characteristics

Hearing loss sufficient to handicap is very common within the general population, with a prevalence of 82.9 per 1000 (U.S. Public Health Service, 1990). The prevalence of severe to profound hearing loss in infants was previously estimated at 1 to 2 in 1000 (Feinmesser, Tell, & Levi, 1982; Martin, Bentzen et al, 1981; Parving, 1985). More recent estimates emanating from newly implemented universal screening programs that have used screening tools sensitive to less severe hearing loss are 5 to 6 per 1000 live births (White, Vohr, & Behrens, 1993). In school-age children the prevalence of severe to profound hearing loss is approximately 8.5 per 1000 (Schein & Delk, 1974), and hearing loss sufficient to limit activities in children under 18 years is estimated at 72 per 1000 (LaPlante, 1988). The inclusion of even milder hearing losses such as hearing loss due to middle ear disease, substantially increases the prevalence of childhood hearing loss, to approximately 1 in 25 (Fria, Cantekin, & Eichler, 1985; Schappert, 1992; Teele, Klein, & Rosner, 1989). With age and exposure to such things as noise and ototoxic agents, the prevalence and incidence of hearing impairment and disability increases substantially to where it is estimated that between 31 and 62% of the geriatric population has a hearing impairment (Bess, Lichtenstein, Logan, & Burger, 1989; Moscicki, Elkins, Baum, & McNamara, 1985) with hearing disability being the third most common chronic condition (after arthritis and hypertension) in persons over 65 (National Center for Health Statistics, 1982).

Speech Characteristics

Although hearing loss is common in the general population, its effects on speech produc-

tion are most pronounced with individuals whose hearing loss is congenital or acquired in early childhood. Only limited effects, if any, are perceptible with most individuals who acquire their hearing losses later in life (Goehl & Kaufman, 1984). Even in cases of complete or nearly complete adventitious hearing loss, speech remains largely intact for most individuals although speaking rate may be reduced, and articulatory and phonatory precision may be compromised (Leder, Spitzer, Kirchner et al, 1987; Lane & Webster, 1991; Waldstein, 1990; Perkell, Lane, Svirsky, & Webster, 1992). The differences largely are similar in nature but not degree to those observed with prelingually deafened speakers.

In addition to there being a relationship between age of onset and degree of speech impairment, there also is a moderately positive relationship between the degree of hearing loss and the severity of the associated speech difficulties (Boothroyd, 1969; Levitt, 1987; Smith, 1975). For example, speech difficulties in children with mild to moderate hearing loss, particularly if well aided, tend to be mild and similar in nature to those of normal-hearing children with developmental articulation disorders (Elfenbein, Hardin-Jones, & Davis, 1994; Oller & Kelly, 1974; West & Weber, 1973). Elfenbein, Hardin-Jones, and Davis (1994) observed that these children are characterized by good intelligibility. The misarticulations that are present tend to be substitutions of affricates and fricatives. In addition, mild hoarseness and resonance problems may be present in 20 to 30% of this subgroup. Their speech problems are usually evaluated and treated in the same manner as hearing speakers because of the mildness of the problems. Therefore, the following discussion of the effects of hearing loss on speech production largely focuses on speakers with congenital or early childhood hearing loss in the severe to profound range.

Individuals with severe to profound prelingual hearing loss are diverse relative to speech production skills. For example, some prelingually impaired speakers with profound hearing loss achieve remarkably high levels of intelligibility. Unfortunately, the majority who are born with a profound hearing loss never acquire the speech skills that permit them to interact easily using spoken language. On average, less than 20% of their words are intelligible to listeners who are not familiar with their speech (Hidgins & Numbers 1942; Markides, 1970; Smith, 1975). Smith (1975) evaluated 40 children with varying levels of hearing impairment, and, on average, only 18.7% (0 to 76%) of their words could be identified by inexperienced listeners. Not surprisingly, there is an inverse relationship between the frequency of segmental and suprasegmental errors and overall intelligibility. Despite a great deal of idiosyncracy with individual speakers, common error and difference patterns emerge when groups of speakers with hearing loss are evaluated. The patterns are similar across the severity range except when comparing the extremes of the range (Levitt & Stromberg, 1983). The following section is an overview of the common patterns observed with hearing-impaired subjects and is summarized by speech production subsystem.

Respiration
The difficulty in controlling respiration for speech has been observed with severely and profoundly hearing-impaired, but rarely in mild to moderately impaired speakers. Forner and Hixon (1977) evaluated the respiratory skills of 10 profoundly hearing-impaired adult speakers and observed that their subjects' vegetative respiratory skills were normal as were their rib cage and abdominal adjustments in anticipation of speech. Nonetheless, respiratory control during speech was faulty. Their subjects often phonated on low lung volumes and spoke within a restricted lung volume range. They also produced fewer syllables per breath unit because of inappropriate pausing either due to inspiration or inefficient air expenditure. Hearing-impaired persons can exhibit mean air volume expenditures as high as 100 cc/syllable with most of the air expended just prior to or during the initial portion of an utterance. In contrast, the normal range is approximately 20 to 40 cc/syllable (Forner & Hixon, 1977; Hardy, 1961; Whitehead, 1983). Whitehead (1982) obtained results similar to Forner and Hixon; however, subjects were grouped according to intelligibility. Whitehead observed that the intelligible hearing-impaired speakers had respiratory patterns more similar to normal hearing speakers and that the less intelligible speakers tended to initiate speech at low lung volumes and continued speaking at levels well below functional residual capacity.

The ability to control the airflow through the glottis is a major contributing factor in the speech breathing difficulties exhibited by some hearing-impaired speakers. It has been proposed that the differences are a reflection of abnormal laryngeal postures and reduced control of intrinsic laryngeal muscles. Mixed laryngeal patterns have been observed within and across studies with both hyper- and hypoabduction of the glottis. Hearing-impaired speakers are usually able to maintain, although inconsistently, an appropriately open and closed vocal tract with the less intelligible speakers exhibiting poorer control of laryngeal valving (Hutchinson & Smith, 1976; Whitehead, 1982; Whitehead & Barefoot, 1980). Using transillumination of the glottis, McGarr and Löfqvist (1982) found that some hearing-impaired speakers exhibit inappropriate glottal abduction between words. McGarr and Löfqvist suggested that these postures result in inefficient air expenditure although they did not simultaneously measure airflow in their study. Others have reported high airflow rates during the production of some consonants and vowels with subjects having difficulty maintaining prolonged continuous phonations (Gilbert, 1974; Hutchinson & Smith, 1976; Itoh, Horii, Daniloff, & Binnie, 1982; Whitehead & Barefoot, 1983). In other conditions such as with voiceless fricatives in VCV syllable contexts, reduced airflow has been observed suggesting excessive restriction of the airway

(Whitehead & Barefoot, 1983). Higgins, Carney, and Schulte (1994) also found evidence of hyperconstriction of the airway. In an aerodynamic and electroglottographic study of phonatory, velopharyngeal, and articulatory function, they found that early deafened adults with intelligible speech exhibited higher than normal subglottal pressures, fundamental frequencies, and laryngeal resistances. Some of their hearing-impaired subjects also exhibited low laryngeal abduction quotients and low phonatory airflows. The indication was that these speakers tended to overdrive and overconstrict their vocal folds during phonation. Higgins et al (1994) postulated that the hyperconstriction of the glottis was adopted to increase tactile feedback. They also suggested that intelligible hearing-impaired speakers are more likely to use a constricted laryngeal posture while less intelligible speakers tend to adopt a hyperabducted posture.

Voice

Given the respiratory and laryngeal valving difficulties that some speakers with hearing loss experience, it is not surprising that vocal abnormalities have been observed in this population. Their instances of hyper and hypoabduction of the larynx can result in voicing and other phonation errors particularly when poorly timed with upper airway articulation. Differences in vocal quality, pitch, and loudness have been reported as well as associated perturbation of the glottal waveform. The vocal quality of hearing-impaired speakers is typically described as breathy, hoarse, or strained (Hudgins & Numbers, 1942; Markides, 1970). As with perceptual judgments of hearing speakers' voice quality, the interjudge agreement on voice quality is good when using extreme samples but less reliable in the middle ranges. In addition, acoustic glottal measurements of perturbation, such as shimmer and jitter, are much less predictive of perceptual judgments of vocal quality in hearing-impaired speakers than for hearing patients with vocal pathologies (Arends, Povel, Van Os, & Speth, 1990). It

should be noted that the use of perceptual judgments of vocal quality and glottal acoustic perturbation measures have restricted applicability even with the normal-hearing population (Martin, Fitch, & Wolf, 1995; Wolfe, Cornell, & Palmer, 1991).

Although common, the pitch and loudness characteristics of hearing-impaired speakers vary within and across speakers (Higgins et al, 1994). Some hearing-impaired speakers use an excessively high habitual fundamental frequency (F0) (Angelocci, Kopp, & Holbrook, 1964; Horii, 1982). It has been suggested that male youths may have problems lowering their habitual fundamental frequency to acceptable levels as they progress through puberty (Boone, 1977, Chapter 6), although Osberger (1981) found that adolescent girls with hearing impairment produced higher fundamental frequencies than did adolescent boys with comparable hearing losses, indicating that elevated fundamental frequency was not isolated to males in this age range. Some hearing-impaired speakers are monopitch in their speech while others' exhibit excessive pitch variations. Diplophonia can be present and is likely due to excessive tension of the intrinsic laryngeal muscles. Not surprisingly, difficulty producing contextually appropriate (socially and linguistically) intensity levels is common in profoundly hearing-impaired speakers. Some speak at excessively high intensity levels (Calvert & Silverman, 1975), others at low levels (Penn, 1955). This difficulty with intensity control may be due, in part, to problems monitoring environmental sounds and the acoustics of a speaker's own voice but a portion is likely due to inefficient speech breathing and laryngeal control. For a number of possible pragmatic, linguistic or speech motor-control reasons, difficulties in modulating intensity and fundamental frequency, substantially interferes with intelligibility (Monsen, 1979).

Resonance

There are two resonance characteristics associated with speakers with prelingual severe to profound hearing loss. One is the cul-de-sac, or pharyngeal, resonance, and the other is the presence of improper nasalization, resulting in hyper- and hyponasality. Pharyngeal resonance is highly salient perceptually and commonly identified with deaf speech. It is not well understood but appears to be the result of improper lingual and pharyngeal posturing. In a radiographic study of 10 normal-hearing and 4 deaf women with pharyngeal resonance, Subtelny, Li, Whitehead, and Subtelny (1989) found that the deaf subjects' tongues tended to function from a more neutral position when producing vowels than did those of the hearing subjects. A neutralized tongue position was observed even though the speech of the deaf subjects was intelligible, and their vowel productions were considered distinct and correct. While producing high vowels the deaf subjects also were identified with elevated hyoids, large vertical dimensions of the laryngeal pharynx, retracted tongue roots, and retruded tongue dorsums that were associated with substantive epiglottis deflections toward the pharyngeal walls.

The nasality problems of hearing-impaired speakers can be due to structural limitations of the velopharyngeal mechanisms, but more commonly they are the result of improper velopharyngeal timing. Stevens, Nickerson, Boothroyd, and Rollins (1976) evaluated a group of 25 deaf children, measuring nasality as vibration transduced from the lateral surface of the nose with an accelerometer. They found that the children showed substantively more instances of vowel nasalization than did groups of normal-hearing children and adults. They also found that it was not uncommon for nasal consonants to be denasalized and for nonnasal consonants to be nasalized by the hearing-impaired children. In addition, a relationship between the degree of inappropriate nasality and intelligibility was observed, and listener judgments of nasality were consistent with the accelerometric findings.

Segmental Characteristics

Vowels. Vowels are usually more intact than consonants for speakers with hearing impairment. Germane to error pattern, hearing-impaired speakers tend to produce low vowels more correctly than high and midvowels, and back vowels more correctly than front vowels (Nober, 1967; Smith, 1975) although Angelocci et al's (1964) data obtained from early adolescent males indicated more errors on low vowels than high vowels. Typical vowel errors include substitutions, neutralizations, prolongations, nasalizations, and diphthongizations (Hidgins & Numbers, 1942; Markides, 1970; McGarr, 1987; Smith, 1975; Tye-Murray & Kirk, 1993). Omissions are more rare with vowels than with consonants, but substitutions and neutralizations are especially common, with substitutions going toward a more central and lax vowel. Angelocci et al's (1964) data show that vowel place errors occur more frequently than height errors, although McCaffrey and Sussman (1994) found that as the degree of hearing loss increases from severe to profound, the likelihood of vowel height errors increases.

The neutralization of vowels also affects the suprasegmental aspects of speech by shortening the vowel and reducing stress. Vowel prolongation and diphthongization also are commonly observed and contribute to reduced speaking rate. Together, the abnormal temporal patterns of vowels likely result in inappropriate linguistic and coarticulatory cues. In addition to singleton vowels being diphthongized, diphthongs are frequently reduced. For example, the intended word "boy" might be produced as /bɪ/. Further, diphthong elements can be produced as abutting single vowels. Prolongation and nasalization are common diphthong errors as well (Smith, 1975).

The perceptual findings of vowel neutralization have been corroborated with acoustic and movement data. For instance, spectrographic analyses of the speech of deaf speakers indicate a tendency for their first (F1) and second (F2) vowel formants to be centralized when compared to normal-hearing talkers (Monsen, 1976a) although excessively high second formants also have been observed, particularly with high back vowels (Angelocci et al, 1964; Stein, 1980). In a study of 17 adolescent hearing-impaired speakers with good vowel intelligibility, McCaffrey and Sussman (1994) found that the F0–F1 and F2–F3 differences (measured in Bark) of their severely hearing-impaired subjects tended to be consistent with those produced by their normal-hearing subjects. The intelligibility of their profoundly hearing-impaired subjects, however, was less than that of the severely hearing-impaired subjects, and their formant differences were significantly reduced. If the severely hearing-impaired subjects showed a reduction in formant space, it was usually with F2 and F3. McCaffrey and Sussman argued that the F2–F3 difference was more susceptible to reduction because F2 and F3 are less audible than F0 and F1. The reduced space between formants is evident as an overlap in vowel targets, which is consistent with neutralization, perceptual ambiguity, and vowel substitutions. It also suggests abnormal lingual posture and/or restricted mobility (Monsen, 1978; Osberger, Levitt, & Slosberg, 1979; Subtelny, Whitehead, & Samar, 1992).

Along with an overlap in vowel target space it has been reported that hearing-impaired speakers often use an elevated fundamental frequency when producing vowels and that fundamental frequency varies more across vowels produced by hearing-impaired speakers than by normal-hearing speakers (Angelocci et al, 1964). They also exhibit reduced variability in their second formants suggesting restricted anterior movement of the tongue (Monsen, 1976a). In addition, it has been hypothesized that changes in F0 and F1 are the primary means with which vowels are differentiated productively by hearing-impaired speakers (Angelocci et al, 1964; Monsen, 1976a; Stein, 1980).

Using glossometry, Dagenais and Critz-Crosby (1992) assessed tongue position and shape during vowel production. Ten profoundly hearing-impaired children with unintelligible speech were compared to 10 normal-hearing children. The hearing-impaired children tended to assume a flat tongue shape with a high back posture. There was less variability in tongue shape and position across vowels, all of which was consistent with vowel neutralization and reduced formant variability. The normal-hearing children, in contrast, exhibited a greater range of lingual postures and tongue shapes across vowels. They also used more discrete tongue positions and less token-to-token variability.

In a cineographic study of two normal-hearing adults and five deaf adults with varying degrees of intelligibility, Stein (1980) found that the deaf subjects produced reasonable tongue height distinctions between high and mid vowels but that posterior-anterior distinctions were lacking. The movement of the subjects' tongue bodies was limited, and the height distinctions may have been mediated by the mandible. Tye, Zimmerman, and Kelso (1983) observed with cinefluorography that their two prelingually deafened adults had similar tongue positions for /u/ and /æ/ unlike their postlingually impaired and normal-hearing subjects. Zimmerman and Rettaliata (1981) evaluated a deaf adult with a childhood-onset progressive hearing loss. This subject's cinefluorographic results, when referenced to the mandible, indicated reduced distinction in tongue shape between vowels and syllable context. Zimmerman and Rettaliata concluded that the distinctions made in the subject's steady-state vowel postures were established with excessive jaw displacement. Tye-Murray (1991), in a microbeam and cinefluorographic study, observed that her three deaf subjects exhibited somewhat reduced tongue mobility but that their mandibles were not excessively mobile in an absolute sense. They did, however, displace their jaws excessively relative to the mobility of the tongue body. In addition, the deaf subjects moved their tongues in a similar fashion regardless of the vowel being produced, whereas her normal sub-jects showed vowel-distinct movement tra-jectories.

Consonants. Speakers with severe to pro-found hearing loss typically produce a myriad of consonantal errors. Omissions are very common and have a profound negative impact on intelligibility. Other common er-rors include voiced-voiceless confusions, substitutions, distor-tions, and errors in con-sonant clusters (Hidgins & Numbers, 1942; Smith, 1975; Tye-Murray, Spencer, & Bedia, in press). Further, consonant errors are somewhat more common in the final than initial syllable position, particularly if they are voiced (Markides, 1970; Osberger, Robbins, Lybolt, Kent, & Peters, 1986; Smith, 1975) although Hidgins and Numbers (1942) observed more errors in the initial position.

One of the most frequent consonant errors is one of voicing. Hidgins and Numbers (1942), in their classic study, found that hear-ing impaired children tend to devoice voiced consonants. Markides (1970) observed a similar pattern, and Nober (1967) observed that voiceless sounds are more often correct than are voiced sounds. In contrast, Smith (1975) observed a pattern of voiced produc-tion of voiceless sounds. Heider, Heider, and Sykes (1940) as well as Carr (1953) observed that hearing-impaired children are more likely to use a voiced as opposed to a voice-less cognate, suggesting that voiced sounds may be easier to produce. Both types of voic-ing errors can be observed in some children. Millin (1971) suggested that the voiced for voiceless errors are likely due to a mistiming of the initiation and termination of phona-tion and can be associated with continuous voicing throughout an utterance. Further, both voicing and devoicing are likely due to inappropriate temporal coordination of the larynx with the upper airway articulators and not phonologic differences. Further, it has been suggested that listener perceptions of the voicing distinctions may be miscued by the durations of the preceding vowels or

durations of segments themselves (Gold, 1980; Osberger & McGarr, 1982; Tobey, Pancamo, Staller, Brimacombe, & Beiter, 1991). For example, stop consonants are per-ceived as voiceless more frequently when preceded by vowels of shorter duration and voiced when preceded by vowels of longer duration (Raphael, 1972). Also, fricatives prolonged relative to a preceding vowel have an increased likelihood of being perceived as voiceless (Denes, 1955).

The instrumental measurements of voicing are consistent with the perceptions of irregu-lar voicing. In a spectrographic study of voice-onset-time (VOT), Monsen (1976b) ob-served a tendency for profoundly hearing-impaired children to reduce the VOTs of their initial voiceless stop consonants al-though the more intelligible children pro-duced VOT in a manner consistent with hearing children. The less intelligible chil-dren had considerable overlap in their VOTs for the voiced and voiceless sounds, with most of their stops produced within the voiced portion of the VOT continuum. They also failed to show differences in VOT rela-tive to place of articulation. McGarr and Löfqvist (1982) obtained results consistent with Monsen. McGarr and Löfqvist (1982) also found that some of their adult subjects had VOTs within the perceptual boundary region for voicing resulting in increased per-ceptual confusion.

Consonant differences related to place of articulation are evident in the speech of per-sons with hearing loss. Consonants that are associated with visible facial movements, such as bilabials, are more likely to be spoken accurately than consonants that are less vis-ible, such as /k/ and /g/. For instance, Kirk and Tye-Murray (1992) analyzed the frequency with which nine prelingually deafened children correctly produced the following consonantal place features in spontaneous speech: bilabial, labiodental, linguadental, alveolar, palatal, velar, and glottal. Their subjects produced the bilabial consonants correctly significantly more often than any other place feature, although they produced bilabial consonants poorly too.

These findings intimate that deaf speakers utilize visual cues from their surrounding language community during speech acquisition. It should be noted though that McCaffrey and Sussman (1994) did not find this consistently with vowels. In addition, Osberger, Robbins, Lybolt, Kent, and Peters (1986) argued that the superiority of bilabials may be a function of the lips being more constrained in their movements as compared to other articulators such as the tongue, and that visibility may not be the key or only factor. In support Osberger et al's argument, consonants made in the middle of the mouth often are in error more than sounds made toward the back of the mouth even though they are more visible (Osberger et al, 1986; Smith, 1975).

Talkers with hearing loss also make manner of articulation errors. Characteristically, deaf and hard-of-hearing individuals are more likely to produce plosive consonants more accurately than nasals, fricatives, glides, or laterals—with affricates being particularly difficult (Nober, 1967; Osberger et al, 1986; Smith, 1975). Manner of articulation also interacts with place of articulation and syllable/word position. For example, the fricatives /z/, /ʃ/, and /s/ are difficult to produce but the fricative /f/ is usually produced correctly nearly as often as the plosives /b/ and /p/. In addition, Osberger et al (1986) found that although plosives were more often correct than fricatives and nasals in the prevocalic position these types of sounds have similar error rates in the postvocalic position.

Finally, a speech error frequently associated with speakers with limited residual hearing is glottalization. It is usually expressed by substituting other sounds with glottal stops, particularly back consonants (Levitt, Smith, & Stromberg, 1976). Glottalization may be used as a mechanism to control the airflow through the glottis and not necessarily as a phonological marker. Further, speakers who use glottalization tend to have relatively poor speech intelligibility (Stevens, Nickerson, & Rollins, 1978).

Suprasegmental

As suggested in the previous discussion, the suprasegmental production of deaf speaker often is aberrant. It clearly is not independent of respiratory and laryngeal function nor is it independent of the segmental aspects of speech. Listeners who hear deaf speech for the first time might describe it as sounding labored, effortful, and lacking in rhythm. Speakers with profound hearing loss tend to speak slowly; they may speak at only half the syllable rate of the normal-hearing population (John & Howarth, 1965; Voelker, 1935). The reduced rate may be due to sound prolongations, excessive and inappropriate pauses, and insertion of adventitious sounds between phonemes. Inappropriate pausing can occur due to either poor linguistic awareness of where to insert pauses or poor breath control. Although the slow rate of hearing-impaired speakers calls attention to itself, Osberger and Levitt (1979) suggested that not all of the factors that contribute to slow rate significantly interfere with intelligibility. They took samples of speech from hearing-impaired speakers and digitally altered the timing by correcting for pauses, relative timing, and absolute syllable duration. They found that only correction for relative timing improved intelligibility, and the improvement was small. Correcting for pauses and syllable duration worsened intelligibility, and when the samples were corrected for both relative timing and pauses, intelligibility was substantially worse than for the uncorrected samples. Although not a direct confirmation, the Osberger and Levitt results are consistent with the assertion of Parkhurst and Levitt (1978) that long pauses, if appropriately placed, may improve intelligibility for hearing-impaired speakers by allowing more listener processing time. Maassen (1986) found that when pauses were inserted at word boundaries, the intelligibility of deaf speech improved slightly. He postulated that longer pauses at word boundaries may make the boundaries more salient and ease word recognition. He further postulated that treatment of pauses, other than within word pauses, would not likely result in improved intelligibility. Osberger and Levitt (1979) also intimated that targeting syllable duration in therapy may decrease, rather than improve, intelligibility.

Poor fundamental frequency and intensity control contributes to the suprasegmental difficulties of hearing-impaired speakers. The fundamental frequency of hearing-impaired speakers, aside from being higher than normal, also can sound monotonic or fluctuate inappropriately within words and across utterances (Formby & Monsen, 1982; Monsen, 1979; Parkhurst & Levitt, 1978). They also do not show the increased fundamental frequency variations normally associated with reading (Horii, 1982); that is, their fundamental frequency variations tend to be similar regardless of whether the speech is spontaneous or read. Further, it is not unusual for hearing-impaired speakers to produce excessively high fundamental frequencies when they initiate utterances. The elevated F0 can then suddenly drop within the first few hundred milliseconds of the production as if correcting for overshoot. The lack of laryngeal control across utterances also is illustrated by their differential performance with variations in fundamental frequency contour. For example, declining fundamental frequency contours tend to be easier for hearing-impaired speakers to produce than are rising or complex contours (Most & Frank, 1991; Rubin-Spitz & McGarr, 1990).

As indicated previously, the vocal intensity of hearing-impaired speakers has been described as both excessively low and excessively high. Like fundamental frequency, it may not vary appropriately with the demands of context or environmental conditions (Hood & Dixon, 1969). Further, the prosody of hearing-impaired persons, as reflected in stress and phrasing, often is sufficiently impaired so as to interfere with the conveyance of meaning. When asked to produce stressed and unstressed CV syllables, Sussman and Hernandez (1979) found that hearing-impaired subjects increased their vocal intensity on stressed syllables but not their fundamental frequency. Some hearing-impaired speakers also have difficulty producing contrastive stress consistently (Murphy, McGarr, & Bell-Berti, 1990; Sussman & Hernandez, 1979). When asked to produce contrastive stress, hearing-impaired subjects often fail to adjust either fundamental frequency or intensity. Osberger and Levitt (1979) observed that some of their hearing-impaired speakers failed to produced durational differences for stressed and unstressed syllables. In contrast, Weiss, Carney, and Leonard (1985) found that hearing-impaired children with intelligible speech were able to produce perceptually adequate contrastive stress if allowances are made for expressive language skill. Tye-Murray and Folkins (1990) also observed that deaf adult speakers are able to make the necessary articulatory adjustments to produce known stress patterns, further indicating that difficulties with stress production may be related to linguistic knowledge.

Coarticulation

Although it is unclear how articulatory gestures are established and controlled in normal-hearing speakers, movement tends to proceed continuously from one open posture to the next (Fowler, 1986; Ohman, 1966). In contrast, many speakers with severe to profound hearing loss, particularly those with reduced intelligibility, may not move their articulators in a continuous, cyclical fashion but as a series of discrete events. For example, in a cinefluorographic study Tye-Murray (1987) observed that during stop consonant production only two of her five hearing-impaired subjects adjusted their tongue and jaw postures adequately in anticipation of following vowels, and these two subjects had relatively high intelligibility. Tye-Murray argued that a lack of distinctiveness between open postures likely contributed to the other subjects' coarticulatory difficulties. Although Stein (1980) and Zimmermann and Rettaliata (1981) suggested that speakers with profound hearing loss distinguish between open postures by altering jaw height, Tye-Murray's less intelligible subjects exhibited no vowel context effects in either jaw or tongue postures. In addition, Tye-Murray, Zimmermann, and Folkins (1987) found that sometimes deaf speakers do not move toward the open posture during the closed portions of articulations.

Acoustic studies have tended to support the movement data. Consonant-vowel transitions are more restricted in frequency for hearing-impaired than normal-hearing speakers, which can be attributed to vowel neutralization (Monsen, 1976c; Rothman, 1976). Most hearing-impaired speakers reduce the duration of the transitions, although some produce excessively lengthened transitions. The formant transitions also vary little with respect to phonetic context suggesting reduced coarticulatory effects. Further, vowel length is inconsistently adjusted in the postvocalic position relative to voicing for many hearing-impaired speakers (Monsen, 1974; Whitehead & Jones, 1978), and difficulties adjusting vowel duration in response to changes in syllable number have been observed (Tye-Murray & Woodworth, 1989). That is, as syllable number increases speakers with hearing impairment are inconsistent in their reductions of vowel duration. Even intelligible speakers may have some difficulty coordinating their speech movements over time. Waldstein and Baum (1991) and Baum and Waldstein (1991) measured both the anticipatory and the perseveratory speech behaviors of a group of intelligible profoundly hearing-impaired children using temporal and spectral acoustic measures (centroid and F2). Their hearing-impaired subjects produced both types of coarticulatory behaviors but to a lesser extent than their normal-hearing subjects.

Viewing the speech of hearing-impaired persons as discrete articulatory events is not supported by an acoustic study by Robb and Pang-Ching (1992). They analyzed the absolute and relative speech timing of 31 young adults with hearing impairment who varied with regard to overall intelligibility. Thir-

teen normal-hearing adults served as controls. Robb and Pang-Ching followed the measurement procedures of Weismer and Fennell (1985) and found that although their hearing-impaired subjects were slower and produced greater absolute durations, their relative timing was no different from that of the normal-hearing subjects. Robb and Pang-Ching also found no relationship between relative timing and speaker intelligibility or degree of hearing loss. If the hearing-impaired speakers produced their speech segments as linearly sequenced independent units, it is unlikely that relative timing would hold across utterances. Similar results have been observed with the speech of other groups associated with temporal disturbances such as people with dysarthria, apraxia, and stuttering (Prosek, Montgomery, & Walden, 1988; Weismer & Fennell, 1985), although McNeil, Liss, Tseng, and Kent (1990) observed irregularities in groups of apraxic and conduction aphasic subjects. Robb and Pang-Ching argued that the temporal differences observed with hearing-impaired speakers is one of degree and not abnormality. They also suggested that their data are consistent with the temporal properties of speech being biologically constrained and independent, to some extent, of auditory feedback. The data of Tye-Murray (1984) and Tye-Murray and Folkins (1990) support this notion. They observed that when speech tasks require alterations such as changes in rate or stress, deaf speakers are able to make the necessary articulatory adjustments (ie, jaw and lower lip displacements) online.

Developmental Speech Characteristics
Some investigators have examined the speech of children with severe to profound hearing loss in longitudinal studies. The evidence suggests that these children demonstrate different developmental patterns from normal-hearing children, and that they reach a plateau in their speech skills relatively early in their development. The phonetic repertoires of infants with severe to profound hearing loss have been found to be

restricted when compared to their normal-hearing peers (Lach, Ling, Ling, & Ship, 1970; Stoel-Gammon & Otomo, 1986). Although individual variability is noted, the early speech of infants with severe to profound hearing loss is dominated by sounds that are motorically less demanding to produce. They also tend to produce sounds that contain more low-frequency information, sounds that tend to be the most auditory salient for children who have substantive hearing impairments. For example, Stoel-Gammon (1988) found that the babbling of her group of hearing-impaired infants contained mainly low-frequency consonants that can be prolonged such as, nasals and glides. Canonical (well-formed and temporally consistent with adult speech) babbling in babies has been observed as late as 31 months (Lynch, Oller, & Steffens, 1989) and generally does not appear before 12 months of age (Oller & Eilers, 1988; Oller, Eilers, Bull, & Carney, 1985).

Several studies have examined the speech characteristics of children aged 8 years and older, and examined performance as a function of age. Hudgins and Numbers (1942) included subjects aged 8 to 20 years in their study. They found little improvement in speech performance as a function of age, as did Smith (1975) in a similar study performed 30 years later. McGarr (1987) studied children longitudinally between the ages of 11 and 14 years. She found little change in the average number and types of vowel and diphthong errors over time.

Many factors probably contribute to the development of speech errors that have been reviewed in this section. These factors include a child's home environment, educational placement, quality and quantity of direct speech intervention received, personality and interest in acquiring spoken language, and other individual characteristics. However, the most predominant factor is probably the amount and quality of residual hearing and the age-of-onset. There is some indication that age-of-onset is a critical factor even with adventitiously hearing-impaired speakers (Lane et al, 1995).

The Role of Audition in Development

Tye-Murray (1992) proposed that auditory information plays five important roles during the acquisition of speech. First, audition allows the child to develop specific principals of articulatory organization. By listening to other members of the language community, a child learns to regulate speech breathing, learns how to flex and extend the tongue body, and learns how to rhythmically alternate between vowels and consonants (ie, open and closed vocal tract positions). The second role of audition is to allow children to learn how to produce specific speech events. For instance, a child might learn to distinguish /t/ with a rapid downward tongue movement, and /l/ with a gesture of slower velocity. Thirdly, children utilize auditory information to develop a system of phonological performance. That is, they learn the phonemes of their language by listening to others use them in speech production. They also learn the rules of acceptability for combining phonemes and syllable structures. The fourth role of auditory information is to inform a child about the consequences of a particular articulatory gesture, and to allow the child to compare those consequences with the speech outputs of other talkers. Finally, when attending to auditory signals, a child may learn to monitor ongoing speech production, and detect and correct speech errors. In subsequent sections of this chapter teaching methods will be considered that may influence a child's acquisition of speech production skills and how the influences of the auditory system in speech production might be augmented or assumed by other mechanisms.

Concomitant Nonspeech Characteristics

Hearing loss may or may not be associated with concomitant deficits. Whether deficits are associated with a hearing loss is largely dependent on the cause of the hearing loss, the site of the lesion, and the developmental status at insult. For example, a noise-induced hearing loss occurring in a young adult has a more limited likelihood of concomitant deficits than a hearing loss in a young child due to bacterial meningitis or a genetic disorder. There are a large number of conditions known to cause, or be associated with, hearing loss, but because approximately 25% of hearing losses are of unknown etiology (Schein & Delk, 1974), it is difficult to clearly associate hearing loss with many co-occurring conditions. The issue becomes more complex with the elderly, in whom hearing loss becomes interrelated with socioeconomic factors as well as cognitive and physical decline (National Center for Health Statistics, 1982).

There are a number of ways in which causes and associated characteristics have been categorized in the literature. Table 15–1 is a simple listing of characteristics that have been acknowledged as coexisting with hearing loss. Some co-occur due to shared causative or predisposing factors, while others are a result of the hearing loss. Many of these characteristics occur in constellations or syndromes. Some of the genetic syndromes commonly associated with hearing loss are listed in Table 15–2. As there are over 400 such identified syndromes associated with hearing loss readers are encouraged to refer to Gorlin, Toriello, and Cohen

Table 15–1. Some nonspeech deficits associated with hearing loss.

A. Cognitive deficits
  1. Mental retardation
  2. Dementia
B. Behavioral disorder
C. Psychiatric disorder
D. Language delay and disorder
E. Learning disability
  1. Reading deficits
  2. Writing deficits
F. Nervous system disease
  1. Motor disturbances
  2. Seizures
  3. Glioma or neuroma
  4. Spina bifida
  5. Impaired taste and smell
  6. Vestibular disturbances
G. Eye disease
  1. Optic degeneration and atrophy
  2. Ocular lens abnormalities
  3. Retinitis pigmentosa
    a. Night blindness
    b. Tunnel vision
    c. Blindness
  4. Oculomotor disturbances
H. Renal disease
I. Musculoskeletal disease
  1. Head and neck abnormalities
    a. Abnormalities of the skull
    b. Malformations of the lip and palate
    c. Eyelid malformations
    d. Abnormal facial features
    e. Malformations of the outer ear
    f. Malformations of the middle ear
    g. Mandible and maxillary malformations

    h. Dental abnormalities
    i. Nasal abnormalities
  2. Digital anomalies
  3. Limb abnormalities
  4. Joint abnormalities
  5. Limb and joint pain
  6. Bone disease
  7. Growth retardation
  8. Vertebral abnormalities
  9. Shoulder abnormalities
  10. Winged scapula
J. Skin disease
  1. Pigmentary disorder
    a. Albinism
    b. White forelock
    c. Vitiligo
    d. Leukonychia
    e. Cafe-au-lait spots
    f. Axillary freckling
    g. Iris bicolor or heterochromia
    h. Salt and pepper retinal pigmentation
  2. Lichenfield skin eruptions
  3. Recurrent urticaria
  4. Keratosis
  5. Sun sensitivity
  6. Thick, coarse hair
  7. Abnormal whorl patterns on hands
  8. Malformed fingernails and toenails
K. Metabolic disease
  1. Diabetes
  2. Goiter
  3. Liver and spleen enlargement
  4. Impaired metabolism of carbohydrates
L. Cardiac and vascular disease
M. Urogenital malformations

(1995) and Konigsmark and Gorlin (1976) for characteristics specific to particular syndromes.

Evaluation Procedures

Sensory

The first step in the evaluation process is the determination of the speaker's sensory skills. In particular, the determination of aided auditory sensitivity and acuity is important because these measures provide an anchor for predicting what further tests and evaluation procedures would be most appropriate. They also may provide a basis for selecting the most advantageous treatment approach. In addition to auditory testing, visual, tactile, proprioceptive, and kinesthetic perceptual testing may provide useful information relative to treatment, especially if a multisensory treatment approach is used (see Kent, this volume). It cannot be assumed that a person with a hearing loss can compensate easily through other modalities such as vision or taction. From what is known about syndromes associated with and causes of hearing loss, a higher likelihood of multimodality impairment should be expected.

Structural

After sensory status has been determined, the integrity of the speech apparatus should be assessed via an age-appropriate oral peripheral examination. The *Oral Speech Mechanism Screening Examination-Revised* (St. Louis & Ruscello, 1987) is an example of a format that can be used with adults. The protocol described by Robbins and Klee (1987) is an example of a protocol that can be used with children. Along with other sensory deficits, people with hearing impairment have a high risk of concomitant oral-facial anomalies such as cleft palate. In addition, it is generally believed that people with hearing loss have a higher prevalence of dysarthria and apraxia of speech, although there is very little documentation to support this belief. Confirming an apraxia of speech in a hearing-impaired person, particularly a child, can be difficult because they often have restricted phonologic and phonetic repertoires, making the distinction between an apraxic effect and a hearing loss effect problematic.

Speech

Speech production can be assessed perceptually as well as instrumentally. The human ear remains the most powerful tool for separating normal from abnormal speech production. It can perceive acoustic nuances associated with abnormalities that are often obscured by noise or complexity in instrumental recordings. However, as with many other sensorimotor speech disorders, some hearing-impaired speakers' errors are so unusual or difficult to explain that the added information provided by instruments may assist in the diagnostic process.

Perceptual

When hearing-impaired speakers exhibit mild segmental differences, it is usually acceptable to use assessment protocols developed for hearing individuals. Using articulation and phonology assessment tools that were standardized on hearing individuals is reasonable, particularly if the hearing loss is mild to moderate and the person is well aided. To assess people who are more impaired, there are a number of assessment protocols that have been developed and standardized to guide the perceptual analysis. Some of the tools are structured to evaluate segmental and suprasegmental aspects of speech; others are used to assess overall intelligibility.

An evaluation approach commonly used with young children includes the Phonetic Level and Phonologic Level Speech Evaluation protocols developed by Ling (1976). They are criterion-referenced procedures that companion Ling's treatment approach, which will be discussed later. In the Phonetic Level Speech Evaluation the children's imitative vocal characteristics are judged for presence, pitch, duration, and intensity. Vowels and diphthongs are elicited as single syllables, repeated, alternated, and produced

357

Table 15–2. Some syndromes commonly associated with hearing loss according to major systems affected.

Syndrome/disease	Type & degree of hearing loss	Oral	Cognitive/learning	Psychiatric	Nervous system	Vesti-bular	Pul-monary	Eye	Renal	Musculo-skeletal	Integu-mentary	Endocrine/metabolic	Cardio-vascular	Uro-genital	Inheritance
Familial streptomycin ototoxicity	S-1 to 4*					X									AD (?)
Ataxia, hypogonadotrophic hypogonadism, mental retardation & sensorineural hearing loss (Richards-Rundle)	S-1 to 3-p		X		X*			X		X	X	X		X	AR
Ataxia and sensorineural hearing loss (Lichtenstein-Knorr)	S-4-c/p/dp	X			X*			X		X			X		AR
Cockayne	S-1 to 3-dp	X	X		X*			X	X	X	X			X	AR
Hallgren	s-3-dp		X	X	X*			X		X				X	AR (?)
Motor & sensory neuropathy, optic atrophy, & sensorineural hearing loss—X-linked (Rosenberg-Chutorian)	S-3-dp				X*			X		X					XR
Motor & sensory neuropathy with sensorineural hearing loss—autosomal dominant (AD Charcot-Marie-Tooth)	S-3-p				X*										AD
Motor & sensory neuropathy with sensorineural hearing loss—autosomal recessive (AR Charcot-Marie-Tooth; Bouldin)	S-1 to 4-c/p				.X*					X					AR
Motor & sensory neuropathy with sensorineural hearing loss—X-linked (X-L Charcot-Marie-Tooth; Cowchock)	S-3-d		X		X*					X					XR
Myoclonus epilepsy, ataxia, & sensorineural hearing loss (May-White)	S-2 to 3-dp	X			X*	X		X				X	X		AR
Myoclonus epilepsy, dementia, & sensorineural hearing loss (Latham-Munro)	S-4-c	X	X	X	X*			X					X		AR
Neurofibromatosis, Type II (Vestibular schwanomas & neural hearing loss)	S-4-dp	X			X*	X		X			X				AD
Infantile Refsum	S-4-c		X		X			X*		X					AR

358

Syndrome	Code	1	2	3	4	5	6	7	8	9	10	Inheritance
Pigmentary retinopathy, diabetes mellitus, hypogonadism, mental retardation, & sensorineural hearing loss (Edwards)	S-2 to 3-dp	X		X		X*		X	X	X	X	AR
Pigmentary retinopathy, diabetes mellitus, obesity, & sensorineural hearing loss (Alström)	S-3-dp	X		X		X*		X	X	X	X	AR
Norrie (Oculo-acousticocerebral dysplasia)	S-1 to 4-c	X	X	X		X*		X				XR
Refsum (heredopathia atactica polyneuritiformis)	S-1 to 3-dp	X		X		X*	X*	X	X	X	X	AR
Usher, Types I & II	S-1 to 4-c/p	X	X	X		X*	X*	X				AR
Adolescent renal tubular acidosis	S-2-p						X*					AR
Alport (nephritis & sensorineural hearing loss)	S-1 to 4-dp	X	X			X	X*	X	X			AD, AR or XR
Infantile renal tubular acidosis & congenital sensorineural hearing loss	S-2 to 4-c/p	X		X			X*	X	X			AR
Macrothrombocytopathia, nephritis & sensorineural hearing loss (Epstein)	S-2 to 3-dp						X*		X	X		AD (?)
Nephritis, motor & neuropathy with sensorineural hearing loss (Lemieux-Neemeh)	S-1 to 3-dp	X		X		X*	X*	X		X		AD
Nephritis, urticara, amyloidosis & sensorineural hearing loss (Muckle-Wells)	S-3-dp	X				X*	X*	X				AD
Renal, genital, & middle ear (Winter)	C-1 to 2-c/p			X		X	X*	X	X		X*	AR
Apert (craniosynostosis)	C-1 to 2-c	X	X	X	X	X	X*	X*				AD
Branchio-oto-renal (BOR; brachio-oto; ear-pit hearing loss)	C/S/M-1 to 4-c/d	X	X	X	X	X	X	X*	X		X	AD
CHARGE	C/S/M-1 to 4-c	X	X	X	X	X	X*	X		X	X	AD or AR
Otofaciocervical	C-1 to 3-c	X	X	X		X*	X*	X*				AD
Crouzon	C-1 to 2-c	X	X	X		X*	X*					AD
Craniodiaphyseal dysplasia	M-1 to 4-p	X		X		X*	X*				X	Unknown
Craniotubular (Pye)	M-1 to 3-dp	X		X		X*	X*					AD or AR
DiGeorge	C/M-1 to 4-c	X	X	X		X*	X*		X			AD, AR or Ch
Ectrodactyly-ectodermal-dysplasia-clefting (EEC)	C/S/M-1 to 4-c	X	X	X	X	X	X*	X			X	AD
Fibrodysplasia ossificans progressiva (FOP)	C/S-1 to 3-dp	X		X			X*	X				AD
Hyperphosphatasemia (Juvenile Paget's)	M-2 to 3-dp	X		X		X	X*	X*		X		AR

Table 15-2. *Continued*

Syndrome/disease	Type & degree of hearing loss	Oral	Cognitive/ learning	Psychiatric	Nervous system	Vestibular	Pulmonary	Eye	Renal	Musculoskeletal	Integumentary	Endocrine/ metabolic	Cardiovascular	Urogenital	Inheritance
Joint fusion, mitrial insufficiency & conductive hearing loss (Formey)	C-1 to 2-c									X^α	X		X		AD
Kniest (metatropic dysplasia, Type II)	C/S/M-1 to 3-dp	X						X		X*			X		AD
Lacrimoauriculodentodigital (LADD; Levy-Hollister)	M-1 to 3-C	X						X	X	X^α					AD
Lop ears, micrognathia, and conductive loss	C/M-1 to 3-c	X								X^α					AD
Mandibulofacial dysostosis (Treacher Collins)	C/M-1 to 4-c	X			X		X		X^α						AD
Oculoauriculvertebral (Goldenhar)	C/S-1 to 3-c	X	X		X		X	X	X	X*			X		AD
Osteogenesis imperfecta, Types I–IV	C/M-1 to 3-dp	X						X		X*			X		AD
Otopalatodigital, Types I & II	C/M-1 to 3-c	X	X		X			X		X*					XR
Severe autosomal-recessive osteopetrosis (Albers-Schönberg)	C/M-1 to 2-dp	X	X		X			X	X	X*		X			AR
Stickler (Marshall-Stickler, Hereditary arthro-ophthalmopathy)	C/S/M-1 to 3-p	X						X		X*			X		AD
Van Buchem's (generalized cortical hyperostosis)	S/M-1 to 3-dp	X			X			X		X*		X			AR
Wildervanck (cervico-oculoacoustic; Klippel-Feil Anomoly Plus)	C/S/M-1 to 4-c/d	X	X		X	X		X	X	X*				X	Unknown
Dominant onychodystrophy, coniform teeth, & sensorineural hearing loss (Robinson)	S-1 to 4-c	X								X	X*	X			AD
Dominant onychodystropy, triphalangeal thumbs, & sensorineural hearing loss (Goodman-Moghadam)	S-2 to 3-c									X*	X*				AD
Dominant piebald trait & sensorineural hearing loss (Telfer)	S-1 to 4-p		X		X						X*				AD

Syndrome									Inheritance
Multiple lentigines (LEOPARD)	S-1 to 3-c/p	X			X	X*	X	X	AD
Pili torti and sensorineural hearing loss (Björnstad)	S-1 to 4-c					X*			AR (?)
Recessive piebaldness (Woolf)	S-4-C					X*	X		AR or XR
Waardenburg, Types I & II	S-1 to 3-c/p	X	X	X	X	X*	X	X	AD
Diabetes insipidus, diabetes mellitus, optic atrophy, and sensorineural hearing loss (DIDMOAD; Wolfram)	S-2 to 3-dp	X	X	X		X*	X		AR
Goiter & profound congenital sensorineural hearing loss (Penred)	S-1 to 4-p?	X		X	X*				AR
Mucopolysaccharidosis I-H (MPS I-H; Hurler)	C/S/M-1 to 3-p	X	X	X	X*	X	X		AR
Mucopolysaccharidosis I-S (MPS I-S; Scheie)	M-1 to 2-p	X		X	X*	X	X		AR
Mucopolysaccharidosis I-H/S (MPS I-H/S; Hurler-Scheie)	C/S/M-1 to 3-p	X	X	X	X*	X	X		AR
Mucopolysaccharidosis II (MPS II; Hunter)	S/M-1 to 2-p	X	X	X	X*	X	X		XR
Mucopolysaccharidosis III (MPS III; Sanfilipo)	S/M-1 to 2-dp	X	X	X	X*	X	X		AR
α-D-Mannosidosis	S/3-dp	X	X	X	X*	X	X		AR
Electyrocardographic abnormalities, fainting spells & sudden death with sensorineural hearing loss (Jervell Lange-Nielsen; cardioaudition; surdocardiac; Long Q-T)	S-3 to 4-c		X		X		X*	X	AR
Sickle Cell	C/S/M-1 to 4-p	X		X	X	X	X*	X	AR
Trisomy 21	C/S/M-1 to 4-c	X	X	X	X	X	X	X	Ch*
Turner (Ullrich-Turner)	C/S/M-1 to 2-c	X	X	X	X	X	X	X	Ch*

Note. An X designates each major system that is characteristically affected with each syndrome. The asterisk (*) is used to indicated the major system that is most likely involved and best characterizes the syndrome. Under the system Musculoskeletal the superscript ex designates the musculoskeletal malformations are primarily limited to the external ear. Under type and degree of hearing loss C = conductive hearing loss, S = sensorineural hearing, and M = mixed hearing loss. The numbers 1 through 4 refer to the degree of hearing loss with 1 being a mild loss, 2 a moderate loss, 3 a severe loss, and 4 a profound loss. The small letters refer to the time course of the hearing loss; the letter c = congenital hearing loss, d = delayed onset, p = progressive loss, and dp = progressive hearing loss with delayed onset.
The information in this table was modified from Gorlin, Toriello and Cohen (1995).

with varying pitch. Simple consonants and blends are evaluated primarily at a structured syllabic-unit level. The syllables are initially elicited as isolated syllables then repeated, alternated, and produced at varying loudness and pitch levels. Word position effects also are assessed. In contrast, the Phonologic Level Speech Evaluation focuses on the quality and complexity of the children's speech at the discourse level. It is a check list of the children's vocal control, linguistic structure, phonemic inventory, and intelligibility when speaking voluntarily in a nonstructured situation.

The strength of Ling's two assessment procedures is that they relate directly to his treatment program. They also include tasks that are simple enough so that very young and very involved children can be assessed. Problematic for the procedures is that no normative data accompany the protocols which are published in the book describing the Ling treatment approach. In addition, the reliability and linearity of the protocols has been questioned (Dunn & Newton, 1986; Shaw & Coggins, 1991).

The *CID Phonetic Inventory* (Moog, 1988) is similar to the Phonetic Level Speech Evaluation in structure and also is based largely on a syllable unit. It was developed primarily for young children or children with severe speech difficulties. In this test, the children are shown a series of printed cards along with spoken models for imitation. The areas tested include suprasegmentals, vowels, diphthongs, and consonants in various syllable configurations. The results are plotted in percent correct per category and are profiled. However, like the Ling assessment procedures, the *CID Phonetic Inventory* is lacking in normative and validation data. The manual also lacks information for interpreting the profiles and there is no indication that the percentages are equivalent across the categories assessed.

The *Fundamental Speech Skills Test* (Levitt, Youdelman, & Head, 1990) also is similar to Ling's two assessment procedures in orientation but is more contained and streamlined. It was developed to test children above five

years through adults who have severe to profound hearing loss. It was structured to evaluate phonatory, suprasegmental, and segmental aspects of speech at varying levels of complexity. Speech behaviors are elicited with picture plates containing symbols, syllable strings, words, and pictures. Although not required, patients who can read are at an advantage. The test results are compared to norms based on age and degree of hearing loss, although the derivations of the norms are not made explicit and there is no documentation of reliability or validity.

Unlike the above-mentioned evaluation protocols, the Speech Intelligibility Evaluation (SPINE) (Monsen, 1981) is not an assessment of isolated speech skills but a means to document the overall intelligibility of a speaker's productions at the single-word level. It was developed for individuals with severe to profound hearing loss who had at least single-word reading skills. The test is not commercially available so the materials, consisting of 40 cards with single words printed on them, must be constructed by the examiner. The cards are arranged into 10 phonemically contrastive sets of four cards. The contrasts are primarily of vowel characteristics and voicing. For each set, the cards are individually directed toward the patient and away from the examiner. The patient is asked to produce the word aloud and the examiner records what he or she thinks the patient said. The percentage of words correctly identified by the examiner is the patient's intelligibility score. Although usable normative data have not been reported for the SPINE, validity and reliability results have been published and were acceptably high.

The *CID Picture SPINE* (Monsen, Moog, & Geers, 1988) was developed to assess speech intelligibility in young children and children who have poor reading skills. It was constructed and administered in the same way as the SPINE except that pictures rather than printed words are used. The materials are commercially available and a standardized format is used. Norms are available and measures of reliability and validity are provided. One limitation of the *CID Picture SPINE* is that the use of simple pictures reduces the types of contrasts that can be tested. In addition, the vocabulary level of the pictures is uneven and can interact with the results. It is not unusual to have to train young children to recognize some of the pictures.

Subtelny and her associates developed a set of rating scales often referred to as the NTID Speech and Voice Rating Scales (or NTID Rating Scales). Although they are described in a number of publications they are published in their most complete form as part of a perceptual training program called the *Speech and Voice Characteristics of the Deaf* (Subtelny, Orlando, & Whitehead, 1981). The training program includes a series of audio tapes that are used to train judgments of overall intelligibility, pitch, resonance, voice quality, and rate. The rating scales, as part of the training program, include categories for intelligibility, pitch register, pitch control, rate, air expenditure, prosodic features, a breathy-weak voice dimension, a tense-harsh vocal dimension, nasal resonance, and pharyngeal resonance. Each category is assessed with a 5-point scale with descriptors applied to each point per category. The speaker reads the rainbow passage (Fairbanks, 1960, p 127) or the CID Everyday Sentences (Silverman & Hirsh, 1955), and the examiner judges the speech according to all 10 categories. Its use with spontaneous speech also has been described (Subtelny, 1977). Although the training program is an attempt to increase rater reliability, there is some indication that multiple raters should be used when assessing a person's speech with these scales making the scales somewhat impractical.

Of all the NTID speech and voice scales, the intelligibility scale has received the greatest amount of attention partly because intelligibility is an overall characteristic of speech, but also because of the multiple factors that can affect intelligibility ratings. For example, experienced raters tend to score speech as more intelligible than inexperienced listeners (Monsen, 1978, 1983; McGarr, 1983). Context

and predictability of speech materials tend to affect all listeners similarly regardless of level of experience although better speakers benefit from increased context while poorer speakers perform less well when context is increased (McGarr, 1983; Sitler, Schiavetti, & Metz, 1983). Further, Schiavetti, Metz, and Sitler (1981) questioned the use of interval scaling procedures when assessing speech intelligibility. Samar and Metz (1988) supported this claim. They found that the validity of the midrange of the NTID intelligibility scale was compromised because of extreme confidence intervals despite acceptable reliability and validity quotients. They recommended the use of write-down procedures like the SPINE which tend to be more accurate in the midskill range.

Instrumental

As with perceptual tools, the selection of instruments for use in an assessment depends on the characteristics of the patient, the questions needing to be addressed, and the specific purpose of the assessment. For example, if the purpose is to document to a third party that respiratory function for speech is abnormal and needs to be treated, then normative data should be available on the tool selected. The tool also must be sensitive and reliable enough to differentiate normal from abnormal function. For many of the instrumental tools available to clinicians, these types of data are not available, which limits their applicability, particularly with the pediatric population.

Pragmatically, there also is the issue of tool availability, practicality and ease of use. With the advances in digital signal processing, the increased availability of low-cost computers, and the commercial introduction of user-friendly speech analysis software systems, the options for assessing patients are substantial. Some systems are dedicated to a particular parameter of speech such as fundamental frequency or nasality, but many of the systems are multimodular and include modules that can be used for treatment as well as assessment and are therefore more cost-effective for many clinicians. All of these instrumental measures are addressed in detail in earlier chapters in this volume. Those specific tools and measurement parameters most applicable and most frequently used with deaf and hearing-impaired individuals (acoustic, kinematic, and aerodynamic) are reviewed below.

Acoustic

Acoustic analyses can be done in a number of ways and can target various speech characteristics. Wideband spectrograms have been used to look at the center frequencies of vowel formants, formant transitions, and VOT (McCaffrey & Sussman, 1994; Monsen, 1976a, 1976b, 1976c; Waldstein, 1990), but wideband spectrograms can be problematic if the bandwidth of the analysis system is not adjustable. This is particularly true when measuring vowel formants. Speakers with excessively high fundamental frequencies will produce spectrograms that represent multiple harmonics rather than formants. In addition to being observed in some hearing-impaired speakers, this is commonly observed with hearing infants, young children, and women. This phenomenon is due to the harmonics being excessively spaced relative to the filter bandwidths and can be compensated for by increasing the bandwidth of the analysis filters. Kent and Read (1992) recommended that the bandwidth of the analyzing filter be two to three times as large as the fundamental frequency. If adjusting the bandwidth of the analysis system is not an option or is not practical (as in the case of extremely high fundamental frequencies), then the speed of taped speech samples can be reduced on playback. Another suggested method for measuring formant frequencies has been to use spectra derived from linear predictive coding because, unlike spectra derived with a Fourier analysis, it does not represent the harmonics of the fundamental but rather the formant frequencies and amplitudes. It is therefore less directly dependent on the fundamental frequency and the integrity of the harmonic structure. However, when the reliability of measuring formant frequencies derived with linear predictive coding was compared to analogous measurements from spectrograms, both types of analyses became unstable with samples having fundamental frequencies above 350 Hz (Monsen & Engebretson, 1983). Further, most linear predictive coding algorithms do not account for antiresonances in their models so the introduction of nasalization and lateralization can be problematic (Kent & Read, 1992).

Fundamental frequency is a common acoustic feature measured with hearing-impaired speakers because of their difficulties with habitual fundamental frequency and F0 control. There are a number of extractions methods available. They vary from measuring waveforms and narrowband spectrograms by hand to digital computational methods. In addition, many digital acoustic analysis systems providing more than one extraction option. Some of the problems associated with measuring fundamental frequency with hearing-impaired speakers are the same as those encountered when measuring the fundamental frequency of women and children. Many of the algorithms have difficulty processing high frequency signals accurately as reflected in frequency doubling, halving, and dropouts. The problem can be compounded by the presence of irregularities in the glottal waveform that are commonly associated with hearing-impaired speakers, irregularities that also often preclude the use of fine-grained vocal acoustic analyses such as shimmer and jitter. Electroglottographic, accelerometric, and inverse filtering methods can be used to avoid some of these problems and are becoming increasingly more available to clinicians.

Problems associated with nasal resonance can be assessed by viewing palatal movement and by direct measures of inappropriate absence or presence of nasal emission (eg, nasal mirror, nasal airflow) but acoustically, nasal resonance is often measured with a nasometer such as the Kay Nasometer (Kay Elemetrics, 1992). It measures the relative intensity of sound coming through the nose and the mouth. Normative data are available for standard speech samples but are limited for very young children and speakers who have low language and reading skills (Dalston & Seaver, 1990; Seaver, Dalston, Leeper, & Adams, 1991). In addition, the headsets are heavy and cumbersome for very young children. An alternative is to use an accelerometer attached to the side of the nose. It can be input to many of the analysis systems that read simple voltages. For example, it can be put into the microphone ports of many computer-based speech training systems. Accelerometers have the advantages of being small, noninvasive, and relatively inexpensive. There are data supporting the validity of using them to measure nasality in hearing-impaired speakers (Stevens, Nickerson, Boothroyd, & Rollins, 1976), and some normative data have been collected on normal-hearing adults (Lippmann, 1981). Placement and degree of contact on the nose are major considerations, however, when obtaining accelerometric results (Lippmann, 1981).

Movement

Some data are available on speech movements, but most have been collected on a small number of intelligible adult speakers with concentration on the tongue (eg, Tye et al, 1983; Tye-Murray, 1991; Zimmerman & Rettaliata, 1981). In addition, most of the data have been collected with systems that require exposure to radiation and/or are not commercially available (ie, x-ray microbeam, cinefluoroscopy, glossometry). However, methods are readily available with which clinicians can assess laryngeal and palatal movements as well as lingual-palatal contact. Electroglottography and videostroboscopy can be used to provide information about laryngeal movements and postures. Nasal endoscopy and photodetection methods can be used to assess palatal movements (Dalston, 1989; Dalston & Seaver, 1990; Karnell, Seaver, & Dalston, 1988). Although not providing direct information about movement, palatometry has been applied to speakers with hearing impairment and can be used to provide information about pat-

terns of lingual-palatal contact. Dagenais and Critz-Crosby (1991) identified five patterns commonly associated with deaf speakers. The patterns included an open configuration with little or no contact, a closed configuration with full lingual-palatal contact, front occlusion with lingual contact around the entire alveolar ridge, back occlusion with contact only toward that back of the palate, and a grooved configuration. Dagenais and Critz-Crosby observed that these patterns often are used idiosyncratically by deaf speakers, particularly those with poor intelligibility. One difficulty associated with the use of the palatometer is that it is difficult to quantify the data, although Byrd, Flemming, Mueller, and Tan (1995) recently reported on a data reduction method for the palatometer.

Airflow

Because many hearing-impaired speakers, even intelligible speakers, have difficulty with speech breathing and articulatory control of the airstream, measurement of breathing and airflow may be warranted in many cases. Respiratory and aerodynamic measures are not commonly used clinically with hearing-impaired speakers, although Whitehead (1991) applied oral airflow tools with hearing-impaired subjects to measure the closure durations of stop consonants, and Higgins et al (1994) reported that airflow measures were easily used even with young children. Nasal and oral airflow can be measured with a number of commercially available systems, and phonatory airflow, subglottal pressure, and laryngeal resistance can be estimated from these two airflow measures (Smitheran & Hixon, 1981). Interested readers should refer to Warren, Rochet, and Hinton in this volume for more on the application of aerodynamic measures.

Treatment Approaches

The treatment approaches for speech impairment secondary to hearing loss have been largely developed according to input and feedback modality rather than process, particularly when it comes to the treatment of children. With adults and older children exhibiting isolated deficits (ie, elevated pitch), treatments are somewhat more process-based. Nonetheless, most treatment approaches remain largely focused on getting sufficient feedback and/or input to the speaker so that normal speech can be acquired or impaired speech modified. Because hearing loss occurring in childhood has a more profound effect on speech than does adventitious hearing loss (Goehl & Kaufman, 1984), most of the treatment approaches described in the literature have been developed for children. However, the speech training of children with hearing loss is often interwoven with language, sensory, and academic training, making it difficult to evaluate the effects of the speech training per se. Compounding the problem is that many of the older, more traditional approaches have been only vaguely described in the literature. What has been published for many of the approaches functions more as philosophies for treatment and not operationalized treatment guidelines or curricula. How they are implemented may vary widely across clinicians and settings. In addition, there are very few treatment efficacy data available for most of the approaches, making statements about their effectiveness limited. Clinicians are therefore encouraged to choose approaches that theoretically best fit a particular client and then collect the needed treatment efficacy data for that and other patients.

Auditory Stimulation Approaches

Auditory approaches have been used extensively and for many years, but they have surprisingly little documentation. Terms such as Acoupedic, Auditory-Global, Auditory-Oral, Aural-Oral, and Unisensory have been applied to these approaches with little differentiation between the terms. Davis and Hardick (1981, p 272) referred to these approaches generically as Auditory Stimulation Methods.

The Auditory Stimulation Approaches tend to be synthetic and are largely restricted to use with preschool children. The goal of these approaches is to train impaired listeners to glean as much from the auditory signal as possible with the rationale that speech is best learned via the auditory modality. The hallmark of these approaches is extensive auditory stimulation and training used in an effort to get early and consistent use of audition. Critical to the present day implementation of these approaches is that acoustic signals are optimized through amplification or other auditory prostheses. The reliance on other modalities is minimized because it is argued that they can interfere with audition and therefore interfere with the auditory system developing to its fullest potential. However, some auditory approaches, such as Northcott's (1977) *Curriculum Guide,* propose that natural communication should be promoted with young hearing-impaired children and natural facial cues and gestures should not be inhibited because they co-occur with oral communication. Common to all of the auditory approaches, speech is not treated directly, but its development is encouraged through auditory stimulation with connected speech produced in context. Naturally occurring strings with natural sounding prosody are promoted, although direct imitation of speech is encouraged and reinforced (Lowell & Pollack, 1974). Training of segmental aspects of speech does not occur in the early years. It is reserved for when the children reach school age. At that time, they continue to receive extensive auditory stimulation but are taught correct speech production with a multisensory approach (Lowell & Pollack, 1974). Other than anecdotal reports and case studies, there is little evidence that these approaches are effective or ineffective in promoting speech production.

Analytic Auditory-Oral Approaches

Ling (1976) and Boothroyd (1982) described in detail two very similar approaches, although Ling's approach is much more detailed and structured than Boothroyd's. In both approaches the auditory modality is the modality of choice for input and sensory feedback when training speech in children with hearing impairment. No attempts are made, however, to restrict the use of naturally occurring nonauditory cues. Auditory training is encouraged, but it is not a focus of treatment and it is acknowledged that many hearing-impaired children need supplemental cues such as visual and tactile cues to more easily acquire speech. These modalities are not targeted in therapy unless needed, and their artificial use is extinguished as quickly as possible. Ling is very specific about what speech sounds might need supplementary cues when training. He also is specific about how nonauditory cues may facilitate treatment and establish usable feedback. The Ling and Boothroyd approaches are initially analytic, output-based, and involve extensive use of imitation. They start by training basic skills such as respiration and voicing for speech, and developing skeletal vowel and consonant repertoires. The basic skills are trained simultaneously and interwoven, and once acquired are expanded in developmental and structural complexity with the syllable as the basic unit of training. The order of the segments taught and the syllabic complexity is clearly specified in both approaches.

A deviation from the analytic format is that both approaches encourage the use of newly acquired skills in meaningful, communicative contexts which Ling refers to as the Phonologic Level. The Phonologic Level is in contrast to the initial analytical training level which Ling refers to as the Phonetic Level. For all levels, Ling suggests that training occur in short intervals multiple times a day. Ling also provides suggestions for training various skills and includes lists of subskills that should be learned in order to get systematic approximation of target sounds.

Neither Ling nor Boothroyd has provided direct empirical evidence that their treatment approaches are efficacious. However, Perigoe and Ling (1986) compared two matched groups of hearing-impaired children relative to the role of grammatical category in generalization training from Phonetic to Phonologic Level productions. One group received speech training with content words (nouns and verbs), the other with function words (pronouns and prepositions). The children received 40 sessions of training over a course of 9 months, and their performance at both the Phonetic and Phonologic Levels was assessed four different times (1 pretreatment, 2 during treatment, and 1 at the end of treatment). Although there were no substantive differences between the groups, both groups showed gains but primarily on the final assessment. However, because of inadequate experimental control, and the duration over which treatment occurred, the question remains whether the gains were a product of the training or other factors such as maturation or concurrent educational/therapeutic activities.

In a study designed to assess generalization of voicing (+ and −) to cognates, McReynolds and Jetzke (1986) used an imitative syllabic training procedure similar to those suggested by Ling and Boothroyd. A single-subject, multiple-baseline across behaviors design was employed with counterbalancing and replication. Eight school-age children with severe or profound hearing losses served as subjects and were trained to produce either /t/ or /d/ and /k/ or /g/ in VC nonsense syllables. All eight of the children in the study improved from a baseline of 15% correct production or less to a criterion of 85% correct over two consecutive 20-item trials. Six of the eight children also exhibited significant generalization to the cognates of the sounds with which they were trained. More generalization occurred with voiced target-sound training than with voiceless target-sound training. These data suggest that imitative procedures are effective when correcting speech production in children with hearing impairment and that, like normal-hearing children, they exhibit generalization within phoneme classes.

Visual Methods

Visual methods are rarely used in isolation to treat the speech of persons with hearing loss. Visual methods are typically supplemental to other approaches or they are used as part of the general speech, language, and reading instruction. Visual methods include the use of speech reading, mirrors, cued speech, and graphic symbol systems to teach the proper production of individual speech sounds or prosodic elements. They also include the bulk of the computer-based feedback systems that will be discussed later in this chapter.

The primary goals of speechreading and cued speech are not proper sound production but improved speech reception for oral communication. However, they are frequently used in the initial training of sounds to indicate proper articulatory placements and movements (Jenson, 1971). The use of the hand cues provided in cued speech are particularly useful in providing location information for difficult-to-view articulations. The hand cues are relatively easy to learn and can be used in speech training even if a child does not use cued speech in his or her daily communications.

The graphic symbols employed in speech instruction vary from pictorial representations to phonetic symbols and diacritical marks. These graphic symbol systems are frequently integrated with reading instruction. The Alcorn symbols (Streng, 1955) are a rather simple set of graphic representations of vowels and diphthongs. They were developed for very young children and roughly reflect mouth configurations during vowel and diphthong productions. For example, the vowel /i/ is depicted by a long horizontal line to represent lip retraction, and the vowel /o/ is represented by two concentric circles, one circle for the labial opening and the other to represent lip rounding. The symbols can be used in isolation or they can be represented on a line drawn face in an

attempt to provide more meaning to children. Because they only represent vowels, it is at times useful to combine them with orthographic symbol systems to form words.

The English alphabet is a graphic symbol system commonly used in speech instruction; however, there is no direct correspondence between the English alphabet and the English sound system. As a result, a number of modifications of the alphabet have been employed in speech instruction such as the Northampton Charts, International Phonetic Alphabet, Initial Teaching Alphabet, and dictionary diacritics.

The Northampton Charts, or Yale Spellings, were developed at the Clark School for the Deaf in 1885 and revised in 1925 with much of the work attributable to Yale (1946). Its primary purpose in speech training is to provide a pronunciation guide and to assist with the association of speech to text when children are introduced to reading. It can act as a guide while a sound or spelling is being taught or used as a visual monitoring device (Davis & Hardick, 1981, p 268). The phonetic symbols employed in the Northampton Charts are based on the English alphabet in order to ease the transfer to standard English orthography. Each sound is associated with a letter or letter combination with most of the symbols corresponding to common English spellings. Secondary spellings and diacritics are added to disambiguate sounds that have multiple representations in English or when an English letter represents various sounds. Cues for word position constraints are provided as well. The phonetic symbols are arranged on two separate charts; consonants on one, and vowels and diphthongs on the other. The consonant chart is arranged in five columns (Fig. 15–1). The first column consists of voiceless sounds, the second includes voiced cognates of the sounds found in the first column, and the third column primarily consists of nasal sounds. The fourth and fifth columns include symbols for \l\, \ks\, \kwʰ\, and \r\. Consonants with similar place of articulation are also arranged in the same rows. The vowels in the vowel chart are arranged in a less straightforward

h- wh p t k 　c 　ck f $_1$ph $_1$th $_1$s 　c(e) 　c(i) 　cy sh ch 　tch	w- b d g v $_2$th z 　$_2$s zh 　$_3$s 　z j 　$_2$g- 　-ge 　-dge	m n 　kn ng 　n(k)	l y- x=ks	r- 　wr qu=kwh

Figure 15–1. The Northampton consonant chart. (Adapted from Berg, 1976; Davis & Hardick, 1981.)

	$_1$ oo	$_2$ oo	o-e	aw	-o-
			oa $_2$-o ow	au o(r)	
	(l)u-e (r)u-e (l)ew (r)ew				
	ee $_2$-e ea e-e	-i- -y	a-e ai ay	-e- $_2$ea	-a-
		a(r)	-u- -a -ar -er -ir -or -ur -re	ur er ir	
a-e ai ay	i-e igh -y	o-e oa -o ow	ou $_1$ow	oi oy	u-e

Figure 15–2. The Northampton vowel chart. (Adapted from Berg, 1976; Davis & Hardick, 1981.)

Table 15–3. Comparison of different phonetic symbol systems

Key words	IPA	ITA	Northampton	Dictionary
*h*at	h	h	h	h
*wh*en	hw	ɯh	wh	wh
*w*as	w	w	w	w
*p*ig	p	p	p	p
*b*ig	b	b	b	b
*m*om	m	m	m	m
*t*ail	t	t	t	t
*d*og	d	d	d	d
*n*o	n	n	n	n
*l*ine	l	l	l	l
*r*un	r	r	r	r
*f*ace, lau*gh*, *ph*one	f	f	f	f
*v*oice	v	v	v	v
*th*ink	θ	tʰ	th^1	th
*th*e	ð	ɟʰ	th^2	*th*
*s*un, *c*ent	s	s	s	s
*z*ebra, i*s*	z	z	z	z
*sh*ake, *s*ugar	ʃ	ʃʰ	sh	sh
a*z*ure, vi*s*ion	ʒ	ʒ	zh	zh
*ch*air, wa*tch*	tʃ	cʰ	ch	ch
*j*u*dg*e, ba*dg*e	ʤ	j	j	j
*y*ellow, on*i*on	j	y	y	y
si*ng*	ŋ	ŋ	ng	ng
m*e*	i	єє	ee	ē
h*i*t	ɪ	i	-i-	ĭ
b*ai*t, s*ay*, l*a*te	e	æ	a-e	ā
b*e*t	ɛ	e	-e-	ĕ
b*a*t	æ	a	-a-	ă
b*oo*t	u	ω	oo^1	o͞o
t*oo*k	ʊ	ω	oo^2	o͝o
b*o*ne, b*oa*t, t*ow*	o	œ	o-e	ō
s*aw*	ɔ	ɑu	aw	ŏ
*f*ather, *o*n	ɑ	ɑ	a(r)	ä
*u*nder, *a*bove	ʌ, ə	u	-u-	ə
h*er*, s*ir*, b*urr*	ɝ, ɚ	r	ur	ur
*tigh*t, m*y*	aɪ	ie	i-e	ī
c*ow*, m*ou*se	au	ɑu	ou	ou
b*oy*, *oi*l	ɔɪ	oi	oi	oi
you, c*u*te	ɪu	ɯe	u-e	ū

Note. IPA = International Phonetic Alphabet; ITA = Initial Teaching Alphabet; Northampton = symbols from the Northampton Charts; Dictionary = symbols from the American Heritage Dictionary.

manner but are roughly arranged according to place, liprounding, and diphthongization (Fig. 15–2).

The International Phonetic Alphabet (IPA) and the Initial Teaching Alphabet (ITA) (Pitman, 1967) have limited utility with young hearing impaired-children because they do not transfer easily to English text. These two very similar phonetic symbol systems require the learning of two different symbol systems if a child is simultaneously learning to read. These symbol systems, however, have use with older children and adults in situations in which therapy is restricted to a few sounds or features. In such cases a limited set of the IPA or ITA symbols and diacritics may be useful as a pronunciation guide or in providing feedback. Dictionary diacritics and symbols have the same limitations but may be more applicable to the school and reading environment. For comparison, a listing of the various phonetic symbols for the different systems is shown in Table 15–3.

Speakers with severe or profound hearing loss often have difficulty with the prosodics of speech, and graphic symbols are commonly used to facilitate the learning of appropriate production. As found in McGarr, Youdelman, and Head's (1992) curriculum for pitch remediation, variations of lines with arrows are frequently used to illustrate durational and frequency aspects of speech. For example, a rising line with an arrow is used to depict a rising pitch contour, a flat line is an uninflected contour, and a dotted line indicates an interrupted production. In addition, some systems code intensity by line width. These lines also can be imposed with text to match the prosodic cues with the intended speech sounds. There are several of these systems (although similar in structure), and readers should refer to Berg (1976) for a more complete review.

Multisensory Approaches

Multisensory Syllabic Unit Approach
Carhart (1947, 1963) advocated a multisensory procedure for teaching speech to children with hearing impairment. He suggested that the performance of the auditory system should be optimized via auditory training and appropriate amplification, particularly with children who have substantial residual hearing. He also suggested visual training in which children are taught to focus on the face first for gestural cues, then speech articulator cues. Vibrotactile and kinesthetic information also should be used to train the production of particular sounds as well as train children to monitor their own productions. Therefore, children are taught to monitor their speech not only by how it sounds but also how it feels. Silverman (1971) expanded Carhart's description of the multisensory approach by including the use of other visual and tactile systems such as orthography, graphic displays, cued speech, fingerspelling, visual displays of acoustic signals, and tactile aids.

The multisensory syllabic unit approach, often referred to as the traditional approach, is largely analytic. As the name would suggest, the basic unit of treatment is the syllable although speakers are given feedback about individual phonemes as well as prosody. Phonemes are taught in a predetermined sequence with most therapists beginning with bilabial consonants in conjunction with mid and back vowels (Davis & Hardick, 1981, p 272). A visual system is usually associated with the sounds taught and other sensory cues are emphasized during the instruction. All phonemes are first taught in isolation or CV and VC syllables. The training then proceeds to CVC, CCVC and finally CVCCC patterns. In addition, natural voice and prosody is promoted and children are encouraged to use newly acquired speech skills in context. Especially with children, Carhart (1947) suggested that the social act of speech, not the precise articulation of segments, be the emphasis of speech in context. However, prosody is treated in a very analytic fashion once the children have acquired a sizable phoneme repertoire.

Lexington School for the Deaf Approach
A multisensory approach used at the Lexington School for the Deaf and described by

371

Vorce (1971, 1974) is somewhat more eclectic. The basic philosophy is that speech training should be synthetic and stimulated in naturally occurring contexts whenever possible with emphasis on the whole unit rather than its parts. However, it is acknowledged that many hearing-impaired children, particularly school-age children, benefit from more analytic and structured instruction. Instruction starts with the most natural of environments and stimuli, regardless of age, and becomes more analytic and structured as needed. Magner (1979) suggested that the analytic component should be added when a child indicates an interest in oral expression. The analytic instruction is segmented according to voice/resonance, articulation, and prosody. Somewhat antithetical to the basic philosophy, however, is that artificial feedback and cueing systems are utilized even with infants.

Association Method

The Association Method is one of the most analytic of the multisensory approaches used with hearing-impaired children. It was developed by McGinnis (1963) at the Central Institute for the Deaf for children termed aphasic, but it has been used with children referred to as centrally deaf and children with peripheral hearing loss who appear to have difficulty in more traditional therapeutic and educational settings. These children have been described as having sequencing, memory, perceptual motor, and attention difficulties in addition to their sensory deficits (Davis & Hardick, 1981, p 264). The Association Method starts at the phoneme level where the children learn to produce individual sounds. These individual sounds are then combined into CV syllables and gradually built into words, phrases, and sentences. All the while the sounds are associated with one another and blended, as well as associated with auditory cues, lipreading, objects, pictures, reading, and writing. Speech is not the sole purpose of the treatment approach. It is a core component associated with other elements of the communicative process. Like many of the other older treatment approaches, there is very little evidence to document the effectiveness of the Association Method with hearing-impaired children.

Verbotonal Method

In contrast to the other multisensory approaches, the Verbotonal Method (developed by Petar Guberina in the 1950s) does not initially stress the use of the auditory system (Craig, Craig, & Burke, 1973). Amplification is introduced gradually and only after the child has associated various prosodic patterns of speech with large body movements. At this early stage, vibratory input rather than auditory input is used and is introduced by way of vibratory floor panels, vibratory benches and/or a personal vibrator placed on the wrist. The stress and rhythmic patterns of speech introduced via vibration are associated with body movements through structured play, role playing, stories, and verbal games. The patterns are ultimately associated with oral speech gestures. Spontaneous speech is encouraged but not demanded with the primary emphasis on natural sounding prosody. Suprasegmental and segmental aspects of speech are always introduced within the confines of whole body activities with the utterance being the unit of interest.

Auditory amplification is introduced when the children have developed an awareness of the vibratory patterns and the oral and gestural activities that accompany them. It is usually introduced under earphones with a group or desktop auditory trainer. These auditory trainers (Suvag I and Suvag II, respectively) house filters that are adjusted to match the frequency response of the child's region(s) of usable hearing. For example, a child with residual hearing restricted in the low frequencies is amplified using an extended low-frequency response. After the child has adjusted to amplification and the optimal frequency response has been determined, he or she is transitioned to a wearable device called the Mini Suvag or a hearing aid that can match the desired frequency response. Even after a child has been amplified, vibratory input is often retained.

Craig, Craig, and DiJohnson (1972) assessed the effectiveness of the Verbotonal Method in training early speech skills by comparing it to what they labeled as the Traditional Method although their implementation of the Traditional Method was not specified. Two groups of preschool-age children who were hearing-impaired served as subjects. The children were randomly assigned to the two different groups with the group compositions comparable relative to age, intelligence, hearing, lipreading skills, and social skills. One group was trained with the Verbotonal Method, the other with the Traditional Method. Using a pretest/posttest design, Craig et al found that both groups of children showed significant improvements in their speech intelligibility, loudness, and pitch. The groups did not differ as a whole, but the higher-functioning children in the Verbotonal group made substantially greater gains than those in the Traditional group. The lower-functioning children in both groups made similar gains.

Todoma Method
One final multisensory approach, the Todoma, or Vibration, Method, was originally developed for individuals who are deaf-blind. It's was formally developed in Norway in the 1890s by Hofguaard (Hansen, 1930) and introduced to the United States in the 1920s by Sophia Alcorn. She first used the approach with two deaf-blind children named Tad Chapman and Oma Simpson after whom she named the technique. Alcorn later developed guidelines for using the method with children who are sighted but hearing-impaired (Alcorn, 1932). The Todoma Method was used most widely from 1920 to 1960 and is presently used in roughly 10% of the educational institutions for deaf and deaf-blind children in the United States and Canada. In most settings it is used as a supplementary treatment tool and not a primary means of communication (Schultz, Norton, Conway-Fithian, & Reed, 1984). Reed et al (1985) estimated that there were only 15 to 20 individuals in the United States who use the Todoma method as their primary means of communication.

With the Todoma Method children are taught to receive speech, and ultimately produce it, by lightly placing their thumbs on a speaker's lips and then fanning their fingers across the speaker's face and neck with individual variations in hand and finger positioning allowed (Vivian, 1966). For example, a sighted hearing-impaired person my want to use a more lateral thumb position on the lips to reduce the interference to lipreading. From this basic hand position Todoma users learn, with extensive training, to extract information from changes in the breath stream, movements of the lips and jaw, and laryngeal vibration (Reed, Durlach, Braida, & Schultz, 1989). Training begins by drawing the children's attention to movements and vibrations in their environment (Vivian, 1966). Then the children work on imitation of movement; first through gross-motor activities then gradually by imitating movements specific to speech. For example, children are encouraged to explore the movement of their clinician's tongue during nonspeech and then speech activities. With refinement of the perception of vibration and movement, prosodic skills and breathing for speech are introduced. When the children are able to recognize a few initial sounds and whole words then active speech reception training starts with vowels, voiceless consonants, and then voiced consonants. As the individual sounds are introduced they are associated with braille or a visual symbol system such as the Alcorn or Northampton Charts (Vivian, 1966) The first introduction of each sound is in isolation or in a CV syllable, but after limited exposure the children are asked to attend to sounds in more complex and varied contexts. Speech reception training with the hands is first associated with visual lipreading in those children who are sighted and hearing-impaired. Later the visual lipreading is eliminated during training sessions. Speech production training is usually begun about 3 months after the speech reception training is initiated. It is first begun holistically at the simple sentence level

373

(three- to four-word commands), then segmental aspects of speech are introduced starting with vowels and then consonants.

In recent years Reed and his associates have studied the Todoma communication approach extensively as a first step in the development of a tactile speech communication aid. As a result, Reed et al (1992) found that speech reception through Tadoma is comparable to auditory reception of speech transmitted at a 0 to 6 dB speech-to-noise ratio. Reed, Durlach, Delhorne, Rabinowitz, and Grant (1985) assessed nine deaf-blind skilled users of Todoma and found that they could identify consonant segments with 52 to 69% accuracy; vowels with 25 to 56% accuracy. In open-set single words, performance ranged from 26 to 56% correct, while identification of key words from the CID Everyday Sentences varied from 0 to 85% correct when speaking rate was 2.5 syllables per second (approximately half the normal speaking rate). Seven of the 9 subjects performed in the 65 to 85% range on the CID Everyday Sentences. As expected, performance improved if supplementary cues were used. Although these data do indicate that people can learn to use the Tadoma method of communicating, the efficacy of using this method has not been documented.

Sensory Aids

Auditory Aids

As indicated previously, many speech training approaches are dependent on optimizing the use of residual hearing. Correspondingly, it is generally believed that speech is learned easiest if speakers can monitor their productions via their auditory systems. Therefore, the proper fit and use of hearing aids, as well as auditory training, could be argued as being important components of speech production training. In support of this argument is the relationship between the degree of prelingual hearing loss and the extent of delay found in children (Boothroyd, 1969; Levitt, 1987; Smith, 1975). So also is the relationship between the degree of hearing loss and the amount of speech impairment

found in older children and adults with prelingual hearing loss, although, surprisingly, most studies assessing the relationship of speech intelligibility to hearing make the comparisons with unaided puretone averages. Aided thresholds and the extent of amplification have not been taken into account. High-frequency hearing and hearing configuration across the frequency range largely has been ignored, although Levitt (1987) and Osberger, Maso, and Sam (1993) found that audiometric configuration had a substantive bearing on speech intelligibility. Despite the indications of a relationship, the empirical data directly relating speech production to the use of hearing aids, hearing aid fitting procedures, hearing aid configurations, or auditory training are limited at best. For example, Novelli-Olmstead and Ling (1984) found that children show more improvement when speech and auditory training are combined than when auditory training is used alone. However, the combined training was not compared to speech training in the absence of auditory training, so it is not known whether the auditory training augmented the speech training or if the effect was solely the result of the speech training. Yoshinaga-Itano, Apuzzo, Coulter, and Stredler-Brown (1995) found that infants who are identified by 3 months, fit early with auditory prostheses, and placed into intervention programs shortly after identification are more advanced in consonant and vowel production when tested at later months than are children identified even as early as 7 or 8 months. However, it is difficult to separate the effects of fitting the prostheses early from other aspects of early intervention. Higgins, Carney, and Schulte (1994) tested intelligible prelingually hearing-impaired adults with and without their hearing aids and observed a trend toward increased lip closure, voicing durations, intraoral pressure, and decreased nasal air flow when their subjects were unaided. Subtle changes in phonation also were noted. Although these were not significant differences, Higgins et al argued that the changes were a result of the subjects' increased tactile feedback used to compensate for the reduced auditory feedback.

Cochlear Implants

In contrast to hearing aids, there is a growing body of literature associating cochlear implants with improved speech production in adventitiously hearing-impaired persons and long-term speech improvement in children with profound hearing impairment. The assessment of speech changes of adventitiously hearing-impaired adults following the insertion of cochlear implants has largely been instrumental in nature because the subjects tend to be intelligible and their speech differences are more subtle in nature. The results also have stimulated discussion over the role of audition in speech motor-control.

With an onset of complete or near complete loss of hearing in adulthood, many speakers exhibit slightly decreased speaking rates relative to normal (Leder, Spitzer, Milner, et al, 1987). Adventitiously hearing-impaired speakers have been found to increase their sentence and pause durations as well as their word, syllable, and vowel durations (Kirk & Edgerton, 1983; Leder et al, 1986, 1987; Waldstein, 1990). Movement durations associated with articulatory gestures also have been observed as being prolonged. Changes in respiratory and vocal control have been noted as reflected in differences in airflow, reduced F0, jitter and vocal intensity, and increased fundamental frequency and breathiness (Lane, Perkell, Svirsky, & Webster, 1991; Leder, Spitzer, & Kirchner, 1987; Leder et al, 1987; Perkell, Lane, Svirsky, & Webster, 1992; Waldstein, 1990). Lane, Wozniak, Matthies, Svirsky, and Perkell (1995) observed that VOT tends to decrease for both voiced and voiceless stop consonants while Waldstein (1990) observed this only with voiceless stop consonants. Finally, the spectral peaks become less distinct and the formant spacing becomes somewhat more restricted (Lane et al, 1995; Waldstein, 1990). All of these changes, although subtle in most cases, are consistent with many of the speech differences common to prelingually hearing-impaired speakers. They also are

more pronounced if the hearing loss occurs in the later teens and early 20s. One difference from prelinguistically impaired speakers is that the suprasegmental aspects of speech that are linguistically bound, such as final pitch contour and contrastive stress, appear to be retained (Waldstein, 1990). In addition, recovery often is observed with implantation and can be reversed by turning off and on the implant (Perkell et al, 1992; Lane et al, 1995). Quite surprising, the degree of decline and recover is not related to the amount of time a person has been deafened prior to implantation; however, it may be related to the age of onset. All of these results imply that audition contributes to speech motor-control even after speech has matured although those aspects of speech strongly tied to linguistic meaning may be resistant to auditory deprivation. The results also indicate that the speech mechanism tends to recalibrate relatively quickly with the return of auditory feedback.

The data collected on children are quite different from those collected from adventitiously hearing-impaired adults. Osberger, Maso, and Sam (1993) observed that children with profound congenital hearing loss or hearing loss occurring in infancy tend to exhibit only limited improvement in speech intelligibility within the first 2 years after implantation and exhibit slight but notable increases after 2 years. Tobey, Angelette et al (1991) observed gains in intelligibility within the first year following implantation although the gains observed were relatively small; 18.1% preoperatively to 33.5% at 1 year postoperatively. During the first 2 years postfitting, children with cochlear implants do, however, increase the number of vocalizations that can be classified as speech sounds (Osberger et al, 1990), and they adopt a more auditory-oral communicative style rather than the visual-gestural style common to children with limited residual hearing (Tait & Lutman, 1994). They also exhibit modest increases in correct vowel production and the diversity of their consonant inventories (Tye-Murray & Kirk, 1993; Tobey, Pancamo, Staller, Brimacombe, & Beiter,

1991) with bilabials and nasals most frequent, and glides and liquids least frequent (Miyamoto et al, 1992). Very young implant users are more likely to show gains in anterior stop consonants while children 6 to 11 are more likely to show gains in velar stops (Tobey et al, 1991). Miyamoto et al (1992) found that by 1.5 years postimplantation, most of their young cochlear implant subjects could produce all manner of articulation whereas prior to implantation they were largely limited to bilabial and nasal sounds. They also found that children implanted with multichannel devices made greater gains in manner of articulation than did those with single-channel devices. Further, children with early onset of hearing loss performed better with an implant if they were implanted early. Osberger et al (1993) suggested that children implanted after 10 years of age were more disadvantaged than children implanted at a younger age, while Tye-Murray, Spencer, and Woodworth (1995) found 5 years to be the cutoff age. However, children implanted in their teens show pre/postimplantation changes in speech intelligibility and consonant production (Dawson et al, 1995). In addition, children who have intact speech skills prior to the onset of their hearing loss typically show substantial deterioration in intelligibility subsequent to their hearing loss but regain much it following implantation (Osberger et al, 1993).

A number of major weaknesses exist in the literature on the treatment effects of cochlear implants. The first is that adequate pretreatment baselines have not been established in most of the published studies. Most of the studies are based on one preimplantation data point which is insufficient to capture the extreme variability characteristics of hearing impaired subjects. Without a measure of the subjects' variability over time it is difficult to determine if the modest gains observed in the literature are true, regardless of their statistical significance. Many of the studies also have been treated as group designs but the inclusion of reasonable, if any, control groups and random assignment has been limited. This largely is due to the small number of subjects available and other clinical constraints of the population, but it nonetheless limits interpretability of the data collected. Further, the postimplantation data points have been obtained at extremely large intervals (eg, 6 months and greater), which precludes eliminating maturation and speech and language therapy as factors influencing the results. The further the measurements of treatment are from the onset of treatment and from one another the less able a researcher is to attribute change to the treatment, particularly with children. Thus, the results described above should be viewed with caution.

Cutaneous Aids

Cutaneous devises come in various forms (See Reed, Durlach, & Braida, 1982; Roeser, 1989). They all provide either vibratory or electrical stimulation to the skin but can vary in the number of channels and transducers used and how the signals are processed and displayed on the skin relative to level, frequency, and time. They can be as simple as a single-channel device driving a bone conduction vibrator that is strapped to the sternum, or as complex as a multichannel electocutaneous device with the electrodes arranged in a spectrogram-like display attached to the forearm or abdomen. The speech cues provided by these devices are limited by their development and by the sensory properties of the skin. There also is some agreement that optimal perception with cutaneous aids require longterm use and instruction (Brooks, Frost, Mason, & Gibson, 1986; Sherrick, 1986; Weisenberger & Percy, 1995). Studies with hearing adults indicate that single-channel tactile aids primarily provide waveform-envelope and prosody cues such as syllable number and stress patterns and they are superior to multichannel devices in transmitting these cues (Carney & Beachler, 1986). It has been suggested that multifrequency devices, by virtue of the complexity of their coding configuration, are better at transmitting segmental information such as voicing and manner cues, but in a training study with artificially deafened adults, Carney (1988) found no difference between a single-channel and a multichannel tactile aid. With both types of tactile aids voicing was perceived better than manner cues, and place cues were the most difficult to perceive. When testing a seven-channel vibrocutaneous aid, Weisenberger and Percy (1995) found that vowel context effects were present in the vibrotactile signal and that discrimination was notably easier if multiple rather than single segmental features differed between the stimuli. It also has been consistently observed that deaf children can perceive a wider array of speech cues with multichannel cochlear implants than with cutaneous aids, although the results are similar with single-channel cochlear implants. For example, Osberger, Carney, Robbins, Renshaw, and Miyamoto (1993) found that children with multichannel cochlear implants performed better than children with one- and two-channel vibrotactile devices on both segmental and suprasegmental discrimination. The three groups of children were most similar on syllable duration, consonant manner of articulation, and vowel height/place discrimination.

Cutaneous aids can be used as longterm wearable devices or as a supplementary tools for speech training. Wearable cutaneous aids for longterm use are most appropriate for individuals who are profoundly impaired and have minimal or no usable hearing. Hearing aids are not effective with these individuals, and many, although not all, of the candidates for cutaneous aids also are candidates for cochlear implants. At present, cutaneous aids are one of the few options for acoustic input to individuals with central deafness or central auditory neuropathy resulting in hearing loss. Nonetheless, as indicated previously, cutaneous aids are a major component of the Verbotonal Method and can be included in other multisensory training approaches as well. The use of cutaneous aids as supplementary tools in speech training sessions has some supporting docu-

mentation as does some modest speech improvement with continuous use of cutaneous aids.

McGarr, Youdelman, and Head (1989) found that using multichannel tactile aids during ongoing speech training was effective in remediating abnormal pitch in older hearing-impaired children. However, Youdelman, MacEachron, and Behrman (1988) found that training pitch control with visual feedback was superior to training in a similar fashion with a tactile aid, although they argued that the lack of improvement associated with the tactile aid reflected a ceiling effect. Geers and Tobey (1992) followed a group of deaf children longitudinally, some fit with cochlear implants and others with tactile aids. Although the cochlear implant children performed superiorly, the children fit with tactile aids made some gains in segmental production. Nonetheless, both groups failed to show substantive increases in intelligibility. Weisenberger (1989) reported on three adolescent boys who had experience wearing multichannel tactile aids during an experimental perceptual task and speech training. The boys produced better speech when they wore the tactile aids in conjunction with their hearing aids than when they wore their hearing aids alone. Eilers, Fishman, Oller, and Steffens (1993) followed two different groups of profoundly hearing-impaired children. One group wore tactile aids while the other wore hearing aids. Eilers et al (1993) obtained speech samples from the children prior to fitting the aids and 3 years later. They determined that the children fit with the tactile aids showed greater gains in their speech than did the children fit with hearing aids, especially in consonant production. However, the two groups of children were in different educational settings over the three period so other factors likely confounded the results. Although the few studies published on the effects of cutaneous stimulation on speech production suggest that cutaneous aids can provide benefit, they can be criticized for many of the same weakness found in the cochlear implant studies—that is, most of the studies were insufficiently controlled experimentally.

Computer-Based Visual Aids

As the quantity, complexity, and digital signal processing capabilities have increased in the last decade so have computer-based speech feedback systems. Correspondingly, their costs have decreased as their accessibility to clinicians has increased. In addition, most of the commercially available systems run on desktop computers, incorporate only a limited number of peripherals, and are multimodular, making them more appealing to clinicians who have limited resources and time, and varied caseloads. The different modules usually respond to various acoustic aspects of speech (eg, fundamental frequency, voicing, vowel production) although one system, the Kay Elemetrics Palatometer (Kay Elemetrics, 1993), uses lingual-palatal contact as well as acoustic input. The modules of most systems also vary according to the instructional nature of the feedback and the interest level of the speaker (Pratt & Hricisak, 1995). For example, some modules may display characteristics of the acoustic input but provide the speaker with little in the way of information about accuracy or correctness. Other modules may indicate if a target has been reached or they may inform the speaker of the goodness of fit between a production and a target. In addition, many of the systems include game-like activities to heighten and maintain the interest of young children. Most of these systems were not developed specifically for hearing-impaired speakers, but because they predominately use vision as the modality for feedback they have a great deal of face validity for use with the hearing-impaired population. None of the systems are wearable, and they are therefore useful primarily in the initial training or correction of productions. Eventually, the speaker must be able to make the target productions without feedback from the computer.

The early treatment applications of computer-based feedback systems with hearing-impaired speakers were mixed (Osberger, Moeller, Kroese, & Lippman, 1981). Most treatment studies were done on prototypes which restricts their application to current commercially available systems. In addition, most of the treatment studies used pretest/posttest designs without adequate controls. For example, Fletcher and Higgins (1980) did not use a control group when assessing the treatment efficacy of TONAR II for improving nasal resonance in children with a profound hearing loss. Fletcher and Hasegawa (1983) treated a young child who had a profound hearing loss with the simultaneous use of palatometry and glossometry. They concluded that the child's productions of the /i/, /ɑ/, and /t/ improved with treatment but they did not establish an adequate pretreatment baseline, and their design was insufficient to document that their system was the sole source of any progress made. More recently Ryalls, Michallet, and Le Dorze (1994) used a group design to compare vowel treatment using the Ling (1976) approach to treatment with the Vowel Accuracy Module of the IBM SpeechViewer (IBM, 1988). They treated two randomly assigned groups of profoundly hearing-impaired school-age children over a 7-week period. No substantive changes in performance were observed over the course of treatment for either group, but no pretreatment measures were obtained and the groups were too small (n = 4) to adequately test for differences between the groups. In contrast, Dagenais, Critz-Crosby, Fletcher, and McCutcheon (1994) recently compared Ling's approach to treating consonants with treatment via palatometry. They used a pretest/posttest group design. An adequate number of subjects were used with random assignment to the two treatment groups. Dagenais et al (1994) observed gains in both groups on target productions and intelligibility, and they concluded that palatometry was as effective as, possibly more so than, Ling's approach for the treatment of consonant production in school-age children with profound hearing loss. Other recent studies have also supported the effectiveness of computer-based feedback systems with this population. Using a single subject design, Pratt, Heintzelman, and Deming (1993) found that the Vowel Accuracy Module of the IBM SpeechViewer was effective in the treatment of vowels in young children with hearing impairment although their results were vowel and subject dependent. Rainier and Pratt (1994) also used a single subject design and found that the Loudness Awareness Module of the SpeechViewer with accelerometric input was effective in treating nasal resonance in a school-age child with a profound hearing loss. Therefore, the computer-based treatment research suggests that this type of feedback can be effectively used with hearing-impaired patients.

Conclusion

As indicated at the beginning of this chapter, the literature on the effects of hearing loss on speech development and production is vast. Much is known about the consequences of hearing loss on speech production when the hearing loss occurs early in life and is severe to profound in degree. However, the information on mild to moderately hearing-impaired persons is scant, particularly if the hearing loss occurs in childhood or is progressive in nature. Previously, there was limited information on the effects of adventitious hear loss on speech production, but with the introduction of cochlear implants this population has received concentrated investigation, and the results suggest a role for audition in speech regulation after the motor speech system has matured. The research has indicated that speech may not be fully mature in early adulthood, that language may influence the role of audition as a sensory feedback mechanism, that speech is affected relatively quickly by auditory deprivation and recovery is equally as quick, and that the duration of the deprivation is not as critical a factor as the age of onset.

In addition to our increased knowledge of the effects of hearing loss on speech production, a number of assessment tools, both perceptual and instrumental, have become available, although most lack adequate

standardization and norms. Further, there are many treatment approaches available but the efficacy data are limited because few studies have been conducted, and of those that have been, adequate experimental control largely has been inadequate. The few well-controlled treatment studies that have been published are promising, however. They tend to indicate that speech treatment is effective with the hearing-impaired population. Finally, the treatment area most notably lacking in efficacy research is the use of hearing aids to promote speech development and preservation. The lack of research in this area is glaring because wearable electroacoustic hearing aids have been available for over 50 years (Lybarger, 1988) and are a fundamental component for many of the direct speech treatment approaches. It is critical that more work be done in this area given the expansion of universal infant hearing screening programs. More infants with hearing loss will be identified shortly after birth, and to effectively treat them more needs to be known about the effects of hearing aids on speech and auditory development.

References

Alcorn S. (1932). The Todoma method. *Volta Rev* 34:195–198.

Angelocci A, Kopp G, Holbrook A. (1964). The vowel formants of deaf and normal-hearing eleven to fourteen year old boys. *J Speech Hear Dis* 29:156–170.

Arends N, Povel D, Van Os E, Speth L. (1990). Predicting voice quality of deaf speakers on the basis of glottal characteristics. *J Speech Hear Res* 33:116–122.

Baum S, Waldstein R. (1991). Perseveratory coarticulation in the speech of profoundly hearing-impaired and normally hearing children. *J Speech Hear Res* 34:1286–1292.

Berg F. (1976). *Educational Audiology: Hearing and Speech Management.* New York: Grune & Stratton.

Bess F, Lichtenstein M, Logan S, Burger M. (1989). Comparing criteria of hearing impairment in the elderly: A functional approach. *J Speech Hear Res* 32:795–802.

Boone D. (1977). *The Voice and Voice Therapy*, 2nd ed. Englewood Cliffs, NJ: Prentice-Hall.

Boothroyd A. (1969). Distribution of hearing levels in the student population of the Clarke School for the Deaf. Northampton, MA: Clarke School for the Deaf.

Boothroyd A. (1982). *Hearing Impairments in Young Children.* Englewood Cliffs, NJ: Prentice-Hall.

Brooks P, Frost B, Mason J, Gibson D. (1986). Continuing evaluation of the Queen's University tactile vocoder I: Identification of open-set words. *J Rehabil Res Dev* 23:119–128.

Brooks P, Frost B, Mason J, Gibson D. (1986). Continuing evaluation of the Queen's University tactile vocoder II: Identification of open-set sentences and tracking narrative. *J Rehabil Res Dev* 23:129–138.

Byrd D, Flemming E, Mueller C, Tan C. (1995). Using regions and indices in EPG data reduction. *J Speech Hear Res* 38:821–827.

Calvert D, Silverman R. (1975). Speech and Deafness. Washington, DC: Alexander Graham Bell Association for the Deaf.

Carhart R. (1947). Conservation of speech. In: Davis H, ed. *Hearing and Deafness, a Guide for Laymen.* New York: Murray Hill Books, pp 300–317.

Carhart R. (1963). Conservation of speech. In Davis H, Silverman SR, eds. *Hearing and Deafness,* Rev Ed. New York: Holt, Rinehart and Winston, pp 387–402.

Carney A. (1988). Vibrotactile perception of segmental features of speech: A comparison of single-channel and multichannel instruments. *J Speech Hear Res* 31:438–448.

Carney A, Beachler C. (1986). Vibrotactile perception of suprasegmental features of speech: A comparison of single-channel and multichannel instruments. *J Acoust Soc Am* 79:131–140.

Carney A, Osberger MJ, Carney E, Robbins A, Renshaw J, Miyamoto R. (1993). A comparison of speech discrimination with cochlear implants and tactile aids. *J Acoust Soc Am* 94:2036–2049.

Carr J. (1953). An investigation of the spontaneous speech sounds of five-year-old deaf-born children. *J Speech Hear Disord* 18:22–29.

Cowie R, Douglas-Cowie E, Kerr A. (1982). A study of speech deterioration in post-lingually deafened adults. *J Laryngol Otol* 96:101–112.

Craig W, Craig H, DiJohnson A. (1972). Preschool verbo-tonal instruction for deaf children. *Volta Rev* 74:236–246.

Craig W, Craig H, Burke R. (1974). Components of verbotonal instruction for deaf students. *Lang Speech Hear Serv Schools* 5:38–42.

Dagenais P, Critz-Crosby P. (1992). Comparing tongue positioning by normal hearing and hearing-impaired children during vowel production. *J Speech Hear Res* 35:5–44.

Dagenais P, Critz-Crosby P, Fletcher S, McCutcheon M. (1994). Comparing abilities of children with profound hearing impairments to learn consonants using electropalatography or traditional aural-oral techniques. *J Speech Hear Res* 37:687–699.

Dalston R. (1989). Using simultaneous photodetection and nasometry to monitor velopharyngeal behavior during speech. *J Speech Hear Res* 32:195–202.

Dalston R, Seaver E. (1990). Nasometric and phototransductive measurements of reaction times among normal adult speakers. *Cleft Palate J* 27:61–67.

Davis J, Hardick E. (1981). *Rehabilitative Audiology for Children and Adults.* New York: John Wiley & Sons.

Davis H, Silverman S. (1978). *Hearing and Deafness.* New York: Holt, Rinehart & Winston.

Dawson P, Blamey P, Dettman S, et al. (1995). A clinical report on speech production of cochlear implant users. *Ear Hear* 16:551–561.

Denes P. (1955). Effect of duration on the perception of voicing. *J Am Acoust Soc* 27:761–764.

Dunn C, Newton L. (1986). A comprehensive model for speech development in hearing-impaired children. *Topics Lang Disord* 6(3):25–46.

Eilers R, Fishman L, Oller K, Steffens M. (1993). Tactile vocoders as aids to speech production in young hearing-impaired children. *Volta Rev* 95:265–293.

Elfenbein J, Hardin-Jones M, Davis J. (1994). Oral communication skills of children who are hard of hearing. *J Speech Hear Res* 37:216–226.

Fairbanks G. (1960). *Voice and Articulation Drill Book,* 2nd ed. New York: Harper & Row.

Feinmesser M, Tell L, Levi H. (1982). Follow-up of 40,000 infants screened for hearing defect. *Audiology* 21:197–203.

Fletcher S, Hasegawa A. (1983). Speech modification by a deaf child through dynamic orometric modeling and feedback. *J Speech Hear Disord* 48:179–185.

Fletcher S, Higgins J. (1980). Performance of children with severe to profound auditory impairment in instrumentally guided reduction of nasal resonance. *J Speech Hear Disord* 45:181–194.

Formby C, Monsen R. (1982). Long-term average speech spectra for normal and hearing-impaired adolescents. *J Acoust Soc Am* 71:196–202.

Forner L, Hixon T. (1977). Respiratory kinematics in profoundly hearing-impaired speakers. *J Speech Hear Res* 66:373–408.

Fowler C. (1986) An event approach to the study of speech perception from a direct-realist perspective. *J Phonet* 14:3–28.

Fria T, Cantekin E, Eichler J. (1985). Hearing acuity of children with otitis media with effusion. *Arch Otolaryngol* 111:10–16.

Geers A, Tobey E. (1992). Effects of cochlear implants and tactile aids on the development of speech production skills in children with profound hearing impairment. *Volta Rev* 94:135–163.

Gilbert H. (1974). Simultaneous oral and nasal airflow during stop consonant production by hearing-impaired speakers. *Folia Phoniatr* 27:423–437.

Goehl H, Kaufman D. (1984). Do the effects of adventitious deafness include disordered speech? *J Speech Hear Disord* 49:58–64.

Gold T. (1980). Speech production in hearing-impaired children. *J Commun Disord* 13:397–418.

Gorlin R, Toriello H, Cohen MM. (1995). *Hereditary Hearing Loss and Its Syndromes.* Oxford Monographs on Medical Genetics, No. 28. New York: Oxford University Press.

Hansen A. (1930). The first case in the world: Miss Petra Heiberg's report. *Volta Rev* 32:223.

Hardy J. (1961). Intraoral breath pressure in cerebral palsy. *J Speech Hear Disord* 126:310–319.

Heider F, Heider G, Sykes J. (1941). A study of the spontaneous vocalizations of fourteen deaf children. *Volta Rev* 43:10–14.

Higgins M, Carney A, Schulte L. (1994). Physiological assessment of speech and voice production of adults with hearing loss. *J Speech Hear Res* 37:510–521.

Hood R, Dixon R. (1969). Physical characteristics of speech rhythm of deaf and normal-hearing speakers. *J Commun Disord* 2:20–28.

Horii Y. (1982). Some voice fundamental frequency characteristics of oral reading and spontaneous speech by hard-of-hearing young women. *J Speech Hear Res* 25:608–610.

Hudgins C, Numbers F. (1942). An investigation of the intelligibility of speech of the deaf. *Genet Psychol Monogr* 25:289–392.

Hutchinson J, Smith L. (1976). Aerodynamic functioning in consonant production by hearing-impaired adults. *Audiol Hear Ed* 2:16–19, 22–25, 34.

IBM. (1988). IBM Personal System/2 Independence Series. SpeechViewer Application Software User's Guide. Boca Raton, FL: Author.

Itoh M, Horii Y, Daniloff R, Binnie C. (1982). Selected aerodynamic characteristics of deaf individuals' various speech and nonspeech tasks. *Folia Phoniatr* 34:191–209.

Jenson P. (1971). The relationship of speechreading and speech. In: Connor LE, ed. *Speech for the Deaf Child: Knowledge and Use.* Washington, DC: A.G. Bell Association for the Deaf, pp 265–279.

John J, Howarth J. (1976). The effect of time distortions on the intelligibility of deaf children's speech. *Lang Speech* 8:127–134.

Karnell M, Seaver E, Dalston R. (1988). A comparison of photodetector and endoscopic evaluations of velopharyngeal functions. *J Speech Hear Res* 31:503–510.

Kay Elemetrics. (1992). Nasometer model 6200-2 instruction manual. Pine Brook, NJ: Author.

Kay Elemetrics. (1993). Palatometer model 6300 instruction manual. Pine Brook, NJ: Author.

Kent R, Read C. (1992). *The Acoustic Analysis of Speech.* San Diego, CA: Singular Publishing Group.

Kirk K, Edgerton B. (1983). The effects of cochlear implant use on voice parameters. *Otolaryngol Clin North Am* 16:281–292.

Konigsmark B, Gorlin R. (1976). *Genetic and Metabolic Deafness.* Philadelphia: W.B. Saunders Co.

Lach R, Ling D, Ling L, Ship N. (1970). Early speech development in deaf infants. *Am Ann Deaf* 115:522–526.

Lane H, Perkell J, Svirsky M, Webster J. (1991). Changes in speech breathing following cochlear implant in postlingually deafened adults. *J Speech Hear Res* 34:526–533.

Lane H, Webster JW. (1991). Speech deterioration in postlingually deafened adults. *J Acoust Soc Am* 89:859–866.

Lane H, Wozniak J, Matthies M, Svirsky M, Perkell J. (1995). Phonemic resetting versus postural adjustments in the speech of cochlear implant users: An exploration of voice-onset-time. *J Acoust Soc Am* 98:3096–3106.

LaPlante M. (1988). Data on disability from the National Health Interview Survey, 1983-85. An Info Use Report. Washington, DC: National Institute on Disability and Rehabilitation Research.

Leder S, Spitzer J, Kirchner JC, Flevaris-Phillips C, Milner P, Richardson F. (1987). Speaking rate of adventitiously deaf male cochlear implant candidates. *J Acoust Soc Am* 82:843–846.

Leder S, Spitzer J, Milner P, Flevaris-Phillips C, Richardson F, Kirchner J. (1986). Reacquisition of contrastive stress in an adventitiously deaf speaker using a single-channel cochlear implant. *J Acoust Soc Am* 79:1967–1974.

Leder S, Spitzer J, Kirchner J. (1987). Speaking fundamental frequency of postlingually profoundly deaf adult men. *Ann Otol Rhinol Laryngol* 96:322–324.

Leder S, Spitzer J, Milner P, Flevaris-Phillips C, Kirchner J, Richardson F. (1987). Voice intensity of prospective cochlear implant candidates and normal-hearing adult males. *Laryngoscope* 97:224–227.

Levitt H. (1987). Interrelationships among the speech and language measures. In: Levitt H, McGarr N, Geffner D, eds. *Development of Language and Communication Skills of Hearing-Impaired Children. ASHA Monogr* 26:123–139.

Levitt H, Youdelman K, Head J. (1990). *Fundamental Speech Skills Test.* Englewood, CO: Resource Point, Inc.

Levitt H, Smith C, Stromberg H. (1976) Acoustical, articulatory and perceptual characteristics of the speech of deaf children. In: Fant G, ed. *Proceedings of the Speech Communication Seminar.* New York: Wiley, pp 129–139.

Levitt H, Stromberg H. (1983). Segmental characteristics of the speech of hearing-impaired children: factors affecting intelligibility. In: Hochberg I, Levitt H, Osberger MJ, eds. *Speech of the Hearing Impaired: Research, Training and Personnel Preparation.* Baltimore: University Park Press, pp 53–73.

Ling D. (1976). *Speech and the Hearing-Impaired Child: Theory and Practice.* Washington, DC: A.G. Bell Association for the Deaf.

Lippmann R. (1981). Detecting nasalization using a low-cost miniature accelerometer. *J Speech Hear Res* 24:314–317.

Lowell E, Pollack D. (1974). Remedial practices with the hearing impaired. In: Dickson S, ed. *Disorders Remedial Principles and Practices.* Glenview, IL: Scott, Foresman and Company, pp 440–497.

Lybarger S. (1988). A historical overview. In: Sandlin R, ed. *Handbook of Hearing Aid Amplification,* Vol I. Boston: College-Hill Press, pp 1–30.

Lynch M, Oller K, Steffens M. (1989). Development of speech-like vocalizations in a child with congenital absence of cochleas: The case of total deafness. *Appl Psycholinguist* 10:315–333.

Maassen B. (1986). Marking word boundaries to improve the intelligibility of the speech of the deaf. *J Speech Hear Res* 29:227–230.

Magner M. (1971). Techniques of teaching. In: Connor LE, ed. *Speech for the Deaf Child: Knowledge and Use.* Washington, DC: A.G. Bell Association for the Deaf, pp 245–264.

Markides A. (1970). The speech of deaf and partially hearing children with special reference to factors affecting intelligibility. *Br J Disord Commun* 5:126–140.

Martin J, Bentzen O, Colley J, et al. (1981). Childhood deafness in the European community. *Scand Audiol* 10:165–174.

Martin D, Fitch J, Wolfe V. (1995). Pathologic voice type and the acoustic prediction of severity. *J Speech Hear Res* 38:765–771.

McCaffrey H, Sussman H. (1994). An investigation of vowel organization in speakers with severe and profound hearing loss. *J Speech Hear Res* 37:938–951.

McGarr N. (1983). The intelligibility of deaf speech to experienced and inexperienced listeners. *J Speech Hear Res* 26:451–458.

McGarr N. (1987). Communication skills of hearing-impaired children in schools for the deaf. In: Levitt H, McGarr N, Geffner D, eds. Development of Language & Communication in Hearing Impaired Children. *ASHA Monogr* 26:91–107.

McGarr N, Löfqvist A. (1982). Obstruent production in hearing-impaired speakers: Interarticulator timing and acoustics. *J Acoust Soc Am* 72:34–42.

McGarr N, Youdelman K, Head J. (1989). Remediation of phonation problems in hearing-impaired children: Speech training and sensory aids. *Volta Rev* 91:7–18.

McGarr N, Youdelman K, Head J. (1992). *Guidebook of Voice Pitch Remediation in Hearing-Impaired Speakers.* Englewood, CO: Resource Point, Inc.

McGinnis M. (1963). Aphasic Children: *Identification and Education by the Association Method.* Washington, DC: A.G. Bell Association for the Deaf.

McNeil M, Liss J, Tseng C, Kent R. (1990). Effects of speech rate on the absolute and relative timing of apraxic and conduction aphasic sentence production. *Brain Lang* 38:135–158.

McReynolds L, Jetzke E. (1986). Articulation generalization of voiced-voiceless sounds in hearing-impaired children. *J Speech Hear Disord* 51:348–355.

Metz D, Whitehead R, Whitehead B. (1984). Mechanics of vocal fold vibration and laryngeal articulatory gestures produced by hearing-impaired speakers. *J Speech Hear Res* 27:6269.

Millin J. (1971). Therapy for reduction of continuous phonation in the hard-of-hearing population. *J Speech Hear Disord* 36:496–498.

Miyamoto R, Osberger MJ, Robbins A, Myres W, Kessler K, Pope M. (1992). Longitudinal evaluation of communication skills of children with single or multichannel channel cochlear implants. *Am J Otol* 13:215–222.

Monsen R. (1974). Durational aspects of vowel production in the speech of deaf children. *J Speech Hear Res* 17:386–398.

Monsen R. (1976a). Normal and reduced-phonological space: The production of English vowels by deaf adolescents. *J Phonet* 4:189–198.

Monsen R. (1976b). The production of English stop consonants in the speech of deaf children. *J Phonet* 4:29–42.

Monsen R. (1976c). Second formant transitions of selected consonant-vowel combinations in the speech of deaf and normal-hearing children. *J Speech Hear Res* 19:279–290.

Monsen R. (1978). Toward measuring how well hearing-impaired children speak. *J Speech Hear Res* 21:197–219.

Monsen R. (1979). Acoustic qualities of phonation in young hearing-impaired children. *J Speech Hear Res* 22:270–288.

Monsen R. (1981). A usable test for the speech intelligibility of deaf talkers. *Am Ann Deaf* 126:845–852.

Monsen R. (1983). The oral intelligibility of hearing-impaired talkers. *J Speech Hear Disord* 48:286–296.

Monsen R, Engebretson A. (1983). The accuracy of formant frequency measurements: A comparison of spectrographic analysis and linear prediction. *J Speech Hear Res* 26:89–97.

Monsen R, Moog J, Geers A. (1988). *CID Picture SPINE.* St. Louis, MO: Central Institute for the Deaf.

Moog J. (1981). *CID Phonetic Inventory.* St. Louis, MO: Central Institute for the Deaf.

Moscicki E, Elkins E, Baum H, McNamara P. (1985). Hearing loss in the elderly: An epidemiologic study of the Framingham Heart Study Cohort. *Ear Hear* 6:184–190.

Most T, Frank Y. (1991). The relationship between the perception and the production of intonation by hearing-impaired children. *Volta Rev* 12:301–309.

Murphy A, McGarr N, Bell-Bert F. (1990). Acoustic analysis of stress contrasts produced by hearing-impaired children. *Volta Rev* 92:80–91.

National Center for Health Statistics, Ries PW. (1982). Hearing ability of persons by sociodemographic and health characteristics: United States. Vital and health statistics (Series 10, N. 140, DHHS Publications No. PHS 82-1568. Public Health Service). Washington, DC: U.S. Government Printing Office.

Nober E. (1967). Articulation of the deaf. *Except Child* 33:611–621.

Northcott W. (1977). *Curriculum Guide, Hearing-Impaired Children (0–3) and Their Parents.* Washington, DC: A.G. Bell Association for the Deaf.

Novelli-Olmstead T, Ling D. (1984). Speech production and speech discrimination by hearing-impaired children. *Volta Rev* 76:72–80.

Ohman S. (1966). Coarticulation in VCV utterances: Spectrographic measurements. *J Acoust Soc Am* 39:151–198.

Oller K, Eilers R. (1988). The role of audition in infant babbling. *Child Dev* 59:441–449.

Oller D, Eilers R, Bull D, Carney A. (1985). Prespeech vocalizations of a deaf infant: a comparison with normal metaphonological development. *J Speech Hear Res* 28:47–63.

Oller D, Kelly C. (1974). Phonological substitution processes of a hard-of-hearing child. *J Speech Hear Disord* 39:65–74.

Osberger MJ. (1981). Fundamental frequency characteristics of the speech of the hearing impaired. *J Acoust Soc Am* 69:S69(A).

Osberger MJ, McGarr N. (1982). Speech production characteristics of the hearing impaired. *Speech Lang* 8:221–283.

Osberger MJ, Maso M, Sam L. (1993). Speech intelligibility of children with cochlear implants, tactile aids, or hearing aids. *J Speech Hear Res* 36:186–203.

Osberger MJ, Miyamoto R, Robbins AM, et al. (1990). Performance of deaf children with cochlear implants and vibrotactile aids. *J Am Acad Audiol* 1:7–10.

Osberger MJ, Moeller M, Kroese J, Lippmann R. (1981). Computer-assisted speech training for the hearing impaired. *J Acad Rehabil Audiol* 14:145–158.

Osberger MJ, Levitt H. (1979). The effect of timing errors on the intelligibility of deaf children's speech. *J Acoust Soc Am* 66:1316–1324.

Osberger MJ, Levitt H, Slosberg R. (1979). Acoustic characteristics of correctly produced vowels. *J Acoust Soc Am* 66:S13(A).

Osberger MJ, Robbins AM, Lybolt J, Kent R, Peters J. (1986). Speech evaluation. In: Osberger MJ, ed. *Language and Learning Skills of Hearing-Impaired Students. ASHA Monogr* 23:24–31.

Parkhurst B, Levitt H. (1978). The effect of selected prosodic errors o the intelligibility of deaf speech. *J Commun Disord* 11:249–256.

Parving A. (1985). Hearing disorders in childhood; some procedures for detection, identification and diagnostic evaluation. *Int J Paediatr Otorhinolaryngol* 9:31–57.

Penn J. (1955). Voice and speech patterns of the hard-of-hearing. *Acta Otolaryngol* (suppl 124).

Perkell J, Lane H, Svirsky M, Webster J. (1992). Speech of cochlear implant patients: A longitudinal study of vowel production. *J Acoust Soc Am* 91:2961–2978.

Perigoe C, Ling D. (1986). Generalization of speech skills in hearing-impaired children. *Volta Rev* 88:351–366.

Pittman J. (1967). Can I.T.A. help the deaf child, his parents and his teacher? Washington, DC: A.G. Bell Association for the Deaf, pp 514–542.

Pratt S, Heintzelman A, Deming S. (1993). The efficacy of using the IBM SpeechViewer Vowel Accuracy Module to treat young children with hearing impairment. *J Speech Hear Res* 36:1063–1074.

Pratt S, Hricisak I. (1994). Commercially available computer-based speech feedback systems. *J Acad Rehabil Audiol* 27:89–106.

Prosek R, Montgomery A, Walden B. (1988). Constancy of relative timing for stutterers and nonstutterers. *J Speech Hear Res* 31:654–658.

Rainier S, Pratt S. (1994). Treating hypernasality: Nasal accelerometry and the SpeechViewer

Loudness Awareness Module. Paper presented at the 1994 annual convention of the American Speech-Language-Hearing Association, New Orleans, LA.

Raphael L. (1972). Preceding vowel duration as a cue to the perception of the voicing characteristic of word-final consonants in American English. *J Acoust Soc Am* 51:1296–1303.

Reed C, Durlach N, Braida L, eds. (1982). Research on tactile communication of speech: A review. *ASHA Monogr* 20:1–23.

Reed C, Rabinowitz W, Durlach N, et al. (1985). Research on the Todoma method of speech communication. *J Acoust Soc Am* 77:247–257.

Reed C, Rabinowitz W, Durlach N, et al. (1992). Analytic study of the Tadoma method: Improving performance through the use of supplementary tactual displays. *J Speech Hear Res* 35:450–465.

Robb M, Pang-Ching G. (1992). Relative timing characteristics of hearing-impaired speakers. *J Acoust Soc Am* 91:2954–2960.

Robbins J, Klee T. (1987). Clinical assessment of oropharyngeal motor development in young children. *J Speech Hear Disord* 52:271–277.

Roeser R. (1989). Tactile aids: Developmental issues and current status. In: Owens E, Kessler D, eds. *Cochlear Implants in Young Deaf Children.* Boston: College-Hill Press, pp 101–136.

Rothman H. (1976). A spectrographic investigation of consonant-vowel transitions in the speech of deaf adults. *J Phonet* 4:129–136.

Rubin-Spitz J, McGarr N. (1990). Perception of terminal fall contours in speech produced by deaf persons. *J Speech Hear Res* 33:174–180.

Ryalls J, Michallet B, Le Dorze G. (1994). A preliminary evaluation of the clinical effectiveness of vowel training for hearing-impaired children on IBM's SpeechViewer. *Volta Rev* 96:19–30.

Samar V, Metz D. (1988). Criterion validity of speech intelligibility rating-scale procedures for the hearing-impaired population. *J Speech Hear Res* 31:307–316.

Sapir S, Canter G. (1991). Postlingual deaf speech and the role of audition in speech production: Comments on Waldstein's paper (1990). *J Acoust Soc Am* 90:1672.

Schappert SM. (1992). Office visits for otitis media: United States, 1975–90. Advance Data from Vital and Health Statistics of the Centers for Disease Control/National Center for

Health Statistics. U.S. Department of Health Services, No. 214.

Schein J, Delk M. (1974). *The Deaf Population of the United States.* Silver Spring, MD: National Association of the Deaf.

Schultz M, Norton S, Conway-Fithian S, Reed C. (1984). A survey of the use of the Todoma method in the United States and Canada. *Volta Rev* 86:282–92.

Seaver E, Dalston R, Leeper H, Adams L. (1991). A study of nasometric values for normal nasal resonance. *J Speech Hear Res* 34:715–721.

Shaw S, Coggins T. (1991). Interobserver reliability using the phonetic level evaluation with severely and profoundly hearing-impaired children. *J Speech Hear Res* 34:989–999.

Sherrick C. (1984). Basic and applied research on tactile aids for deaf people: Progress and prospectus. *J Acoust Soc Am* 75:1325–1342.

Silverman S. (1971). The education of deaf children. In: Travis LE, ed. *Handbook of Speech and Language Pathology.* Englewood Cliffs, NJ: Prentice-Hall, pp 399–430.

Silverman S, Hirsh I. (1955). Problems related to the use of speech in clinical audiometry. *Ann Otol Rhinol Laryngol* 64:1234–1244.

Sitler R, Schiavetti N, Metz D. (1983). Contextual effects in the measurement of hearing-impaired speakers' intelligibility. *J Speech Hear Res* 26:30–34.

Smith C. (1975). Residual hearing and speech production in the deaf. *J Speech Hear Res* 19:795–811.

Smitheran J, Hixon T. (1981). A clinical method for estimating laryngeal airway resistance during vowel production. *J Speech Hear Disord* 46:138–146.

Stein D. (1980). A study of articulatory characteristics of deaf talkers. *Dissert Abstr Int* 41:1327B.

Stevens K, Nickerson R, Rollins A. (1978). On describing the suprasegmental properties of the speech of deaf children. In: McPherson D, Davids M, eds. *Advances in Prosthetic Devices for the Deaf: A Technical Workshop.* Rochester, NY: National Technical Institute for the Deaf, pp 134–155.

Stevens K, Nickerson R, Rollins A, Boothroyd A. (1974). Assessment of nasalization in the speech of deaf children. *J Speech Hear Res* 19:393–416.

St. Louis K, Ruscello D. (1987). *Oral Speech Mechanism Screening Examination,* Revised. Austin, TX: Pro-Ed, Inc.

Stoel-Gammon C. (1988). Prelinguistic vocalizations of hearing-impaired & normally hearing subjects: A comparison of consonantal inventories. *J Speech Hear Disord* 53:302–315.

Stoel-Gammon C, Otomo K. (1986). Babbling development of hearing-impaired and normally hearing subjects. *J Speech Hear Disord* 5:33–41.

Streng A. (1955). *Hearing Therapy for Children.* New York: Grune and Stratton.

Subtelny J. (1977). Assessment of speech with implications for training. In: Bess F, ed. *Childhood Deafness.* New York: Grune & Stratton, pp 183–194.

Subtelny J, Orlando N, Whitehead R. (1981). *Speech and Voice Characteristics of the Deaf.* Washington, DC: A.G. Bell Association for the Deaf.

Subtelny J, Li W, Whitehead R, Subtelny JD. (1989). Cephalometric and cineradiographic study of deviant resonance in hearing-impaired speakers. *J Speech Hear Disord* 54:249–263.

Subtelny J, Whitehead R, Samar V. (1992). Spectral study of deviant resonance in the speech of women who are deaf. *J Speech Hear Res* 35:574–579.

Sussman H, Hernandez M. (1979). A spectrographic analysis of the suprasegmental aspects of the speech of hearing-impaired adolescents. *Audiol Hear Educ* 5:12–16.

Tait M, Lutman M. (1994). Comparison of early communicative behavior in young children with cochlear implants and with hearing aids. *Ear Hear* 15:352–361.

Teele D, Klein J, Rosner B. (1989). Epidemiology of otitis media during the first seven years of life in children in greater Boston. *J Infect Dis* 160:83–94.

Tobey E, Pancamo S, Staller S, Brimacombe J, Beiter A. (1991). Consonant production children receiving a multichannel cochlear implant. *Ear Hear* 12:23–31.

Tobey E, Angelette S, Murchison C, et al. (1991). Speech production in children receiving a multichannel cochlear implant. *Am J Otol* 12(suppl):164–172.

Tye N, Zimmerman G, Kelso J. (1983). "Compensatory articulation" in hearing impaired speakers: A cinefluorographic study. *J Phonet* 11:101–115.

Tye-Murray N. (1984). Articulatory behavior of deaf and hearing speakers over changes in rate and stress: A cinefluorographic study. *Dissert Abstr Int* 45:2128B.

Tye-Murray N. (1987). Effects of vowel context on the articulatory closure postures of deaf speakers. *J Speech Hear Res* 30:90–104.

Tye-Murray N. (1990). Jaw and lip movements of deaf talkers producing utterances with known stress patterns. *J Acoust Soc Am* 87:2675–2683.

Tye-Murray N. (1991). The establishment of open articulatory postures by deaf and hearing talkers. *J Speech Hear Res* 34:453–459.

Tye-Murray N. (1992). Articulatory organizational strategies and the role of audition. *Volta Rev* 94:243–260.

Tye-Murray N, Folkins J. (1990). Jaw and lip movements of deaf talkers producing utterances with known stress patterns. *J Acoust Soc Am* 87:2675–2683.

Tye-Murray N, Kirk K. (1993). Vowel and diphthong production by young cochlear implant users and the relationship between the phonetic level evaluation and spontaneous speech. *J Speech Hear Res* 36:488–502.

Tye-Murray N, Spencer L, Bedia E. (In press). Speaking with the cochlear implant turned on and turned off and allophonic variations. *J Speech Hear Res*.

Tye-Murray N, Spencer L, Woodworth G. (1995). Acquisition of speech by children who have prolonged cochlear implant experience. *J Speech Hear Res* 38:327–337.

Tye-Murray N, Woodworth G. (1989). The influence of final-syllable position on the vowel and word duration of deaf talkers. *J Acoust Soc Am* 75:629–632.

Tye-Murray N, Zimmerman G, Folkin J. (1987). Movement timing in deaf and hearing speakers: Comparison of phonetically heterogeneous syllable strings. *J Speech Hear Res* 30:411–417.

U.S. Public Health Service. (1990). *Healthy People 2000*. Washington, DC: U.S. Government Printing Office.

Vivian R. (1966). The Todoma method: A tactual approach to speech and speech reading. *Volta Rev* 68:733–737.

Voelker C. (1938). An experimental study of the comparative rate of utterance of deaf and normal-hearing speakers. *Am Ann Deaf* 83:274–284.

Vorce E. (1971). Speech curriculum. In: Connor LE, ed. *Speech for the Deaf Child*. Washington,

DC: A.G. Bell Association for the Deaf, pp 221–224.

Vorce E. (1974). *Teaching Speech to Deaf Children*. Washington, DC: AG Bell Association for the Deaf.

West J, Weber J. (1973). A phonological analysis of the spontaneous language of a four-year-old hard-of-hearing child. *J Speech Hear Disord* 38:25–35.

Waldstein R. (1990). Effects of postlingual deafness on speech production: Implications for the role of auditory feedback. *J Acoust Soc Am* 88:2099–2114.

Waldstein R, Baum S. (1991). Anticipatory coarticulation in the speech of profoundly hearing-impaired and normally hearing children. *J Speech Hear Res* 34:1276–1285.

Weisenberger J. (1989). Tactile aids for speech perception and production by hearing-impaired people. *Volta Rev* 91:79–100.

Weisenberger J, Percy M. (1995). The transmission of phoneme-level information by multi-channel tactile speech perception aids. *Ear Hear* 16:392–405.

Weismer G, Fennell A. (1985). Constancy of (acoustic) relative timing measures in phrase-level utterances. *J Acoust Soc Am* 78:49–57.

Weiss A, Carney A, Leonard L. (1985). Perceived contrastive stress production in hearing-impaired and normal hearing children. *J Speech Hear Res* 28:26–35.

White K, Vohr B, Behrens T. (1993). Factors affecting the interpretation of transient evoked otoacoustic emission results in neonatal hearing screening. *Semin Hear* 14:57–72.

Whitehead R. (1982). Some respiratory and aerodynamic patterns in the speech of the hearing impaired. In: Hochberg I, Levitt H, Osberger MJ, eds. *Speech of the Hearing Impaired: Research, Training, and Personnel Preparation*. Baltimore: University Park Press.

Whitehead R. (1991). Stop consonant closure durations for normal-hearing and hearing-impaired speakers. *Volta Rev* 93:145–153.

Whitehead R, Barefoot S. (1980). Some aerodynamic characteristics of plosive consonants produced by hearing-impaired speakers. *Am Ann Deaf* 125:366–373.

Whitehead R, Barefoot S. (1983). Airflow characteristics of fricative consonants produced by normally hearing and hearing-impaired speakers. *J Speech Hear Res* 26:185–194.

Whitehead R, Jones K. (1978). The effect of vowel environment on duration of consonants produced by normal-hearing, hearing-impaired and deaf adult speakers. *J Phonet* 6:77–81.

Wolfe V, Cornell R, Palmer C. (1991). Acoustic correlates of pathologic voice types. *J Speech Hear Res* 34:509–516.

Yale C. (1946). *Formation and Development of Elementary English Sounds.* Northampton, MA: Metcalf.

Yoshinaga-Itano C, Apuzzo M, Coulter D, Stredler-Brown A. (1995). The effect of early identification of hearing loss on development. Presented at the Annual Convention of the American Academy of Audiology, Dallas, TX.

Youdelman K, MacEachron M, Behrman AM. (1988). Visual and tactile sensory aids: Integration into an ongoing speech training program. *Volta Rev* 90:197–207.

Zimmermann G, Rettaliata P. (1981). Articulatory patterns of an adventitiously deaf speaker: Implications for the role of auditory information in speech production. *J Speech Hear Res* 24:169–178.

Index

Numbers in italic indicate references to figures. Numbers followed by a t *indicate references to tables.*